Differential Diagnoses in Surgical Pathology:

Pulmonary Pathology

Differential Diagnoses in Surgical Pathology:

Pulmonary Pathology

Rosane Duarte Achcar, MD, FCAP, FASCP
Assistant Professor
Pathology Division
Department of Medicine
National Jewish Health
Denver, Colorado

Steve D. Groshong, MD, PhD
Chief of Pathology Division
Department of Medicine at National Jewish Health
Associate Professor of Medicine
National Jewish Health and the University of Colorado
Denver, Colorado

Carlyne D. Cool, MD
Clinical Professor
Department of Pathology
University of Colorado Denver School of Medicine
National Jewish Health
Denver, Colorado

SERIES EDITOR

Jonathan I. Epstein, MD
Professor of Pathology, Urology and Oncology
The Reinhard Professor of Urological Pathology
Director of Surgical Pathology
The Johns Hopkins Medical Institutions
Baltimore, Maryland

Wolters Kluwer

Philadelphia • Baltimore • New York • London
Buenos Aires • Hong Kong • Sydney • Tokyo

Acquisitions Editor: Ryan Shaw
Product Development Editor: Kate Heaney
Production Project Manager: Alicia Jackson
Manufacturing Coordinator: Beth Welsh
Marketing Manager: Dan Dressler
Design Coordinator: Teresa Mallon
Production Service: S4Carlisle Publishing Services

9 8 7 6 5 4 3 2 1

Printed in China

Library of Congress Cataloging-in-Publication Data
Names: Duarte Achcar, Rosane, author. | Groshong, Steve D., author. | Cool, Carlyne D., author.
Title: Pulmonary pathology / Rosane Duarte Achcar, Steve Groshong, Carlyne Cool.
Other titles: Differential diagnoses in surgical pathology series.
Description: Philadelphia: Wolters Kluwer Health, [2017] | Series: Differential diagnosis in surgical pathology | Includes index.
Identifiers: LCCN 2016021553 | ISBN 9781451195279 (hardback)
Subjects: | MESH: Lung Diseases—diagnosis | Lung Diseases—pathology | Pulmonary Surgical Procedures—methods | Diagnosis, Differential
Classification: LCC RC711 | NLM WF 141 | DDC 616.2/407—dc23
LC record available at https://lccn.loc.gov/2016021553

LWW.com

CCS0816

DEDICATION

This book is dedicated to my mother Eurydice, in loving memory, and to my father Nival, with heartfelt gratitude and deepest love for all their unconditional love, guidance, sacrifice, and support. I would also like to dedicate this work to my significant other Wesley, to my brothers Marcos and Marcelo, and to all close family members and wonderful friends in the United States and Brazil, whose love, support, encouragement, and infinite optimism over the years carried me through this and many other projects.

Rosane Duarte Achcar

This work is dedicated to the memory of my parents, Dale and Audrey.

Steve D. Groshong

To my husband, J. Scott Stewart, for his support and encouragement, to my children, Ian and Jacob, for their understanding, and to my coauthors for their friendship.

Carlyne D. Cool

PREFACE

Lung pathology is a highly specialized area of surgical pathology, which encompasses many unique diseases and is more than ever an essential part of clinical decision-making and patient management. Despite many advances, interpretation of lung pathology remains a significant source of diagnostic difficulty encountered by surgical pathologists every day. "Is this UIP or NSIP?" and "Is this malignant mesothelioma or reactive mesothelial hyperplasia?" are common dilemmas and questions faced on a daily basis. This book is intended to offer practicing pathologists, pathologists-in-training, residents and medical students a succinct and comprehensible reference with key clinical and microscopic findings of the most common to selected less frequently seen challenging disorders in neoplastic and non-neoplastic lung pathology. Our objective is to provide, through an appealing format of side by side tables and histopathology color images, a quick and user-friendly summary of information, which will assist in distinguishing challenging entities that have overlapping morphologic features in pulmonary pathology. The book is oriented primarily towards adult pulmonary pathology and a small array of references are supplied so that the reader can obtain more in depth material if desired. Writing a textbook is an immense undertaking and we sincerely hope that you will find this volume of *Differential Diagnosis In Surgical Pathology* enjoyable to read and a valuable consultative tool in the evaluation of pulmonary pathology specimens for study and for practice.

Rosane Duarte Achcar
Steve D. Groshong
Carlyne D. Cool

ACKNOWLEDGMENTS

I would like to express my deep gratitude to Dr. Jeff Kern for his friendship, mentorship, good advice, and constant good humor. I would like to extend my sincerest thanks and appreciation to Dr. Phillip Cagle for his generous review and constructive comments. Gratitude and appreciation is also extended to Dr. Yale Rosen and UPMC department of pathology for their illustrative material contribution from personal files and archival cases. Finally, I also would like to heartily thank my colleagues Dr. Carlyne D. Cool and Dr. Steve D. Groshong for their friendship, for sharing their expertise in pulmonary pathology on a daily basis in our practice, and for their hard work during the preparation of this book.

Rosane Duarte Achcar

Table of Contents

1 ASTHMA VS. CELLULAR (CHRONIC) BRONCHIOLITIS

	Asthma	Cellular (Chronic) Bronchiolitis
Age	Any age. Extrinsic asthma (allergy to exogenous substances is recognized), usually begins in childhood. Intrinsic asthma (no exogenous factors can be identified) more often has its onset in adult life.	Any age. Age predilection depends on etiologic factors.
Location	Large and small airways.	Small airways including small bronchi, less than 2–3 mm in diameter, and membranous bronchioles (terminal and respiratory bronchioles). Terminal bronchioles are less than 1 mm in diameter and are just proximal to the respiratory bronchioles, the first airways that have alveoli budding from their walls.
Symptoms	Recurrent episodes of wheezing, coughing, chest tightness, and shortness of breath.	It varies depending on the causative agent. Dyspnea and usually nonproductive cough are common.
Signs	Increase in respiratory rate, end-expiratory wheezing, and peripheral blood eosinophilia. Spirometry shows reduced FEV1/FVC ratio that improves with bronchodilators.	High-resolution computed tomography (HRCT) scans may show centrilobular nodularity or tree-in-bud pattern.
Etiology	Genetic and environmental factors play a role. Extrinsic (atopic) asthma, the most common type, involves stimulation of Th2 responses by inhaled antigens, leading to type I immunoglobulin E-mediated hypersensitivity reactions. Symptoms may be triggered by exposure to allergens, respiratory tract infections, exercise, medications, gastroesophageal reflux, air pollution, cold, stress, and occupational exposure. Asthma can be associated with other diseases including allergic bronchopulmonary fungal disease, eosinophilic pneumonia, and Churg–Strauss syndrome.	Infection (e.g., virus and *Mycoplasma* infection); connective tissue disorders, especially rheumatoid arthritis and Sjögren syndrome; inherited or acquired immunodeficiency syndromes, extraintestinal manifestation of inflammatory bowel disease, graft-vs.-host disease, transplant-associated cellular bronchiolitis, lymphoproliferative diseases, or idiopathic. It may also occur secondary to large airways disease, particularly in small airways distal to markedly dilated large airways (bronchiectasis).
Histology	Luminal mucous plugs admixed with eosinophils, epithelial cells, and Charcot–Leyden crystals *(Fig. 1.1)*. Airway with submucosal eosinophil-rich inflammatory cell infiltrate, goblet cell hyperplasia, subbasal lamina thickening due to collagen deposition, and submucosal smooth muscle prominence *(Figs. 1.2–1.4)*.	Infiltration of the walls of small airways by chronic inflammatory cell infiltrate *(Figs. 1.5–1.7)*.
Special studies	Gomori methenamine silver (GMS) special stain is used to exclude bronchial colonization by fungal organisms.	Tissue cultures and appropriate molecular testing are used to exclude infectious etiology.

	Asthma	Cellular (Chronic) Bronchiolitis
Prognosis	Symptoms usually improve or disappear as children become adults. Most patients respond to treatment with anti-inflammatory agents, bronchodilators, and avoidance of potential trigger factors, although some individuals will have persistent asthma even though exposure to causative agent has stopped. Complications include pneumonia, pneumothorax, pneumomediastinum, and respiratory distress, requiring intubation and mechanical ventilation.	It varies depending on the causative agent. May progress to constrictive bronchiolitis.

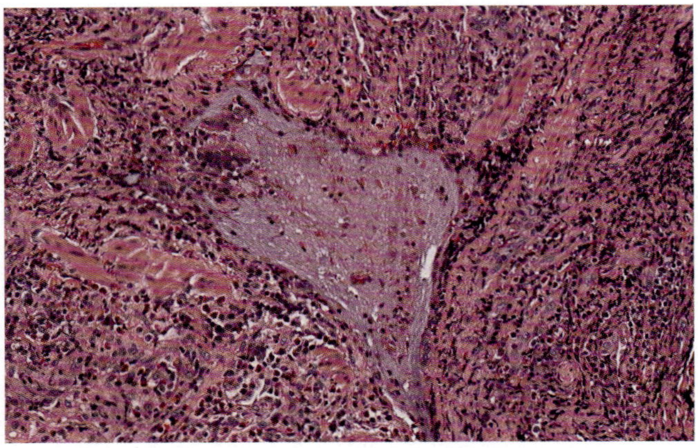

Figure 1.1 Asthma: Largely denuded bronchial wall showing luminal mucous plug admixed with eosinophils and Charcot–Leyden crystals. The airway is infiltrated by mixed eosinophil-rich inflammatory cell infiltrate.

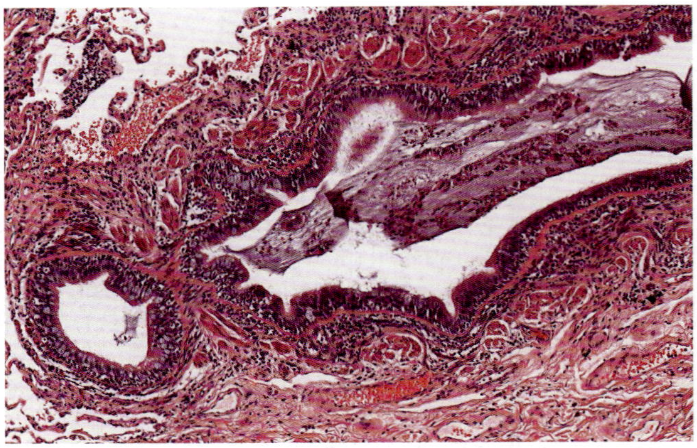

Figure 1.2 Asthma: The lumen is filled with eosinophil-rich mucous plug (*right*), the epithelium shows goblet cell hyperplasia, and the subbasal lamina is expanded.

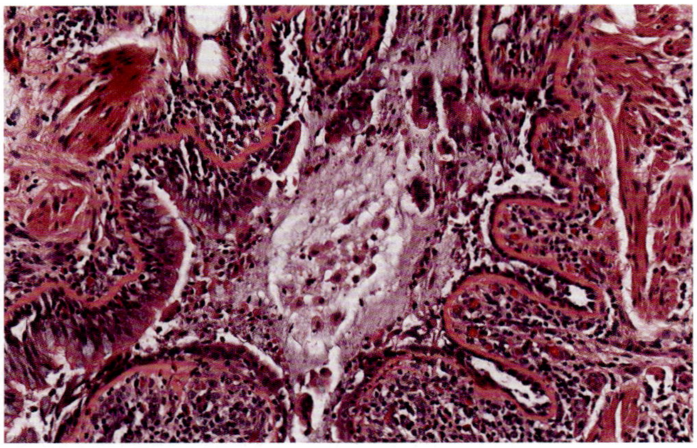

Figure 1.3 Asthma: Mucous plug, bronchiolar tortuosity, diffuse expansion of the subbasal lamina, and eosinophil-rich airway wall infiltrate.

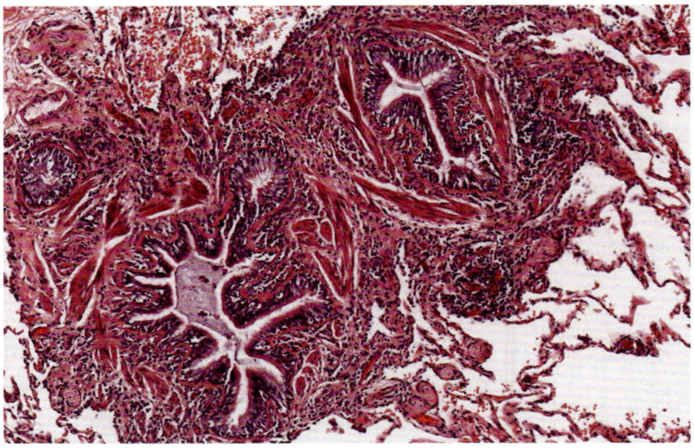

Figure 1.4 Asthma: Bronchiolar tortuosity, expansion of the subbasal lamina, and submucosal smooth muscle prominence.

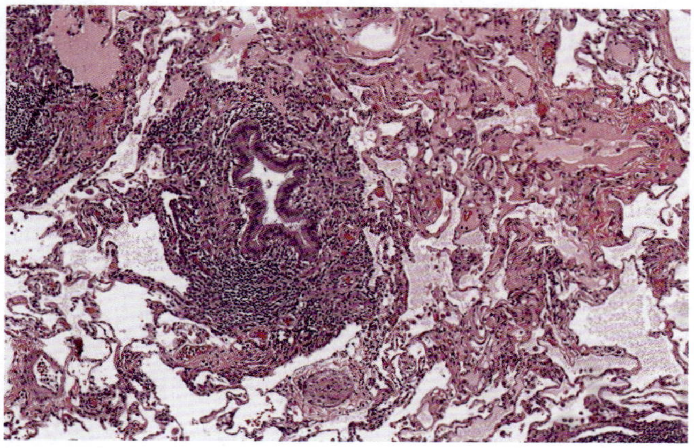

Figure 1.5 Cellular (chronic) bronchiolitis: Small airway wall with concentric infiltration by chronic inflammatory cell infiltrate.

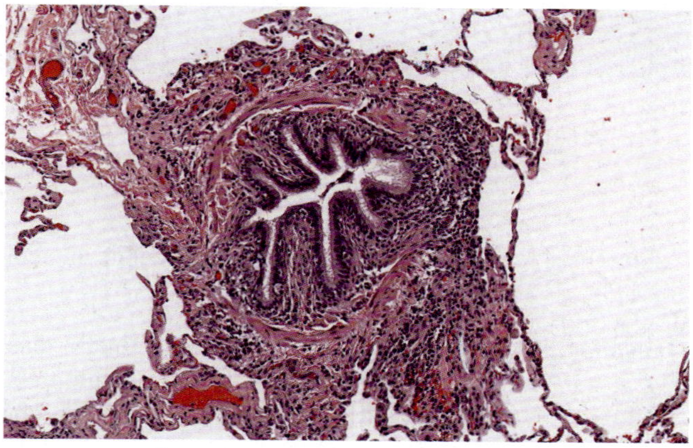

Figure 1.6 Cellular (chronic) bronchiolitis: Papillary epithelial hyperplasia and concentric bronchiolar wall infiltration by chronic inflammatory cell infiltrate.

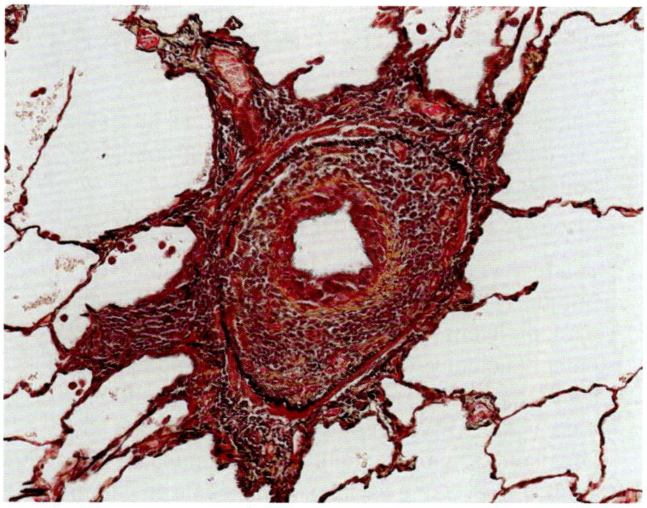

Figure 1.7 Cellular (chronic) bronchiolitis: Pentachrome special stain: Bronchiolar and peribronchiolar circumferential chronic inflammatory cell infiltrate promoting luminal narrowing of the airway in a 35-year-old woman with rheumatoid arthritis.

2 CELLULAR (CHRONIC) BRONCHIOLITIS VS. FOLLICULAR BRONCHIOLITIS

	Cellular (Chronic) Bronchiolitis	Follicular Bronchiolitis
Age	Any age. Age predilection depends on etiologic factors.	May occur in children and adults, but adults are affected most often (median age is 44 y).
Location	Small airways including small bronchi, less than 2–3 mm in diameter, and membranous bronchioles (terminal and respiratory bronchioles). Terminal bronchioles are less than 1 mm in diameter and are just proximal to the respiratory bronchioles, the first airways that have alveoli budding from their walls.	Small airways.
Symptoms	It varies depending on the causative agent. Dyspnea and usually nonproductive cough are common.	Dyspnea, cough, fever, and symptoms related to associated underlying diseases.
Signs	High-resolution computed tomography (HRCT) scans may show centrilobular nodularity or tree-in-bud pattern.	Spirometry may demonstrate obstructive or restrictive defects. HRCT shows bilateral centrilobular nodular or reticulonodular opacities.
Etiology	Infection (e.g., virus and *Mycoplasma* infection); connective tissue disorders, especially rheumatoid arthritis and Sjögren syndrome; inherited or acquired immunodeficiency syndromes, extraintestinal manifestation of inflammatory bowel disease, graft-vs.-host disease, transplant-associated cellular bronchiolitis, lymphoproliferative diseases, or idiopathic. It may also occur secondary to large airways disease, particularly in small airways distal to markedly dilated large airways (bronchiectasis).	Most of the cases are associated with an underlying connective tissue disease (e.g., rheumatoid arthritis or Sjögren syndrome); or congenital or acquired immunodeficiency states such as common variable immunodeficiency (CVID), acquired immunodeficiency syndrome (AIDS) related to human immunodeficiency virus (HIV) infection, or hypogammaglobulinemia (e.g., immunoglobulin A deficiency). It may also be seen at the periphery of a localized infectious process or be associated with some occupational exposure settings, such as in the case of nylon flock workers. Some cases are idiopathic.
Histology	Infiltration of the walls of small airways by chronic inflammatory cell infiltrate *(Fig. 2.1)*.	Numerous lymphoid follicles with well-formed germinal centers surrounding a bronchiolar wall *(Fig. 2.2)*. The hyperplastic lymphoid tissue may distort and narrow the bronchiolar lumen *(Fig. 2.3)*. The lymphoid infiltrate may extend into alveolar septa adjacent to the bronchiolar wall without significant extension into more distal lung parenchyma. The airspaces are uninvolved *(Figs. 2.4 and 2.5)*.
Special studies	Tissue cultures and appropriate molecular testing are used to exclude infectious etiology.	Special stains are usually not required. The lymphoid follicles should demonstrate a mixture of B (CD20 positive) and T (CD3 and CD5 positive) cell markers expression. The B cell–rich germinal center cells stain for CD20 and BCL6, while the interfollicular lymphoid cells stain for CD3 and CD5. The germinal center should be negative for BCL-2 and should be surrounded by immunoglobulin D and BCL2-positive mantle zones.
Prognosis	It varies depending on the causative agent. It may progress to constrictive bronchiolitis.	It varies depending on the underlying cause.

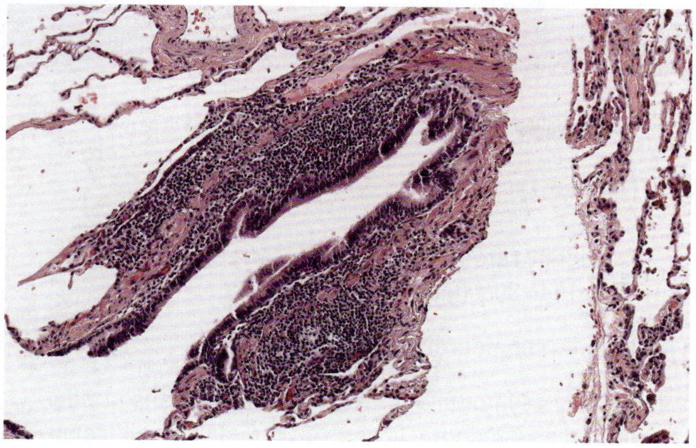

Figure 2.1 Cellular (chronic) bronchiolitis: Small airway wall showing concentric infiltration by chronic inflammatory cell infiltrate.

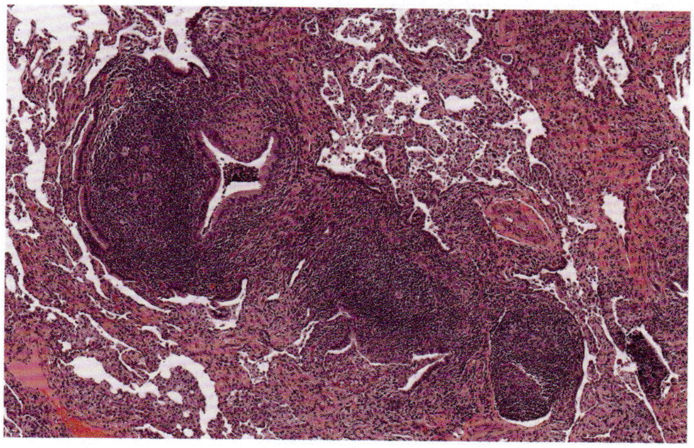

Figure 2.2 Follicular bronchiolitis: Lymphoid follicles with well-formed germinal centers surrounding and within a bronchiolar wall.

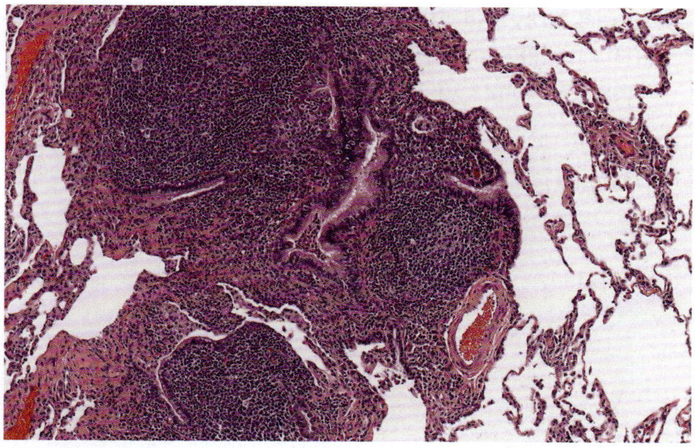

Figure 2.3 Follicular bronchiolitis: Hyperplastic lymphoid follicles compressing bronchiolar lumens.

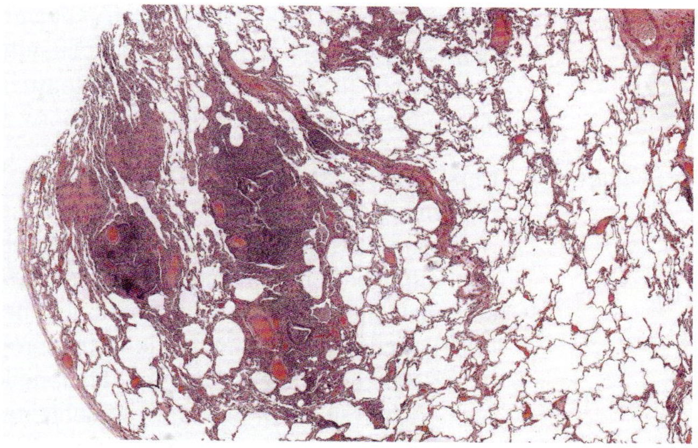

Figure 2.4 Follicular bronchiolitis: The lymphoid infiltrate (low power/2×) may extend into alveolar septa adjacent to the bronchiolar wall without significant extension into more distal lung parenchyma. The airspaces are uninvolved.

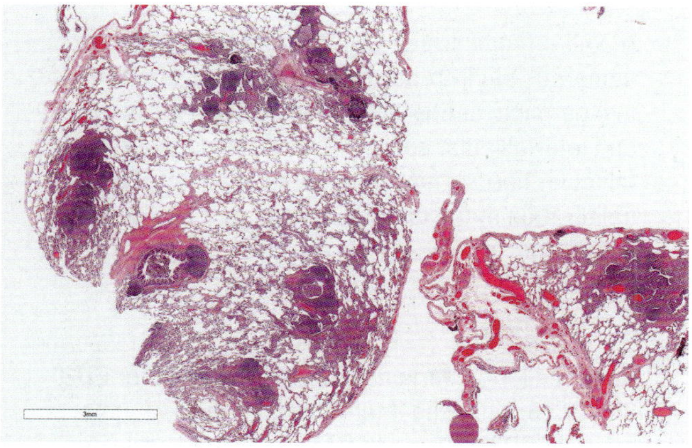

Figure 2.5 Follicular bronchiolitis: These peribronchial lymphoid infiltrates may be seen on HRCT as centrilobular nodules.

3 FOLLICULAR BRONCHIOLITIS VS. NODULAR LYMPHOID HYPERPLASIA

	Follicular Bronchiolitis	Nodular Lymphoid Hyperplasia
Age	May occur in children and adults, but adults are affected most often (median age is 44 y).	Extremely rare condition. It may affect people aged from 19 to 80 y (median, 65 y).
Location	Small airways.	Usually subpleural or peripheral.
Symptoms	Progressive dyspnea and cough occasionally associated with fever.	Usually asymptomatic. The majority of cases are detected as incidental lesions on radiologic studies obtained for other reasons. Symptoms, when present, may include shortness of breath, cough, and pleuritic chest pain.
Signs	Spirometry may demonstrate obstructive or restrictive defects. High-resolution computed tomography (HRCT) shows bilateral centrilobular nodular or reticular nodular opacities.	Chest x-ray and CT typically show a solitary pulmonary nodule or mass usually measuring between 0.5 and 6 cm in greatest dimension.
Etiology	Most of the cases are associated with an underlying connective tissue disease (e.g., rheumatoid arthritis or Sjögren syndrome) or congenital or acquired immunodeficiency state such as common variable immunodeficiency (CVID), acquired immunodeficiency syndrome (AIDS) related to human immunodeficiency virus (HIV) infection, or hypogammaglobulinemia (e.g., immunoglobulin A deficiency). It may also be seen at the periphery of a localized infectious process or be associated with some occupational exposure settings, such as in the case of nylon flock workers. Some cases are idiopathic.	Usually idiopathic.
Histology	Numerous lymphoid follicles with well-formed germinal centers surrounding a bronchiolar wall *(Fig. 3.1)*. The hyperplastic lymphoid tissue may distort and narrow the bronchiolar lumen *(Fig. 3.2)*. The lymphoid infiltrate may extend into alveolar septa adjacent to the bronchiolar wall without significant extension into more distal lung parenchyma. The airspaces are uninvolved *(Figs. 3.3 and 3.4)*.	A well-circumscribed nodule or mass composed of numerous back-to-back lymphoid follicles with reactive germinal center and preserved mantle zones and interfollicular zones. Variable amounts of interfollicular fibrosis may be present and may promote obliteration of the underlying lung parenchyma *(Figs. 3.5 and 3.6)*.
Special studies	Special stains are usually not required. The lymphoid follicles should demonstrate a mixture of B (CD20 positive) and T (CD3 and CD5 positive) cell markers expression.	The B cell–rich germinal center cells stain for CD20 and BCL6, while the interfollicular lymphoid cells stain for CD3, CD5, and CD43 (T-cell markers). The CD20-positive lymphocytes should not coexpress either CD5 or CD43. The germinal center should be negative for BCL2, and should be surrounded by immunoglobulin D and BCL2–positive mantle zones. CD21 should stain the network of follicular dendritic cells.

	Follicular Bronchiolitis	Nodular Lymphoid Hyperplasia
	The B cell–rich germinal center cells stain for CD20 and BCL6, while the interfollicular lymphoid cells stain for CD3 and CD5. The germinal center should be negative for BCL2, and surrounded by immunoglobulin D and BCL2-positive mantle zones.	A polyclonal pattern of kappa and lambda expression is present in the interfoliculllar plasma cells, which should demonstrate bland cytologic features, not associated with Dutcher bodies. Pancytokeratin shows absence of destructive lymphoepithelial lesion. If immunohistochemical stains or flow cytometry studies are not conclusive, follow-up with molecular testing should be pursued to exclude B-cell clonality.
Prognosis	It is variable and depends on the underlying cause.	Benign lesion without risk of recurrence. Surgical excision is required for definite diagnosis.

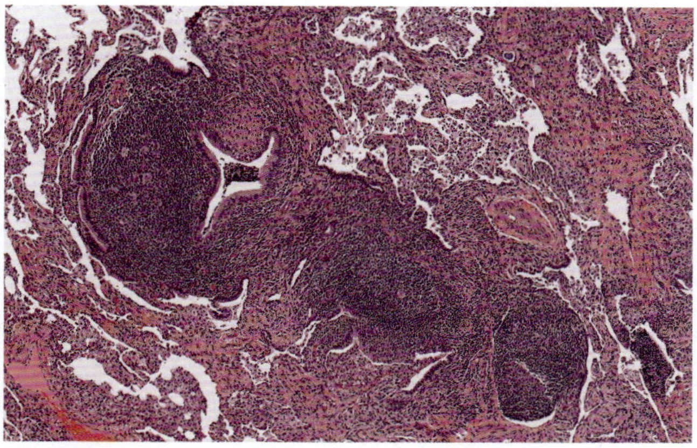

Figure 3.1 Follicular bronchiolitis: Lymphoid follicles with well-formed germinal centers surrounding and within a bronchiolar wall.

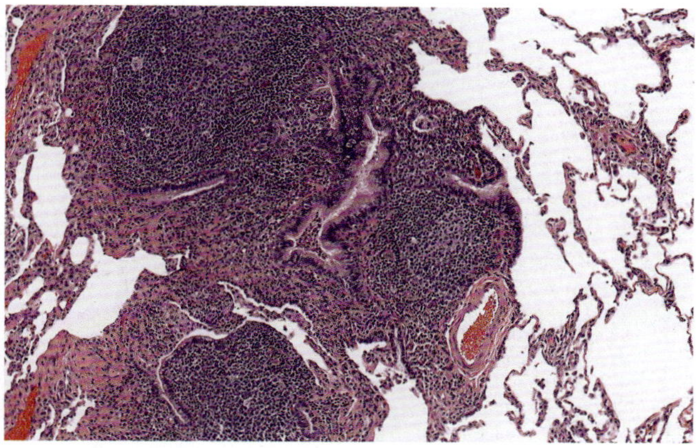

Figure 3.2 Follicular bronchiolitis: Hyperplastic lymphoid follicles compressing bronchiolar lumens.

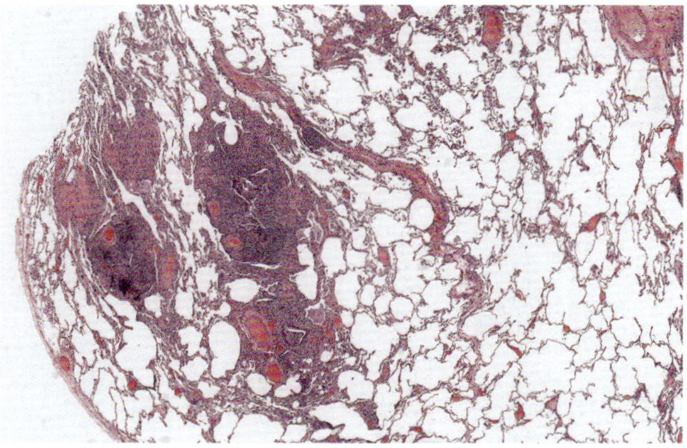

Figure 3.3 Follicular bronchiolitis: The lymphoid infiltrate (low power/2×) may extend into alveolar septa adjacent to the bronchiolar wall without significant extension into more distal lung parenchyma. The airspaces are uninvolved.

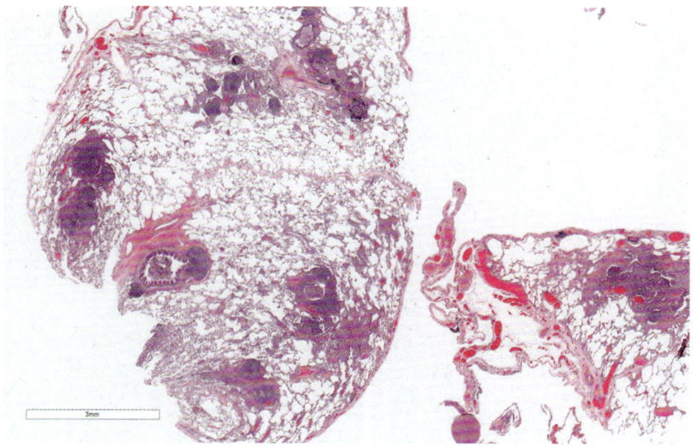

Figure 3.4 Follicular bronchiolitis: These peribronchial lymphoid infiltrates may be seen on HRCT as centrilobular nodules.

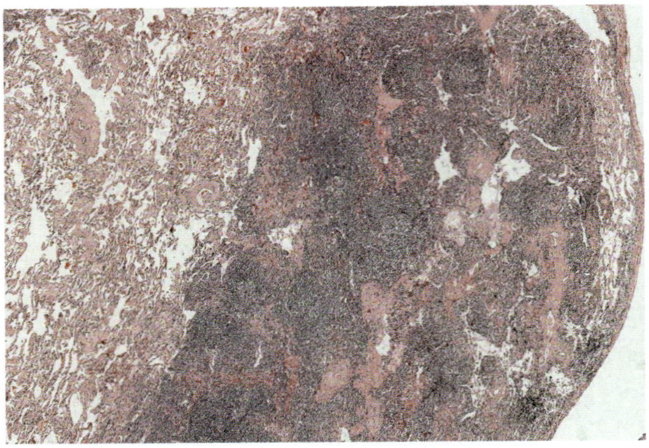

Figure 3.5 Nodular lymphoid hyperplasia: Subpleural well-circumscribed nodular lesion composed of numerous lymphoid follicles.

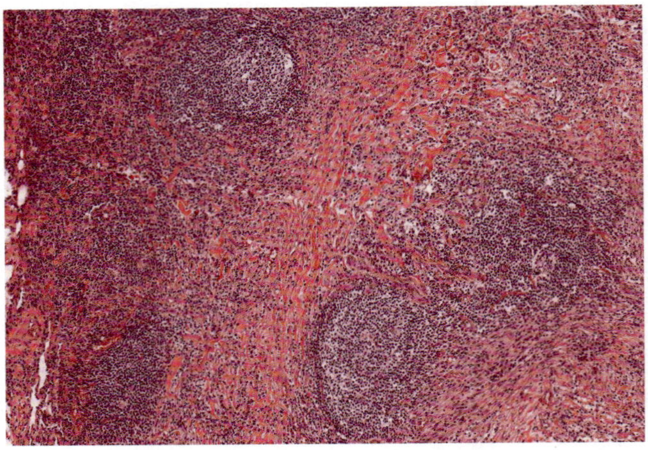

Figure 3.6 Nodular lymphoid hyperplasia: The lesion may be associated with variable amounts of interfollicular fibrosis, which in some cases can promote obliteration of the underlying lung parenchyma.

4 CELLULAR (CHRONIC) BRONCHIOLITIS VS. DIFFUSE PANBRONCHIOLITIS

	Cellular (Chronic) Bronchiolitis	Diffuse Panbronchiolitis
Age	Any age. Age predilection depends on etiologic factors.	Rare disease that usually occurs between the second and seventh decades of life, with mean age of presentation at 50 y, in native East Asian patients, particularly in Koreans, Japanese, and Chinese. Only rare cases have been reported in non-Asian individuals. The male-to-female ratio is usually 2:1.
Location	Small airways including small bronchi, less than 2–3 mm in diameter, and membranous bronchioles (terminal and respiratory bronchioles). Terminal bronchioles are less than 1 mm in diameter and are just proximal to the respiratory bronchioles, the first airways that have alveoli budding from their walls.	Small airways, usually terminal and respiratory bronchioles.
Symptoms	It varies depending on the causative agent. Dyspnea and usually nonproductive cough are common.	Cough, sputum production, dyspnea, fever, and sometimes digital clubbing. History of associated chronic paranasal sinusitis is common. When superimposed infection happens (e.g., *Hemophilius influenza*, *Streptococcus pneumonia*, or *Pseudomonas aeruginosa*), increased dyspnea with increased purulent sputum production occurs.
Signs	High-resolution computed tomography (HRCT) scans may show centrilobular nodularity or tree-in-bud pattern.	Persistent and marked elevation of serum cold hemagglutinins is characteristic. Hypoxemia, leukocytosis, increased sedimentation rate and C-reactive protein, and elevated levels of immunoglobulin G (IgG) and A (IgA). Pulmonary function tests usually show a pattern of obstruction. Chest radiographs demonstrate bilateral diffuse nodular to reticulonodular opacities and hyperinflation. HRCT scans show centrilobular opacities along thickened bronchioles, bronchiolectasis, and air trapping.
Etiology	Infection (e.g., virus and *Mycoplasma* infection); connective tissue disorders, especially rheumatoid arthritis and Sjögren syndrome; inherited or acquired immunodeficiency syndromes, extraintestinal manifestation of inflammatory bowel disease, graft-vs.-host disease, transplant-associated cellular bronchiolitis, lymphoproliferative diseases, or idiopathic. It may also occur secondary to large airways disease, particularly in small airways distal to markedly dilated large airways (bronchiectasis).	Unknown. Genetic susceptibility has been identified on the basis of the observation of familial cases and the association of specific human leukocyte antigen (HLA) haplotypes. HLA-B54 is the haplotype reported in Japanese patients and HLA-A11 is identified in those of Korean ancestry, suggesting that the diffuse panbronchiolitis susceptibility gene might be located between the *HLA-B* and *HLA-A* genes loci, probably residing within the short arm of chromosome 6 (6p21.3).

	Cellular (Chronic) Bronchiolitis	Diffuse Panbronchiolitis
Histology	Infiltration of the walls of small airways by chronic inflammatory cell infiltrate *(Fig. 4.1)*.	Cellular (chronic) bronchiolitis characterized by the presence of thickening of walls of respiratory and terminal bronchioles by inflammatory cell infiltrate composed predominantly of lymphocytes, histiocytes, and plasma cells, which can also be seen in the bronchiolar lumens. Lymphoid aggregates can be seen. Intraluminal neutrophils can be prominent. This is associated with characteristic accumulations of vacuolated or foamy macrophages in the peribronchiolar interstitium *(Figs. 4.2–4.4)*. In advanced stages, constriction of bronchioles and more proximal bronchiolectasis and bronchiectasis can occur. It should be noted that the interstitial accumulation of foamy histiocytes, while highly characteristic of panbronchiolitis, is not unique to this condition. Similar change can be seen associated with other diseases including cystic fibrosis and bronchiectasis. The diagnosis of diffuse panbronchiolitis should be made only when other conditions are absent.
Special studies	Tissue cultures and appropriate molecular testing are used to exclude infectious etiology.	Usually not required.
Prognosis	It is variable depending on the causative agent. It may progress to constrictive bronchiolitis.	Progressive disease with poor prognosis. Debilitating bronchiectasis and cystic lung disease develop in advanced cases. The overall survival is approximately 50% at 5 y and 25% at 10 y. Death is usually due to cor pulmonale and respiratory failure. Long-term low dose of erythromycin has significantly improved the prognosis and constitutes the major form of treatment. Lung transplantation has been performed in some cases.

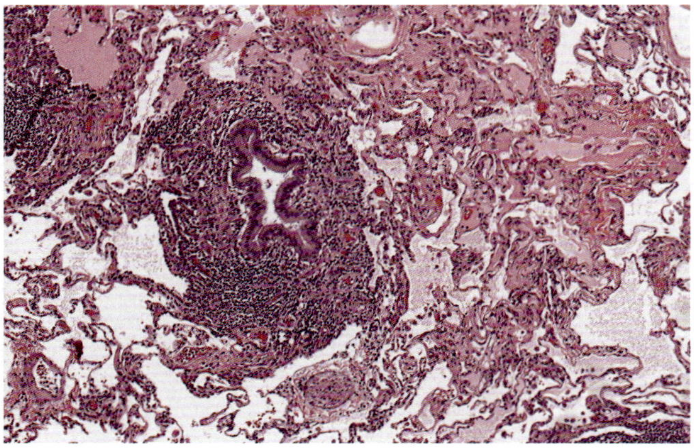

Figure 4.1 Cellular (chronic) bronchiolitis: Small airway wall showing infiltration by chronic inflammatory cell infiltrate.

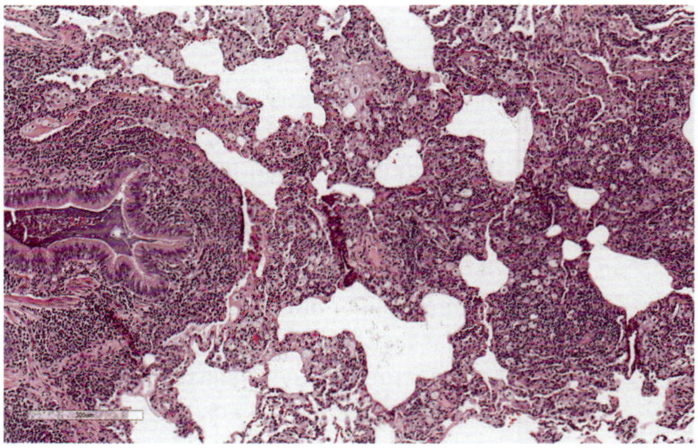

Figure 4.2 Diffuse panbronchiolitis: Cellular bronchiolitis associated with numerous foamy macrophages, which infiltrate the adjacent peribronchial interstitium.

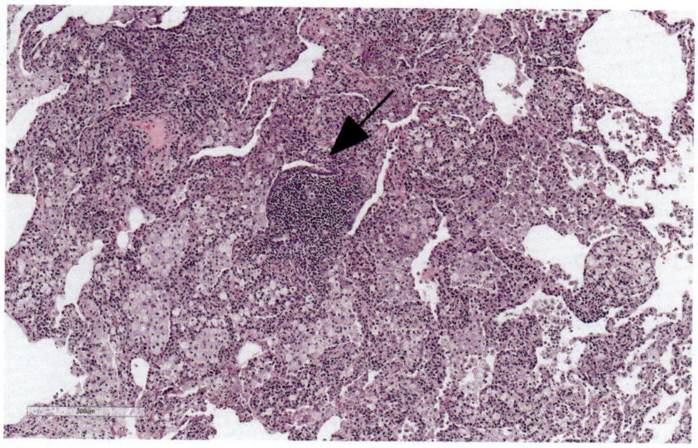

Figure 4.3 Diffuse panbronchiolitis: There is characteristic interstitial bronchiolocentric accumulations of vacuolated or foamy macrophages. Note small airway showing chronic inflammation (*upper center/arrow*).

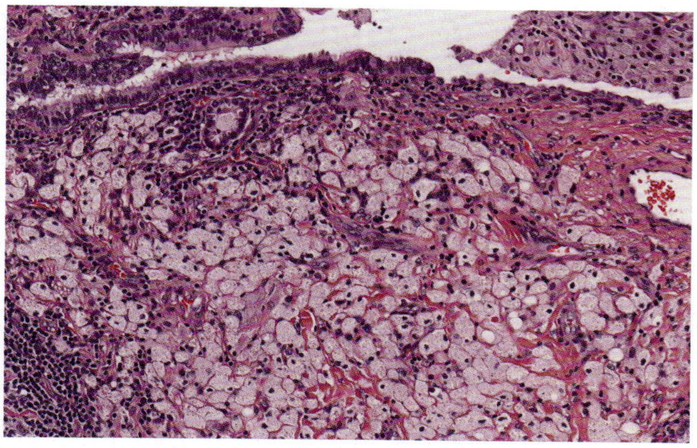

Figure 4.4 Diffuse panbronchiolitis (high power): Peribronchial interstitial macrophages.

5 CELLULAR (CHRONIC) BRONCHIOLITIS VS. CONSTRICTIVE BRONCHIOLITIS

	Cellular (Chronic) Bronchiolitis	Constrictive Bronchiolitis
Age	Any age. Age predilection depends on etiologic factors.	It may affect adults and children of both genders. Age predilection depends on etiologic factors.
Location	Small airways including small bronchi with less than 2–3 mm in diameter and membranous bronchioles (terminal and respiratory bronchioles). Terminal bronchioles are less than 1 mm in diameter and are just proximal to the respiratory bronchioles, the first airways that have alveoli budding from their walls.	Small airways.
Symptoms	It varies depending on the causative agent. Dyspnea and usually nonproductive cough are common.	Chronic cough and dyspnea.
Signs	High-resolution computed tomography (HRCT) scans may show centrilobular nodularity or tree-in-bud pattern.	Pulmonary function tests demonstrate obstructive pattern with lack of response to bronchodilators therapy. Chest x-ray films show lung hyperinflation. HRCT shows air trapping, often associated with ground-glass opacities, mosaic attenuation, and bronchial wall thickening.
Etiology	Infection (e.g., virus and *Mycoplasma* infection); connective tissue disorders, especially rheumatoid arthritis and Sjögren syndrome; inherited or acquired immunodeficiency syndromes, extraintestinal manifestation of inflammatory bowel disease, graft-vs.-host disease, transplant-associated cellular bronchiolitis, lymphoproliferative diseases, or idiopathic. It may also be secondary to large airways disease, particularly in small airways distal to markedly dilated large airways (bronchiectasis).	Unknown. May be seen in the setting of lung transplantation, indicating chronic airway rejection; bone marrow transplantation, representing a manifestation of graft-vs.-host disease; after mycoplasma or viral infections (e.g., cytomegalovirus, adenovirus, influenza virus, parainfluenza virus, varicella virus); in the setting of systemic autoimmune diseases (e.g., rheumatoid arthritis, systemic sclerosis, mixed connective tissue disease, and ankylosing spondylitis); as extraintestinal manifestation of inflammatory bowel disease; after exposure to inhaled toxic agents (e.g., nitrogen dioxide, sulfur dioxide, ammonia, chlorine, phosgene, fly ash, styrene, fire fumes, and possibly after inhalation of certain organic compounds, as described in workers at a microwave popcorn factory who were exposed to volatile butter-flavoring ingredients); after massive dust exposure (e.g., "Ground Zero" dust exposure of the World Trade Center disaster); with some medications (e.g., gold, penicillamine, chemotherapeutic agents such as lomustine and 5-fluorouracil); after consumption of toxins from juice of the plant *Sauropus androgynus* (appetite suppressant); in the setting of dermatologic conditions (e.g., paraneoplastic pemphigus in cases of malignant lymphomas and Castleman disease, Stevens–Johnson syndrome, and toxic epidermal necrolysis); or idiopathic.

	Cellular (Chronic) Bronchiolitis	Constrictive Bronchiolitis
Histology	Infiltration of the walls of small airways by chronic inflammatory cell infiltrate *(Fig. 5.1)*. Pentachrome special stain does not highlight subepithelial collagenization/scarring *(Fig. 5.2)*.	It ranges from variable amounts of eccentric subepithelial collagenization/scarring of bronchioles walls, which may result in luminal constriction, to complete circumferential replacement of the bronchiole wall and lumen by mature dense collagen deposition, which may extend into the peribronchiolar zones *(Figs. 5.3–5.6)*. Subtle findings suggestive of constrictive bronchiolitis include lung hyperinflation, bronchiolar tortuosity, branches of small pulmonary arteries that are not paired with respective bronchioles *(Fig. 5.7)*, and small airways showing decrease in size in comparison with respective accompanying pulmonary arteries, which should be approximately the same size.
Special studies	Tissue cultures and appropriate molecular testing to exclude infectious etiology.	Pentachrome special stain is very useful in assisting in the identification of obliterated bronchioles by highlighting eccentric or concentric luminal and mural collagen deposition/scarring (yellow) with luminal narrowing of the airways and displacement of the single bronchiolar elastic tissue layer (black). Pentachrome and elastic stains are also useful in differentiating airways (single elastic tissue layer) from pulmonary arteries (two elastic tissue layers).
Prognosis	It is variable and depends on the causative agent. It may progress to constrictive bronchiolitis.	Poor prognosis, with progressive disease in most patients that is unresponsive to corticosteroids or cytotoxic therapy. Many patients undergo lung transplantation.

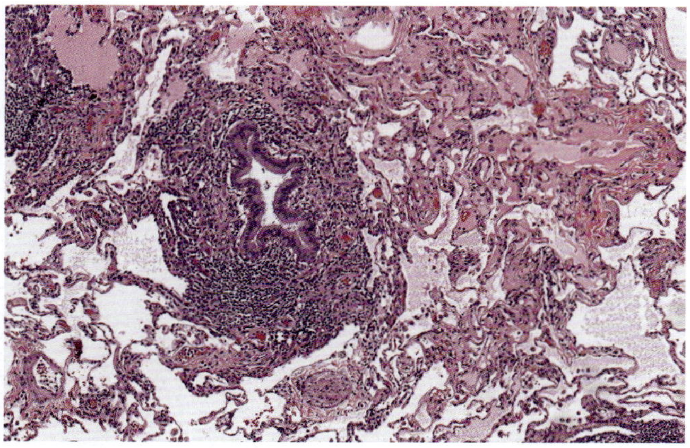

Figure 5.1 Cellular (chronic) bronchiolitis: Small airway wall showing infiltration by chronic inflammatory cell infiltrate.

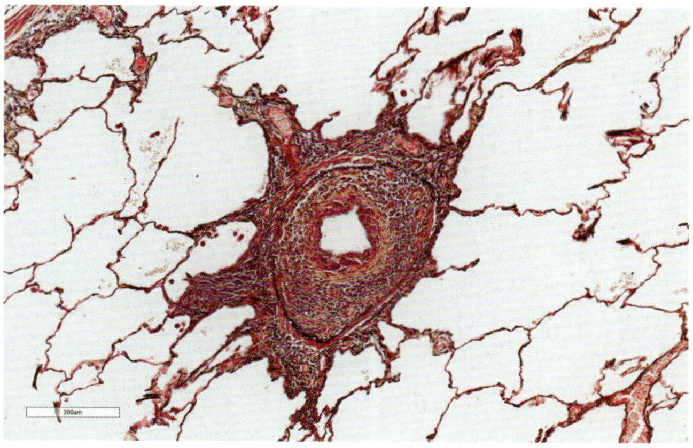

Figure 5.2 Cellular (chronic) bronchiolitis (pentachrome special stain): Bronchiolar and peribronchiolar circumferential chronic inflammatory cell infiltrate causing luminal narrowing of the airway in a 35-year-old woman with rheumatoid arthritis. Note the absence of subepithelial scarring.

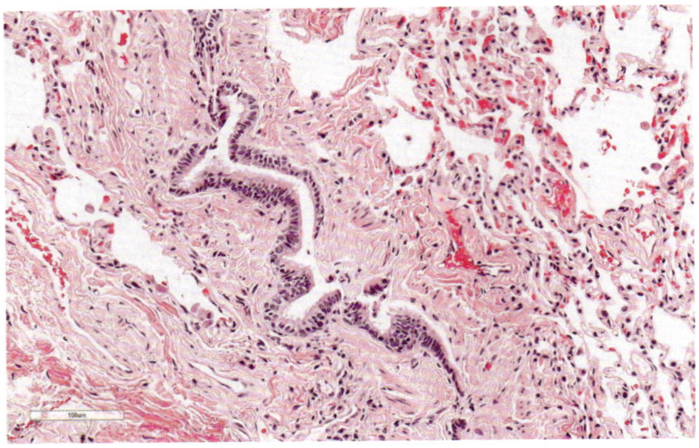

Figure 5.3 Constrictive bronchiolitis: There is bronchiolar tortuosity and subepithelial scarring, which can be confirmed by pentachrome special stain.

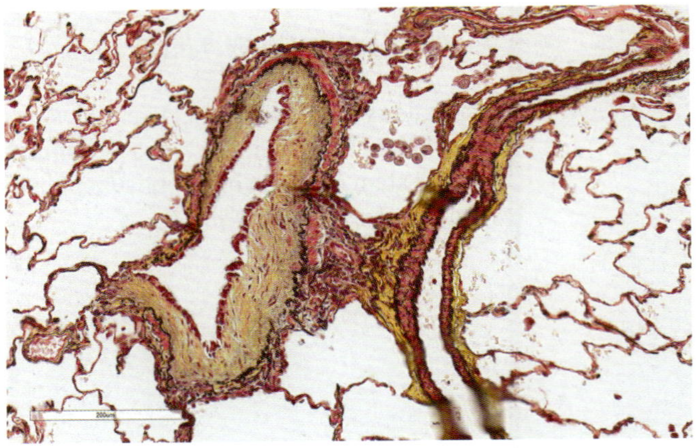

Figure 5.4 Constrictive bronchiolitis: Small airway subepithelial dense collagen deposition (pentachrome, *yellow*, *left*), displaces the bronchiolar single elastic layer (*black*). The adjacent alveolar septa are thin and delicate.

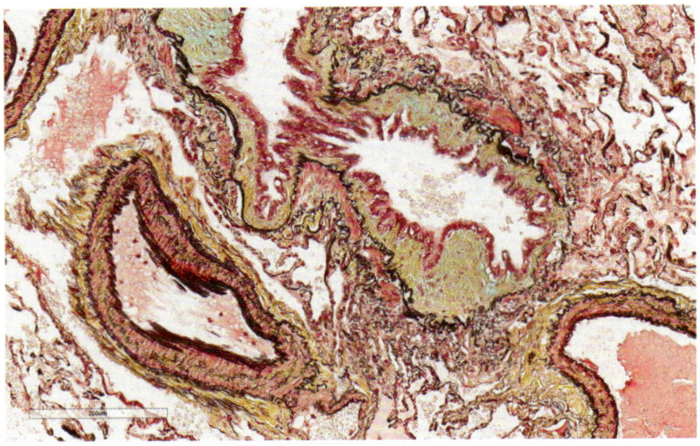

Figure 5.5 Constrictive bronchiolitis: Moderate concentric small airway subepithelial collagenization (pentachrome, *yellow*, *right*), is interposed between epithelium and single elastic layer (*black*). Pentachrome special stain is useful in differentiating airways (single elastic layer, *right*) from pulmonary arteries (two elastic layers, *left*).

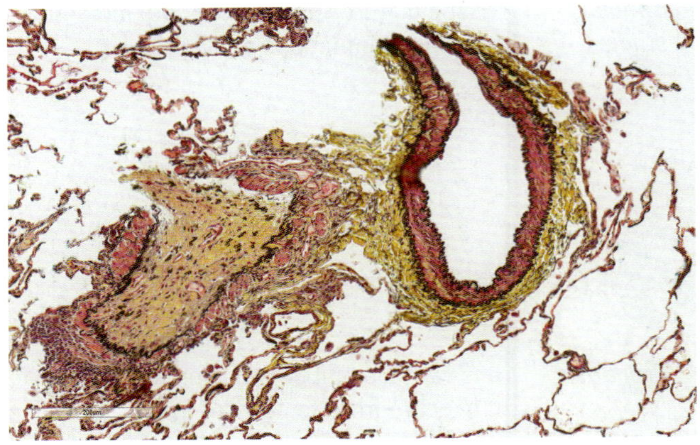

Figure 5.6 Constrictive bronchiolitis: Marked small airway subepithelial collagenization/scarring (pentachrome, *yellow*, *left*) that completely replaces the bronchiole wall and lumen. Note that the corresponding small pulmonary artery (*right*) has double elastic layer (*black*).

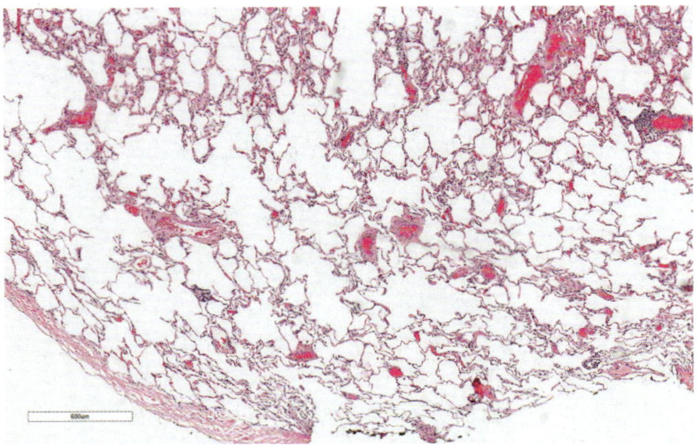

Figure 5.7 Constrictive bronchiolitis: Subtle findings suggestive of constrictive bronchiolitis include lung hyperinflation and small pulmonary artery branches that are not paired with respective bronchioles.

6 CONSTRICTIVE BRONCHIOLITIS VS. ORGANIZING PNEUMONIA

	Constrictive Bronchiolitis	Organizing Pneumonia (OP)
Age	It may affect adults and children of both genders. Age predilection depends on etiologic factors.	Usually seen in the fifth and sixth decades, with mean age of onset at 55 y. Affects men and women equally.
Location	Small airways.	Lumens of distal bronchioles, alveolar ducts, and peribronchiolar alveolar spaces.
Symptoms	Chronic cough and dyspnea.	Subacute illness, characterized by 2–3 mo history of cough and dyspnea, which can be associated with weight loss, fever, sweats, chills, and myalgia.
Signs	Pulmonary function tests demonstrate obstructive pattern with lack of response to bronchodilators therapy. Chest x-ray films show lung hyperinflation. High-resolution computed tomography (HRCT) shows air trapping, often associated with ground-glass opacities, mosaic attenuation, and bronchial wall thickening.	Inspiratory crackles on physical examination. Pulmonary function tests may show mild-to-moderate restrictive pattern. Airflow obstruction is usually absent. Chest x-ray shows patchy airspace consolidation, which is usually bilateral but may be unilateral. Chest CT shows bilateral/unilateral patchy airspace consolidation/ground-glass opacities in a peribronchial distribution.
Etiology	Unknown. May be seen in the setting of lung transplantation indicating chronic airway rejection; bone marrow transplantation, representing a manifestation of graft-vs.-host disease; after mycoplasma or viral infections (e.g., cytomegalovirus, adenovirus, influenza virus, parainfluenza virus, varicella virus); in the setting of systemic autoimmune diseases (e.g., rheumatoid arthritis, systemic sclerosis, mixed connective tissue disease and ankylosing spondylitis); as extraintestinal manifestation of inflammatory bowel disease; after exposure to inhaled toxic agents (e.g., nitrogen dioxide, sulfur dioxide, ammonia, chlorine, phosgene, fly ash, styrene, fire fumes, and possibly after inhalation of certain organic compounds, as described in workers at a microwave popcorn factory who were exposed to volatile butter-flavoring ingredients); after massive dust exposure (e.g., "Ground Zero" dust exposure of the World Trade Center disaster); with some medications (e.g., gold, penicillamine, chemotherapeutic agents such as lomustine and 5-fluorouracil); after consumption of toxins from juice of the plant *Sauropus androgynus* (appetite suppressant); in the setting of dermatologic conditions (e.g., paraneoplastic pemphigus in cases of malignant lymphomas and Castleman disease, Stevens–Johnson syndrome, and toxic epidermal necrolysis); or idiopathic.	OP may occur as a nonspecific reaction around a wide variety of unrelated processes such as distal to airway obstruction (e.g., by tumor or aspirated foreign material); on the periphery of any inflammatory or mass lesions such as edges of granulomas, tumors, abscesses, vasculitis, or infarcts; or as a minor component of other respiratory illnesses (e.g., eosinophilic pneumonia, hypersensitivity pneumonia, Langerhans cell histiocytosis, nonspecific interstitial pneumonia or granulomatosis with polyangiitis [formerly known as Wegener granulomatosis]). OP also may represent the primary cause of respiratory illness (e.g., infection, aspiration, drug reaction, toxic inhalational injury, and connective tissue disease). If an underlying etiology cannot be identified, the process is classified as cryptogenic organizing pneumonia (COP), which was previously referred to as idiopathic bronchiolitis obliterans organizing pneumonia (BOOP).

	Constrictive Bronchiolitis	Organizing Pneumonia (OP)
Histology	It ranges from variable amounts of eccentric subepithelial collagenization/scarring of bronchioles walls, which may result in luminal constriction, to complete circumferential replacement of the bronchiole wall and lumen by mature dense collagen deposition, which may extend into the peribronchiolar zones *(Figs. 6.1–6.4)*. Subtle findings suggestive of constrictive bronchiolitis include lung hyperinflation, bronchiolar tortuosity, small pulmonary artery branches that are not paired with respective bronchioles *(Fig. 6.5)*, and small airways showing decrease in size in comparison with respective accompanying pulmonary arteries.	Airway lumens, alveolar ducts, and alveolar spaces filled in varying proportions by polypoid, elongated, branching, and serpiginous foci of organizing fibroblastic tissue *(Figs. 6.6 and 6.7)* in a patchy, bronchiolocentric distribution, which may be associated with variable, usually mild to moderate, chronic inflammation in the interstitium (alveolar septa). Alveolar macrophage accumulation, usually secondary to some degree of airway obstruction, may be present. The lung architecture is preserved.
Special studies	Pentachrome special stain is very useful in the identification of obliterated bronchioles by highlighting eccentric or concentric luminal and mural collagen deposition/scarring (yellow) with luminal narrowing of the airways and displacement of the single bronchiolar elastic tissue layer (black). Pentachrome and elastic stains are also useful in differentiating airways (single elastic tissue layer) from pulmonary arteries (two elastic tissue layers).	The foci of loosely arranged fibroblastic tissue stains green with pentachrome special stain, compared with the yellow-staining characteristic of dense fibrosis.
Prognosis	Poor prognosis, with progressive disease in most patients that is unresponsive to corticosteroids or cytotoxic therapy. Many patients undergo lung transplantation.	Usually good, with excellent response to corticosteroid therapy.

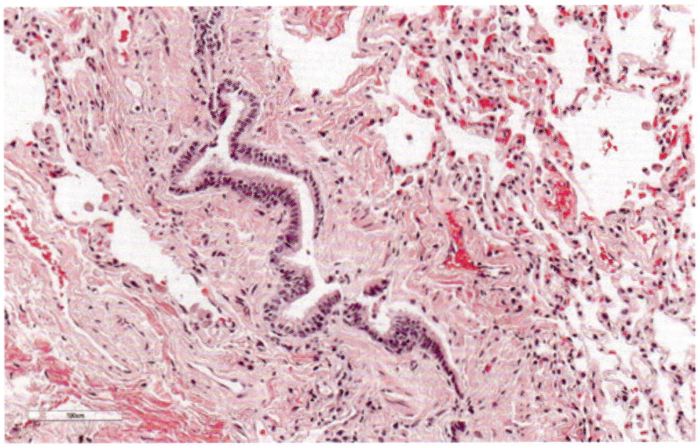

Figure 6.1 Constrictive bronchiolitis: There is bronchiolar tortuosity and subepithelial scarring, which can be confirmed by pentachrome special stain.

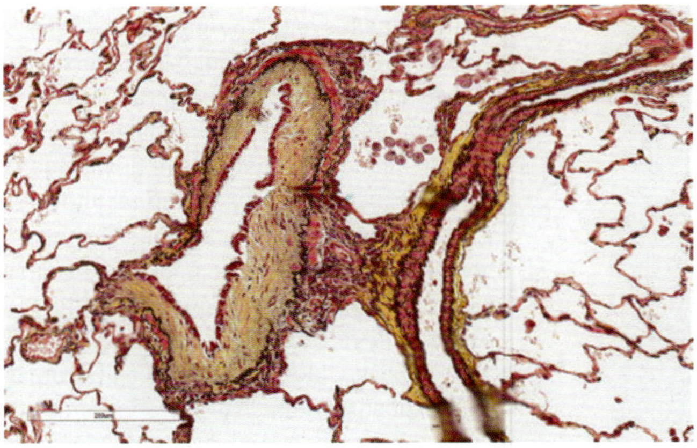

Figure 6.2 Constrictive bronchiolitis: Small airway subepithelial dense collagen deposition (pentachrome, *yellow*, *left*), displaces the bronchiolar single-tissue elastic layer (*black*). The adjacent alveolar septa are thin and delicate.

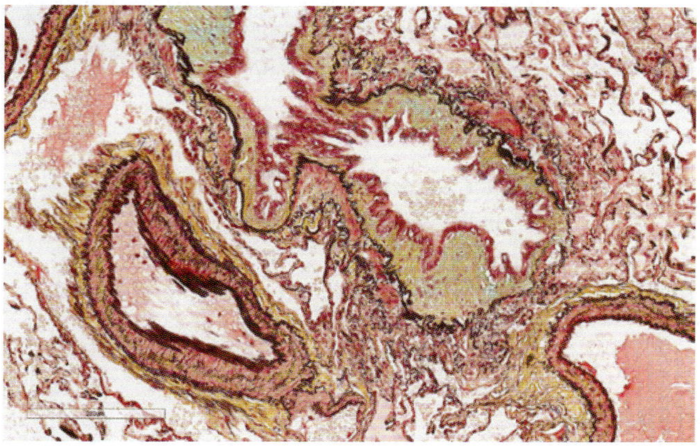

Figure 6.3 Constrictive bronchiolitis: Moderate concentric small airway subepithelial collagenization (pentachrome, *yellow, right*) displaces the bronchiolar single-tissue elastic layer (*black*). Pentachrome special stain is useful in differentiating airways (single elastic tissue layer, *right*) from pulmonary arteries (two elastic tissue layers, *left*).

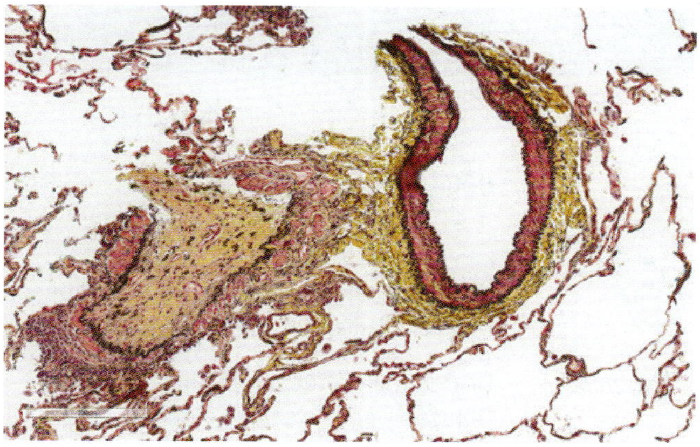

Figure 6.4 Constrictive bronchiolitis: Marked small airway subepithelial collagenization/scarring (pentachrome, *yellow, left*) that completely replaces the bronchiole wall and lumen. Note that the corresponding small pulmonary artery (*right*) has double elastic tissue layer (*black*).

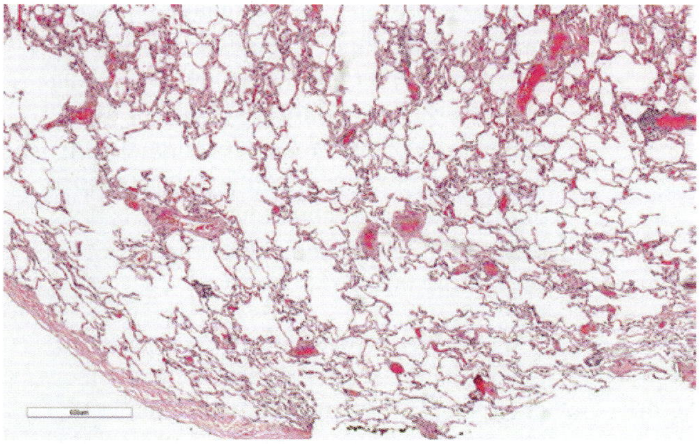

Figure 6.5 Constrictive bronchiolitis: Subtle findings suggestive of constrictive bronchiolitis include lung hyperinflation and small pulmonary artery branches that are not paired with respective bronchioles.

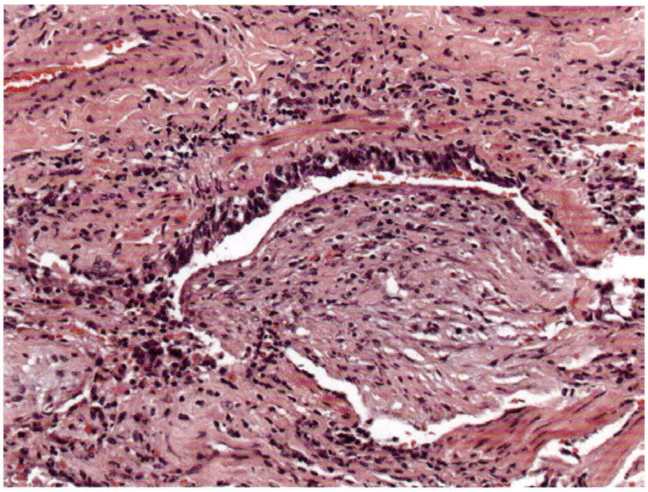

Figure 6.6 OP: Airway lumen filled with polypoid plug of OP. Different from constrictive bronchiolitis, in OP there is no subepithelial collagenization and scar of airways.

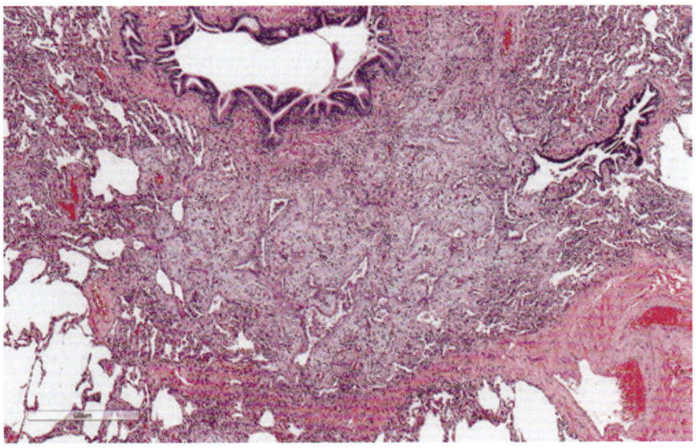

Figure 6.7 OP: OP is a primary airspace-filling process. In the picture, peribronchial alveolar spaces are filled by serpiginous foci of OP.

7 DIFFUSE ALVEOLAR DAMAGE VS. ACUTE EXACERBATION OF USUAL INTERSTITIAL PNEUMONIA

	Diffuse Alveolar Damage (DAD)	Acute Exacerbation of Usual Interstitial Pneumonia (UIP)
Age	Wide age range. Age predilection depends on etiologic factors. No gender predominance.	Patients are usually between 50 and 70 y of age.
Location	DAD usually affects the lungs bilaterally. Diffuse alveolar damage means that the process affects all parts of the alveolus (epithelium, endothelium, and interstitial space).	Same as DAD.
Symptoms	Severe hypoxemia and dyspnea with rapidly progressive respiratory failure, which usually requires mechanical ventilation.	There is abrupt clinical deterioration in patients with established diagnosis of UIP, characterized by sudden unexpected severe worsening of chronic dyspnea and hypoxemia and new opacities on imaging studies without evidence of infection or cardiac failure. It has been reported to occur from 3 mo to near 8 y following the diagnosis of UIP. It can also be the initial manifestation of the disease in patients without a prior diagnosis of UIP, in whom the presence of UIP is first recognized at the time of the biopsy for acute respiratory failure.
Signs	Severe hypoxemia regardless of the positive end-expiratory pressure (PEEP) or inspired oxygen fraction (FIO_2) concentration. The ratio of arterial partial pressure of oxygen to inspired oxygen fraction (PaO_2/FIO_2) is less than 200. Chest x-ray shows bilateral patchy airspace consolidations, which become rapidly confluent and diffuse. The consolidation is usually most severe in the peripheral lung regions. The computed tomography (CT) of the chest often shows bilateral patchy-to-diffuse ground-glass opacities and airspace consolidation.	The chest CT shows typical coarse reticular abnormalities and peripheral honeycomb change of UIP associated with superimposed ground-glass opacities and airspace consolidation.
Etiology	The causes of DAD are numerous, including, but not limited to, infections; shock (traumatic, hemorrhagic, neurogenic, or cardiogenic); sepsis; aspiration of gastric contents; ingestion of paraquat, kerosene, and other substances; inhalational injury, radiation pneumonitis; drugs; metabolic disorders (e.g., pancreatitis, uremia); hematologic disorders (e.g., intravascular coagulation and transfusion-associated acute lung injury); connective tissue disorders; and pulmonary hemorrhage syndrome and vasculitis. In the absence of known etiologies, the case falls under the acute interstitial pneumonia (AIP) category also known as Hamman–Rich syndrome.	Unknown. Presumably immunologic.

	Diffuse Alveolar Damage (DAD)	Acute Exacerbation of Usual Interstitial Pneumonia (UIP)
Histology	The acute/exudative phase (first week after initial injury) demonstrates interstitial and intra-alveolar edema, sparse mononuclear inflammation, hyaline membranes, intravascular fibrin thrombi, and variable amount of type 2 pneumocyte hyperplasia *(Figs. 7.1–7.3)*. In the organizing/proliferative phase (second week after initial injury), edema and hyaline membranes are not prominent and there is prominent fibroblastic and myofibroblastic proliferation mostly seen in the interstitium (alveolar septa), but also noted within airspaces, associated with scattered inflammatory cells and marked type 2 pneumocyte hyperplasia *(Figs. 7.4 and 7.5)*. Squamous cell metaplasia may be present *(Fig. 7.6)*. In the fibrotic phase (late stage), there is variable amount of interstitial scarring/fibrosis, which may progress to extensive remodeling of the underlying lung parenchyma.	Same features of DAD, superimposed on underlying lung parenchyma showing UIP morphology, including patchy or end-stage interstitial scarring (old fibrosis) and honeycomb change. If more than one lobe is biopsied, UIP morphology may be identified in one lobe, while DAD may be noted in another *(Figs. 7.7–7.9)*.
Special studies	Gomori methanamine silver (GMS), acid-fast bacilli (AFB), and Gram special stains, virus immunoperoxidase stains, and tissue cultures should be performed to exclude infectious etiology.	Same as DAD.
Prognosis	High mortality rate, ranging from 40% to 60%.	Same as DAD, with high mortality rate.

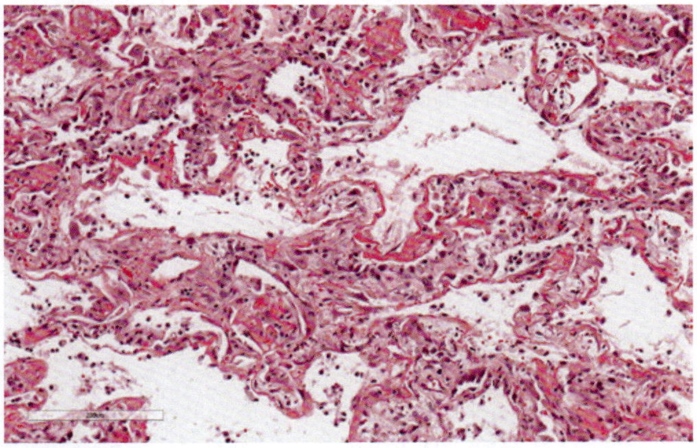

Figure 7.1 DAD (acute/exudative phase): There is alveolar septal (interstitial) thickening by edema and sparse mononuclear inflammation associated with hyaline membranes.

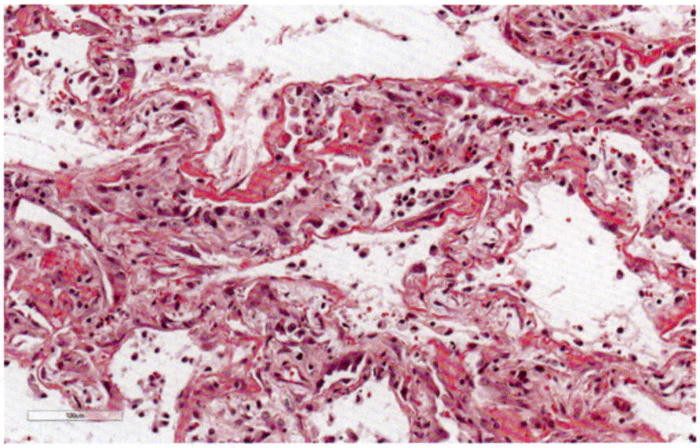

Figure 7.2 DAD (acute/exudative phase): Hyaline membranes (homogeneous, pink fibrinous material) are the hallmark of the acute stage. They are located along the alveolar septa and associated with variable amounts of type 2 pneumocyte hyperplasia.

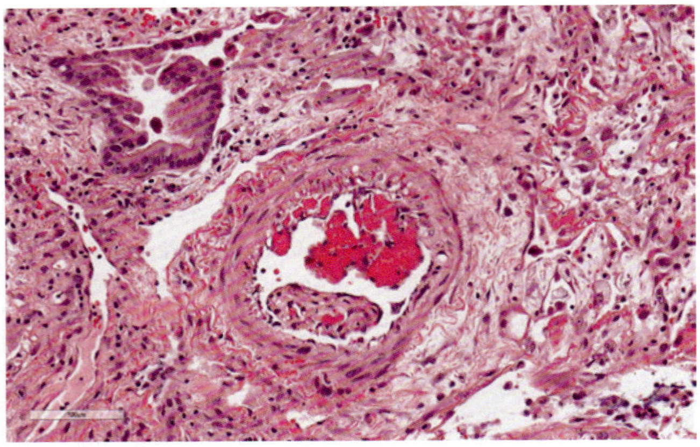

Figure 7.3 DAD (acute/exudative phase): Fibrin thrombi are frequently present in the small pulmonary arteries.

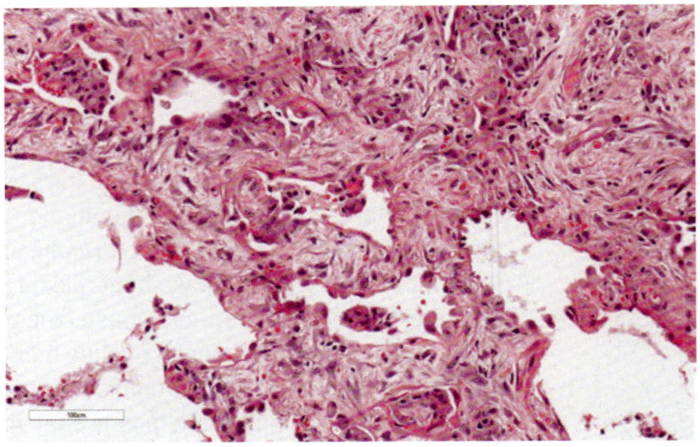

Figure 7.4 DAD (organizing/proliferative): There is prominent fibroblastic and myofibroblastic proliferation mostly seen in the interstitium (alveolar septa), associated with scattered inflammatory cells and marked type 2 pneumocyte hyperplasia.

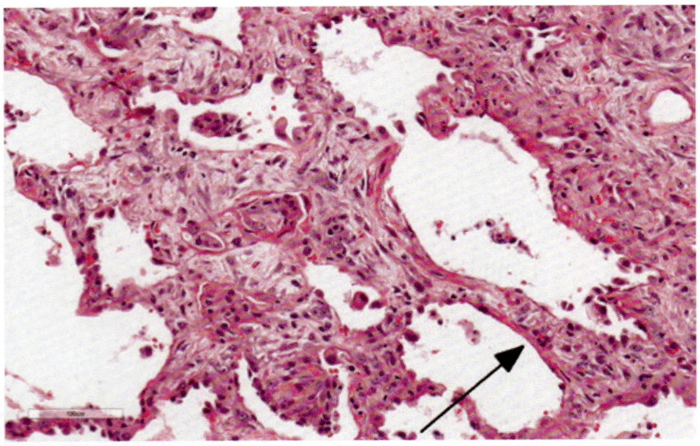

Figure 7.5 DAD (organizing/proliferative): Remnants of hyaline membranes (*arrow*) may be seen in the organizing stage.

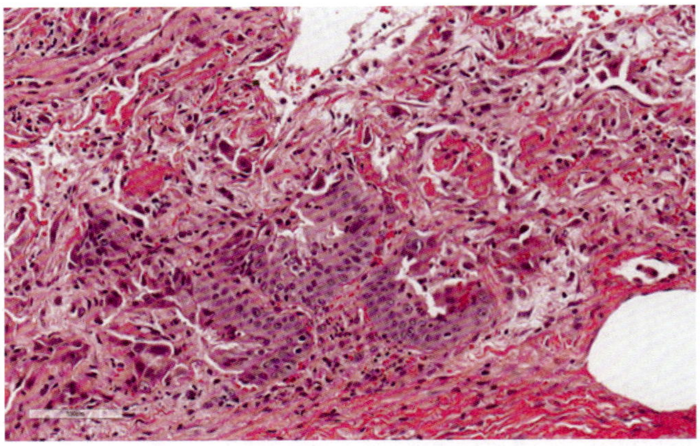

Figure 7.6 DAD (organizing/proliferative): Squamous cell metaplasia may occur in and around terminal bronchioles. Cytologic atypia is common and in some cases may be severe and mimic malignancy.

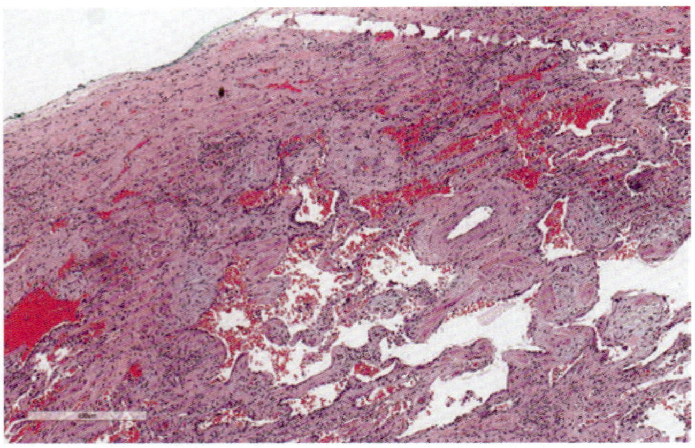

Figures 7.7 UIP morphology: Temporally heterogeneous pattern of interstitial fibrosis composed of dense (old) fibrosis and foci of recent organization (fibroblastic activity) characteristic of UIP.

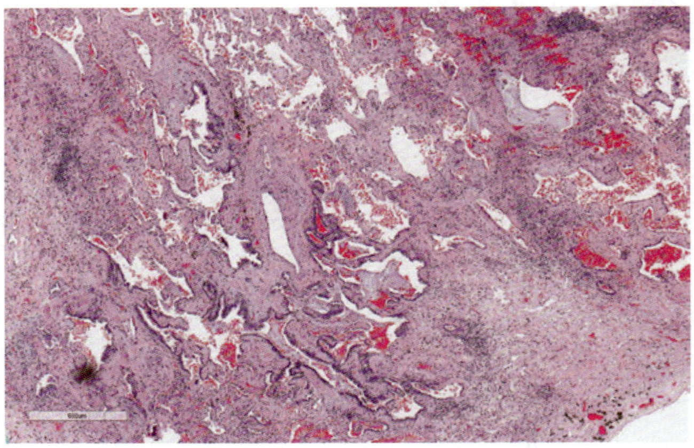

Figure 7.8 UIP morphology: Dense fibrosis and honeycomb change typical of UIP.

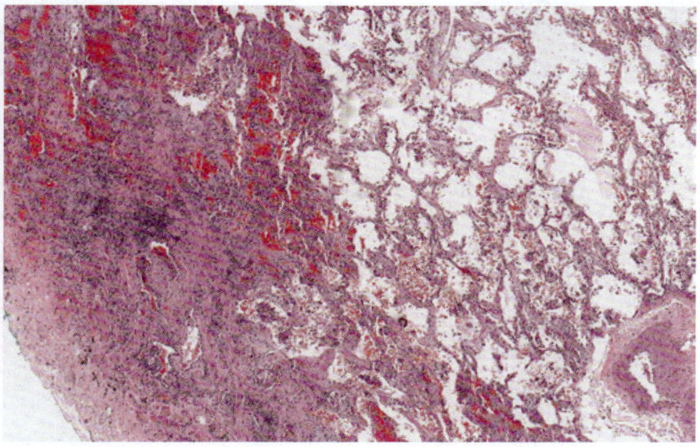

Figure 7.9 Acute exacerbation of UIP: There is acute and organizing lung injury (right) and subpleural dense fibrosis with smooth muscle hyperplasia of UIP (left).

8 DIFFUSE ALVEOLAR DAMAGE VS. NONSPECIFIC INTERSTITIAL PNEUMONIA

	Diffuse Alveolar Damage (DAD)	Nonspecific Interstitial Pneumonia (NSIP)
Age	Wide age range. Age predilection depends on etiologic factors. No gender predominance.	The average age ranges from 40 to 57 y, but is also found in children. It is slightly more common in women.
Location	DAD usually affects the lungs bilaterally. Diffuse alveolar damage means that the process affects all parts of the alveolus (epithelium, endothelium, and interstitial space).	It usually affects the lower lobes, spares subpleural spaces, and tends to be bilateral and symmetrical.
Symptoms	Severe hypoxemia and dyspnea with rapidly progressive respiratory failure, which usually requires mechanical ventilation.	Different from DAD, the symptoms in NSIP develop gradually. Shortness of breath, cough, fatigue, and weight loss are the most common symptoms. Fever and digital clubbing have been reported but are uncommon.
Signs	Severe hypoxemia regardless of the positive end-expiratory pressure (PEEP) or inspired oxygen fraction (FIO_2) concentration. The ratio of arterial partial pressure of oxygen to inspired oxygen fraction (PaO_2/FIO_2) is less than 200. Chest x-ray shows bilateral patchy airspace consolidations that becomes rapidly confluent and diffuse. The consolidation is usually most severe in the peripheral lung regions. The CT of the chest often shows bilateral patchy-to-diffuse ground-glass opacities and airspace consolidations.	High-resolution computed tomography (HRCT) scans show bilateral lower-lobe predominant infiltrates and ground-glass attenuation that evolve into traction bronchiectasis as the disease becomes fibrotic. There is subpleural sparing and honeycombing is generally not present. Volume loss, particularly of the lower lobes, is common. Pulmonary function tests usually reveal a restrictive pattern with decreased diffusing capacity of the lung carbon monoxide (DLCO).
Etiology	The causes of DAD are numerous, including, but not limited to, infections; shock (traumatic, hemorrhagic, neurogenic, or cardiogenic); sepsis; aspiration of gastric contents; ingestion of paraquat, kerosene, and other substances; inhalational injury; radiation pneumonitis; drugs; metabolic disorders (e.g., pancreatitis, uremia); hematologic disorders (e.g., intravascular coagulation and transfusion-associated acute lung injury); connective tissue disorders; and pulmonary hemorrhage syndrome and vasculitis. In the absence of known etiologies, the case falls under the acute interstitial pneumonia (AIP) category, also known as Hamman–Rich syndrome.	Pulmonary manifestation of underlying autoimmune/collagen vascular disease (e.g., rheumatoid arthritis, Sjögren syndrome), immunodeficiency disorders (e.g., acquired immunodeficiency syndrome, common variable immunodeficiency), drug toxicity (e.g., Dilantin), or idiopathic.

	Diffuse Alveolar Damage (DAD)	Nonspecific Interstitial Pneumonia (NSIP)
Histology	The acute/exudative phase (first week after initial injury) demonstrates interstitial and intra-alveolar edema, sparse mononuclear inflammation, hyaline membranes, intravascular fibrin thrombi, and variable amount of type 2 pneumocyte hyperplasia *(Figs. 8.1–8.3)*. In the organizing/proliferative phase (second week after initial injury), edema and hyaline membranes are not prominent and there is prominent fibroblastic and myofibroblastic proliferation mostly seen in the interstitium (alveolar septa), but also noted within airspaces, associated with scattered inflammatory cells and marked type 2 pneumocyte hyperplasia *(Figs. 8.4 and 8.5)*. Squamous cell metaplasia may be present *(Fig. 8.6)*. In the fibrotic phase (late stage), there is variable amount of interstitial scarring/fibrosis, which may progress to extensive remodeling of the architecture of the underlying lung parenchyma.	*Cellular variant*: There is diffuse and uniform interstitial (alveolar septal) expansion by mild-to-moderate chronic inflammatory cell infiltrate containing predominantly small mature lymphocytes and occasional plasma cells associated with alveolar pneumocyte prominence. The inflammatory process may be associated with lymphoid aggregates (with or without germinal centers), chronic pleuritis, and increase in perivascular collagen deposition, which although nonspecific, are features commonly associated with autoimmune disorder/collagen vascular disease manifesting in the lung *(Figs. 8.7–8.10)*. *Fibrosing variant*: There is diffuse and uniform interstitial expansion by dense collagen deposition (fibrosis), few fibroblasts, little amount of inflammation, and alveolar pneumocyte prominence *(Figs. 8.11–8.13)*. *Mixed cellular and fibrosing variant*: There is diffuse and uniform interstitial expansion by similar amounts of inflammation and fibrosis. In all three forms of NSIP, the underlying lung architecture is preserved, with no honeycomb change. Fibroblastic foci may be present, but they are usually inconspicuous and never numerous. Few plugs of organizing pneumonia and variable amounts of peribronchiolar metaplasia may be present. Increased numbers of macrophages are frequently found within the alveolar spaces.
Special studies	Gomori methenamine silver (GMS), acid-fast bacilli (AFB), and Gram special stains; virus immunoperoxidase stains; and tissue cultures to exclude infectious etiology.	None suggested.
Prognosis	High mortality rate, ranging from 40% to 60%.	The prognosis of cellular NSIP is better than that of fibrosing NSIP. The 5-y survival rate for patients with cellular NSIP is nearly 100% with good response to corticosteroid therapy. The 5- and 10-y survival rates for patients with fibrosing NSIP are 90% and 35%, respectively.

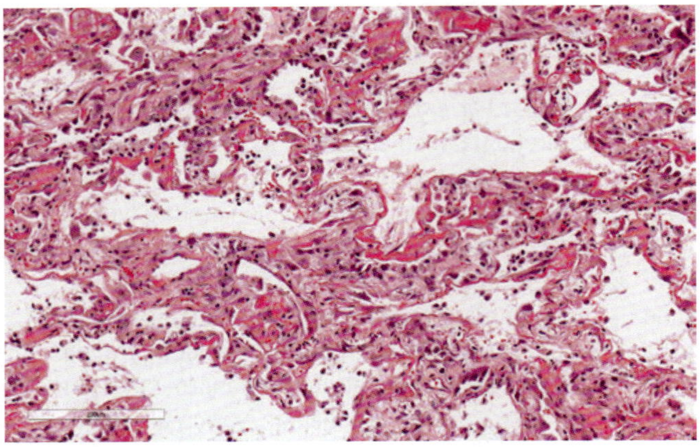

Figure 8.1 DAD (acute/exudative phase): There is alveolar septal (interstitial) thickening by edema and sparse mononuclear inflammation associated with hyaline membranes.

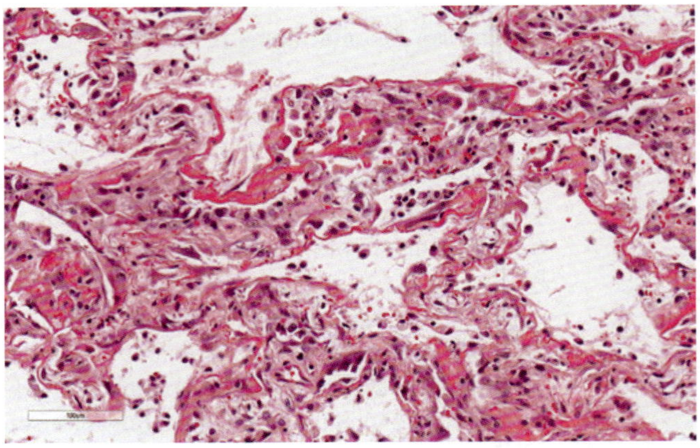

Figure 8.2 DAD (acute/exudative phase): Hyaline membranes (homogeneous, pink fibrinous material) are the hallmark of the acute stage. They are located along the alveolar septa and associated with variable amounts of type 2 pneumocyte hyperplasia.

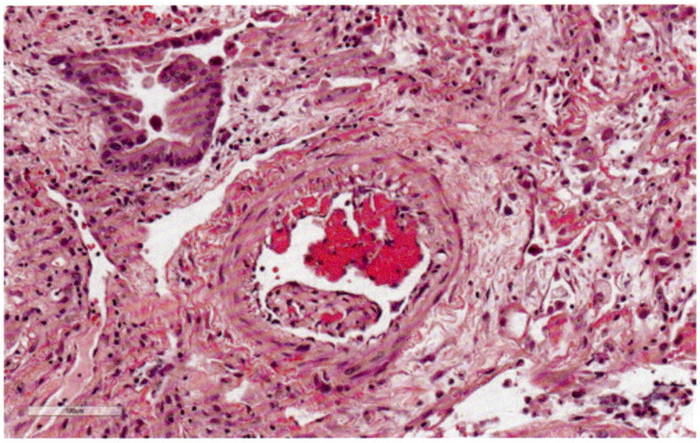

Figure 8.3 DAD (acute/exudative phase): Fibrin thrombi are frequently present in the small pulmonary arteries.

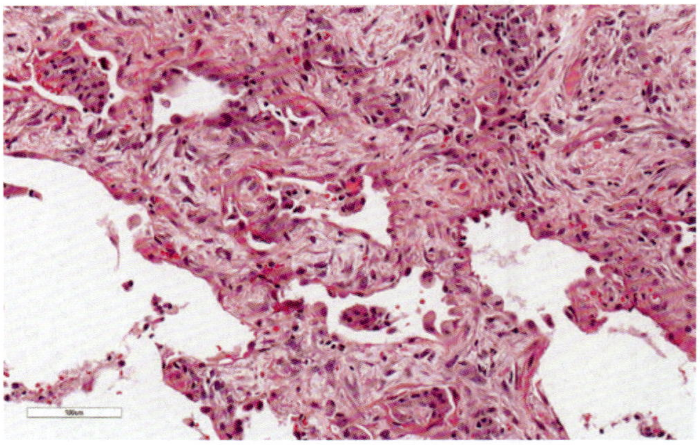

Figure 8.4 DAD (organizing/proliferative): There is prominent fibroblastic and myofibroblastic proliferation mostly seen in the interstitium (alveolar septa), associated with scattered inflammatory cells and marked type 2 pneumocyte hyperplasia.

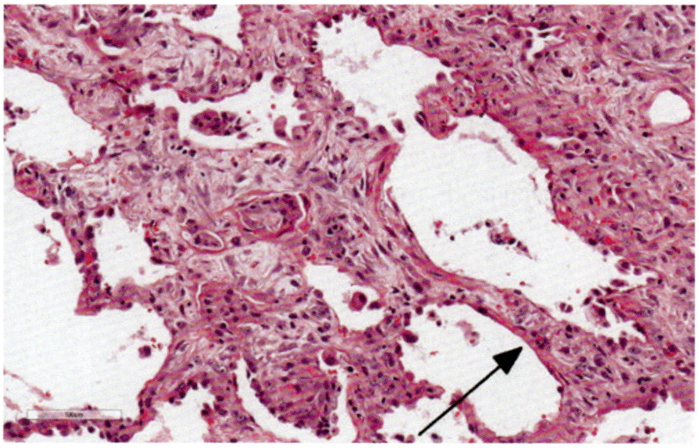

Figure 8.5 DAD (organizing/proliferative): Remnants of hyaline membranes (*arrow*) may be seen in the organizing stage.

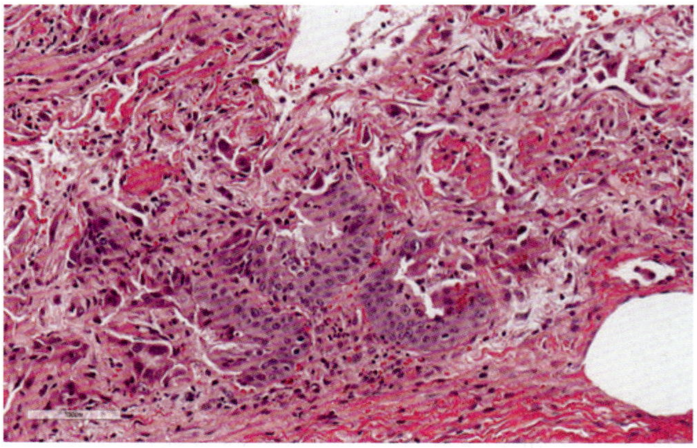

Figure 8.6 DAD (organizing/proliferative): Squamous cell metaplasia may occur in and around terminal bronchioles. Cytologic atypia is common and in some cases may be severe and mimic malignancy.

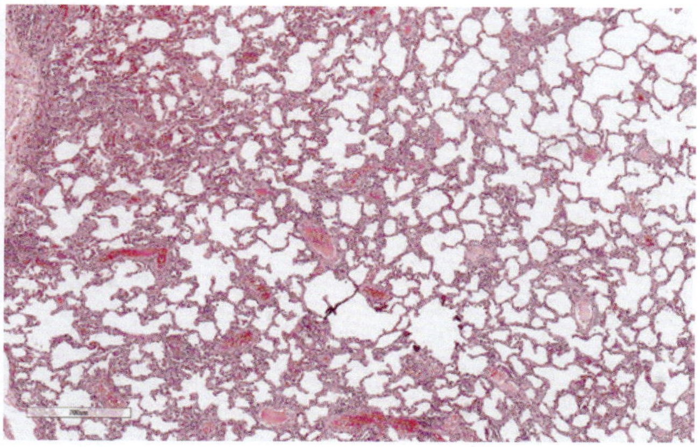

Figures 8.7 Cellular NSIP (low power): There is diffuse and uniform interstitial (alveolar septal) expansion.

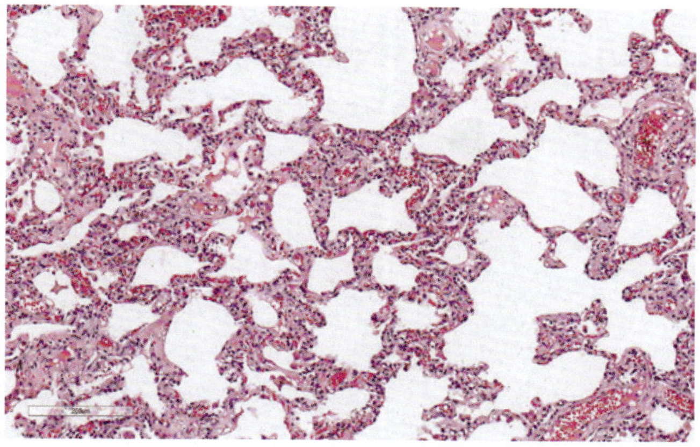

Figure 8.8 Cellular NSIP (high power): The alveolar septal expansion is composed of mild-to-moderate chronic inflammatory cell infiltrate containing predominantly small mature lymphocytes. Different from DAD in NSIP there is no interstitial organization or hyaline membranes.

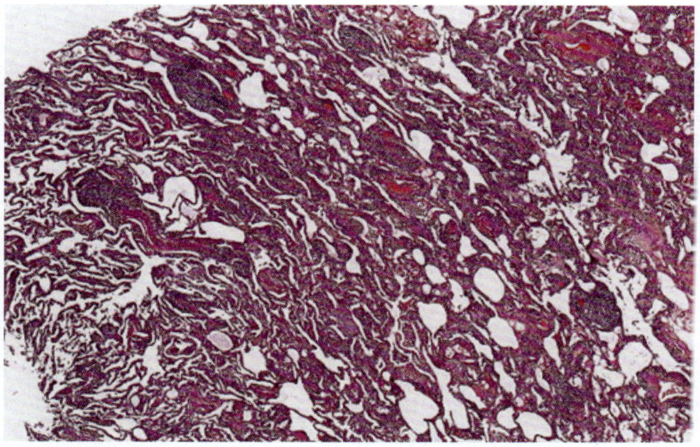

Figure 8.9 Cellular NSIP (low power): NSIP secondary to rheumatoid arthritis in a 62-year-old woman. Note diffuse and uniform septal cellular expansion associated with frequent lymphoid follicles.

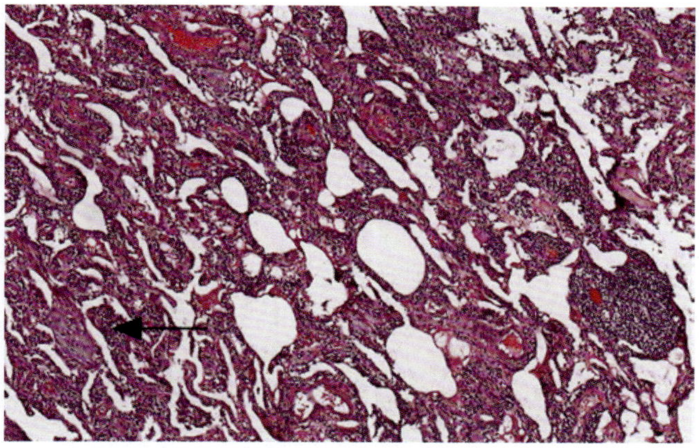

Figure 8.10 Cellular NSIP (high power): Same patient from Figure 8.9. The cellular septal expansion is composed predominantly of lymphocytic inflammatory cell infiltrate. Note small focus of organizing pneumonia (*arrow*).

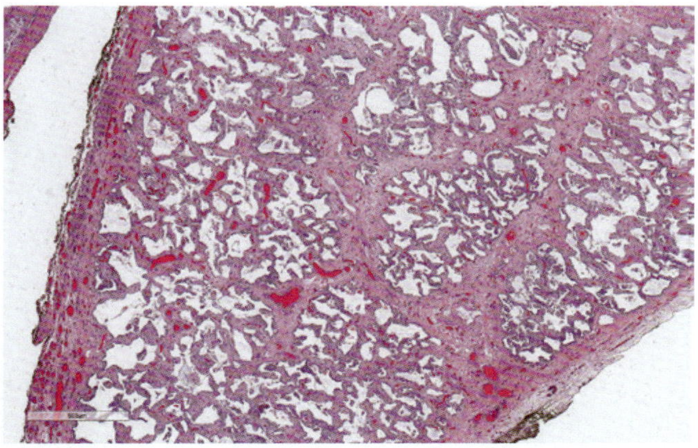

Figure 8.11 Fibrotic NSIP (low power): There is diffuse and uniform interstitial (alveolar septal) expansion by eosinophilic material.

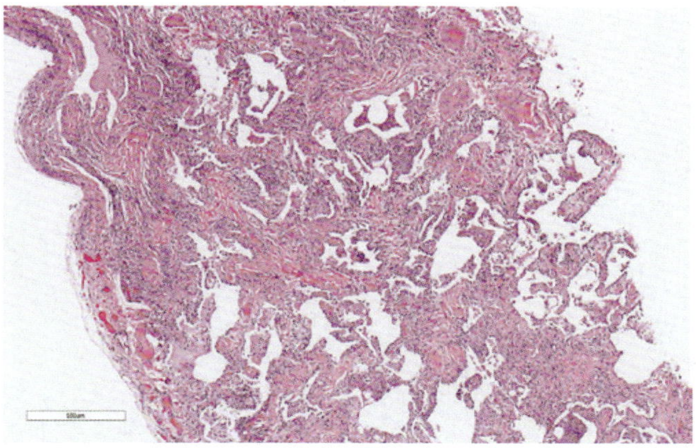

Figure 8.12 Fibrotic NSIP (high power): The interstitial eosinophilic material is composed of dense collagen deposition (fibrosis) and little inflammation.

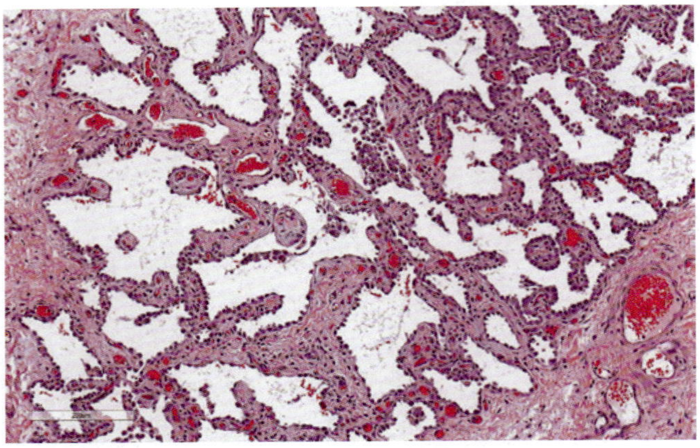

Figure 8.13 Fibrotic NSIP: The alveolar septal scarring is frequently associated with alveolar pneumocyte prominence. Macrophages are frequently found within the alveolar spaces.

9 DIFFUSE ALVEOLAR DAMAGE VS. ORGANIZING PNEUMONIA

	Diffuse Alveolar Damage (DAD)	Organizing Pneumonia (OP)
Age	Wide age range. Age predilection depends on etiologic factors. No gender predominance.	Occurs mostly in the fifth and sixth decades, with mean age of onset at 55 y. Affects men and women equally.
Location	DAD usually affects the lungs bilaterally. Diffuse alveolar damage means that the process affects all parts of the alveolus (epithelium, endothelium, and interstitial space).	Lumens of distal bronchioles, alveolar ducts, and peribronchiolar alveolar spaces.
Symptoms	Severe hypoxemia and dyspnea with rapidly progressive respiratory failure, which usually requires mechanical ventilation.	Subacute illness, characterized by 2-to-3-mo history of cough, dyspnea, which can be associated with weight loss, fever, sweats, chills, and myalgia.
Signs	Severe hypoxemia regardless of the positive end-expiratory pressure (PEEP) or inspired oxygen fraction (FIO_2) concentration. The ratio of arterial partial pressure of oxygen to inspired oxygen fraction (PaO_2/FIO_2) is less than 200. Chest x-ray shows bilateral patchy airspace consolidations, which becomes rapidly confluent and diffuse. The consolidation is usually most severe in the peripheral lung regions. Chest CT often shows bilateral patchy-to-diffuse ground-glass opacities and airspace consolidations.	Inspiratory crackles on physical examination. Pulmonary function tests may show mild-to-moderate restrictive pattern. Airflow obstruction is usually absent. Chest x-ray shows patchy airspace consolidation, which is usually bilateral but may be unilateral. Chest CT shows bilateral/unilateral patchy airspace consolidation/ground-glass opacities in a peribronchial distribution.
Etiology	The causes of DAD are numerous, including, but not limited to, infections; shock (traumatic, hemorrhagic, neurogenic, or cardiogenic); sepsis; aspiration of gastric contents; ingestion of paraquat, kerosene, and other substances; inhalational injury; radiation pneumonitis; drugs; metabolic disorders (e.g., pancreatitis, uremia); hematologic disorders (e.g., intravascular coagulation and transfusion associated acute lung injury); connective tissue disorders; and pulmonary hemorrhage syndrome and vasculitis. In the absence of known etiologies, the case would fall under the acute interstitial pneumonia (AIP) category, also known as Hamman–Rich syndrome.	OP may occur as a nonspecific reaction around a wide variety of unrelated processes such as distal-to-airway obstruction (e.g., by tumor or aspirated foreign material); on the periphery of any inflammatory or mass lesions such as edges of granulomas, tumors, abscesses, vasculitis, or infarcts, or as a minor component of other respiratory illnesses (e.g., eosinophilic pneumonia, hypersensitivity pneumonia, Langerhans cell histiocytosis, nonspecific interstitial pneumonia, or granulomatosis with polyangiitis [formerly known as Wegener granulomatosis]). OP also may represent the primary cause of respiratory illnesses (e.g., infection, aspiration, drug reaction, toxic inhalational injury, and connective tissue disease). If an underlying etiology cannot be identified, the process is classified as cryptogenic organizing pneumonia (COP), which was referred to previously as idiopathic bronchiolitis obliterans organizing pneumonia (BOOP).

	Diffuse Alveolar Damage (DAD)	Organizing Pneumonia (OP)
Histology	The acute/exudative phase (first week after initial injury) demonstrates interstitial and intra-alveolar edema, sparse mononuclear inflammation, hyaline membranes, intravascular fibrin thrombi, and variable amounts of type 2 pneumocyte hyperplasia *(Figs. 9.1–9.3)*. In the organizing/proliferative phase (second week after initial injury), edema and hyaline membranes are not prominent and there is prominent fibroblastic and myofibroblastic proliferation, mostly seen in the interstitium (alveolar septa), but also noted within airspaces, associated with scattered inflammatory cells and marked type 2 pneumocyte hyperplasia *(Figs. 9.4 and 9.5)*. Squamous cell metaplasia may be present *(Fig. 9.6)*. In the fibrotic phase (late stage), there is variable amount of interstitial scarring/fibrosis, which may progress to extensive remodeling of the architecture of the underlying lung parenchyma.	Airway lumens, alveolar ducts, and alveolar spaces are filled in varying proportions by polypoid, elongated, branching, and serpiginous foci of organizing fibroblastic tissue *(Figs. 9.7–9.11)* in a patchy, bronchiolocentric distribution, which may be associated with variable, usually mild to moderate, chronic inflammation in the interstitium (alveolar septa). Alveolar macrophage accumulation, usually secondary to some degree of airway obstruction, may be present. The lung architecture is preserved.
Special studies	Gomori methenamine silver (GMS), acid-fast bacilli (AFB), and Gram special stains; virus immunoperoxidase stains; and tissue cultures are carried out to exclude infectious etiology.	The foci of loosely arranged fibroblastic tissue stains green with pentachrome special stain, compared with the yellow-staining characteristic of dense fibrosis.
Prognosis	High mortality rate, ranging from 40% to 60%.	Usually good, with excellent response to corticosteroid therapy.

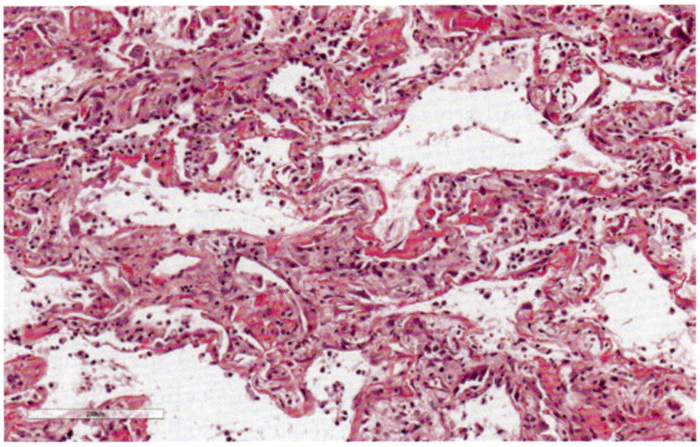

Figure 9.1 DAD (acute/exudative phase): There is *alveolar septal (interstitial)* thickening by edema and sparse mononuclear inflammation associated with hyaline membranes.

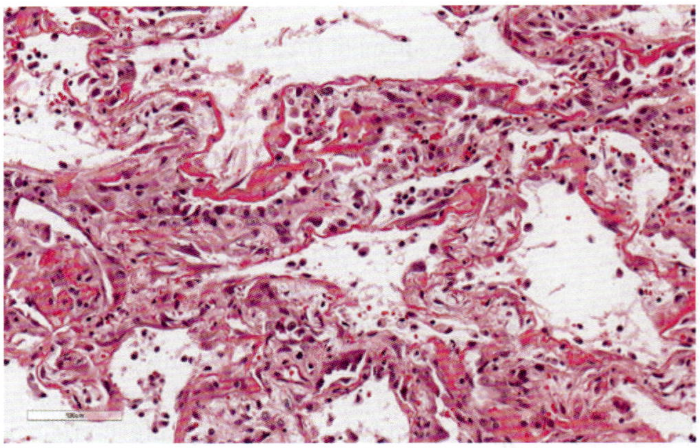

Figure 9.2 DAD (acute/exudative phase): Hyaline membranes (homogeneous, pink fibrinous material) are the hallmark of the acute stage. They are located along the alveolar septa and are associated with variable amounts of type 2 pneumocyte hyperplasia.

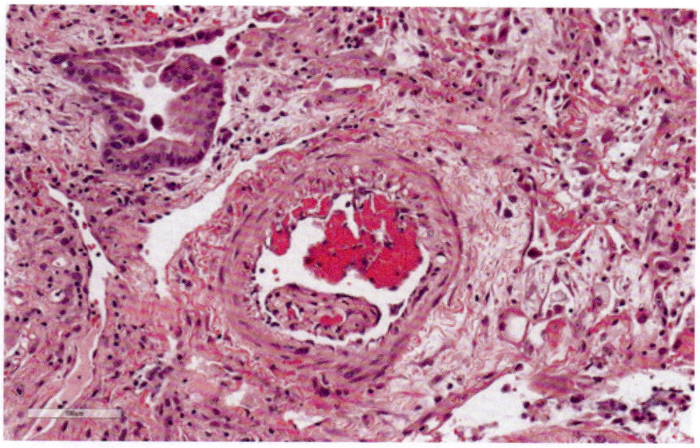

Figure 9.3 DAD (acute/exudative phase): Fibrin thrombi are frequently present in the small pulmonary arteries.

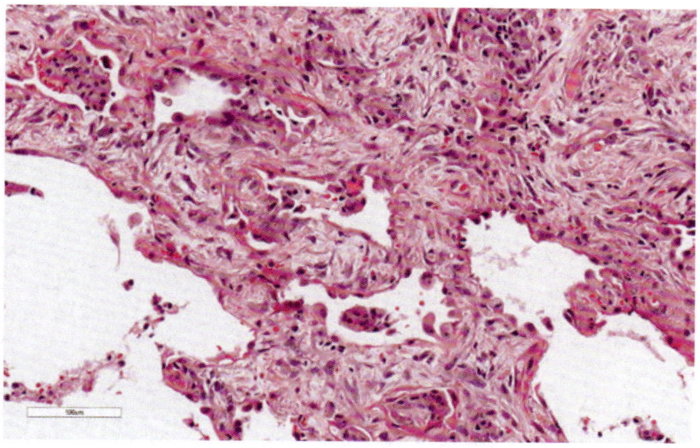

Figure 9.4 DAD (organizing/proliferative): There is prominent fibroblastic and myofibroblastic proliferation mostly seen in the *interstitium* (alveolar septa), associated with scattered inflammatory cells and marked type 2 pneumocyte hyperplasia.

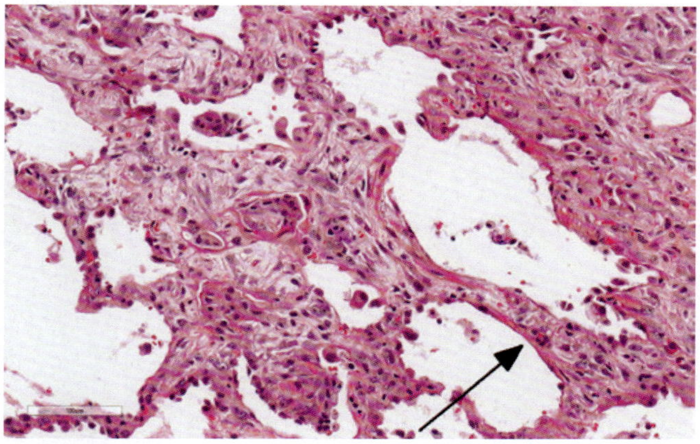

Figure 9.5 DAD (organizing/proliferative): Remnants of hyaline membranes (*arrow*) may be seen in the organizing stage.

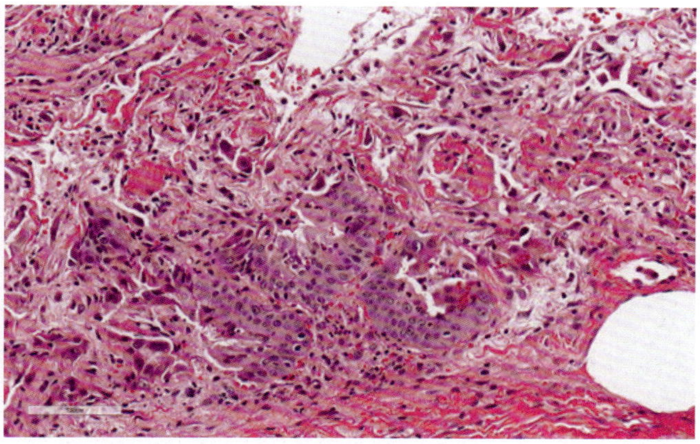

Figure 9.6 DAD (organizing/proliferative): Squamous cell metaplasia may occur in and around terminal bronchioles. Cytologic atypia is common and in some cases may be severe and mimic malignancy.

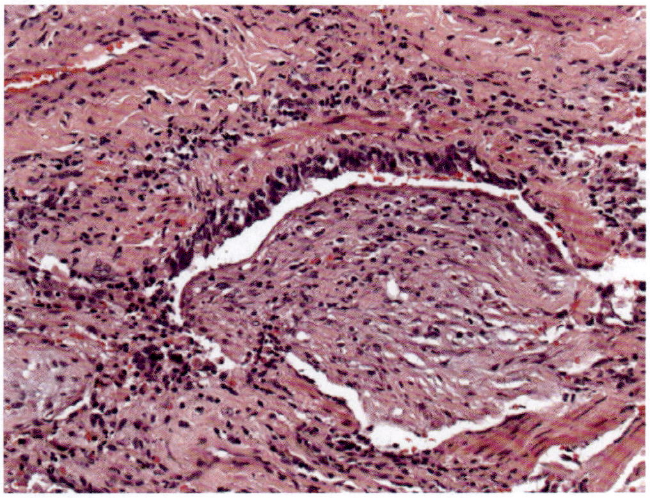

Figure 9.7 OP: Airway lumen filled with polypoid plug of organizing pneumonia.

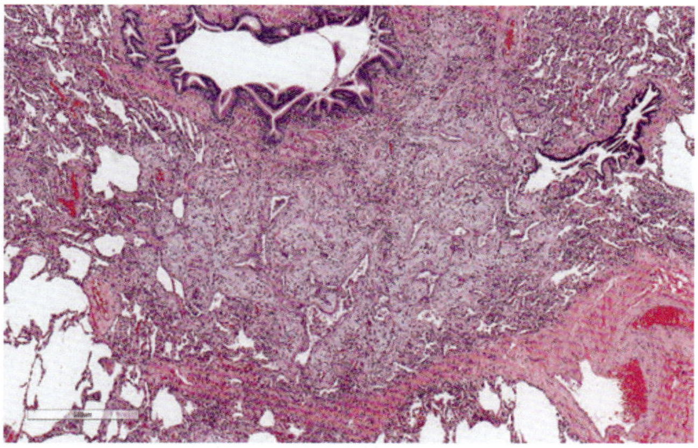

Figure 9.8 OP: Peribronchial alveolar spaces filled by serpiginous foci of OP. In OP, foci of recent organization primarily fill the airspaces, while in DAD the areas of recent organization largely expand the alveolar septa (interstitium).

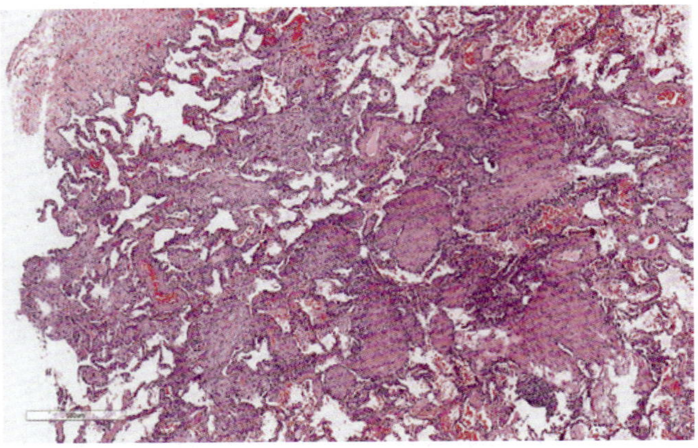

Figure 9.9 OP: Alveolar spaces are filled by polypoid, elongated, and branching foci of organizing fibroblastic tissue associated with mild amounts of chronic inflammation in the interstitium (alveolar septa).

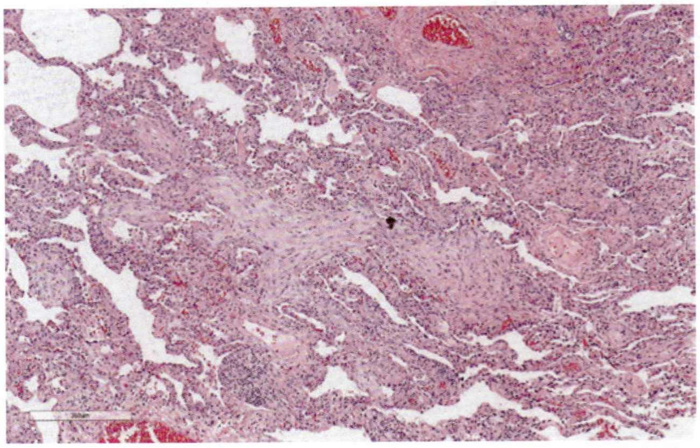

Figure 9.10 OP: Elongated focus of OP (*center*). While DAD affects all parts of the alveolus (epithelium, endothelium, and interstitial space), OP is a primary airspace-filling process, which lacks hyaline membranes and may be associated with mild-to-moderate amounts of chronic inflammation in the interstitium.

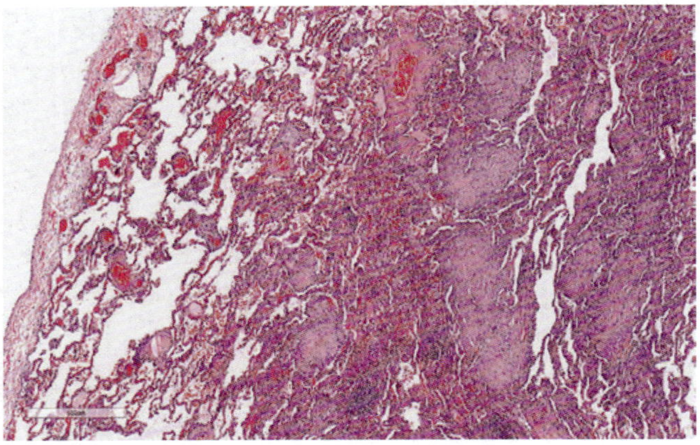

Figure 9.11 OP: Areas of unaffected alveolar spaces (*left*) and areas showing airspace filling by foci of OP (*right*).

10 DIFFUSE ALVEOLAR DAMAGE VS. ACUTE FIBRINOUS AND ORGANIZING PNEUMONIA

	Diffuse Alveolar Damage (DAD)	Acute Fibrinous and Organizing Pneumonia (AFOP)
Age	Wide age range. Age predilection depends on etiologic factors. No gender predominance.	Similar to DAD.
Location	DAD usually affects the lungs bilaterally. Diffuse alveolar damage means that the process affects all parts of the alveolus (epithelium, endothelium, and interstitial space).	It affects the alveolar spaces in a patchy or diffuse distribution.
Symptoms	Severe hypoxemia and dyspnea with rapidly progressive respiratory failure, which usually requires mechanical ventilation.	Acute or subacute onset of dyspnea, fever, cough, or hemoptysis.
Signs	Acute respiratory distress syndrome (ARDS), also known as acute lung injury, manifesting as severe hypoxemia regardless of the positive end-expiratory pressure (PEEP) or inspired oxygen fraction (FIO_2) concentration. The arterial partial pressure of oxygen to inspired oxygen fraction (PaO_2/FIO_2) is less than 200. Chest x-ray shows bilateral patchy airspace consolidations, which becomes rapidly confluent and diffuse. The consolidation is usually most severe in the peripheral lung regions. Chest CT often shows bilateral patchy-to-diffuse ground-glass opacities and airspace consolidations.	The presence of bilateral opacities, with diffuse or patchy distribution, is the most common radiologic pattern in chest high-resolution computed tomography (HRCT), particularly in basilar zones.
Etiology	The causes of DAD are numerous, including, but not limited to, infections, shock (traumatic, hemorrhagic, neurogenic, or cardiogenic), sepsis, aspiration of gastric contents, ingestion of paraquat, kerosene and other substances, inhalational injury, radiation pneumonitis, drugs, metabolic disorders (e.g., pancreatitis, uremia), hematologic disorders (e.g., intravascular coagulation and transfusion-associated acute lung injury), connective tissue disorders, and pulmonary hemorrhage syndrome and vasculitis. In the absence of known etiologies, the case falls under the acute interstitial pneumonia (AIP) category, also known as Hamman–Rich syndrome.	AFOP can occur in an idiopathic setting or can be associated with a large spectrum of clinical conditions, including, but not limited to, infections, collagen vascular disease, drug toxicity, and uremia.

	Diffuse Alveolar Damage (DAD)	Acute Fibrinous and Organizing Pneumonia (AFOP)
Histology	The acute/exudative phase (first week after initial injury) demonstrates interstitial and intra-alveolar edema, sparse mononuclear inflammation, hyaline membranes, intravascular fibrin thrombi, and variable amounts of type 2 pneumocyte hyperplasia *(Figs. 10.1–10.3)*. In the organizing/proliferative phase (second week after initial injury), edema and hyaline membranes are not prominent and there is prominent fibroblastic and myofibroblastic proliferation mostly seen in the interstitium (alveolar septa), but also noted within airspaces, associated with scattered inflammatory cells and marked type 2 pneumocyte hyperplasia *(Figs. 10.4 and 10.5)*. Squamous cell metaplasia may be present *(Fig. 10.6)*. In the fibrotic phase (late stage), there is variable amount of interstitial scarring/fibrosis, which may progress to extensive remodeling of the underlying lung parenchyma architecture.	Alveolar spaces filled by fibrin balls or aggregates *(Figs. 10.7–10.9)*. Classic hyaline membranes, as seen in DAD, are absent. The prominent alveolar fibrin deposition is associated with variable amounts of organizing pneumonia, characterized by the presence of loose organized fibroblastic tissue within the bronchioles, alveolar ducts, and alveolar spaces *(Fig. 10.9)*. The lesion usually has a patchy distribution, although some cases may appear more diffuse. The alveolar septa adjacent to alveolar spaces with fibrin deposition may show changes similar to those of DAD, such as septal edema, type 2 pneumocyte hyperplasia, and acute and chronic inflammatory infiltrates. The intervening lung parenchyma between the affected areas shows minimal changes, such as sparse chronic inflammatory cell infiltrate, but interstitial (alveolar septal) scarring is essentially absent. Vascular thrombi may be present.
Special studies	Gomori methenamine silver (GMS), acid-fast bacilli (AFB), and Gram special stains; virus immunoperoxidase stains; and tissue cultures to exclude infectious etiology.	Same as DAD.
Prognosis	High mortality rate, ranging from 40% to 60%.	The overall mortality rate is similar to DAD, and therefore AFOP may represent a histologic variant of DAD.

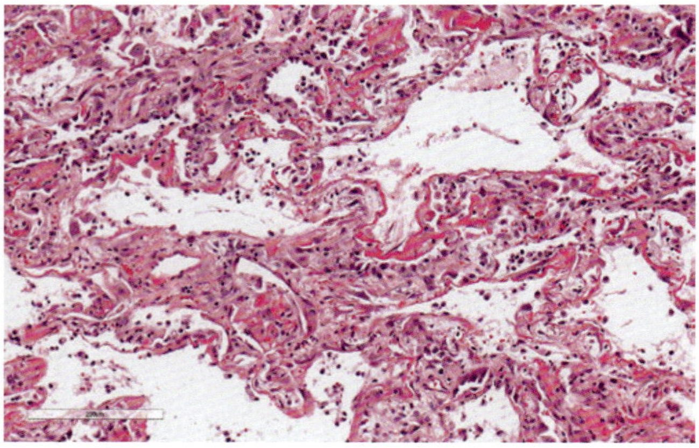

Figure 10.1 DAD (acute/exudative phase): There is alveolar septal (interstitial) thickening by edema and sparse mononuclear inflammation associated with hyaline membranes.

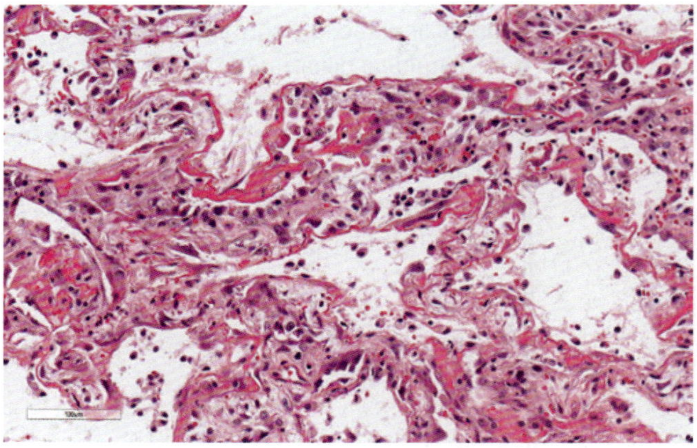

Figure 10.2 DAD (acute/exudative phase): Hyaline membranes (homogeneous, pink fibrinous material) are the hallmark of the acute stage. They are located along the alveolar septa and associated with variable amounts of type 2 pneumocyte hyperplasia.

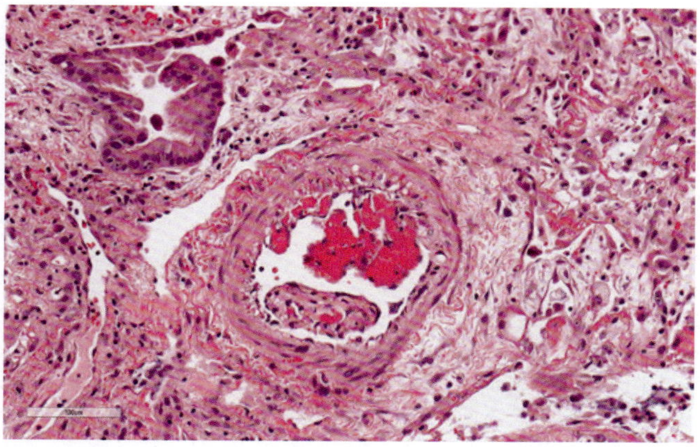

Figure 10.3 DAD (acute/exudative phase): Fibrin thrombi are frequently present in the small pulmonary arteries.

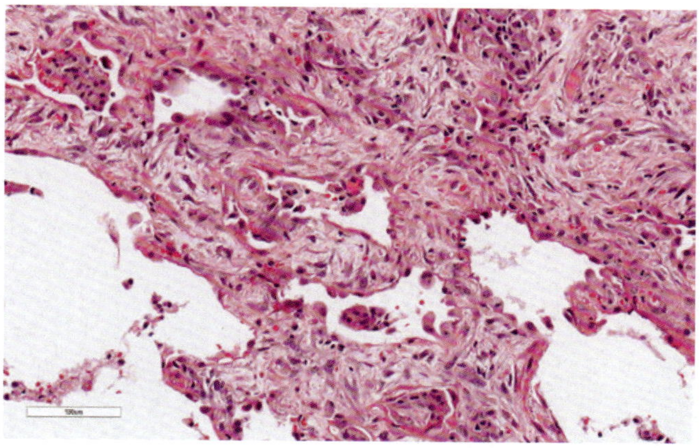

Figure 10.4 DAD (organizing/proliferative): There is prominent fibroblastic and myofibroblastic proliferation mostly seen in the interstitium (alveolar septa), associated with scattered inflammatory cells and marked type 2 pneumocyte hyperplasia.

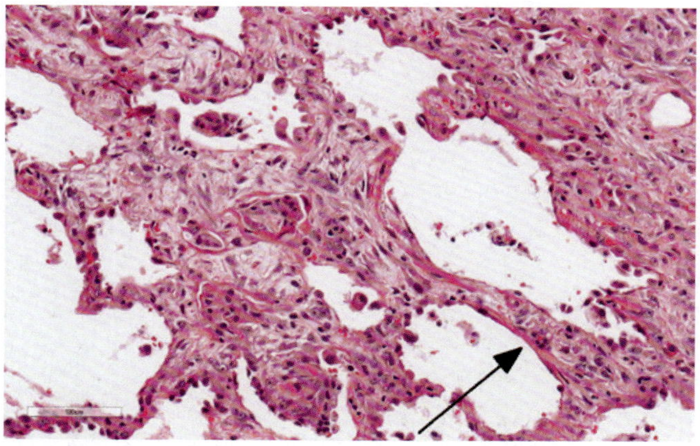

Figure 10.5 DAD (organizing/proliferative): Remnants of hyaline membranes (*arrow*) may be seen in the organizing stage.

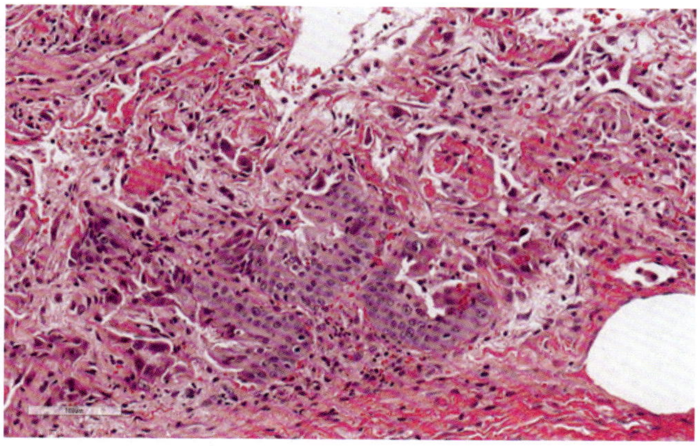

Figure 10.6 DAD (organizing/proliferative): Squamous cell metaplasia may occur in and around terminal bronchioles. Cytologic atypia is common and in some cases may be severe and mimic malignancy.

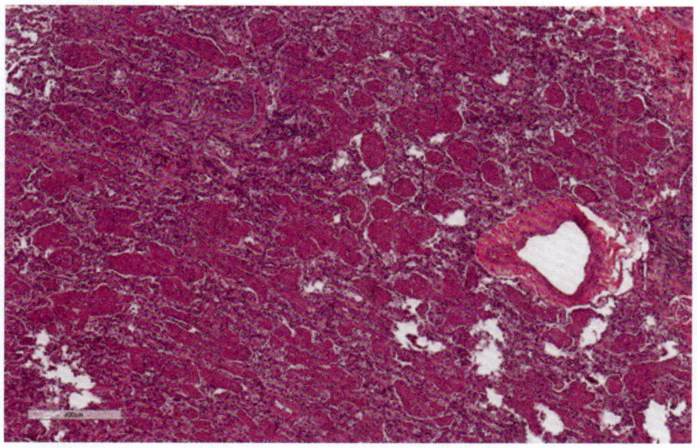

Figure 10.7 AFOP (low power): Alveolar spaces filled by numerous fibrin balls.

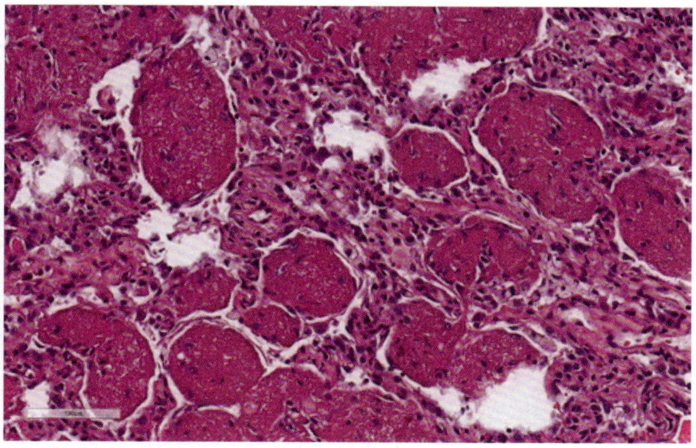

Figure 10.8 AFOP (high power): The fibrin balls are not associated with hyaline membranes.

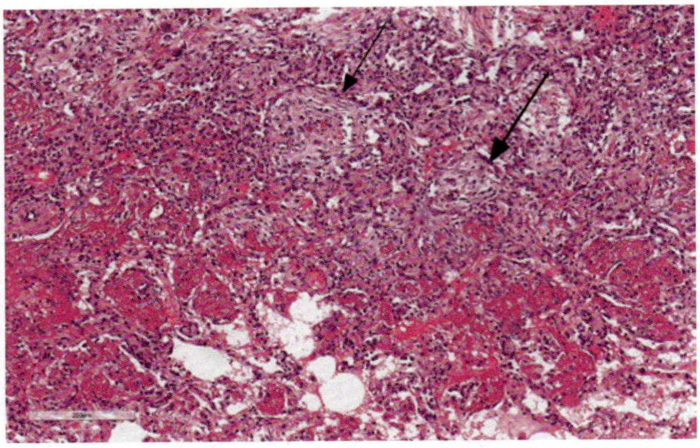

Figure 10.9 AFOP: Foci of organizing pneumonia (*arrows*) may be seen but do not represent the main pattern of injury in AFOP.

11 ORGANIZING PNEUMONIA VS. USUAL INTERSTITIAL PNEUMONIA

	Organizing Pneumonia (OP)	Usual Interstitial Pneumonia (UIP)
Age	Occurs in the fifth and sixth decades, with mean age of onset at 55 y. Affects men and women equally.	Majority of the patients are between 50 and 70 y of age, with an average age of onset at 60 y, and slight male predominance.
Location	Lumens of distal bronchioles, alveolar ducts, and peribronchiolar alveolar spaces.	It usually involves the lung basilar regions bilaterally.
Symptoms	Subacute illness, characterized by 2–3 mo history of cough and dyspnea, which can be associated with weight loss, fever, sweats, chills, and myalgia.	Insidious onset of nonproductive cough and slowly progressive dyspnea. Chest auscultation usually demonstrates bibasilar inspiratory crackles.
Signs	Inspiratory crackles on physical examination. Pulmonary function tests may show mild-to-moderate restrictive pattern. Airflow obstruction is usually absent. Chest x-ray shows patchy airspace consolidation, which is usually bilateral but may be unilateral. Chest CT shows bilateral/unilateral patchy airspace consolidation/ground-glass opacities in a peribronchial distribution.	High-resolution computed tomography (HRCT) of the chest showing patchy, predominantly peripheral (subpleural), bibasilar, and often asymmetrical reticular opacities are characteristic findings. Pulmonary function tests demonstrate a restrictive pattern.
Etiology	OP may occur as a nonspecific reaction around a wide variety of unrelated processes such as distal-to-airway obstruction (e.g., by tumor or aspirated foreign material); on the periphery of any inflammatory or mass lesions such as edges of granulomas, tumors, abscesses, vasculitis, or infarcts; or as a minor component of other respiratory illnesses (e.g., eosinophilic pneumonia, hypersensitivity pneumonia, Langerhans cell histiocytosis, nonspecific interstitial pneumonia or granulomatosis with polyangiitis [formerly known as Wegener granulomatosis]). OP also may represent the primary cause of respiratory illness (e.g., infection, aspiration, drug reaction, toxic inhalational injury, connective tissue disease). If an underlying etiology cannot be identified, the process is classified as cryptogenic organizing pneumonia (COP), which was referred to previously as idiopathic bronchiolitis obliterans organizing pneumonia (BOOP).	Potential etiologies include pulmonary manifestation of systemic autoimmune/connective tissue disease, drug toxicity, pneumoconiosis, familial idiopathic pulmonary fibrosis, and possibly fibrotic phase of chronic hypersensitivity pneumonia. These possibilities should be clinically excluded before placing the case under the idiopathic pulmonary fibrosis (IPF) category.

	Organizing Pneumonia (OP)	Usual Interstitial Pneumonia (UIP)
Histology	Lumens of airways, alveolar ducts, and alveolar spaces filled in varying proportions by polypoid, elongated, branching, and serpiginous foci of organizing fibroblastic tissue *(Figs. 11.1–11.4)* in a patchy, bronchiolocentric distribution, which may be associated with variable, usually mild-to-moderate, chronic inflammation in the interstitium (alveolar septa). Alveolar macrophages accumulation, usually secondary to some degree of airway obstruction may be present. The lung architecture is preserved.	UIP has a typical variegated appearance with subpleural and paraseptal areas of interstitial fibrosis and areas of uninvolved lung *(Fig. 11.5)*. This temporally heterogeneous pattern of interstitial fibrosis is characterized by the presence of dense, pink, mature ("old") interstitial fibrosis and loosely arranged, light blue, immature ("recent") interstitial foci of fibroblastic activity *(Figs. 11.6 and 11.7, arrows)*. Note that both OP and UIP show areas of recent organization. However, while in OP these areas are present filling bronchial lumens and alveolar spaces, in UIP these areas are seen in subepithelial interstitial regions, usually at the transition zones between dense fibrosis and normal lung. The process promotes remodeling of the underlying lung parenchyma architecture associated with peripheral honeycomb change *(Fig. 11.8)*. Interstitial inflammation, if present, is typically patchy and mild, mostly noted in the areas of honeycombing. Usually, there is little or no interstitial inflammation away from the areas of fibrosis. Lymphoid follicles with germinal centers tend to be prominent in cases associated with connective tissue disease particularly rheumatoid arthritis. Secondary traction bronchiectasis/bronchiolectasis, peribronchiolar metaplasia, squamous cell metaplasia, and smooth muscle hyperplasia *(Fig. 11.9)* may be present. Nonspecific interstitial pneumonia (NSIP)-like areas may be present, but the final diagnosis should be based on the histologically worst areas *(Figs. 11.10 and 11.11)*.
Special studies	The foci of loosely arranged fibroblastic tissue stains green with pentachrome special stain, compared with the yellow-staining characteristic of dense fibrosis. Foci of organizing pneumonia are seen filling alveolar spaces and lumen of airways.	The subepithelial loosely arranged foci of fibroblastic activity stains green with pentachrome special stain, compared with the yellow-staining characteristic of dense fibrosis. Foci of fibroblastic activity are located in subepithelial interstitial zones.
Prognosis	Usually good, with excellent response to corticosteroid therapy.	Not good. The cicatricial process is usually progressive and fatal in most cases. The median survival from the time of diagnosis is 2–3 y. UIP associated with an underlying collagen vascular disease tends to have a better clinical course/longer survival.

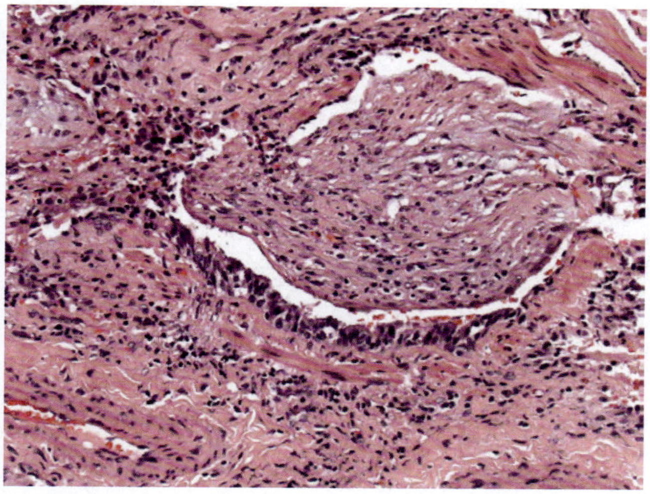

Figure 11.1 OP: Airway lumen filled with polypoid plug of organizing fibroblastic tissue.

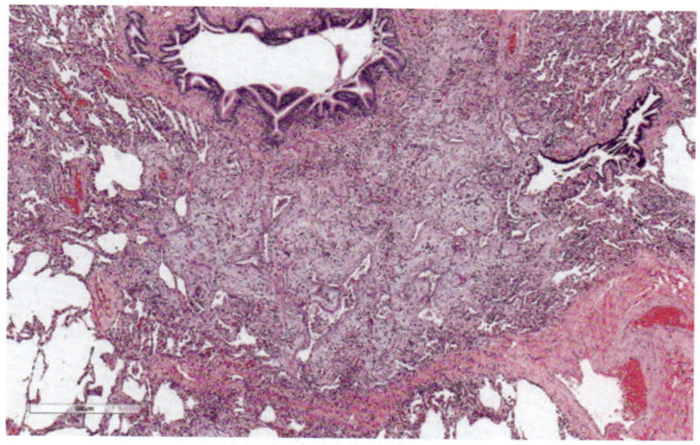

Figure 11.2 OP: Peribronchial alveolar spaces filled by serpiginous foci of organizing fibroblastic tissue.

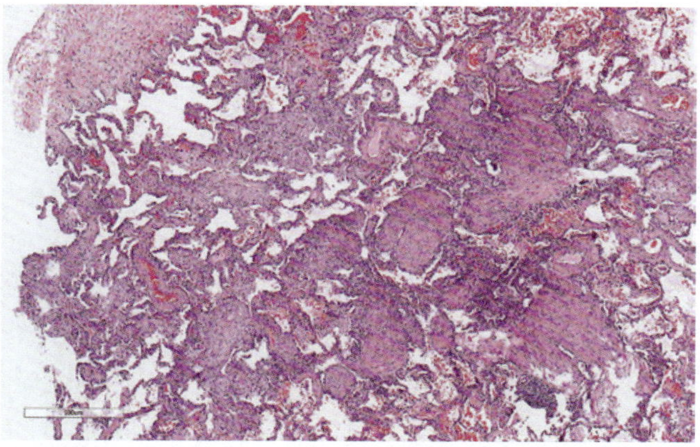

Figure 11.3 OP: There are alveolar spaces filled by polypoid, elongated, and branching foci of organizing fibroblastic tissue associated with mild amount of chronic inflammation in the interstitium (alveolar septa).

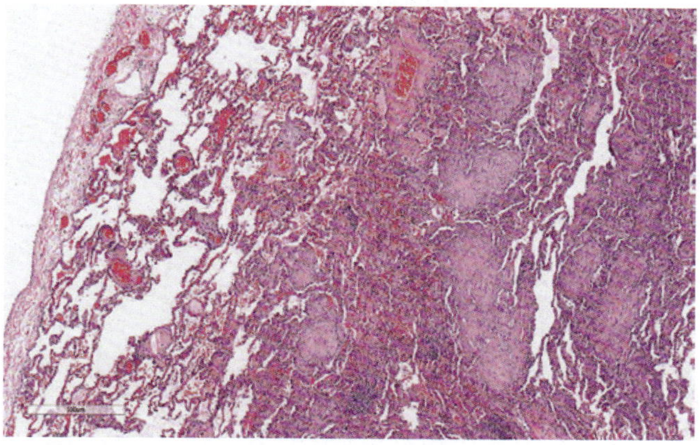

Figure 11.4 OP: Areas of unaffected alveolar spaces (*left*) and areas showing airspace filling by foci of organizing pneumonia (*right*). The overall lung architecture is preserved, lacking interstitial fibrosis or honeycomb change typical of UIP.

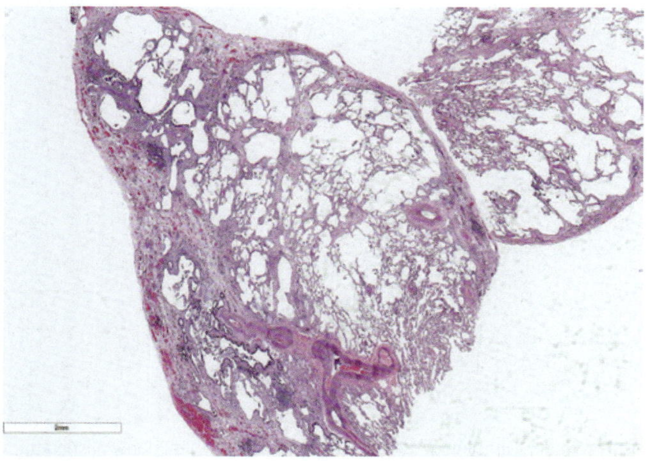

Figure 11.5 UIP: At low power, UIP is characterized by variegated appearance with subpleural and paraseptal areas of interstitial fibrosis and areas of uninvolved lung.

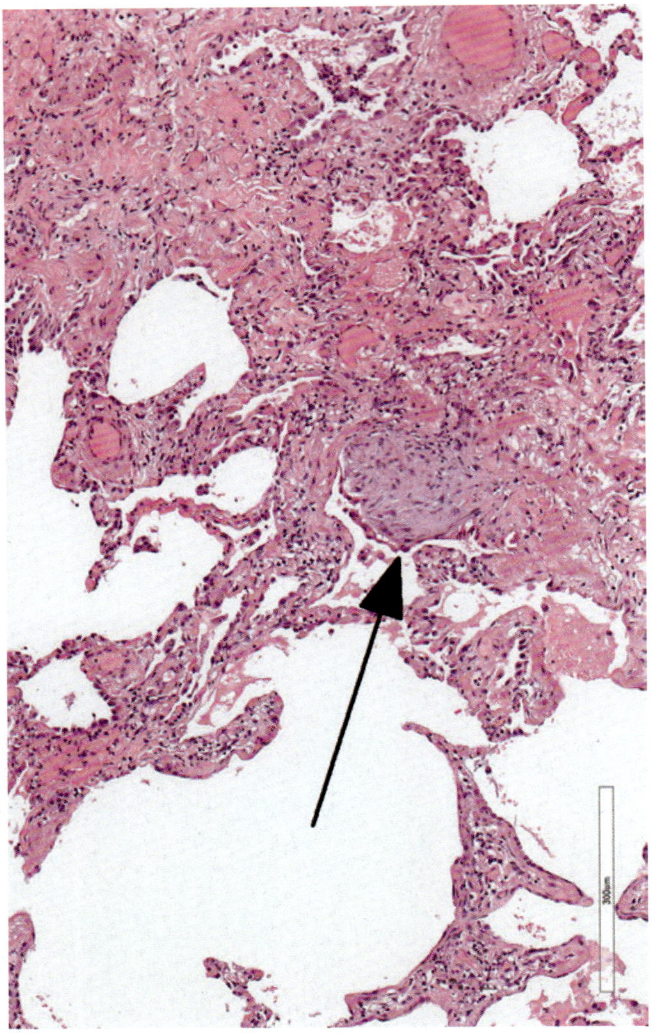

Figure 11.6 UIP: The temporally heterogeneous process is characterized by the presence of dense, pink, mature ("old") interstitial fibrosis (upper field), and loosely arranged, light blue, myxoid, immature ("recent") interstitial foci of fibroblastic activity (*arrow*).

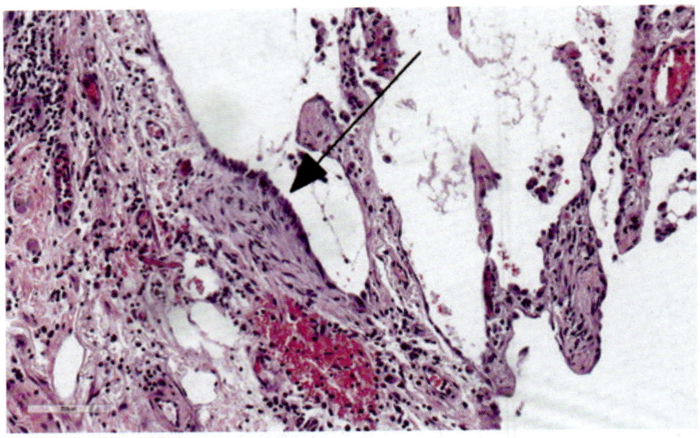

Figure 11.7 UIP: Note that foci of OP are present in airspaces, whereas in UIP foci of fibroblastic activity are interstitial/subepithelial (*arrow*).

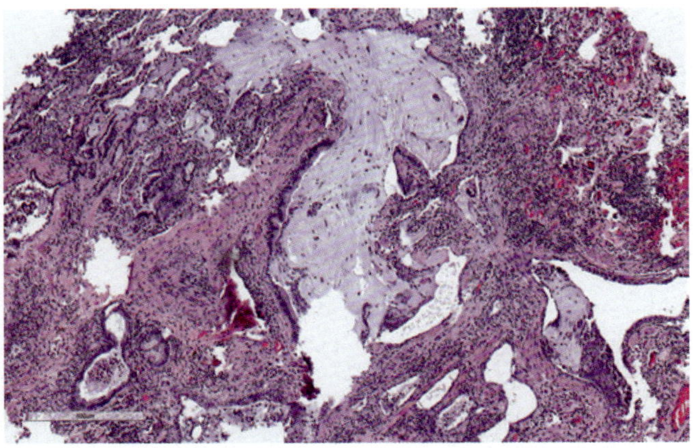

Figure 11.8 UIP: UIP promotes remodeling of the underlying lung architecture with peripheral honeycomb change, characterized by the presence of enlarged irregular spaces lined by bronchiolar type of epithelium containing a mucinous exudate with macrophages and inflammatory cells, which is surrounded by dense fibrosis and chronic inflammation. These are not features of OP. In OP, the lung architecture is preserved.

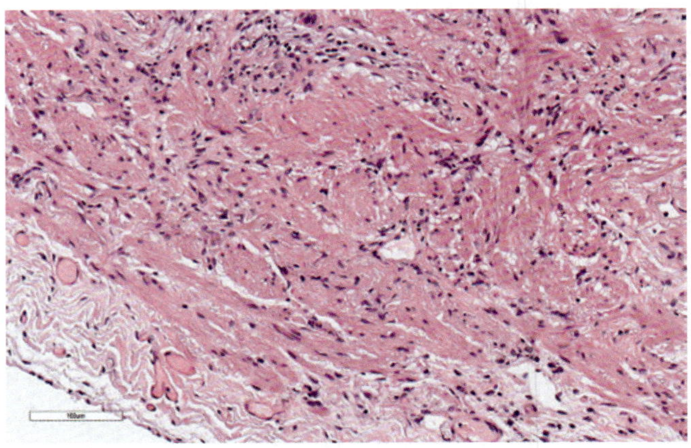

Figure 11.9 UIP: Smooth muscle hyperplasia is a commonly associated feature.

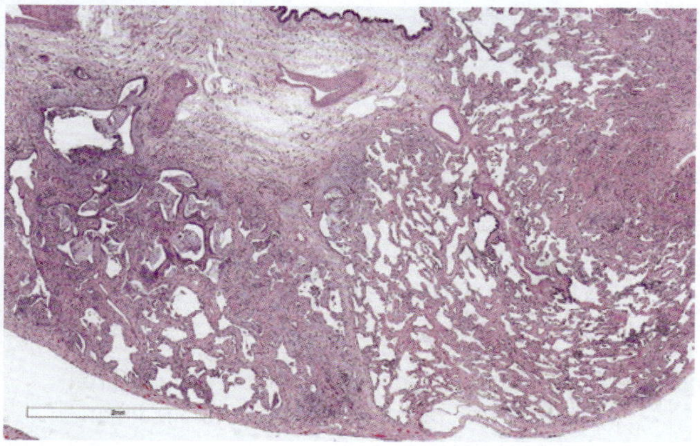

Figure 11.10 UIP: NSIP-like areas may be present (*right*), but the final diagnosis should be based on the histologically worst areas (*left*).

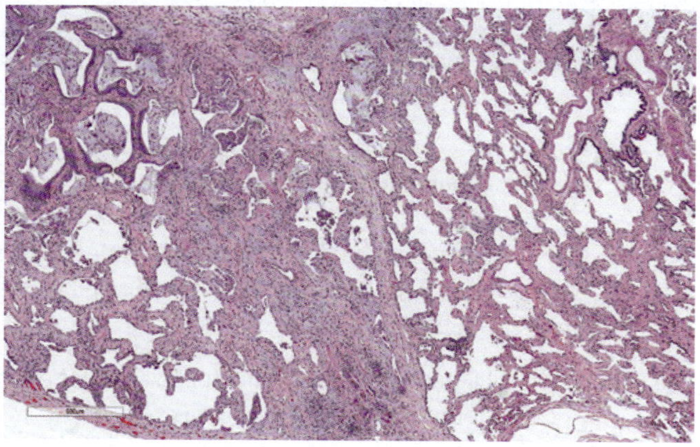

Figure 11.11 UIP: Higher magnification from Figure 11.10. Interstitial areas of recent organization (fibroblastic foci) are present (*center*) and should not be confused with organizing pneumonia.

12 ORGANIZING PNEUMONIA VS. CHRONIC HYPERSENSITIVITY PNEUMONIA

	Organizing Pneumonia (OP)	Chronic Hypersensitivity Pneumonia (HP)
Age	Occurs in the fifth and sixth decades, with mean age of onset at 55 y. Affects men and women equally.	There is no gender or age predilection, although it is uncommon in children.
Location	Lumens of distal bronchioles, alveolar ducts, and peribronchiolar alveolar spaces.	It is usually a predominantly centrilobular/bronchiolocentric process involving the middle and upper lung zones.
Symptoms	Subacute illness, characterized by 2–3 mo history of cough and dyspnea, which can be associated with weight loss, fever, sweats, chills, and myalgia.	Insidious onset of dyspnea, often associated with dry cough, fatigue, and malaise.
Signs	Inspiratory crackles on physical examination. Pulmonary function tests may show mild-to-moderate restrictive pattern. Airflow obstruction is usually absent. Chest x-ray shows patchy airspace consolidation, which is usually bilateral but may be unilateral. Chest CT shows bilateral/unilateral patchy airspace consolidation/ground-glass opacities in a peribronchial distribution.	High-resolution computed tomography (HRCT) of the chest demonstrates mid-to-upper-lobe predominant linear interstitial opacities and small nodules associated with traction bronchiectasis and honeycomb areas. If small airway obstruction is present, air trapping can be seen on expiratory HRCT manifesting as a mosaic attenuation pattern. Bronchoalveolar lavage marked lymphocytosis, although nonspecific, can further support the diagnosis of chronic HP.
Etiology	OP may occur as a nonspecific reaction around a wide variety of unrelated processes such as distal-to-airway obstruction (e.g., by tumor or aspirated foreign material) on the periphery of any inflammatory or mass lesions such as edges of granulomas, tumors, abscesses, vasculitis, or infarcts, or as a minor component of other respiratory illnesses (e.g., eosinophilic pneumonia, HP, Langerhans cell histiocytosis, nonspecific interstitial pneumonia or granulomatosis with polyangiitis [formerly known as Wegener granulomatosis]). OP may also represent the primary cause of respiratory illness (e.g., infection, aspiration, drug reaction, toxic inhalational injury, connective tissue disease). If an underlying etiology cannot be identified, the process is classified as cryptogenic organizing pneumonia (COP), which was referred to previously as idiopathic bronchiolitis obliterans organizing pneumonia (BOOP).	HP represents a combination of immune complex–mediated (type III) and T-cell–mediated, delayed (type IV) hypersensitivity reactions. Exposure to inhaled environmental antigens (e.g., mold, bacteria, animal proteins, avian proteins) or other allergen particles of small size (5 µm or smaller) triggers the disease. Sometimes the causal agent cannot be identified. The disease, which is also called extrinsic allergic alveolitis (EAA), may also be known by a great variety of names depending on the causal agent (farmer's lung, pigeon breeder's disease, ventilation pneumonitis). However, regardless of the pathologic responsible agent, the clinical presentation and pathologic findings are similar.

	Organizing Pneumonia (OP)	Chronic Hypersensitivity Pneumonia (HP)
Histology	Lumens of airways, alveolar ducts, and alveolar spaces filled in varying proportions by polypoid, elongated, branching, and serpiginous foci of organizing fibroblastic tissue *(Figs. 12.1–12.4)* in a patchy, bronchiolocentric distribution, which may be associated with variable, usually mild-to-moderate, chronic inflammation in the interstitium (alveolar septa). Alveolar macrophage accumulation, secondary to some degree of airway obstruction, may be present. The lung architecture is preserved.	Chronic cellular interstitial pneumonia (typically showing bronchiolocentric accentuation), cellular chronic bronchiolitis, and small, predominantly interstitial, nonnecrotizing, poorly formed granulomas composed of loose clusters of epithelioid histiocytes, multinucleated giant cells, and lymphocytes *(Figs. 12.5–12.10)*. Peribronchiolar metaplasia, peribronchiolar fibrosis, and patchy foci of OP are frequently present *(Figs. 12.11 and 12.12)*. Constrictive bronchiolitis may occur, and foamy macrophages related to bronchiolar obstruction may be seen within the nearby alveolar spaces. In the advanced phase of chronic HP, interstitial scarring/fibrosis and honeycomb change may become prominent, resembling UIP.
Special studies	The foci of loosely arranged fibroblastic tissue stains green with pentachrome special stain, compared with the yellow-staining characteristic of dense fibrosis.	Gomori methenamine silver (GMS) and acid-fast bacilli (AFB) special stains and tissue cultures should be performed to exclude infection.
Prognosis	Usually good, with excellent response to corticosteroid therapy.	The prognosis is worse when associated with interstitial scarring. Some patients respond to removal of antigen exposure and corticosteroid therapy, but some cases become self-sustained and progress to fibrotic phase despite removal from the antigen exposure. How much fibrosis is required to move into the poor outcome group is unclear. Overall, once dense fibrosis develops with honeycomb change, the disease is irreversible.

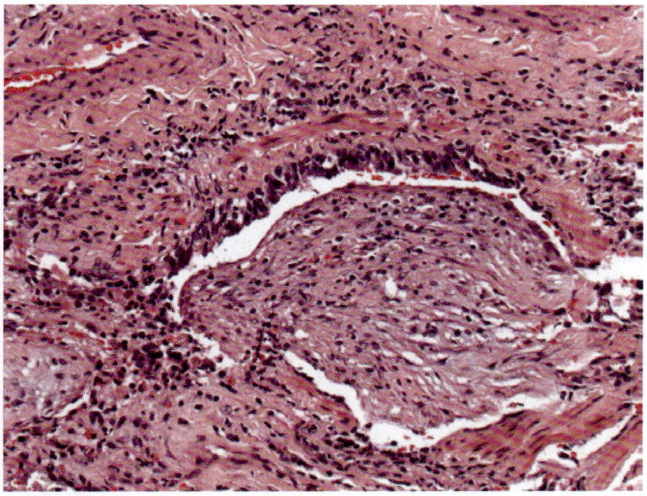

Figure 12.1 OP: Airway lumen filled with polypoid plug of organizing pneumonia.

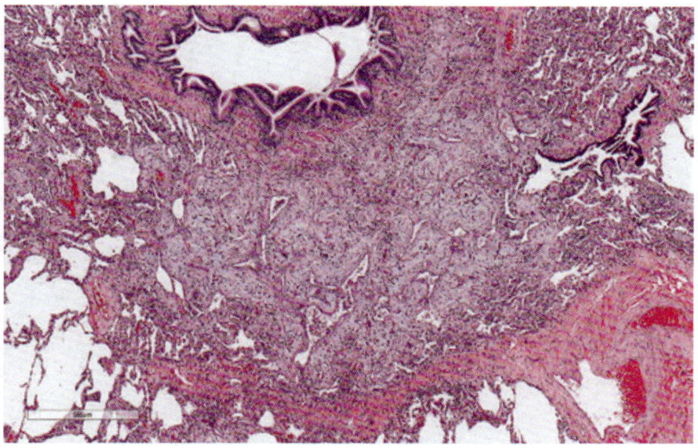

Figure 12.2 OP: Peribronchial alveolar spaces filled by serpiginous foci of organizing pneumonia.

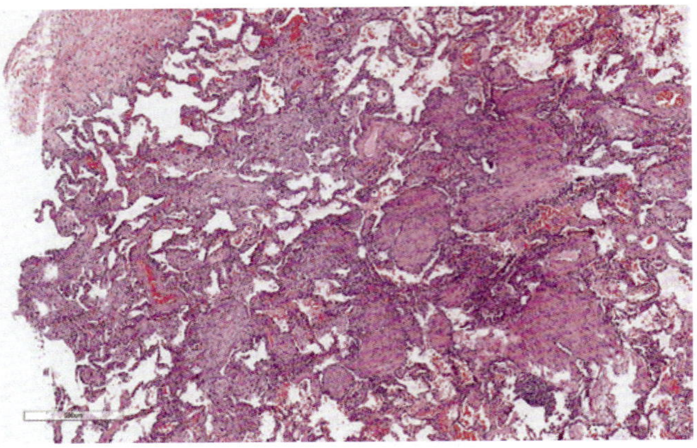

Figure 12.3 OP: Alveolar spaces filled by polypoid, elongated, and branching foci of organizing fibroblastic tissue associated with mild amounts of chronic inflammation in the interstitium (alveolar septa).

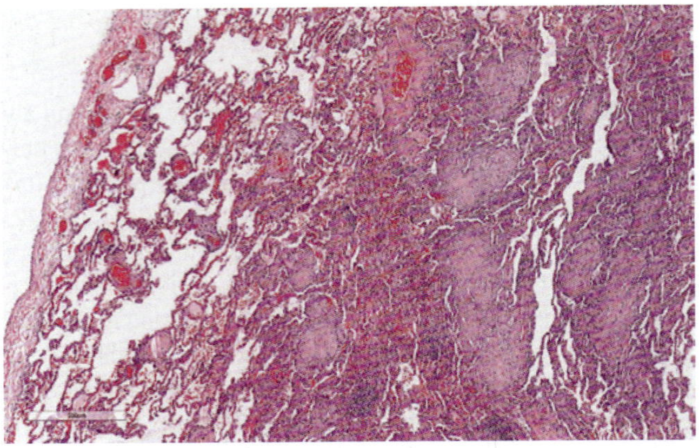

Figure 12.4 OP: Areas of unaffected alveolar spaces (*left*) and areas showing airspace filling by foci of organizing pneumonia (*right*). There is mild-to-moderate amount of chronic inflammation in the interstitium (alveolar septa) in contrast to HP, which usually shows bronchiolocentric chronic interstitial pneumonia.

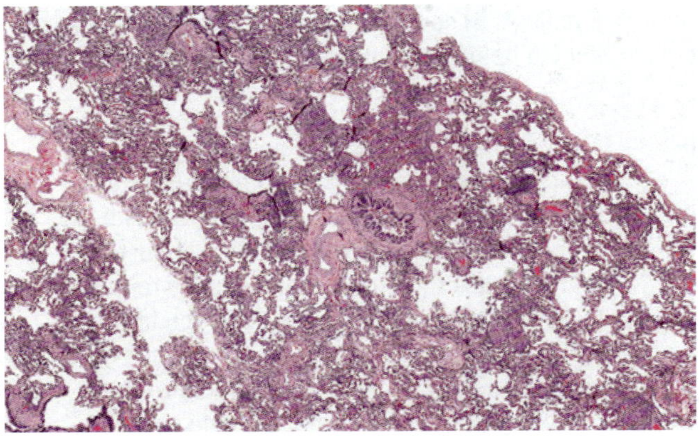

Figure 12.5 HP: While OP is an airspace-filling process, HP is an interstitial process characterized by diffuse chronic cellular interstitial pneumonia with bronchiolocentric accentuation.

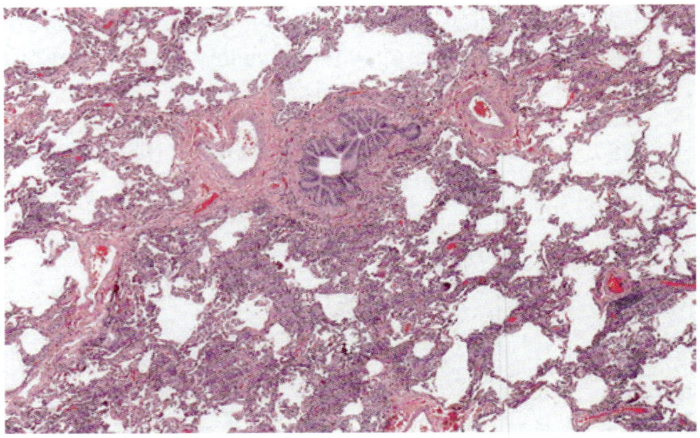

Figure 12.6 HP: There is diffuse expansion of the alveolar septa by chronic inflammatory cell infiltrate, which is more pronounced in the peribronchiolar zones.

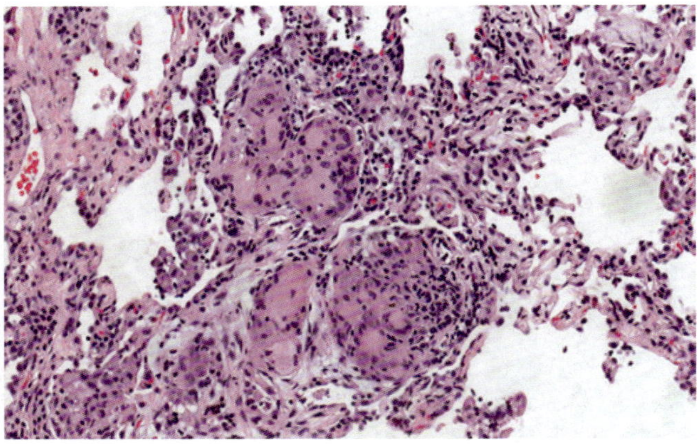

Figure 12.7 HP: The granulomas present in HP are not typically seen in alveolar spaces but in the interstitium (alveolar septa). They are poorly formed and may be composed of giant cells and lymphocytes.

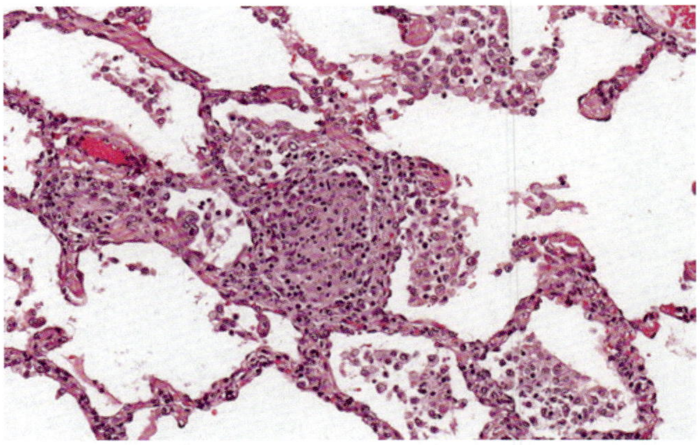

Figure 12.8 HP: Interstitial, nonnecrotizing, poorly formed granuloma composed of loose cluster of epithelioid histiocytes. The granulomas are most commonly seen in the peribronchiolar interstitium.

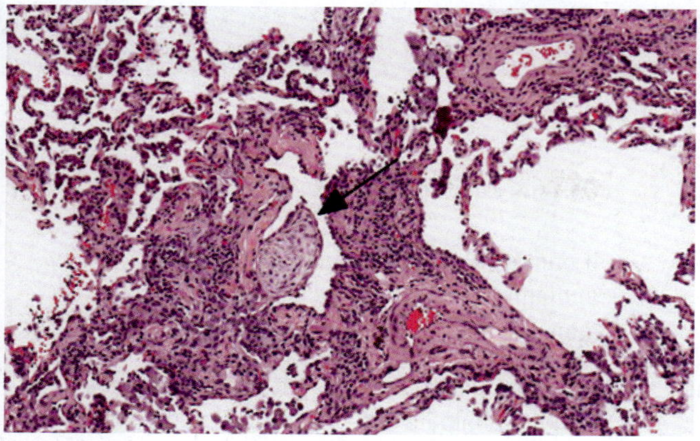

Figure 12.9 HP: Focus of organizing pneumonia in HP (*arrow*). Note peribronchiolar septal expansion by chronic interstitial pneumonia.

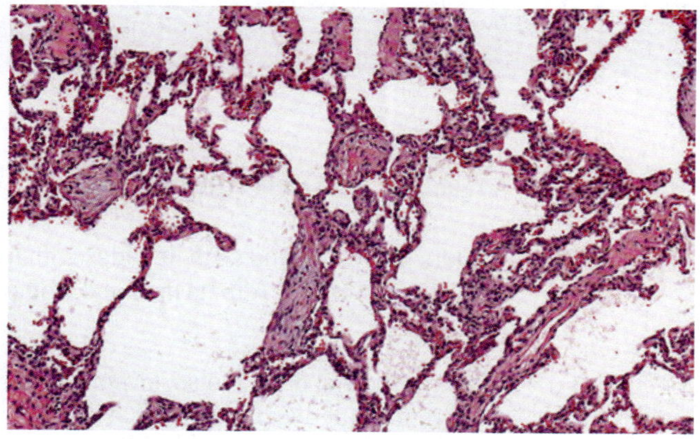

Figure 12.10 HP: Few foci of organizing pneumonia may be present in HP, which do not represent the main pattern of injury in HP.

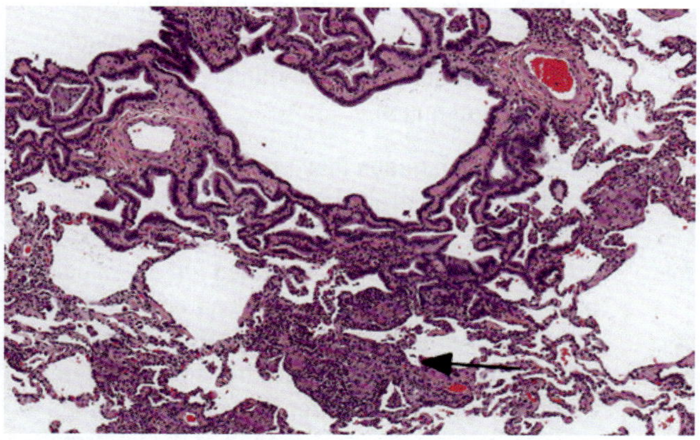

Figure 12.11 HP: Peribronchiolar metaplasia is another feature commonly seen in HP. Note poorly formed peribronchiolar interstitial granuloma (*arrow*).

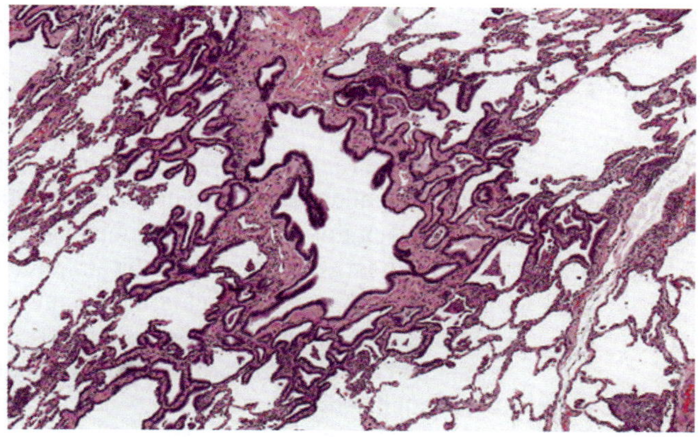

Figure 12.12 HP: Peribronchiolar metaplasia may be extensive in HP.

13 ORGANIZING PNEUMONIA VS. CHRONIC EOSINOPHILIC PNEUMONIA

	Organizing Pneumonia (OP)	Chronic Eosinophilic Pneumonia (EP)
Age	Occurs in the fifth and sixth decades with mean age of onset at 55 y. Affects men and women equally.	It can develop at any age, with mean age of 45 y at diagnosis. Women are more affected than men.
Location	Lumens of distal bronchioles, alveolar ducts, and peribronchiolar alveolar spaces.	Airspace-filling process that usually involves periphery of middle and upper lung zones.
Symptoms	Subacute illness, characterized by 2 to 3 mo history of cough and dyspnea, which can be associated with weight loss, fever, sweats, chills, and myalgia.	Chronic disease characterized by relapsing subacute episodes of dyspnea, cough, and chest pain, which is often associated with fatigue, malaise, fever, chills, and weight loss that may last for several weeks or months. Clinical history of chronic asthma, chronic rhinitis, or chronic sinusitis is common.
Signs	Inspiratory crackles on physical examination. Pulmonary function tests may show mild-to-moderate restrictive pattern. Airflow obstruction is usually absent. Chest x-ray shows patchy airspace consolidation, which is usually bilateral but may be unilateral. Chest CT shows bilateral/unilateral patchy airspace consolidation/ground-glass opacities in a peribronchial distribution.	Physical examination may reveal wheezes or crackles. Peripheral blood, sputum, and bronchoalveolar lavage containing markedly increased eosinophils and elevated IgE are usually present. Chest CT demonstrates patchy, bilateral, often peripheral (subpleural), poorly defined "migratory" infiltrates, which are transient infiltrates that tend to resolve and reappear in the same location or elsewhere. Migration of the infiltrates over time is strongly suggestive of the diagnosis. The predominant dense peripheral distribution of the infiltrates is often referred to as reverse pulmonary edema pattern.
Etiology	Organizing pneumonia may occur as a nonspecific reaction around a wide variety of unrelated processes such as distal-to-airway obstruction (e.g., by tumor or aspirated foreign material); on the periphery of any inflammatory or mass lesions such as edges of granulomas, tumors, abscesses, vasculitis, or infarcts; or as a minor component of other respiratory illnesses (e.g., eosinophilic pneumonia, hypersensitivity pneumonia, Langerhans cell histiocytosis, nonspecific interstitial pneumonia, granulomatosis with polyangiitis [formerly known as Wegener granulomatosis]). Organizing pneumonia also may represent the primary cause of respiratory illness (e.g., infection, aspiration, drug reaction, toxic inhalational injury, connective tissue disease). If an underlying etiology cannot be identified, the process is classified as cryptogenic organizing pneumonia (COP), which was referred to previously as idiopathic bronchiolitis obliterans organizing pneumonia (BOOP).	Potential etiologies would include but not be limited to drug toxicity (e.g., ampicillin, bleomycin, cromoglycate, glafenine, hydralazine, naproxen, nitrofurantoin, para-aminosalicylic acid, penicillin, streptomycin, sulfasalazine, sulfonamides, tetracycline, L-tryptophan); fungal organisms, particularly Aspergillus sp.; parasites; bacteria; viruses; inhalants (e.g., cocaine, nickel, carbonyl vapor); and other allergens. Rare cases of eosinophilic pneumonia may be an initial manifestation of autoimmune disease, and therefore a rheumatologic panel should be indicated. In the absence of known etiologies, the case falls into the cryptogenic eosinophilic pneumonia category.

	Organizing Pneumonia (OP)	Chronic Eosinophilic Pneumonia (EP)
Histology	Lumens of airways, alveolar ducts, and alveolar spaces filled in varying proportions by polypoid, elongated, branching, and serpiginous foci of organizing fibroblastic tissue *(Figs. 13.1–13.4)* in a patchy, bronchiolocentric distribution, which may be associated with variable, usually mild-to-moderate, chronic inflammation in the interstitium (alveolar septa). Alveolar macrophages accumulation, usually secondary to some degree of airway obstruction, may be present. The lung architecture is preserved.	Alveolar spaces filled by eosinophils admixed with variable number of macrophages, proteinaceous-to-fibrinous exudate and frequent foci of organizing pneumonia *(Figs. 13.5–13.7)*. Granulomatous formation may be seen, characterized by dense accumulations of macrophages, sometimes accompanied by multinucleated giant cells. Eosinophilic abscesses may be seen, characterized by the presence of a central area of necrosis surrounded by palisading histiocytes mixed with eosinophils. The predominantly airspace-filling process is usually accompanied by mild-to-moderate interstitial pneumonia characterized by expansion of the alveolar septa by a mixture of eosinophils, lymphocytes, and plasma cells with associated alveolar pneumocytes type II prominence. Necrosis of the intra-alveolar cellular infiltrate is common, but alveolar septal (interstitial) necrosis does not occur. Mild perivascular and transmural infiltration by nonnecrotizing, eosinophil-rich, chronic inflammatory cell infiltrate involving small arteries and venules is often seen *(Figs. 13.8 and 13.9)*. However, this finding does not indicate Churg–Strauss syndrome since necrotizing vasculitis should not be present. Chronicity may be suggested by the presence of variable interstitial fibrosis. Of note, if the patient has received steroids prior to the biopsy, the tissue eosinophilia may be inconspicuous or absent, and the alveolar spaces may be filled with macrophages only, requiring correlation with clinical history and laboratory findings of peripheral eosinophilia to support the diagnosis.
Special studies	The foci of loosely arranged fibroblastic tissue stains green with pentachrome special stain, compared with the yellow-staining characteristic of dense fibrosis.	GMS special stains and tissue cultures to exclude infection.
Prognosis	Usually good, with excellent response to corticosteroid therapy.	The clinical course depends on the underlying causal agent, but overall most patients respond favorably to corticosteroid therapy, although recurrences are common and prolonged therapy may be necessary.

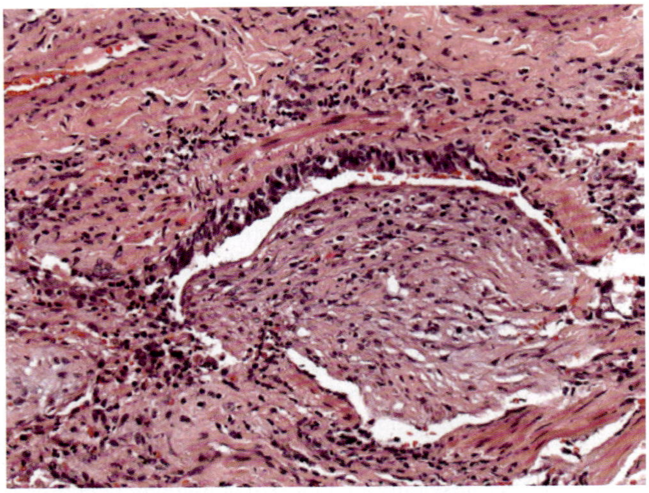

Figure 13.1 OP: Airway lumen filled with polypoid plug of organizing fibroblastic tissue.

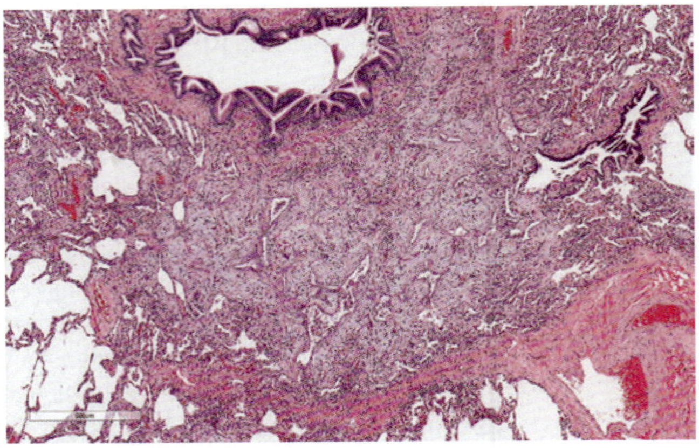

Figure 13.2 OP: Peribronchial alveolar spaces filled by serpiginous foci of organizing fibroblastic tissue.

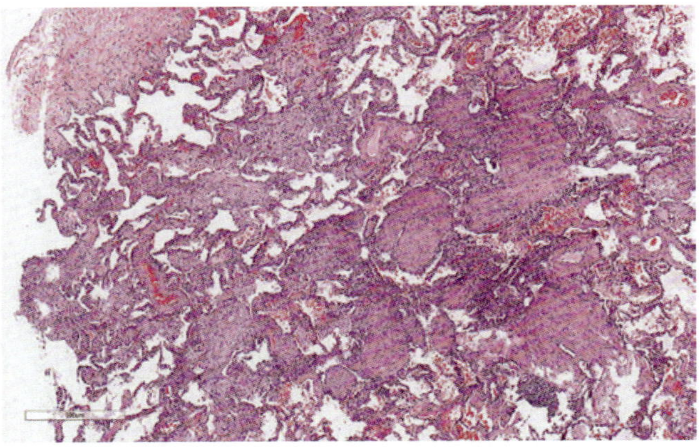

Figure 13.3 OP: Alveolar spaces filled by polypoid, elongated, and branching foci of organizing fibroblastic tissue associated with mild chronic inflammation in the interstitium (alveolar septa).

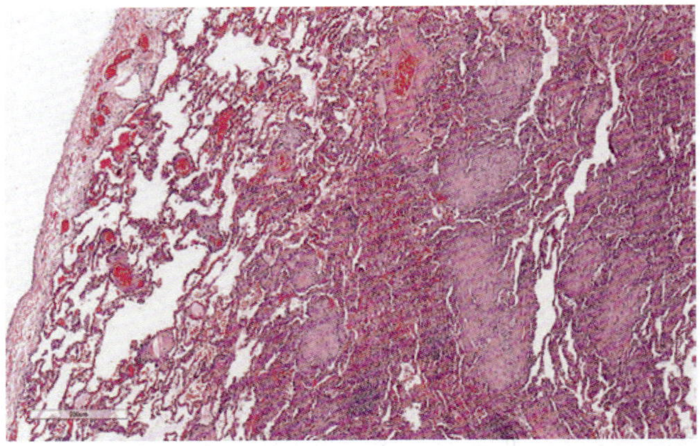

Figure 13.4 OP: Areas of unaffected alveolar spaces (*left*) and areas showing airspace filling by foci of organizing pneumonia (*right*). There is mild-to-moderate chronic inflammation in the interstitium (alveolar septa), lacking airspace eosinophilia, macrophages, and fibrinous exudates characteristic of eosinophilic pneumonia.

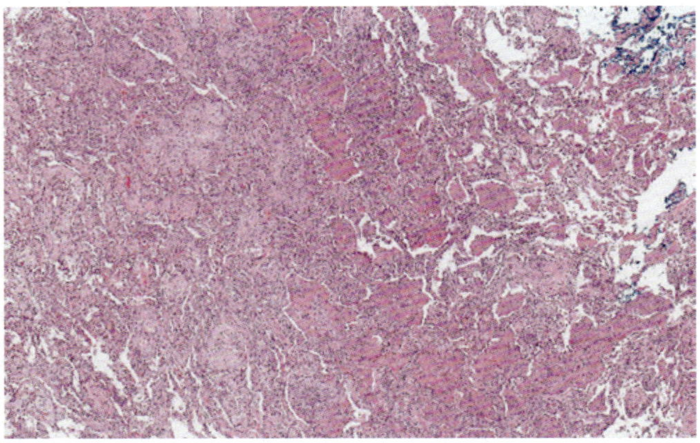

Figure 13.5 EP: There is dense lung parenchyma consolidation, with filling of the alveolar spaces by fibrinous exudates (dark pink material, *middle right*) and polypoid-to-elongated plugs of organizing pneumonia (*middle left*). Foci of organizing pneumonia are frequently seen in EP.

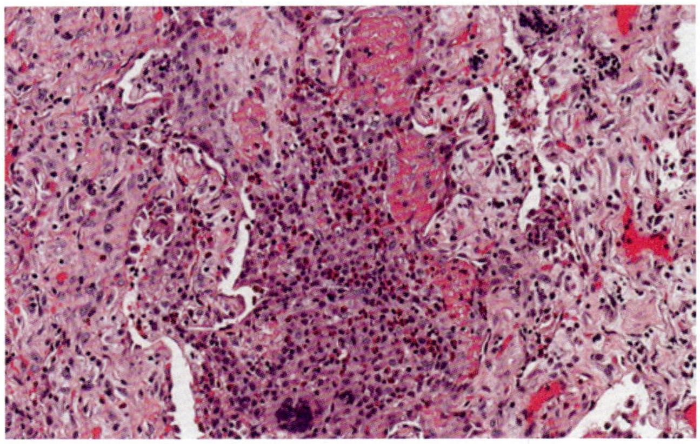

Figure 13.6 EP: Higher power showing airspace filling by fibrinous exudate (*middle right*) and inflammatory cell infiltrate composed of numerous eosinophils and macrophages (*middle left*).

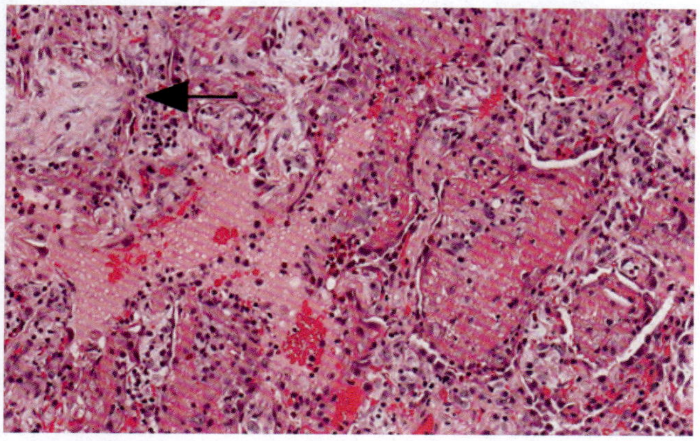

Figure 13.7 EP: In addition to fibrinous exudate (dark pink, *right*), proteinaceous exudates (light pink, *left*) may also be seen. Note focus or organizing pneumonia (*arrow*).

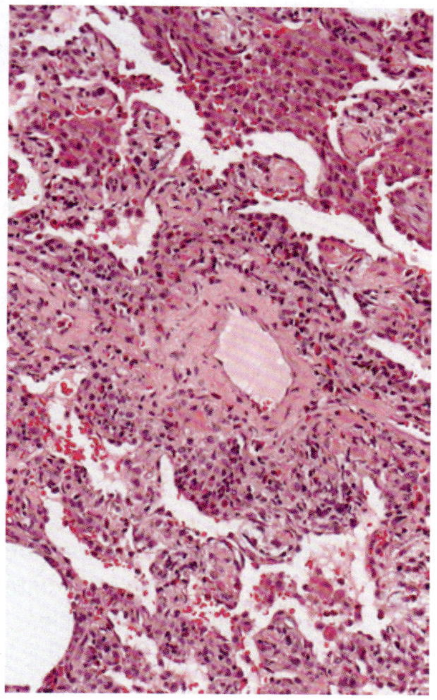

Figure 13.8 EP: Perivascular infiltration by eosinophils. Note associated mild chronic interstitial pneumonia characterized by the presence of adjacent septal expansion by chronic inflammatory cells and eosinophils.

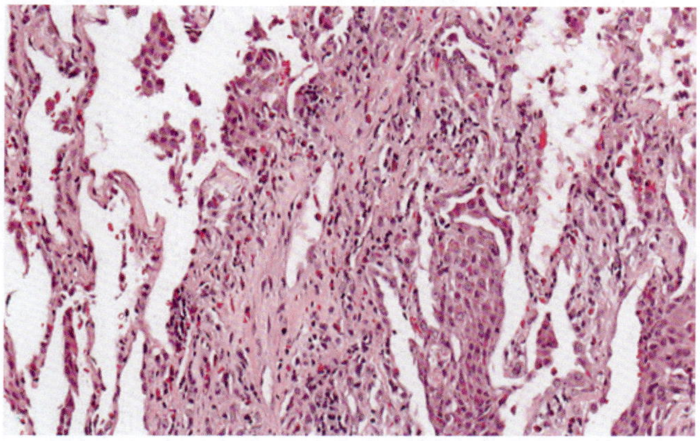

Figure 13.9 EP: Mild transmural infiltration by eosinophils is often seen involving small arteries and venules. This finding does not indicate Churg–Strauss syndrome since necrotizing vasculitis is not present.

14 USUAL INTERSTITIAL PNEUMONIA VS. FIBROTIC NONSPECIFIC INTERSTITIAL PNEUMONIA

	Usual Interstitial Pneumonia (UIP)	**Nonspecific Interstitial Pneumonia (NSIP), Fibrotic Variant**
Age	Majority of the patients are between 50 and 70 y of age, with an average age of onset at 60 y and a slight male predominance.	The average age ranges from 40 to 57 y. It is slightly more common in women.
Location	It usually involves the lung subpleural basilar regions bilaterally.	It usually affects the lower lobes, spares subpleural spaces, and tends to be bilateral and symmetrical.
Symptoms	Insidious onset of nonproductive cough and slowly progressive dyspnea. Chest auscultation usually demonstrates bibasilar inspiratory crackles.	The symptoms in NSIP develop gradually. Shortness of breath, cough, fatigue, and weight loss are the most common symptoms. Fever and digital clubbing have been reported but are uncommon.
Signs	High-resolution computed tomography (HRCT) of the chest shows patchy, predominantly peripheral (subpleural), bibasilar, and often asymmetrical reticular opacities and honeycombing as characteristic findings. Pulmonary function tests demonstrate a restrictive pattern.	Pulmonary function tests demonstrate a restrictive pattern. On chest HRCT, areas of ground-glass attenuation, which are usually extensive, is the predominant finding and is seen in nearly all cases.
Etiology	Potential etiologies include pulmonary manifestation of systemic autoimmune/connective tissue disease, drug toxicity, pneumoconiosis, familial idiopathic pulmonary fibrosis, and possibly fibrotic phase of chronic hypersensitivity pneumonia, and these possibilities should be clinically excluded before placing the case under the idiopathic pulmonary fibrosis (IPF) category.	Pulmonary manifestation of underlying collagen vascular disease (e.g., rheumatoid arthritis, Sjögren syndrome); immunodeficiency disorders (e.g., acquired immunodeficiency syndrome, common variable immunodeficiency); drug toxicity (e.g., Dilantin), or idiopathic.
Histology	Temporally heterogenous pattern of interstitial fibrosis characterized by the presence of dense, pink, mature ("old") interstitial scarring/fibrosis; loosely arranged, light blue, immature ("recent") interstitial foci of fibroblastic activity; and areas of normal-appearing lung *(Fig. 14.1)*. Fibroblastic foci are usually seen at the transition zones between dense fibrosis and normal lung *(Figs. 14.2 and 14.3)*. The process usually has a subpleural and paraseptal distribution and promotes remodeling of the underlying lung parenchyma architecture associated with peripheral honeycomb change *(Fig. 14.4)*. Interstitial inflammation if present is typically patchy and mild, mostly noted in the areas of honeycombing. Usually, there is little or no interstitial inflammation away from the areas of fibrosis. Lymphoid follicles with germinal centers tend to be prominent in cases associated with connective tissue disease, particularly rheumatoid arthritis. Secondary traction bronchiectasis/bronchiolectasis, peribronchiolar metaplasia, squamous cell metaplasia, and smooth muscle hyperplasia *(Fig. 14.5)* may be present. NSIP-like areas may be present but the final diagnosis should be based on the histologically worst areas *(Figs. 14.6 and 14.7)*.	*Fibrosing variant:* There is diffuse and uniform interstitial (alveolar septal) expansion by dense collagen deposition (fibrosis), few fibroblasts, and little amount of inflammation and alveolar pneumocyte prominence *(Figs. 14.8–14.10)*. The underlying lung parenchyma architecture is preserved, with no honeycomb change. Fibroblastic foci may be present, but they are usually inconspicuous and never numerous. Few plugs of organizing pneumonia and variable amounts of peribronchiolar metaplasia may be present. Increased numbers of macrophages are frequently found within the alveolar spaces.

	Usual Interstitial Pneumonia (UIP)	Nonspecific Interstitial Pneumonia (NSIP), Fibrotic Variant
Special studies	The foci of loosely arranged fibroblastic activity stains green with pentachrome special stain, compared with the yellow-staining characteristic of dense fibrosis.	None suggested.
Prognosis	Not good. The cicatricial process is usually progressive and fatal in most cases. The median survival from the time of diagnosis is 2–3 y. UIP associated with an underlying collagen vascular disease tends to have a better clinical course/longer survival.	The prognosis of fibrosing NSIP is usually better than that of UIP. The 5- and 10-y survival rates for patients with fibrosing NSIP are 90% and 35%, respectively.

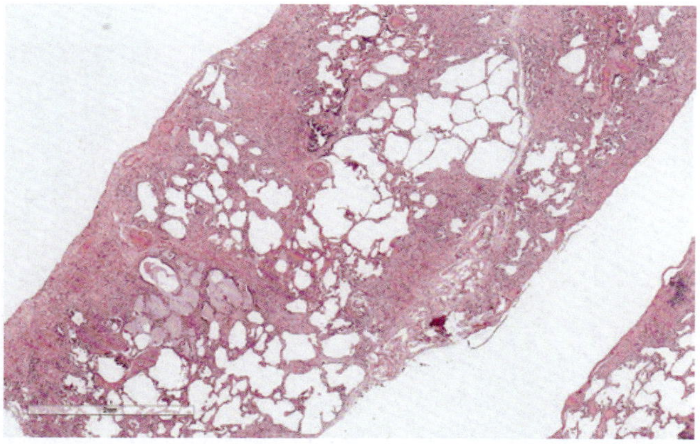

Figure 14.1 UIP: At low power, UIP is characterized by variegated appearance with subpleural and paraseptal areas of interstitial fibrosis and areas of uninvolved lung.

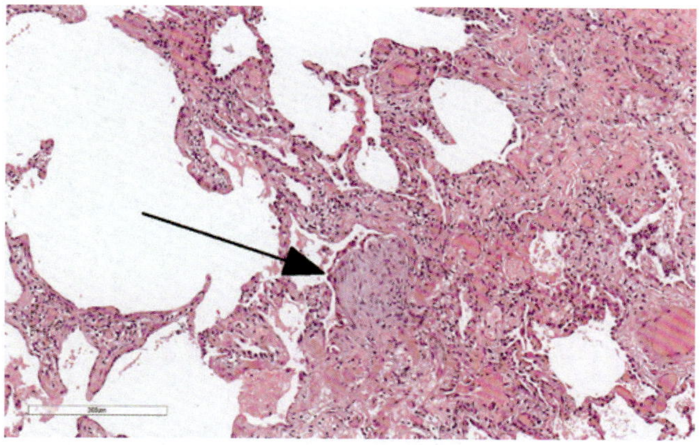

Figure 14.2 UIP: The temporally heterogeneous process is characterized by the presence of dense, pink, mature ("old") interstitial fibrosis (right field) and loosely arranged, light blue, myxoid, immature ("recent") interstitial foci of fibroblastic activity (*arrow*).

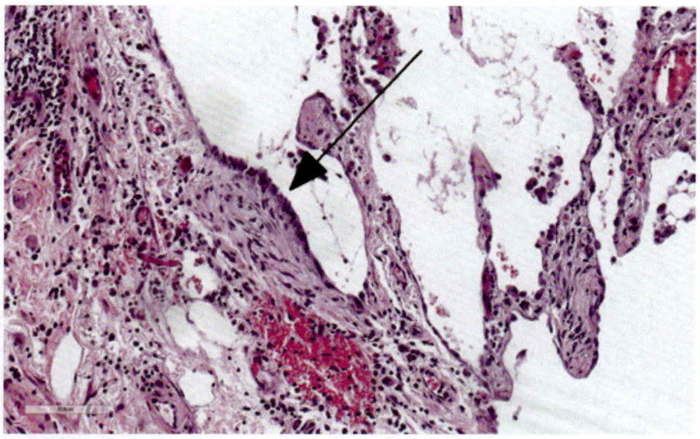

Figure 14.3 UIP: Note that foci of fibroblastic activity are interstitial/subepithelial (*arrow*).

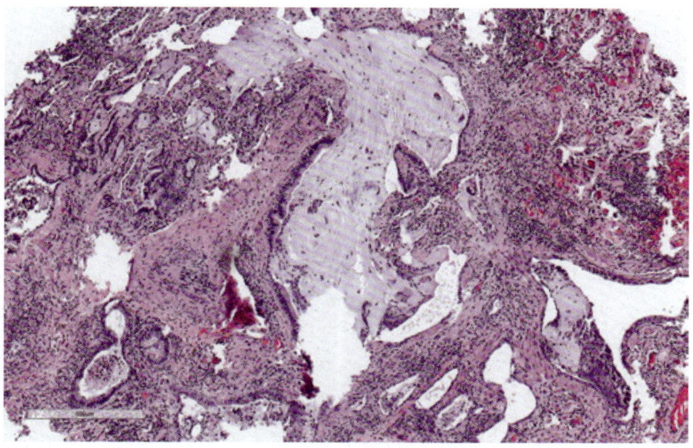

Figure 14.4 UIP: The disease promotes remodeling of the underlying lung architecture associated with peripheral honeycomb change, characterized by the presence of enlarged irregular spaces lined by bronchiolar type of epithelium containing a mucinous exudate with macrophages and inflammatory cells, which is surrounded by fibrosis and chronic inflammation. This is not a feature of NSIP.

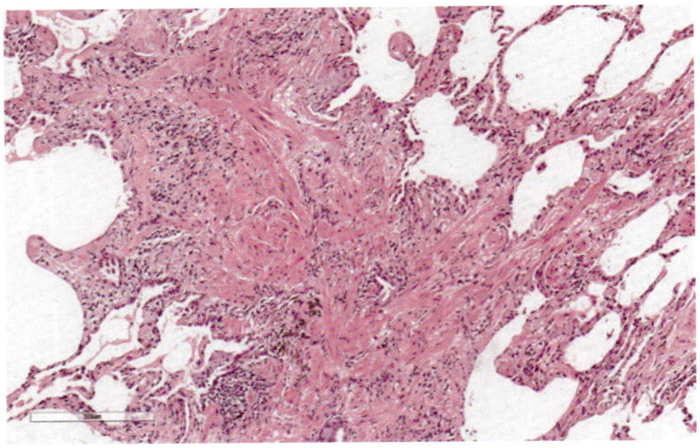

Figure 14.5 UIP: Smooth muscle hyperplasia is a common associated UIP feature.

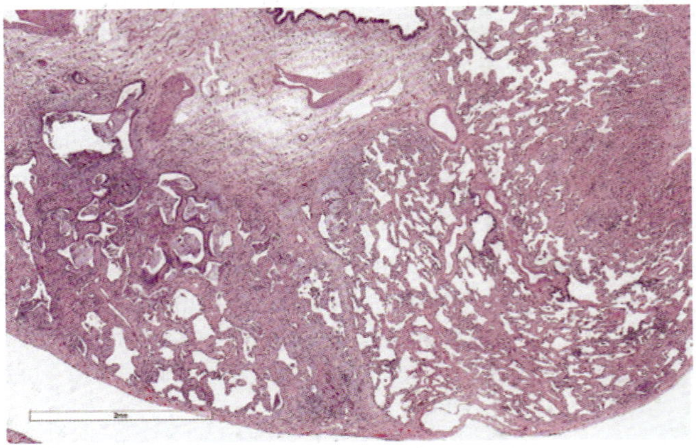

Figure 14.6 UIP: NSIP-like areas may be present (*right*) but the final diagnosis should be based on the histologically worst areas (*left*).

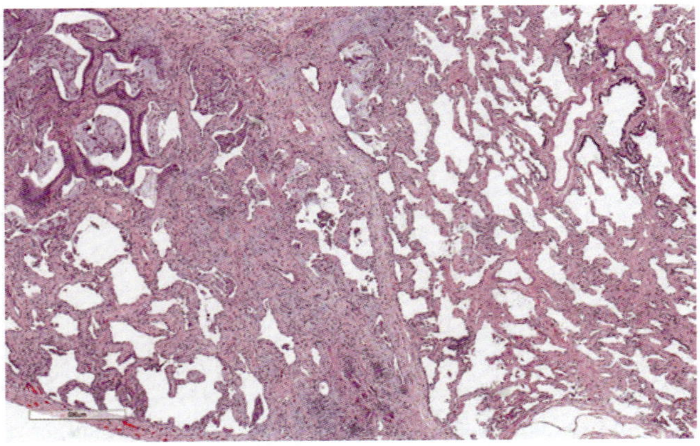

Figure 14.7 UIP: Higher magnification from Figure 14.6. Temporally heterogeneous process with interstitial areas of recent organization a.k.a. fibroblastic activity or fibroblastic foci (*center*).

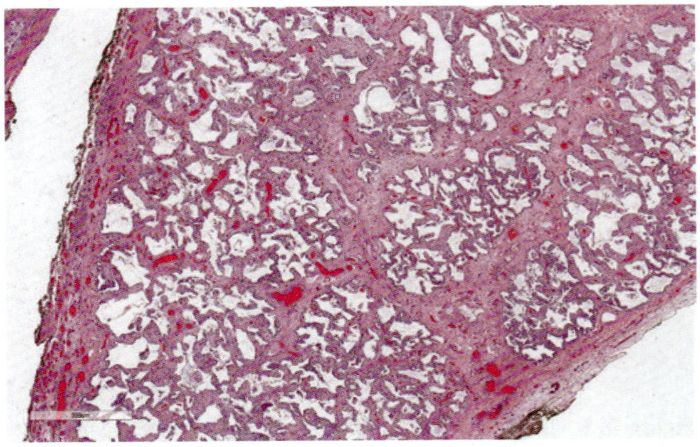

Figure 14.8 Fibrotic NSIP (low power): There is diffuse and uniform interstitial (septal) expansion by fibrosis. The underlying lung architecture is relatively preserved with no honeycombing. Fibroblastic foci may be present, but they are usually inconspicuous and never numerous.

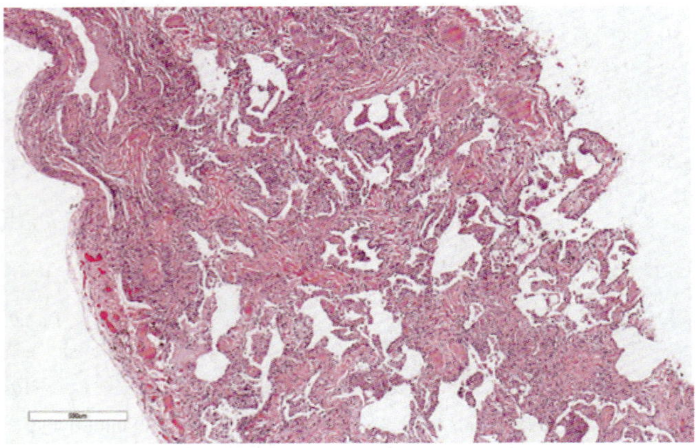

Figure 14.9 Fibrotic NSIP (high power): The interstitial expansion is composed of dense collagen deposition (fibrosis) and little amount of inflammation.

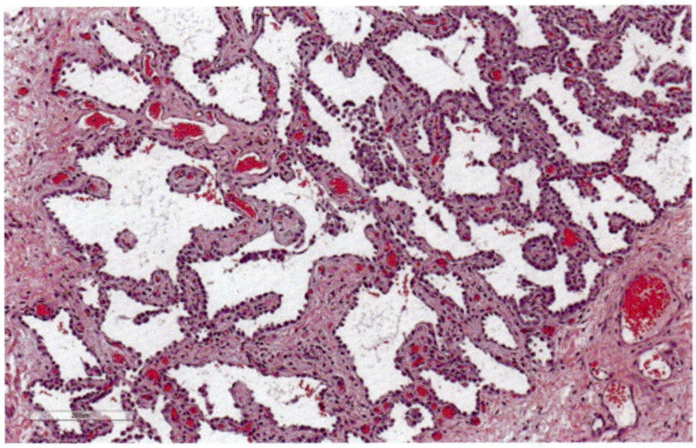

Figure 14.10 Fibrotic NSIP: The septal scarring is frequently associated with alveolar pneumocyte prominence. Macrophages are frequently found within the alveolar spaces.

15 USUAL INTERSTITIAL PNEUMONIA VS. FIBROTIC PHASE OF CHRONIC HYPERSENSITIVITY PNEUMONIA

	Usual Interstitial Pneumonia (UIP)	Fibrotic Phase of Chronic Hypersensitivity Pneumonia (HP)
Age	Majority of the patients are between 50 and 70 y of age, with an average age of onset at 60 y, and a slight male predominance.	There is no gender or age predilection, although it is uncommon in children.
Location	It usually involves the lung basilar regions bilaterally.	Usually, it is a predominantly centrilobular/bronchiolocentric process involving the middle and upper lung zones.
Symptoms	Insidious onset of nonproductive cough and slowly progressive dyspnea. Chest auscultation usually demonstrates bibasilar inspiratory crackles.	Insidious onset of dyspnea, often associated with dry cough, fatigue, and malaise.
Signs	Chest high-resolution computed tomography (HRCT) shows patchy, predominantly peripheral (subpleural), bibasilar, and often asymmetrical reticular opacities as characteristic findings. Pulmonary function tests demonstrate a restrictive pattern.	Chest HRCT demonstrates mid-to-upper lobe predominant linear interstitial opacities and small nodules associated with traction bronchiectasis and honeycomb areas. If small airway obstruction is present, air trapping can be seen on expiratory HRCT, manifesting as a mosaic attenuation pattern. Bronchoalveolar lavage marked lymphocytosis, although nonspecific, can further support the diagnosis of chronic HP.
Etiology	Potential etiologies include pulmonary manifestation of systemic autoimmune/connective tissue disease, drug toxicity, pneumoconiosis, familial idiopathic pulmonary fibrosis, and possibly fibrotic phase of chronic HP, and these possibilities should be clinically excluded before placing the case under the idiopathic pulmonary fibrosis (IPF) category.	HP represents a combination of immune complex–mediated (type III) and T-cell–mediated, delayed (type IV) hypersensitivity reactions. Exposure to inhaled environmental antigens (e.g., mold, bacteria, animal proteins, avian proteins) or other allergen particles of small size (5 μm or smaller) triggers the disease. Sometimes the causal agent cannot be identified. The disease, which is also called extrinsic allergic alveolitis (EAA), may also be known by a great variety of names depending on the causal agent (farmer's lung, pigeon breeder's disease, ventilation pneumonitis). However, regardless of the pathologic responsible agent, the clinical presentation and pathologic findings are similar.

	Usual Interstitial Pneumonia (UIP)	**Fibrotic Phase of Chronic Hypersensitivity Pneumonia (HP)**
Histology	UIP has a typical variegated appearance, with subpleural and paraseptal areas of interstitial fibrosis and areas of uninvolved lung *(Fig. 15.1)*. This temporally heterogenous pattern of interstitial fibrosis is characterized by the presence of dense, pink, mature ("old") interstitial fibrosis, and loosely arranged, light blue, immature ("recent") interstitial foci of fibroblastic activity *(Figs. 15.2 and 15.3, arrows)*. Fibroblastic foci are usually seen at the transition zones between dense fibrosis and normal lung. The process usually has a subpleural and paraseptal distribution and promotes remodeling of the underlying lung parenchyma architecture associated with peripheral honeycomb change *(Fig. 15.4)*. Interstitial inflammation, if present, is typically patchy and mild, mostly noted in the areas of honeycombing. Usually, there is little or no interstitial inflammation away from the areas of fibrosis. Lymphoid follicles with germinal centers tend to be prominent in cases associated with connective tissue disease, particularly rheumatoid arthritis. Secondary traction bronchiectasis/bronchiolectasis, peribronchiolar metaplasia, squamous cell metaplasia, and smooth muscle hyperplasia *(Fig. 15.5)* may be present. Nonspecific interstitial pneumonia (NSIP)-like areas may be present, but the final diagnosis should be based on the histologically worst areas *(Figs. 15.6 and 15.7)*.	In the advanced phase of chronic HP, interstitial scarring/fibrosis and honeycomb change may become prominent, resembling UIP. Features that would suggest the diagnosis of fibrotic phase of chronic HP include the presence of peribronchiolar fibrosis, prominent peribronchiolar metaplasia, residual areas of bronchiolocentric cellular interstitial pneumonia, poorly formed granulomas or giant cells, and few foci of organizing pneumonia *(Figs. 15.8–15.15)*. A small percentage of cases of chronic HP and UIP cannot be separated by pathologic examination.
Special studies	The foci of loosely arranged fibroblastic activity stains green with pentachrome special stain, compared with the yellow-staining characteristic of dense fibrosis.	Noncontributory.
Prognosis	Not good. The cicatricial process is usually progressive and fatal in most cases. The median survival from the time of diagnosis is 2–3 y. UIP associated with an underlying collagen vascular disease tends to have a better clinical course/longer survival.	The prognosis of HP is worse when associated with interstitial scarring. Some patients respond to removal of antigen exposure and corticosteroid therapy but some cases become self-sustained and progress to fibrotic phase despite removal from the antigen exposure. How much fibrosis is required to move into the poor outcome group is unclear. Overall, once dense fibrosis develops with honeycomb change, the disease is irreversible.

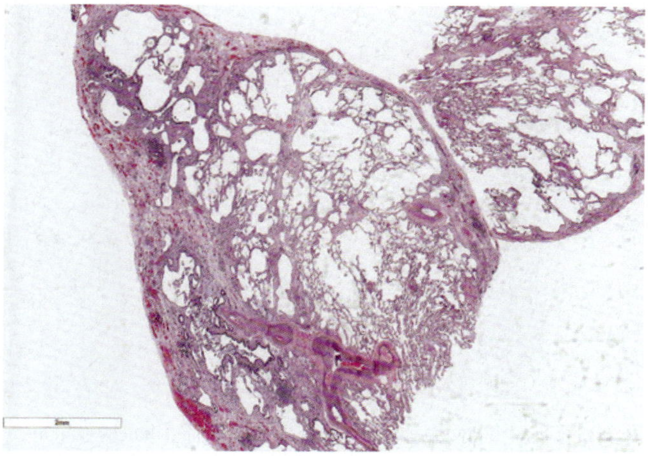

Figure 15.1 UIP: At low power, UIP is characterized by variegated appearance with subpleural and paraseptal areas of interstitial fibrosis and areas of uninvolved lung.

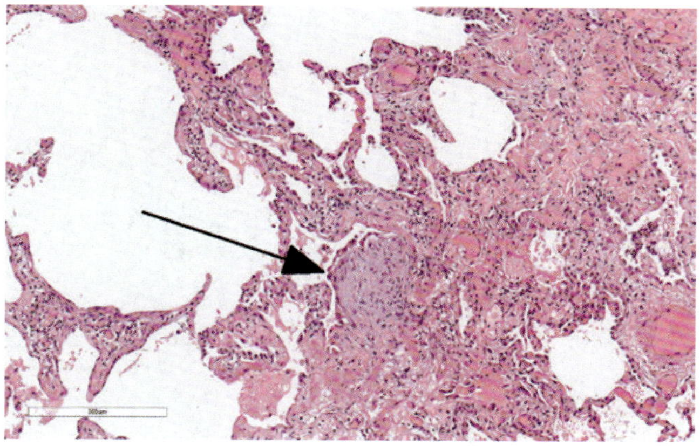

Figure 15.2 UIP: The temporally heterogeneous process is characterized by the presence of dense, pink, mature ("old") interstitial fibrosis (right field) and loosely arranged, light blue, myxoid, immature ("recent") interstitial foci of fibroblastic activity (*arrow*).

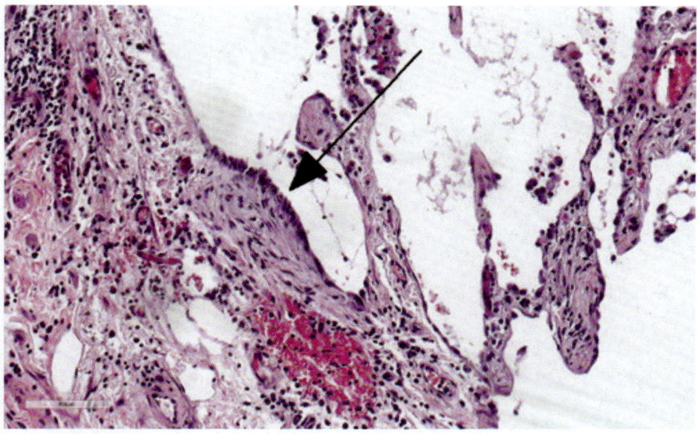

Figure 15.3 UIP: Note that foci of fibroblastic activity are interstitial/subepithelial (*arrow*).

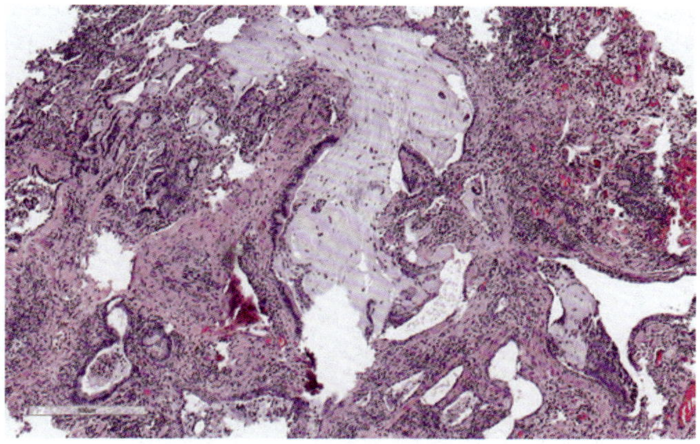

Figure 15.4 UIP: The disease promotes remodeling of the underlying lung parenchyma architecture associated with peripheral honeycomb change, characterized by the presence of enlarged irregular spaces lined by bronchiolar type of epithelium containing a mucinous exudate with macrophages and inflammatory cells, which is surrounded by fibrosis and chronic inflammation. Honeycombing may be also seen in fibrotic phase of HP.

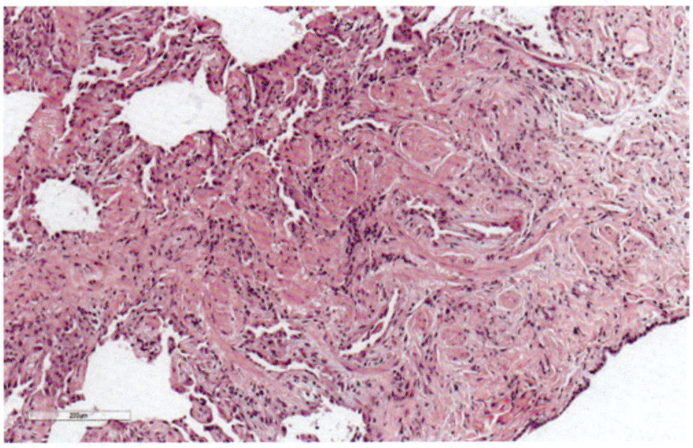

Figure 15.5 UIP: Smooth muscle hyperplasia is a common, associated UIP feature.

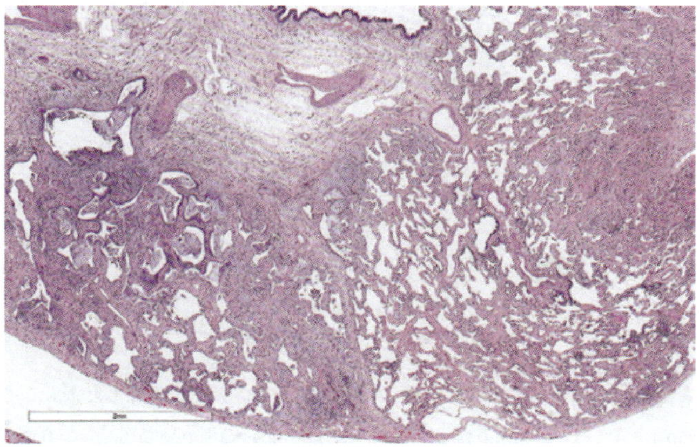

Figure 15.6 UIP: NSIP-like areas may be present (*right*), but the final diagnosis should be based on the histologically worst areas (*left*).

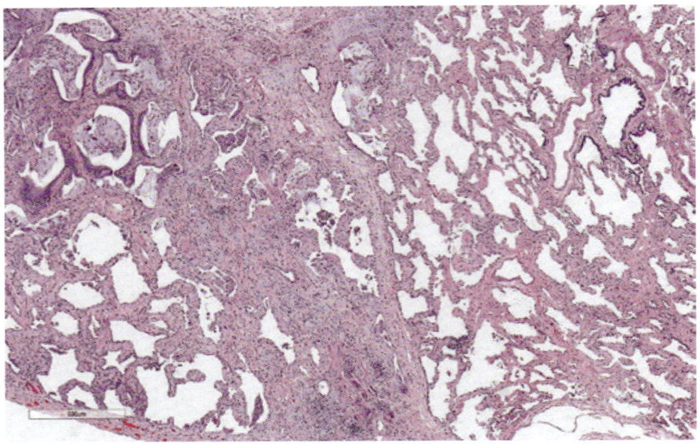

Figure 15.7 UIP: Higher magnification from Figure 15.6. Temporally heterogeneous process with interstitial areas of recent organization a.k.a. fibroblastic activity or fibroblastic foci (*center*).

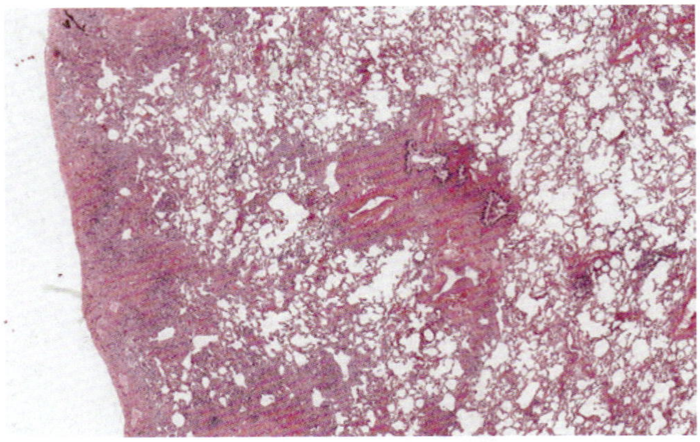

Figure 15.8 Fibrotic phase of HP: The fibrosis in HP is patchy with involvement of peripheral (subpleural) and central (peribronchiolar/airway-centered) zones rather than predominantly subpleural and paraseptal as seen in UIP. Upper- and middle-lobes predominance, air trapping on expiratory HRCT manifesting as a mosaic attenuation pattern, known exposure to offending antigens, and bronchoalveolar lavage lymphocytosis are additional diagnostic criteria that if present would help to make the distinction between UIP and fibrotic phase of HP.

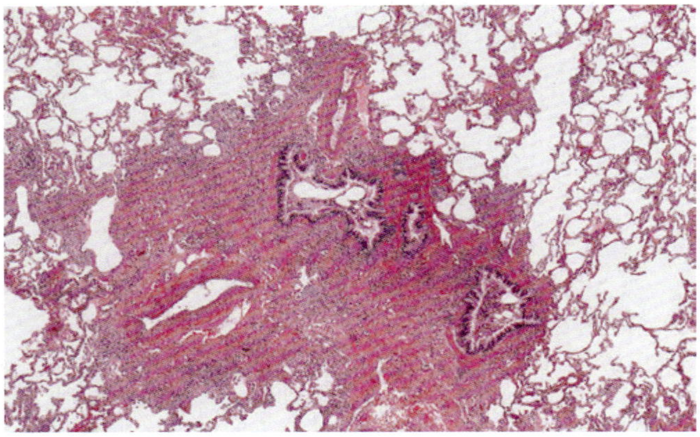

Figure 15.9 Fibrotic phase of HP: High power of Figure 15.8 showing peribronchiolar fibrosis, a feature highly suggestive of fibrotic phase of HP, rather than UIP.

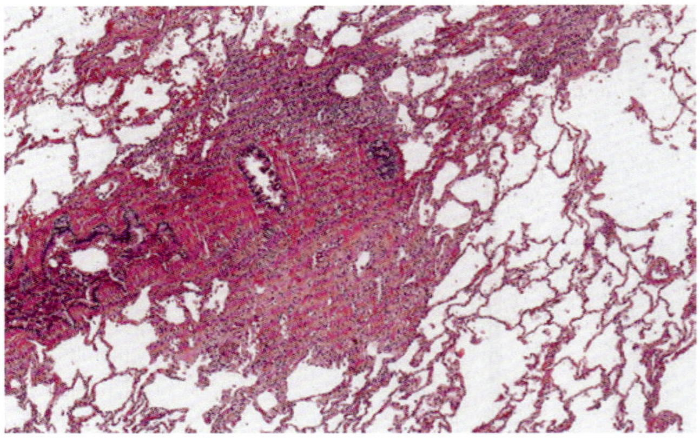

Figure 15.10 HP: Fibrotic phase of the disease may be associated with variable degree of peribronchiolar fibrosis, a characteristic although nonspecific feature.

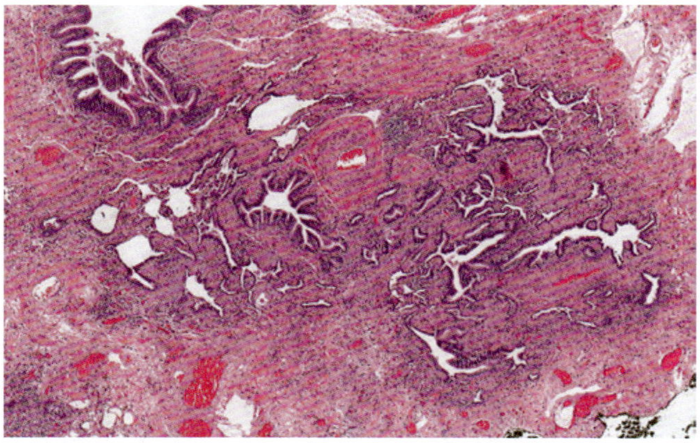

Figure 15.11 Fibrotic phase of HP: Prominent peribronchiolar metaplasia is another feature that suggests fibrotic phase of HP rather than UIP, particularly if associated with peribronchiolar scarring.

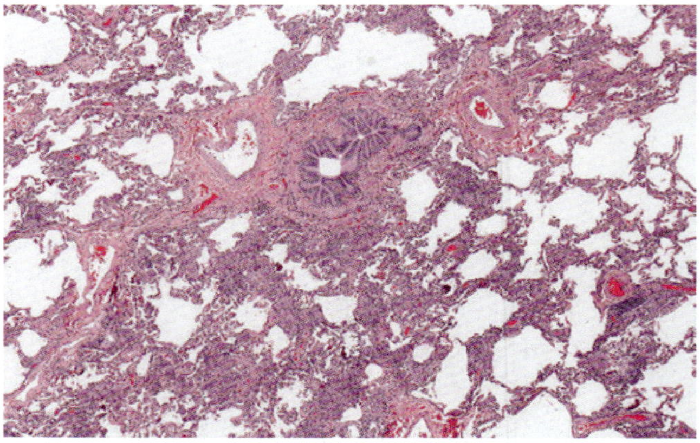

Figure 15.12 Fibrotic phase of HP: *Residual* areas of bronchiolocentric cellular chronic interstitial pneumonia *if present* are helpful in supporting the diagnosis of fibrotic phase of HP.

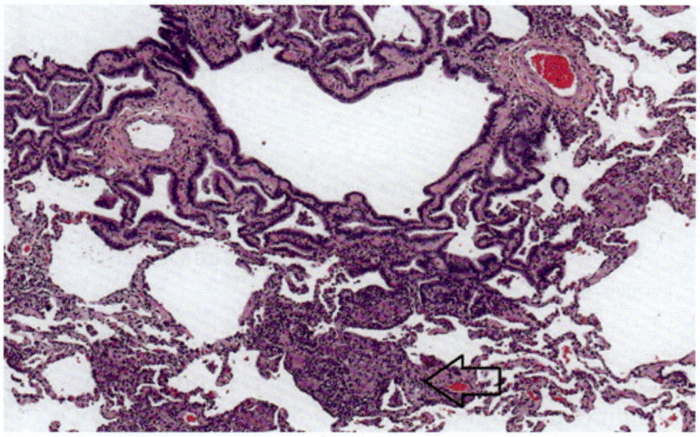

Figure 15.13 Fibrotic phase of HP: Residual area of bronchiolocentric cellular chronic interstitial pneumonia associated with peribronchiolar metaplasia and nonnecrotizing, poorly formed granuloma composed of loosely arranged epithelioid histiocytes (seen in the peribronchiolar interstitium, *arrow*), supportive of HP rather than UIP.

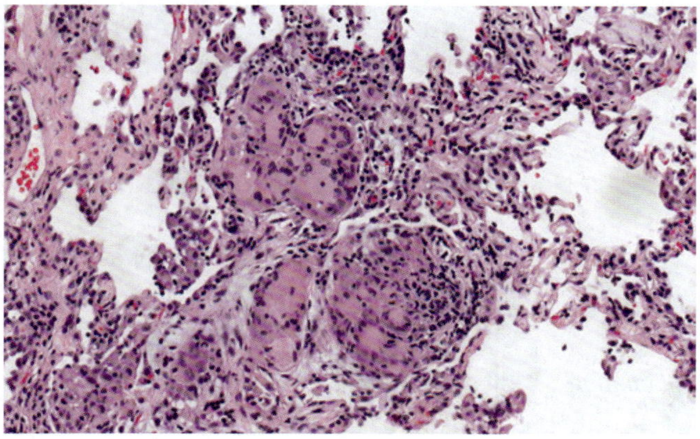

Figure 15.14 Fibrotic phase of HP: Granulomas in HP are characteristically poorly formed and may be composed mostly of multinucleated giant cells and few lymphocytes.

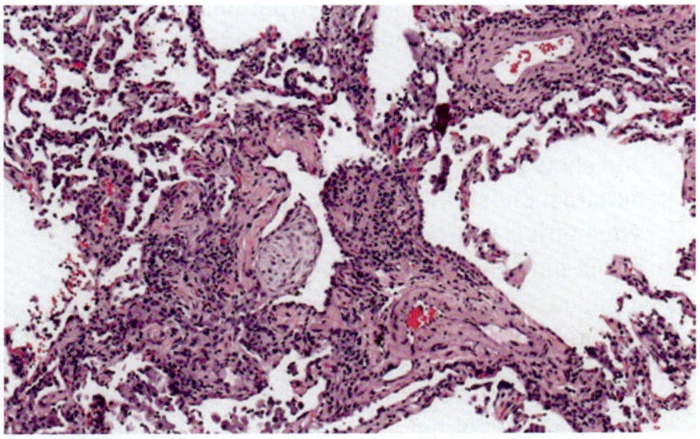

Figure 15.15 Fibrotic phase of HP: Few foci of organizing pneumonia may be seen in *residual areas* of cellular chronic interstitial pneumonia.

16 USUAL INTERSTITIAL PNEUMONIA VS. PULMONARY LANGERHANS CELL HISTIOCYTOSIS

	Usual Interstitial Pneumonia (UIP)	Pulmonary Langerhans Cell Histiocytosis (PLCH)
Age	Majority of the patients are between 50 and 70 y of age, with an average age of onset at 60 y, and a slight male predominance.	Primarily affects young and middle-aged adults between the ages of 20 and 50 y.
Location	It usually involves the lung basilar regions bilaterally, with predominant subpleural and paraseptal distribution.	Mid-lung zones and upper lobes, with predominant centrilobular/peribronchiolar distribution.
Symptoms	Insidious onset of nonproductive cough and slowly progressive dyspnea. Chest auscultation usually demonstrates bibasilar inspiratory crackles.	Chronic cough and dyspnea are the most common presenting complaints. Up to 25% patients are asymptomatic. Systemic symptoms (fever, weight loss, and malaise) occur occasionally. Spontaneous pneumothorax is the initial clinical presentation in about 20% of the cases. Rarely hemoptysis can occur. In advanced cases, pulmonary hypertension and manifestations of cor pulmonale may develop.
Signs	Chest high-resolution computed tomography (HRCT) shows patchy, predominantly peripheral (subpleural), bibasilar, and often asymmetrical reticular opacities and honeycombing as characteristic findings. Pulmonary function tests demonstrate a restrictive pattern.	Reduced diffusing capacity for carbon monoxide is the most common finding. Pulmonary function tests can show normal, obstructive, restrictive, or mixed patterns. Chest HRCT usually demonstrates bilateral symmetrical micronodules and cysts predominantly in mid-lung and upper lobes with centrilobular distribution. When fibrosis occurs, reticular opacities are present. In advanced cases, honeycomb change may be present.
Etiology	Potential etiologies include pulmonary manifestation of systemic autoimmune/connective tissue disease, drug toxicity, pneumoconiosis, familial idiopathic pulmonary fibrosis, and possibly fibrotic phase of chronic hypersensitivity pneumonia, and these possibilities should be clinically excluded before placing the case under the idiopathic pulmonary fibrosis (IPF) category.	Uncertain, but largely seen in smoking individuals.

	Usual Interstitial Pneumonia (UIP)	Pulmonary Langerhans Cell Histiocytosis (PLCH)
Histology	UIP has a typical variegated appearance with subpleural and paraseptal areas of interstitial fibrosis and areas of uninvolved lung *(Fig. 16.1)*. This temporally heterogenous pattern of interstitial fibrosis is characterized by the presence of dense, pink, mature ("old") interstitial fibrosis and loosely arranged, light blue, immature ("recent") interstitial foci of fibroblastic activity *(Figs. 16.2 and 16.3, arrows)*. Fibroblastic foci are usually seen at the transition zones between dense fibrosis and normal lung. The process usually has a subpleural and paraseptal distribution and promotes remodeling of the underlying lung parenchyma architecture associated with peripheral honeycomb change *(Fig. 16.4)*. Interstitial inflammation, if present, is typically patchy and mild, mostly noted in the areas of honeycombing. Usually there is little or no interstitial inflammation away from the areas of fibrosis. Lymphoid follicles with germinal centers tend to be prominent in cases associated with connective tissue disease, particularly rheumatoid arthritis. Secondary traction bronchiectasis/bronchiolectasis, peribronchiolar metaplasia, squamous cell metaplasia, and smooth muscle hyperplasia *(Fig. 16.5)* may be present. NSIP-like areas may be present but the final diagnosis should be based on the histologically worst areas *(Figs. 16.6 and 16.7)*.	*Proliferative (cellular) phase:* Airway-centered stellate to irregular cellular nodules composed of clusters of Langerhans cells (LCs) admixed with variable numbers of eosinophils, lymphocytes, plasma cells, neutrophils, and macrophages *(Figs. 16.8–16.10)*. Respiratory bronchiolitis is typically seen, characterized by the presence of macrophages containing light brown to golden yellow, coarsely granular cytoplasmic pigmentation (smoker's macrophages, *Fig. 16.11*), within bronchioles and peribronchiolar alveolar spaces and within and around the nodules. Variable-sized cysts lacking cell lining are formed at the periphery of the nodules by traction of the adjacent alveolar septa or destructive dilation of bronchioles. Patchy foci of airspace (organizing pneumonia, *Fig. 16.12*, arrow) and interstitial organization may be seen. Other smoking-related lung changes including DIP/RBILD, emphysematous change, small airways disease with mucostasis, and peribronchiolar metaplasia may be present. Vascular changes, such as intimal proliferation and medial thickening, are often present and may account for the clinical finding of pulmonary hypertension. The pleura may show reactive eosinophilic pleuritis if the patient had pneumothoraces. *Fibrotic phase:* The lung cellular nodules can be seen at different stages of cellularity and fibrosis. However, with the aging of the lesions, the LCs and other inflammatory cells become progressively decreased in number and overshadowed by fibrosis *(Fig. 16.13)*, eventually evolving into stellate to irregular scars *(Fig. 16.14)*. The airspaces adjacent to the fibrotic areas become cystically dilated *(Figs. 16.14, star, and 16.15, stars)*. In severe cases, interstitial fibrosis with honeycomb change may develop, mimicking UIP. The bronchiolocentric fibrotic scars often maintain the stellate shape of the cellular lesions, which is a clue that suggests PLCH in cases where only fibrotic lesions are sampled in the biopsy *(Figs. 16.16 and 16.17)*.
Special studies	The foci of loosely arranged fibroblastic activity stains green with pentachrome special stain, compared with the yellow-staining characteristic of dense fibrosis.	Immunoperoxidase stains CD1a *(Fig. 16.18)*, langerin, and S100 decorate small clusters or sheets of LCs in the pulmonary interstitial nodular lesions as well as in adjacent alveoli. It should be noted that LCs can be found in other inflammatory (and neoplastic) lung diseases, where they occur singly. In PLCH, the LCs *aggregate* in *clusters*, usually aggregates of more than 25 LCs. Cytoplasmic Birbeck granules and pentalaminar rod-shaped (or racket-shaped) organelles are identified by electron microscopy study. Some cases have a mutation in BRAF gene (V600E), although at this point relatively few of the tested cases were of lung origin.

	Usual Interstitial Pneumonia (UIP)	Pulmonary Langerhans Cell Histiocytosis (PLCH)
Prognosis	Not good. The cicatricial process is usually progressive and fatal in most cases. The median survival from the time of diagnosis is 2–3 y. UIP associated with an underlying collagen vascular disease tends to have a better clinical course/longer survival.	Variable and unpredictable. Clinical and radiologic stabilization or resolution of the disease occurs in 50% of patients, spontaneous regression in up to 25%, and progression to respiratory failure due to irreversible fibrosis in approximately 25%. In advanced cases, pulmonary hypertension and cor pulmonale may develop. Some patients develop and die of malignancies including lung cancer, lymphoma, and myeloproliferative disorders. The median survival is 12 y, with 5- and 10-y survival rates of 74% and 64%, respectively. Smoking cessation is recommended for all patients. Immunosuppression with corticosteroids, with or without the addition of chemotherapeutic agents, has been used to treat patients with variable results. Lung transplantation has been successful in treating patients with advanced disease, although relapse of PLCH in the transplanted lung has been reported. BRAF target therapy might be useful.

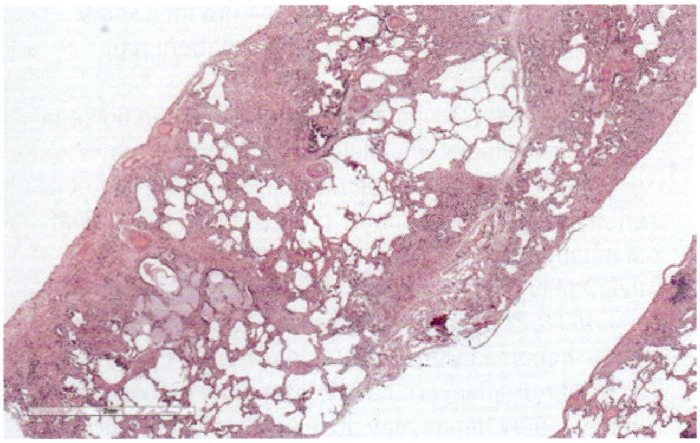

Figure 16.1 UIP: At low power, the disease is characterized by variegated appearance with subpleural and paraseptal areas of interstitial fibrosis and areas of uninvolved lung.

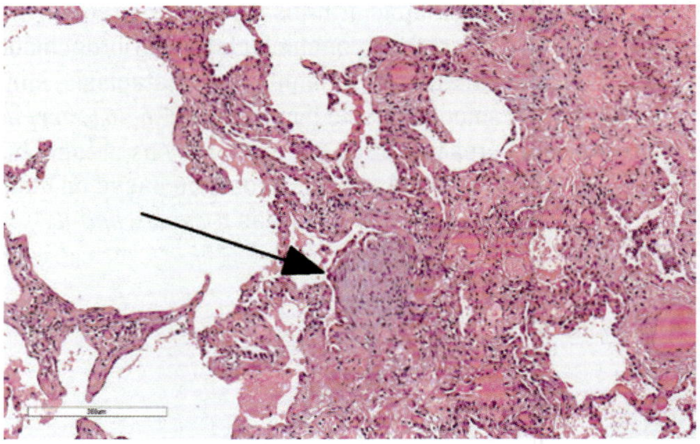

Figure 16.2 UIP: The temporally heterogeneous process is characterized by the presence of dense, pink, mature ("old") interstitial fibrosis (right field), and loosely arranged, light blue, myxoid, immature ("recent") interstitial foci of fibroblastic activity (*arrow*).

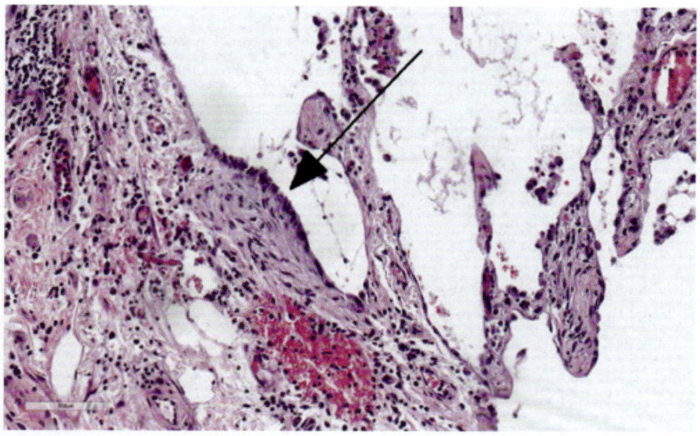

Figure 16.3 UIP: Note that foci of fibroblastic activity are interstitial/subepithelial (*arrow*).

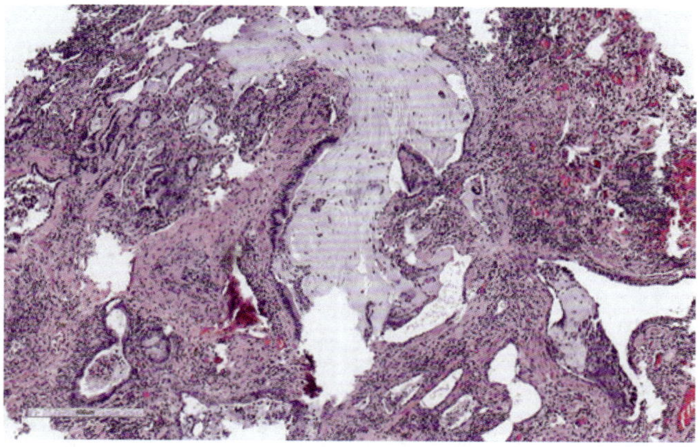

Figure 16.4 UIP: The disease promotes remodeling of the underlying lung parenchyma architecture associated with peripheral honeycomb change, characterized by the presence of enlarged irregular spaces lined by bronchiolar type of epithelium containing a mucinous exudate with macrophages and inflammatory cells, which is surrounded by fibrosis and chronic inflammation. Interstitial inflammation, if present, is typically noted in the areas of honeycombing. In severe cases of PLCH, interstitial fibrosis with honeycomb change may develop.

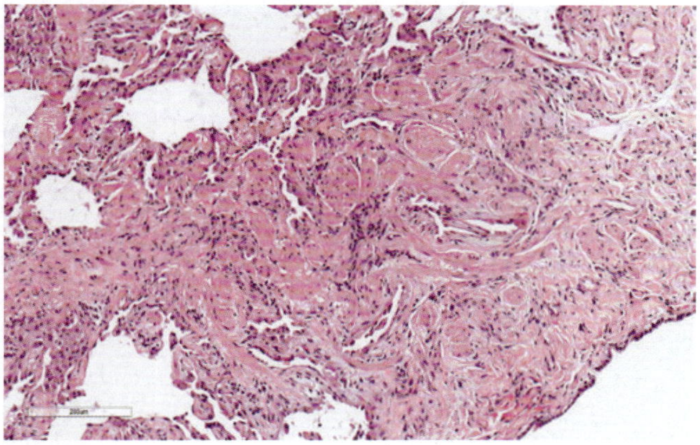

Figure 16.5 UIP: Smooth muscle hyperplasia is a common associated feature.

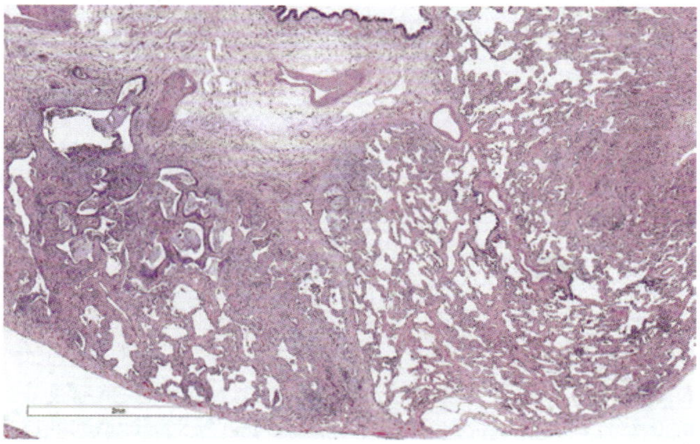

Figure 16.6 UIP: NSIP-like areas may be present (*right*), but the final diagnosis should be based on the histologically worst areas (*left*).

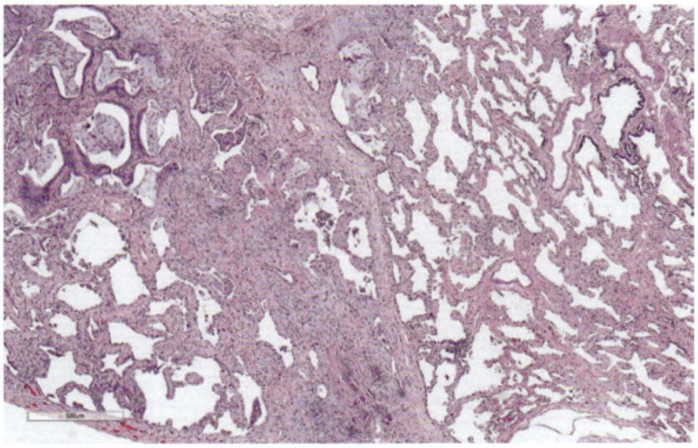

Figure 16.7 UIP (higher magnification from Figure 16.6): Temporally heterogeneous process with interstitial areas of recent organization a.k.a. fibroblastic activity or fibroblastic foci (*center*).

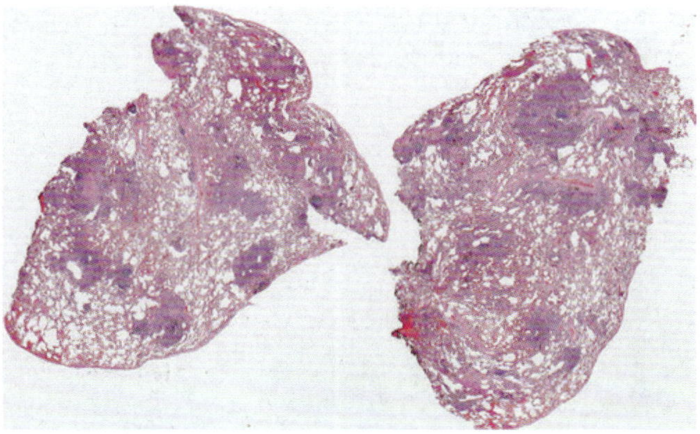

Figure 16.8 PLCH (cellular phase): Airway-centered cellular nodules.

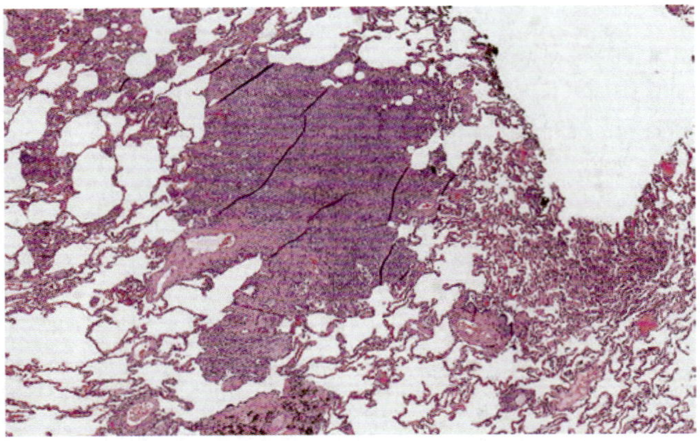

Figure 16.9 PLCH (cellular phase): High magnification of stellate to irregular airway-centered cellular nodule (note pulmonary artery in *middle left*).

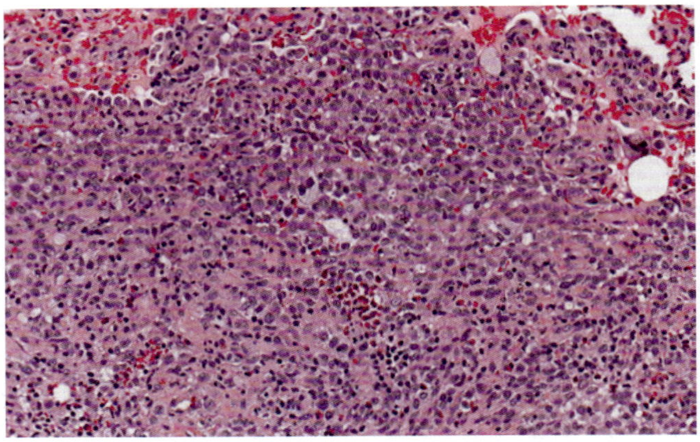

Figure 16.10 PLCH (cellular phase; high power): The cellular nodules are composed of clusters of LCs, admixed with variable number of eosinophils, lymphocytes, plasma cells, neutrophils, and macrophages.

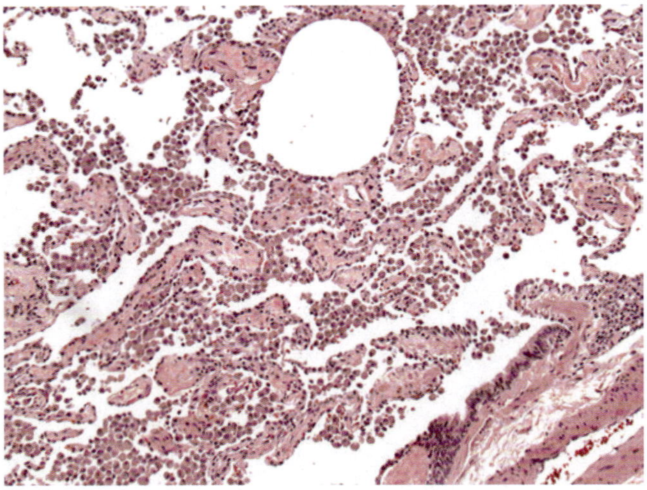

Figure 16.11 PLCH: Respiratory bronchiolitis is typically seen, characterized by the presence of macrophages containing light brown to golden yellow, coarsely granular cytoplasmic pigmentation (smoker's macrophages).

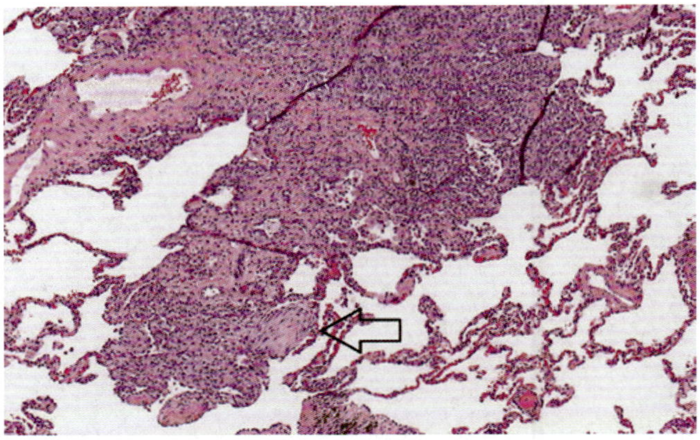

Figure 16.12 PLCH: Small foci of organizing pneumonia (*arrow*) may represent a small component of PLCH.

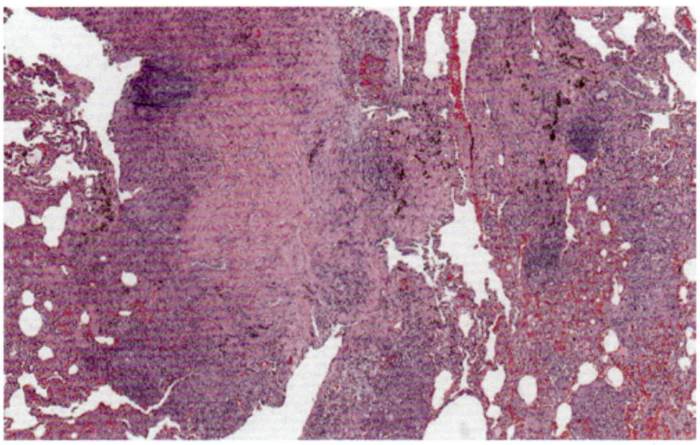

Figure 16.13 PLCH (fibrotic phase): With the aging of the lesions, the LCs and other inflammatory cells become progressively decreased in number and overshadowed by fibrosis.

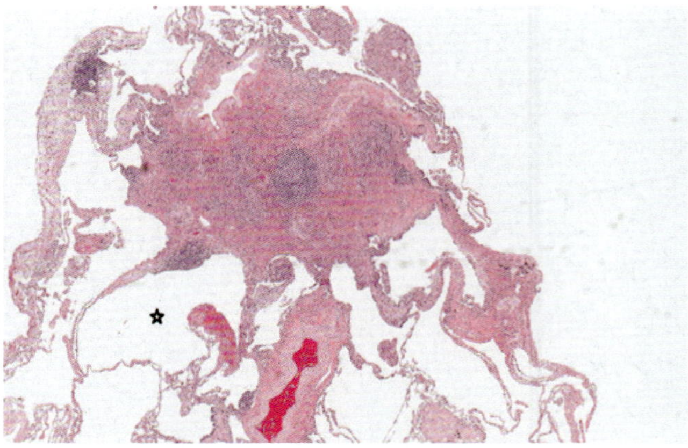

Figure 16.14 PLCH (fibrotic phase): The cellular nodules become progressively overshadowed by fibrosis, eventually evolving into stellate scars. Note cystic dilated alveolar space (*star*) at the periphery of the fibrotic nodular lesion (paracicatricial emphysema).

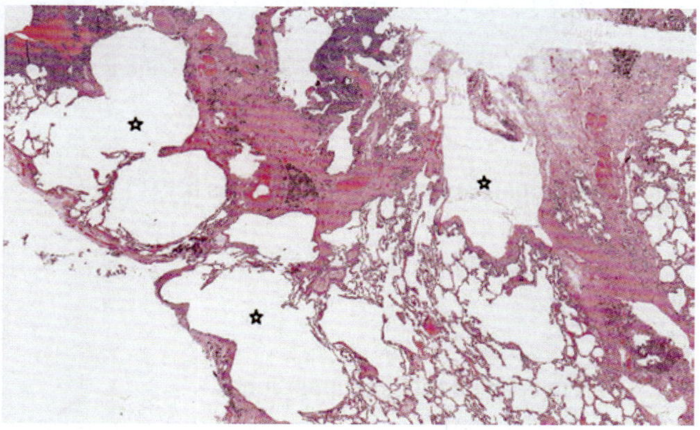

Figure 16.15 PLCH: Variable-sized cysts lacking cell lining are formed at the periphery of the nodules by traction of the adjacent alveolar septa (*stars*), also seen in Figure 16.14.

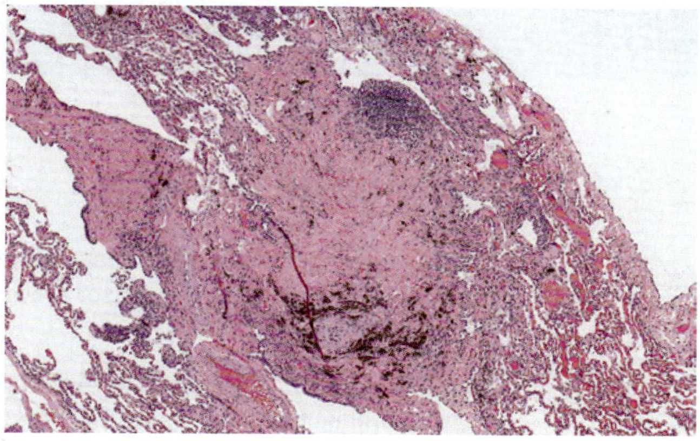

Figure 16.16 PLCH: Fibrotic phase of PLCH may be confused with UIP, but the fibrotic scars in PLCH often retain a stellate shape and show bronchiolocentric distribution, and not a predominantly subpleural and paraseptal temporo heterogenous typical UIP pattern of fibrosis.

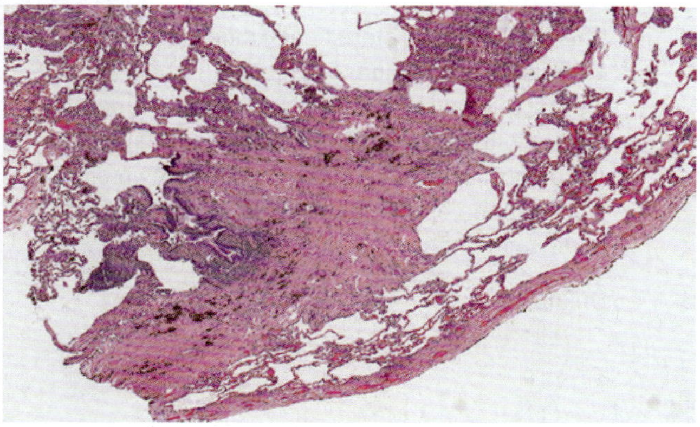

Figure 16.17 PLCH (fibrotic phase): Fibrotic scar with stellate to irregular shape, bronchiolocentric distribution (note bronchovascular bundle, *left middle*).

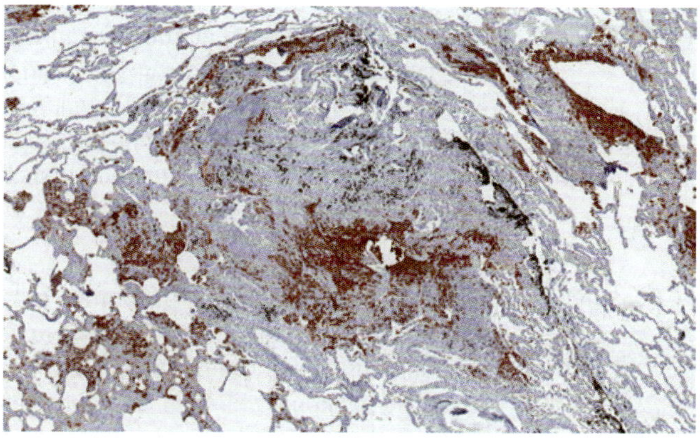

Figure 16.18 PLCH: Immunoperoxidase stain CD1a decorates clusters and sheets of LCs within the cellular nodule, confirming the diagnosis of PLCH.

17 USUAL INTERSTITIAL PNEUMONIA VS. PLEUROPARENCHYMAL FIBROELASTOSIS

	Usual Interstitial Pneumonia (UIP)	**Pleuroparenchymal Fibroelastosis (PPFE)**
Age	Majority of the patients are between 50 and 70 y of age, with an average age of onset at 60 y and a slight male predominance.	The age ranges from 32 to 65 y.
Location	It usually involves the lung basilar regions bilaterally with predominant subpleural and paraseptal distribution.	It typically affects the upper lobes.
Symptoms	Insidious onset of nonproductive cough and slowly progressive dyspnea. Chest auscultation usually demonstrates bibasilar inspiratory crackles.	Dyspnea on exertion and cough. Pneumothorax has been reported in some cases.
Signs	Chest high-resolution computed tomography (HRCT) shows patchy, predominantly peripheral (subpleural), bibasilar, and often asymmetrical reticular opacities and honeycombing as characteristic findings. Pulmonary function tests demonstrate a restrictive pattern.	Chest HRCT characteristically demonstrates marked bilateral upper lung (apical) visceral pleural thickening extending into the lung parenchyma with subpleural reticular abnormalities. Associated features include upper-lobe volume loss, traction bronchiectasis, and in rare cases, honeycombing.
Etiology	Potential etiologies include pulmonary manifestation of systemic autoimmune/connective tissue disease, drug toxicity, pneumoconiosis, familial idiopathic pulmonary fibrosis, and possibly fibrotic phase of chronic hypersensitivity pneumonia, and these possibilities should be clinically excluded before placing the case under the idiopathic pulmonary fibrosis (IPF) category.	Unknown.

	Usual Interstitial Pneumonia (UIP)	**Pleuroparenchymal Fibroelastosis (PPFE)**
Histology	Temporally heterogenous pattern of interstitial fibrosis characterized by the presence of dense, pink, mature ("old") interstitial scarring/fibrosis; loosely arranged, light blue, immature ("recent") interstitial foci of fibroblastic activity; and areas of normal-appearing lung *(Fig. 17.1)*. Fibroblastic foci are usually seen at the transition zones between dense fibrosis and normal lung *(Figs. 17.2 and 17.3)*. The process usually has a subpleural and paraseptal distribution and promotes remodeling of the underlying lung parenchyma architecture associated with peripheral honeycomb change *(Fig. 17.4)*. Interstitial inflammation, if present, is typically patchy and mild, mostly noted in the areas of honeycombing. Usually, there is little or no interstitial inflammation away from the areas of fibrosis. Lymphoid follicles with germinal centers tend to be prominent in cases associated with underlying connective tissue disease, particularly rheumatoid arthritis. Secondary traction bronchiectasis/bronchiolectasis, peribronchiolar metaplasia, squamous cell metaplasia, and smooth muscle hyperplasia *(Fig. 17.5)* may be present. NSIP-like areas may be present, but the final diagnosis should be based on the histologically worst areas *(Figs. 17.6 and 17.7)*.	There is marked thickening of the visceral pleura and remodeling of the subpleural parenchyma architecture by a homogeneous mixture of dense collagen deposition and elastic tissue (fibroelastotic scarring) *(Fig. 17.8)*. Rare fibroblastic activity may be present at the leading edge of the fibroelastotic scarring. Mild chronic inflammation is commonly seen in the fibroelastotic zones, but the uninvolved lung parenchyma is characteristically free of significant inflammation or scarring. The margins between the fibroelastotic zones and the underlying normal lung are typically sharply defined. The uninvolved lung usually shows minimal abnormalities, mainly involving small airways, such as bronchiolectasis or bronchiolar fibrosis *(Figs. 17.9 and 17.10)*. Extensive pleural adhesions may be present, most likely secondary to common history of pneumothorax.
Special studies	The foci of loosely arranged fibroblastic activity stains green with pentachrome special stain, compared with the yellow-staining characteristic of dense fibrosis.	Pentachrome special stain decorates dense collagen deposition (yellow) admixed with elastic fibers (black) *(Fig. 17.11)*.
Prognosis	Not good. The cicatricial process is usually progressive and fatal in most cases. The median survival from the time of diagnosis is 2–3 y. UIP associated with an underlying collagen vascular disease tends to have a better clinical course/longer survival.	Variable. Progressive disease with eventual death within several years has been reported.

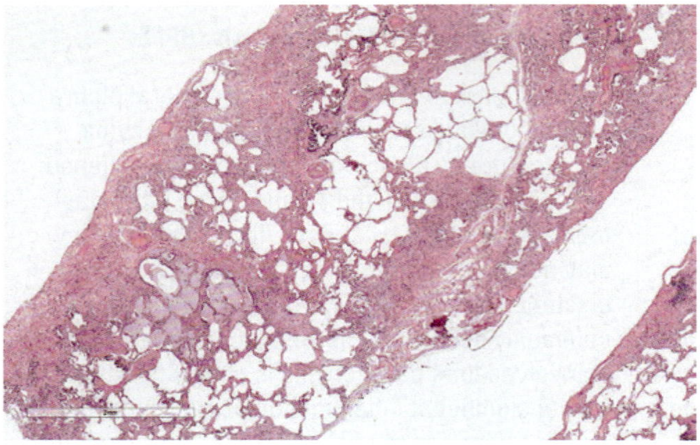

Figure 17.1 UIP: At low power, UIP is characterized by variegated appearance with subpleural and paraseptal areas of interstitial fibrosis and areas of uninvolved lung. Variegated appearance is not a feature of PPFE.

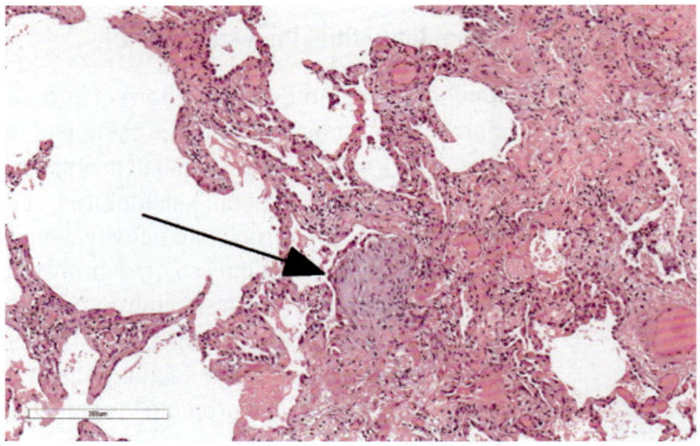

Figure 17.2 UIP: The temporally heterogeneous process is characterized by the presence of dense, pink, mature ("old") interstitial fibrosis (right field) and loosely arranged, light blue, myxoid, immature ("recent") interstitial foci of fibroblastic activity (*arrow*). Temporal heterogeneity is not a characteristic feature of PPFE.

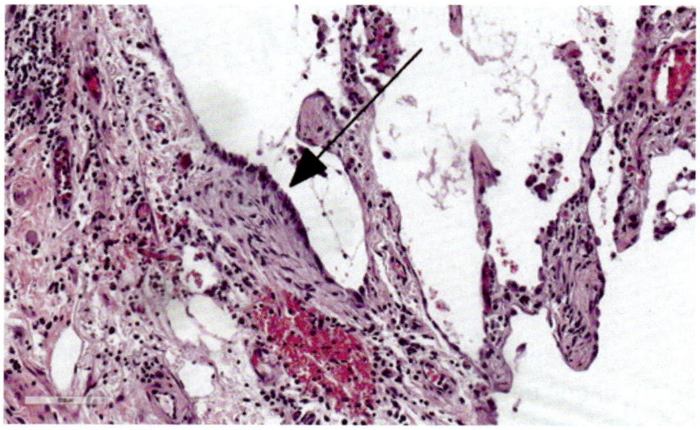

Figure 17.3 UIP: Note that foci of fibroblastic activity are interstitial/subepithelial (*arrow*).

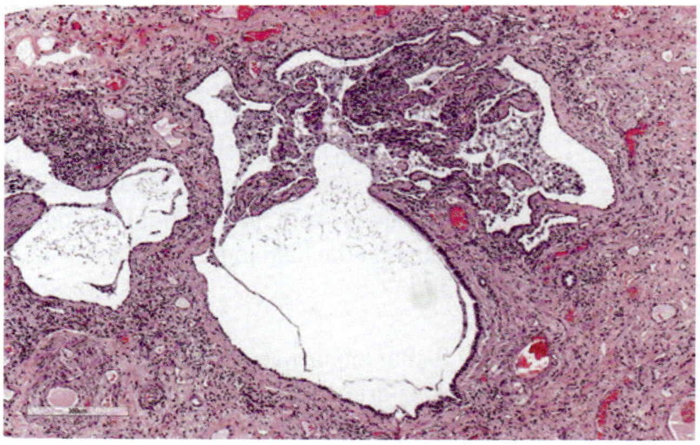

Figure 17.4 UIP: The disease promotes remodeling of the underlying lung architecture associated with peripheral honeycomb change, characterized by the presence of enlarged irregular spaces lined by bronchiolar type of epithelium containing a mucinous exudate with macrophages and inflammatory cells, which is surrounded by fibrosis and chronic inflammation. Honeycombing is not a common feature of PPFE.

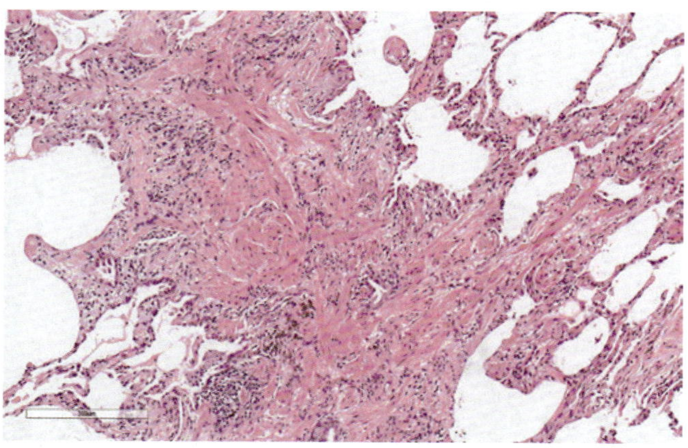

Figure 17.5 UIP: Smooth muscle hyperplasia is a common associated feature, not seen in PPFE.

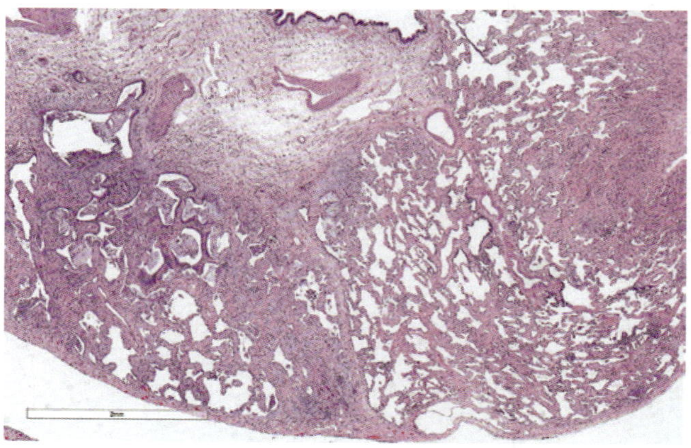

Figure 17.6 UIP: NSIP-like areas may be present (*right*) but the final diagnosis should be based on the histologically worst areas (*left*). NSIP-like areas are not seen in PPFE.

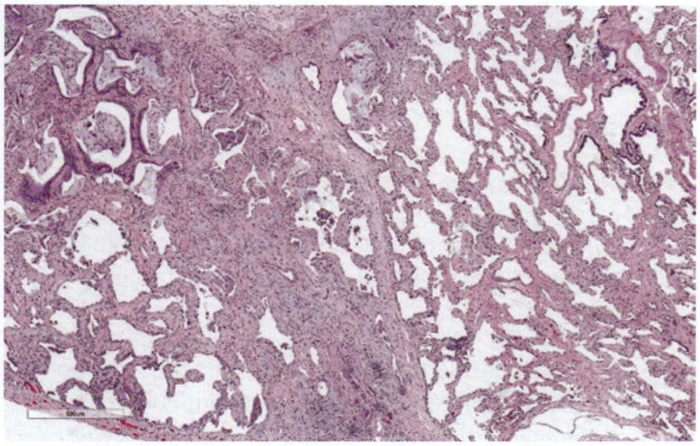

Figure 17.7 UIP (higher magnification from Figure 14.6): Temporally heterogeneous process with numerous interstitial areas of recent organization a.k.a. fibroblastic activity or fibroblastic foci (*center*). Different from UIP, fibroblastic foci in PPFE are never numerous.

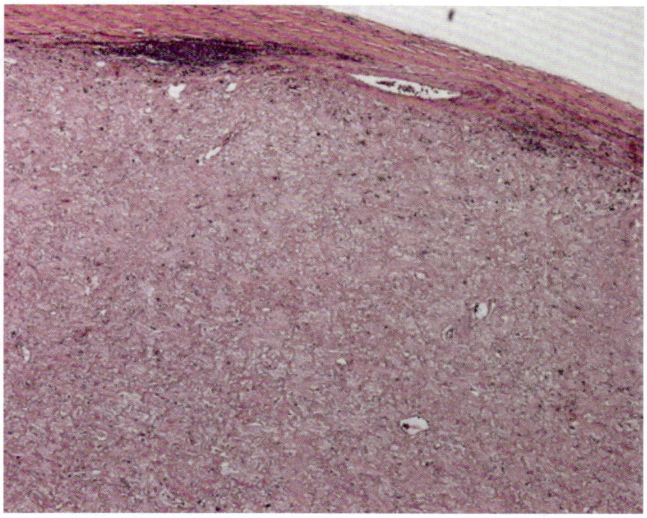

Figure 17.8 PPFE: There is thickening of the visceral pleura and remodeling of the subpleural parenchyma architecture by homogeneous fibroelastotic scarring.

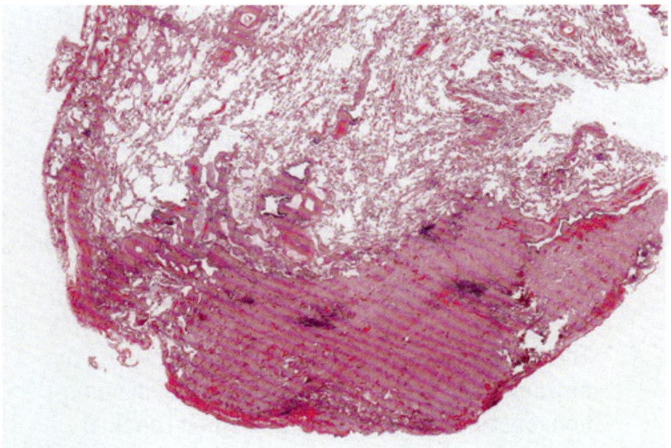

Figure 17.9 PPFE: In contrast to UIP, the subpleural fibroelastotic scarring seen in PPFE is not temporally heterogeneous and is rarely associated with honeycomb change.

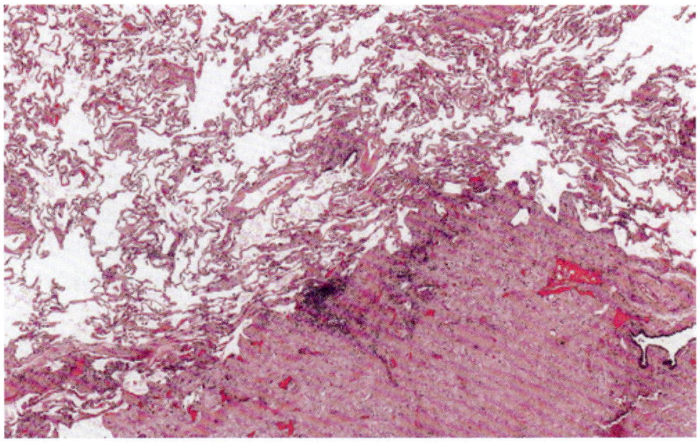

Figure 17.10 PPFE: There is abrupt transition between fibroelastotic and normal lung parenchyma. The uninvolved lung parenchyma is characteristically free of significant inflammation or scarring. PPFE shows rare fibroblastic activity, which may be present at the leading edge of the fibroelastotic scarring. In contrast to UIP, fibroblastic foci in PPFE are never numerous.

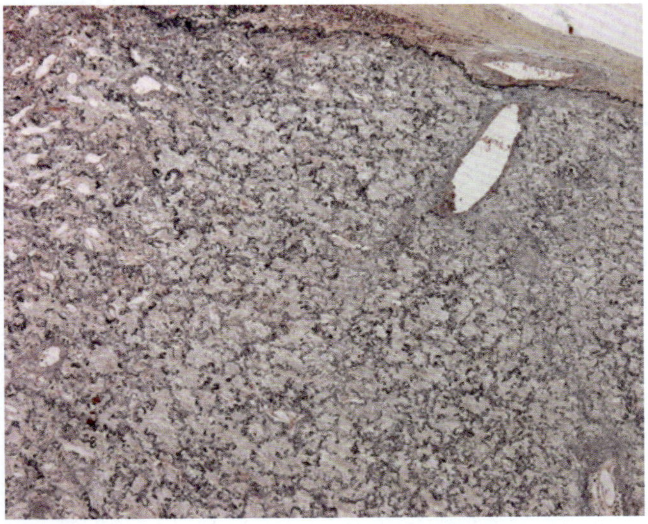

Figure 17.11 PPFE: Pentachrome special stain demonstrates that the subpleural fibroelastotic scarring is composed of a homogeneous mixture of dense collagen deposition (*yellow*) and elastotic fibers (*black*).

18 USUAL INTERSTITIAL PNEUMONIA VS. BRONCHIECTASIS WITH SCARRING

	Usual Interstitial Pneumonia (UIP)	Bronchiectasis with Scarring
Age	Majority of the patients are between 50 and 70 y of age, with an average age of onset at 60 y, and a slight male predominance.	Bronchiectasis affects all ages and both sexes. Age predilection depends on etiologic factors.
Location	It usually involves the lung basilar regions bilaterally with predominant subpleural and paraseptal distribution.	It affects cartilaginous airways (bronchi). Can be localized or diffuse in distribution, depending on etiologic factors. For instance, predilection for upper lobes is noted in tuberculosis and allergic bronchopulmonary fungal disease; lower lobes in bacterial and viral infections; and all lobes in cystic fibrosis and immunodeficiencies.
Symptoms	Insidious onset of nonproductive cough and slowly progressive dyspnea. Chest auscultation usually demonstrates bibasilar inspiratory crackles.	Productive cough with purulent sputum, fever, shortness of breath, and hemoptysis (which can be massive). Clinical course with recurrent exacerbation is common. Many patients have coexisting sinusitis. Hypoxemia may develop in advanced cases.
Signs	Chest high-resolution computed tomography (HRCT) shows patchy, predominantly peripheral (subpleural), bibasilar, and often asymmetrical reticular opacities as characteristic findings. Pulmonary function tests demonstrate a restrictive pattern.	Chest HRCT demonstrates bronchiectasis (cylindrical, varicose, saccular, or cystic), with mucous plugs and thickening of the bronchial wall. Atelectasis and pulmonary infiltrates in the affected lung segment or lobe are commonly seen.
Etiology	Potential etiologies include pulmonary manifestation of systemic autoimmune/connective tissue disease, drug toxicity, pneumoconiosis, familial idiopathic pulmonary fibrosis, and possibly fibrotic phase of chronic hypersensitivity pneumonia, and these possibilities should be clinically excluded before placing the case under the idiopathic pulmonary fibrosis (IPF) category.	The pathogenesis of bronchiectasis is related to any condition that promotes recurrent inflammation, obstruction, and damage of the bronchial walls, resulting in weakening and dilatation over the time. Possible etiologies include, but are not limited to, infections (bacterial, tuberculous and nontuberculous mycobacterial, fungal, viral, and anaerobic due to recurrent aspiration), primary or secondary ciliary dysfunction, cystic fibrosis (inspissated mucous plug) and cystic fibrosis variants, α-1 protease inhibitor deficiency, immunodeficiency, allergic bronchopulmonary fungal disease, obstructing neoplasm, aspirated foreign body, right middle lobe syndrome, congenital anatomic defect (e.g., pulmonary sequestration), pulmonary manifestation of systemic disorders (e.g., rheumatoid arthritis and Sjögren syndrome), extraintestinal manifestation of inflammatory bowel disease, diffuse panbronchiolitis, bone marrow transplantation–associated bronchiolitis obliterans, or idiopathic.

	Usual Interstitial Pneumonia (UIP)	**Bronchiectasis with Scarring**
Histology	UIP has a typical variegated appearance with subpleural and paraseptal areas of interstitial fibrosis and areas of uninvolved lung *(Fig. 18.1)*. This temporally heterogenous pattern of interstitial fibrosis is characterized by the presence of dense, pink, mature ("old") interstitial fibrosis and loosely arranged, light blue, immature ("recent") interstitial foci of fibroblastic activity *(Figs. 18.2 and 18.3, arrows)*. Fibroblastic foci are usually seen at the transition zones between dense fibrosis and normal lung. The process usually has a subpleural and paraseptal distribution and promotes remodeling of the underlying lung parenchyma architecture associated with peripheral honeycomb change *(Fig. 18.4)*. Interstitial inflammation if present is typically patchy and mild, mostly noted in the areas of honeycombing. Usually, there is little or no interstitial inflammation away from the areas of fibrosis. Lymphoid follicles with germinal centers tend to be prominent in cases associated with connective tissue disease, particularly rheumatoid arthritis. Secondary traction bronchiectasis/bronchiolectasis, peribronchiolar metaplasia, squamous cell metaplasia, and smooth muscle hyperplasia *(Fig. 18.5)* may be present. NSIP-like areas may be present, but the final diagnosis should be based on the histologically worst areas *(Figs. 18.6 and 18.7)*.	Airway walls demonstrate marked chronic inflammation, prominent lymphoid follicles, and variable degrees of acute inflammation *(Fig. 18.8)*. There is luminal filling by acute inflammation and mucopurulent or necrotic debris *(Figs. 18.9 and 18.10)*. Fungal organisms, particularly Aspergillus sp., may colonize ectatic bronchi. If secondary to mycobacterial or fungal infections, granulomatous inflammation can be present. Surface epithelium ulceration and replacement by metaplastic epithelium may be present. If the inflammation and obstruction are resolved early in the process, the damage may be reversible. If not, over time in severe cases there will be destruction of all components of the bronchial wall, including mucosa, submucosa, muscularis propria, elastic fibers, and cartilage, with granulation tissue formation and eventually irreversible replacement of the airway wall by dense fibrosis *(Fig. 18.11)*. The bronchial dilatation varies from subtle enlargement that can only be appreciated by comparing the bronchus to its accompanying pulmonary artery (which should be approximately the same size) *(Fig. 18.12)* to massive dilatation *(Figs. 18.10 and 18.13)*. The adjacent alveolated lung parenchyma may show acute pneumonia, organizing pneumonia, and variable amount of alveolar septal fibrosis. Parenchymal scarring secondary to bronchiectasis *(Fig. 18.14)* may mimic interstitial fibrosis of UIP showing all the features of honeycomb change, with metaplastic epithelium and mucous pooling in airspaces. Clinical and radiologic features and the presence of airway-centered scarring are helpful in the diagnosis of bronchiectasis. Obstructive change may be present, manifesting as constrictive bronchiolitis of the distal small airways, foamy macrophages in alveolar spaces, and lung hyperinflation. Pulmonary arteries may show pulmonary hypertension change in advanced cases.
Special studies	The foci of loosely arranged fibroblastic activity stains green with pentachrome special stain, compared with the yellow-staining characteristic of dense fibrosis.	A number of special studies may be required depending on the clinical setting, including tissue cultures, GMS and AFB special stains, ciliary motility and ultrastructural studies, skin tests, sweat test, semen analysis, serum immunoglobulins titers, and rheumatologic workup. Bronchoscopy may detect and remove airway obstruction by foreign body.

	Usual Interstitial Pneumonia (UIP)	Bronchiectasis with Scarring
Prognosis	Not good. The cicatricial process is usually progressive and fatal in most cases. The median survival from the time of diagnosis is 2–3 y. UIP associated with an underlying collagen vascular disease tends to have a better clinical course/longer survival.	The incidence of bronchiectasis appears to have decreased with prevention and treatment of airway infections with immunizations, chest physiotherapy, and antibiotic therapy. Most patients are treated with conservative nonsurgical therapy, but resection may be performed in cases with severely affected lobes. Potential complications include recurrent pneumonia, empyema, pneumothorax, lung abscesses, hemoptysis, and chronic respiratory failure associated with cor pulmonale. Vessel embolization can be performed in cases of significant hemoptysis. Massive hemoptysis may sometimes require emergency surgery. Secondary infection and inflammation in the distal lung (small airways) may cause irreversible constrictive/obstructive bronchiolitis. Lung transplantation can be considered in advanced cases.

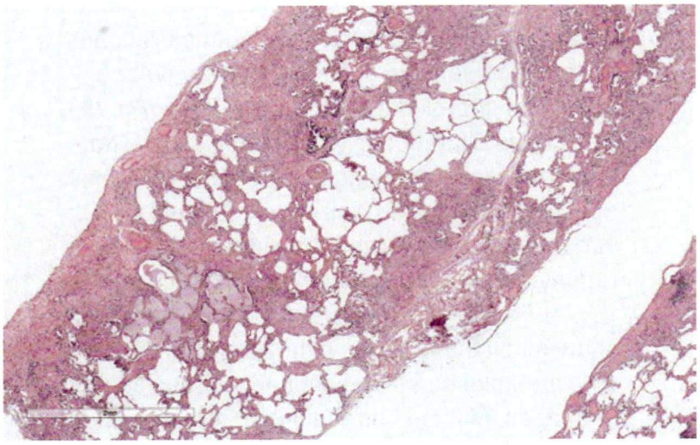

Figure 18.1 UIP: At low power, the disease is characterized by variegated appearance with subpleural and paraseptal areas of interstitial fibrosis and areas of uninvolved lung.

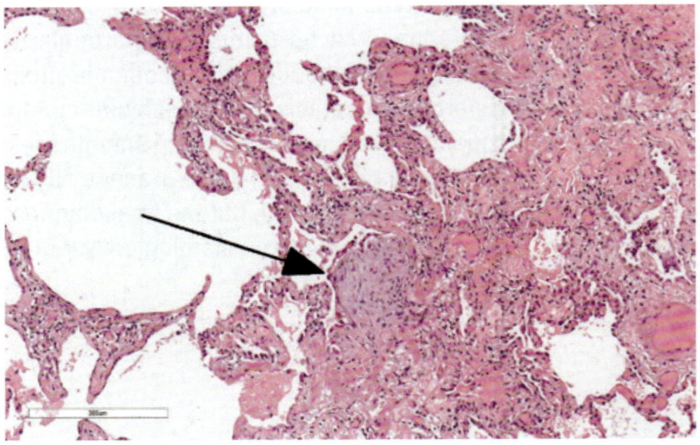

Figure 18.2 UIP: The temporally heterogeneous process is characterized by the presence of dense, pink, mature ("old") interstitial fibrosis (right field) and loosely arranged, light blue, myxoid, immature ("recent") interstitial foci of fibroblastic activity (*arrow*).

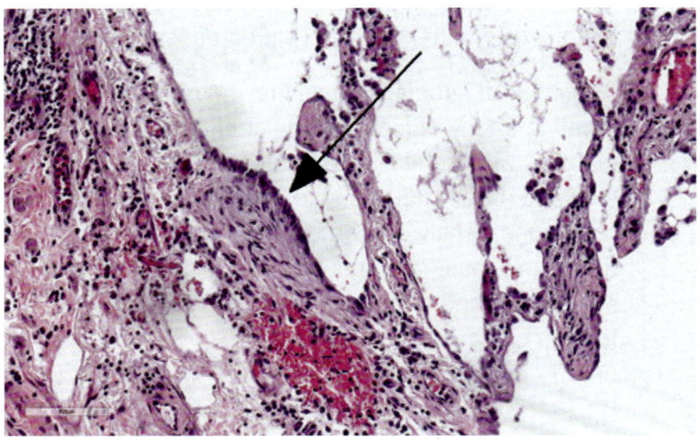

Figure 18.3 UIP: Note that foci of fibroblastic activity are interstitial/subepithelial (*arrow*).

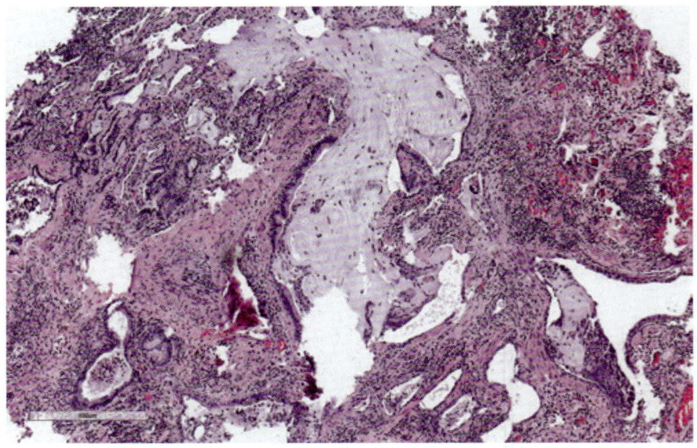

Figure 18.4 UIP: The disease promotes remodeling of the underlying lung architecture associated with peripheral honeycomb change, characterized by the presence of enlarged irregular spaces lined by bronchiolar type of epithelium containing a mucinous exudate with macrophages and inflammatory cells, which is surrounded by fibrosis and chronic inflammation.

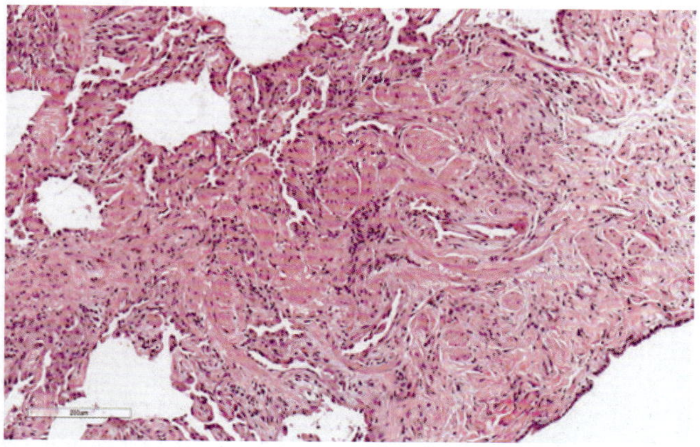

Figure 18.5 UIP: Smooth muscle hyperplasia is a common associated feature.

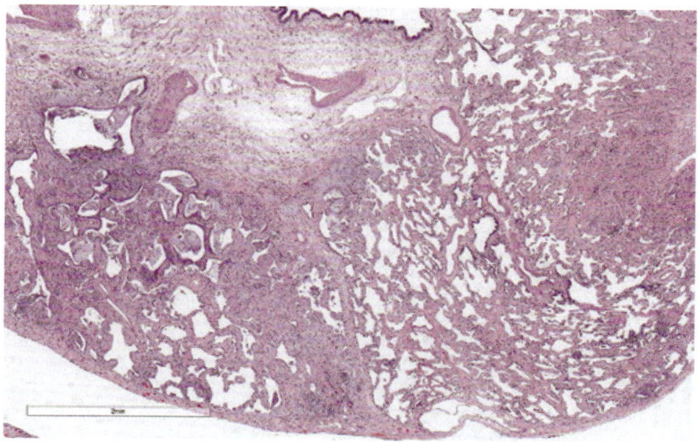

Figure 18.6 UIP: NSIP-like areas may be present (*right*), but the final diagnosis should be based on the histologically worst areas (*left*).

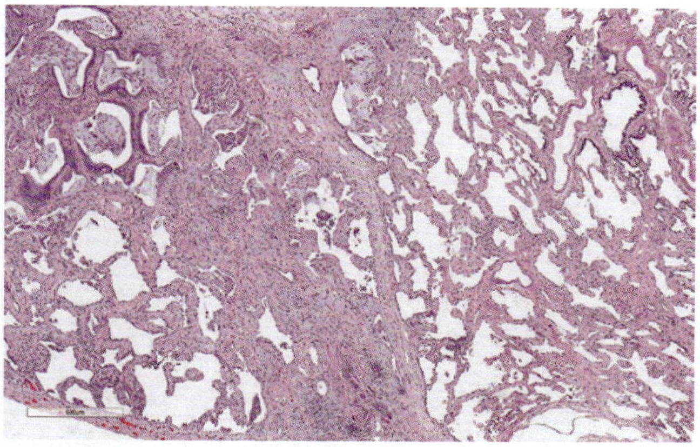

Figure 18.7 UIP: Higher magnification from Figure 18.6. Temporally heterogeneous process with interstitial areas of recent organization a.k.a. fibroblastic activity or fibroblastic foci (*center*).

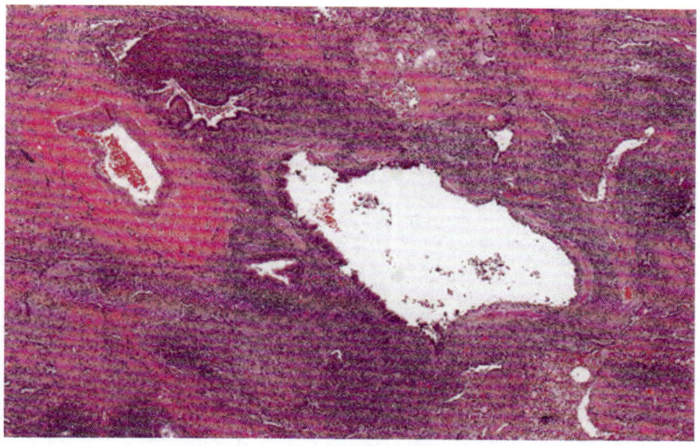

Figure 18.8 Bronchiectasis: There is bronchial luminal ectasia, denudation of the surface epithelium, and irregular wall thickening by marked chronic inflammation and prominent lymphoid follicles.

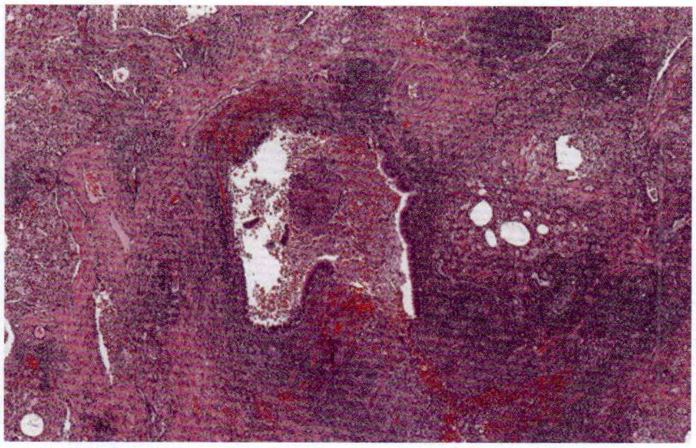

Figure 18.9 Bronchiectasis: Luminal dilatation associated with mucopurulent necrotic debris.

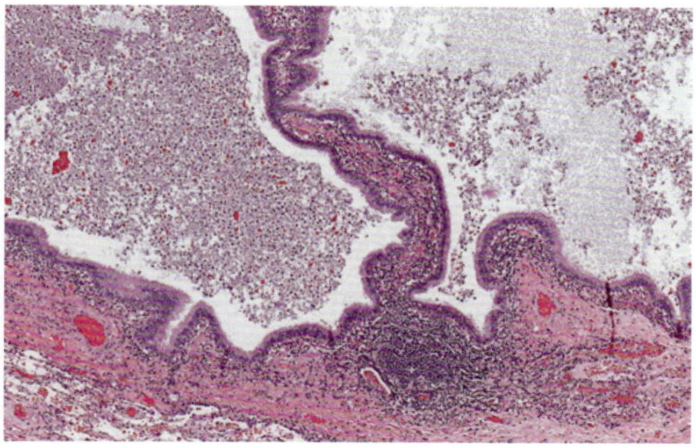

Figure 18.10 Bronchiectasis: Marked luminal dilatation associated with lymphoid follicle and luminal filling by acute inflammation and necrotic debris.

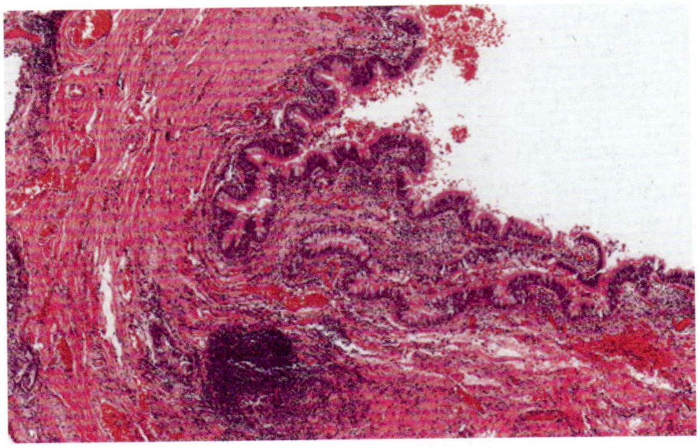

Figure 18.11 Bronchiectasis: There is distortion of the airway wall by chronic inflammation with lymphoid follicle formation and dense fibrosis/scarring (*upper left*). Note the absence of smooth muscle, cartilage, and submucosal glands.

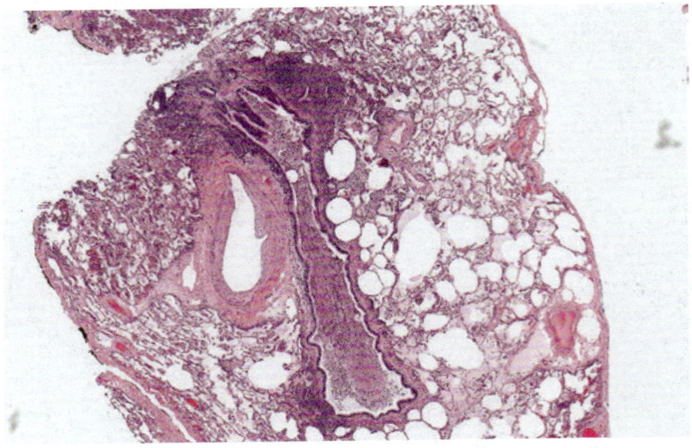

Figure 18.12 Bronchiectasis: The bronchial dilatation can be appreciated by comparing the bronchus to its accompanying pulmonary artery (which should be approximately the same size).

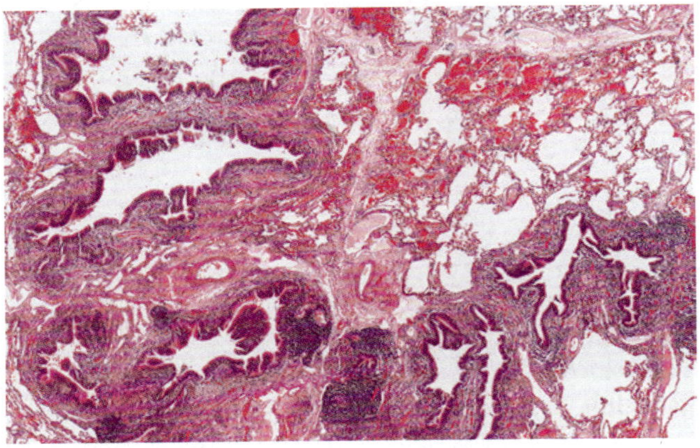

Figure 18.13 Bronchiectasis: Disease involving multiple airways.

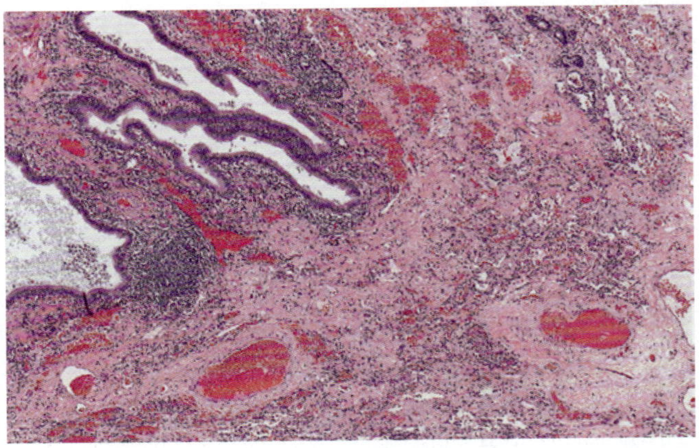

Figure 18.14 Bronchiectasis: In this case, there is secondary parenchymal scarring, which may mimic interstitial fibrosis of UIP. Clinical and radiologic features and the presence of airway-centered scarring (seen in bronchiectasis) rather than temporally heterogenous process with peripheral honeycombing (seen in UIP) are helpful in making the distinction between these diagnoses.

19 USUAL INTERSTITIAL PNEUMONIA VS. END-STAGE HONEYCOMB LUNG

	Usual Interstitial Pneumonia (UIP)	End-Stage Honeycomb Lung
Age	Majority of the patients are between 50 and 70 y of age, with an average age of onset at 60 y, and a slight male predominance.	It varies depending on the etiology.
Location	It usually involves the lung basilar regions bilaterally with predominant subpleural and paraseptal distribution.	Honeycomb areas are usually more prominent in subpleural lung parenchyma and lung bases.
Symptoms	Insidious onset of nonproductive cough and slowly progressive dyspnea. Chest auscultation usually demonstrates bibasilar inspiratory crackles.	Similar to UIP, except in cases secondary to acute interstitial pneumonia (AIP) and diffuse alveolar damage (DAD).
Signs	Chest high-resolution computed tomography (HRCT) shows patchy, predominantly peripheral (subpleural), bibasilar, and often asymmetrical reticular opacities and honeycombing as characteristic findings. Pulmonary function tests demonstrate a restrictive pattern.	Chest HRCT shows honeycomb cysts and traction bronchiectasis.
Etiology	Potential etiologies include pulmonary manifestation of systemic autoimmune/connective tissue disease, drug toxicity, pneumoconiosis, familial idiopathic pulmonary fibrosis, and possibly fibrotic phase of chronic hypersensitivity pneumonia, and these possibilities should be clinically excluded before placing the case under the idiopathic pulmonary fibrosis (IPF) category.	It represents an end-stage pattern of injury and may result from a variety of interstitial inflammatory and fibrosing processes, including usual interstitial pneumonia (UIP), desquamative interstitial pneumonia (DIP), interstitial granulomatous disease (e.g., infections, hypersensitivity pneumonia, sarcoidosis, chronic beryllium disease), pulmonary Langerhans cell histiocytosis, and pneumoconiosis (e.g., asbestosis and hard metal lung disease/giant cell pneumoconiosis). Although most cases of end-stage honeycomb lung take many years to develop, it can also develop in few weeks in patients with AIP and DAD.

	Usual Interstitial Pneumonia (UIP)	End-Stage Honeycomb Lung
Histology	Temporally heterogeneous pattern of interstitial fibrosis characterized by the presence of dense, pink, mature ("old") interstitial scarring/fibrosis; loosely arranged, light blue, immature ("recent") interstitial foci of fibroblastic activity; and areas of normal-appearing lung *(Fig. 19.1)*. Fibroblastic foci are usually seen at the transition zones between dense fibrosis and normal lung *(Figs. 19.2 and 19.3)*. The process usually has a subpleural and paraseptal distribution and promotes remodeling of the underlying lung parenchyma architecture associated with peripheral honeycomb change *(Fig. 19.4)*. Interstitial inflammation, if present, is typically patchy and mild, mostly noted in the areas of honeycombing. Usually, there is little or no interstitial inflammation away from the areas of fibrosis. Lymphoid follicles with germinal centers tend to be prominent in cases associated with connective tissue disease, particularly rheumatoid arthritis. Secondary traction bronchiectasis/bronchiolectasis, peribronchiolar metaplasia, squamous cell metaplasia, and smooth muscle hyperplasia *(Fig. 19.5)* may be present. NSIP-like areas may be present, but the final diagnosis should be based on the histologically worst areas *(Figs. 19.6 and 19.7)*.	The morphology is similar to the honeycombing seen in UIP but lacking the temporally heterogenous pattern of interstitial fibrosis characteristic of UIP. There is extensive remodeling of the underlying lung parenchyma architecture by enlarged/cystic airspaces filled by mucin-containing variable number of inflammatory cells and macrophages, lined by bronchiolar epithelium and surrounded by dense fibrosis/scarring *(Fig. 19.8)*. The honeycomb spaces in end stage of DAD are usually lined by alveolar pneumocytes rather than bronchiolar epithelium, and their walls contain less dense collagen. The microscopic appearance of end-stage honeycomb lung is nonspecific regardless of the etiology. Clinical and radiologic correlation and review of previous/earlier biopsies (if available) may be required to determine the cause.
Special studies	The foci of loosely arranged fibroblastic activity stains green with pentachrome special stain, compared with the yellow-staining characteristic of dense fibrosis.	Noncontributory.
Prognosis	Not good. The cicatricial process is usually progressive and fatal in most cases. The median survival from the time of diagnosis is 2–3 y. UIP associated with an underlying collagen vascular disease tends to have a better clinical course/longer survival.	Same as UIP. Lungs with extensive interstitial fibrosis and honeycomb areas are associated with an increased risk of developing peripheral pulmonary carcinomas.

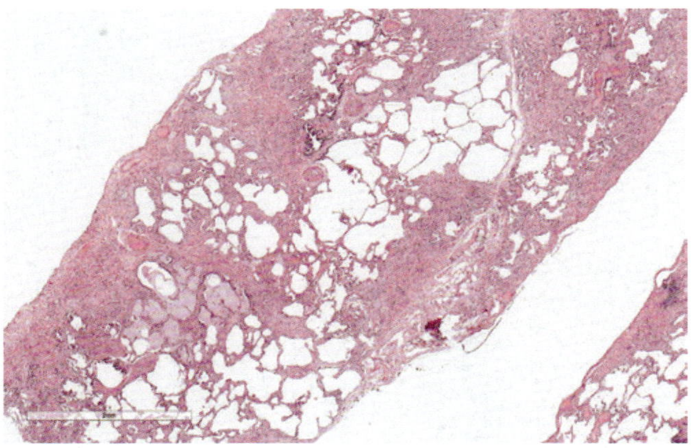

Figure 19.1 UIP: At low power, UIP is characterized by variegated appearance with subpleural and paraseptal areas of interstitial fibrosis and areas of uninvolved lung.

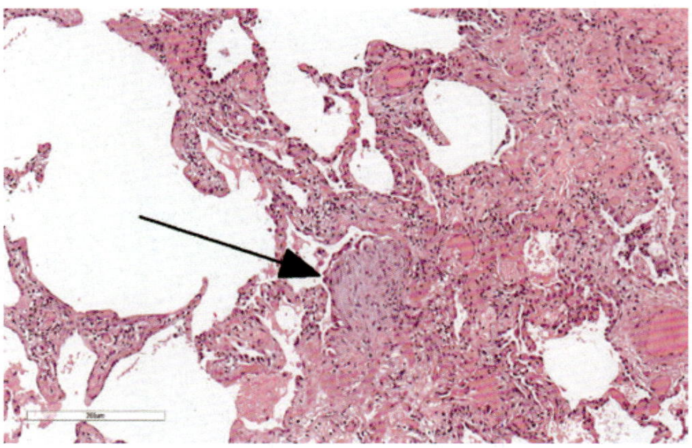

Figure 19.2 UIP: The temporally heterogeneous process is characterized by the presence of dense, pink, mature ("old") interstitial fibrosis (right field) and loosely arranged, light blue, myxoid, immature ("recent") interstitial foci of fibroblastic activity (*arrow*).

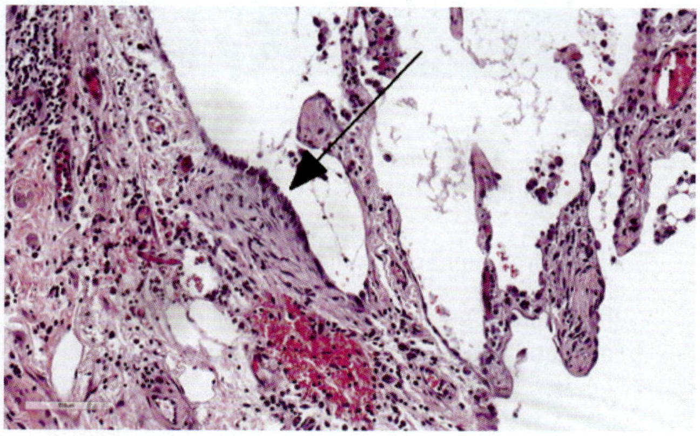

Figure 19.3 UIP: Note that foci of fibroblastic activity are interstitial/subepithelial (*arrow*).

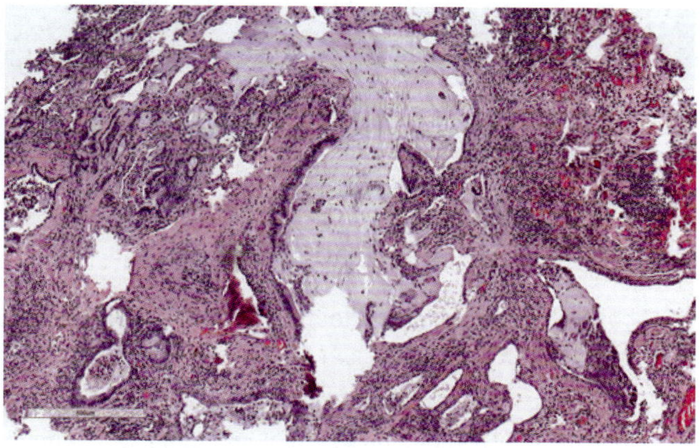

Figure 19.4 UIP: The disease promotes remodeling of the underlying lung architecture associated with peripheral honeycomb change, characterized by the presence of enlarged irregular spaces lined by bronchiolar type of epithelium containing a mucinous exudate with macrophages and inflammatory cells, which is surrounded by fibrosis and chronic inflammation.

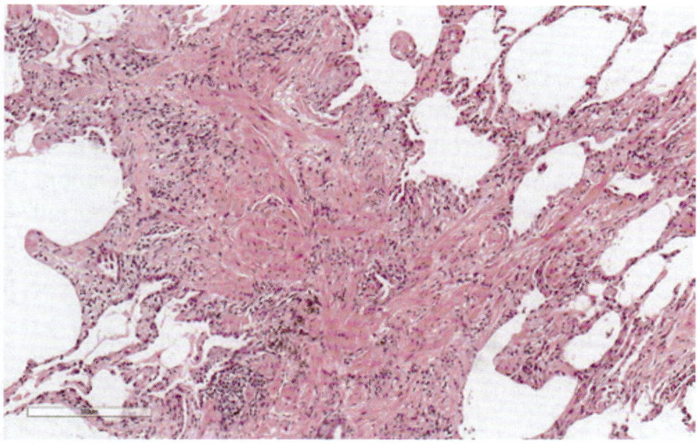

Figure 19.5 UIP: Smooth muscle hyperplasia is a common associated feature.

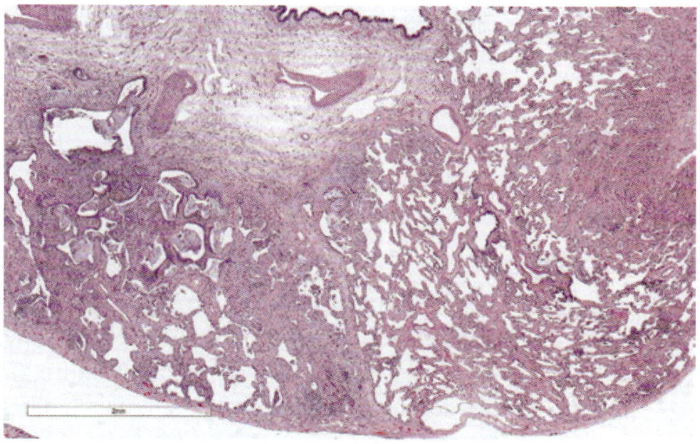

Figure 19.6 UIP: NSIP-like areas may be present (*right*) but the final diagnosis should be based on the histologically worst areas (*left*).

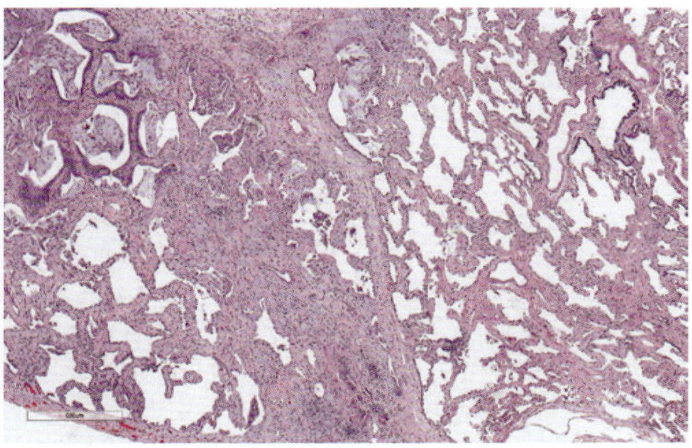

Figure 19.7 UIP: Higher magnification from Figure 19.6. Temporally heterogeneous process with interstitial areas of recent organization a.k.a. fibroblastic activity or fibroblastic foci (*center*).

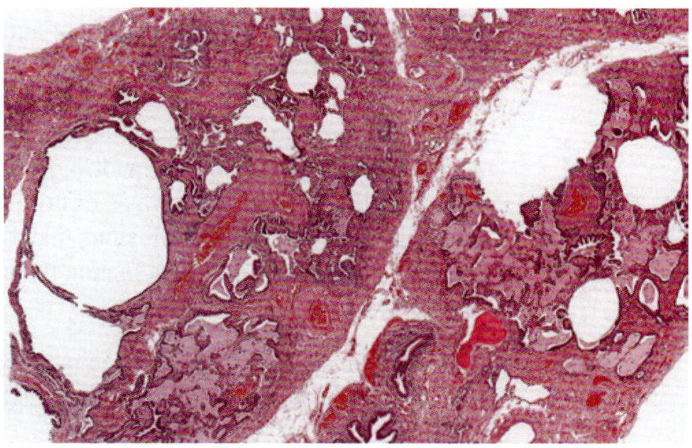

Figure 19.8 End-stage honeycomb lung: The morphology of end-stage honeycomb lung is similar to the honeycombing seen in UIP, but lacking the temporally heterogeneous pattern of interstitial fibrosis characteristic of UIP.

20 PLEUROPARENCHYMAL FIBROELASTOSIS VS. APICAL CAP

	Pleuroparenchymal Fibroelastosis (PPFE)	Apical Cap
Age	The age ranges from 32 to 65 y.	Seen predominantly in older population.
Location	It typically affects the upper lobes.	It usually affects the upper lobes bilaterally. It can also occur in the superior segments of the lower lobes.
Symptoms	Dyspnea on exertion and cough. Pneumothorax has been reported in some cases.	No clinical symptoms are present.
Signs	Chest high-resolution computed tomography (HRCT) characteristically demonstrates marked bilateral upper-lung (apical) visceral pleural thickening extending into the lung parenchyma with subpleural reticular abnormalities. Associated features include upper-lobe volume loss, traction bronchiectasis, and in rare cases, honeycombing.	Chest HRCT demonstrates bilateral upper-lung (apical) visceral pleural thickening extending into the lung parenchyma.
Etiology	Unknown.	It may represent the residua of infection, be secondary to chronic ischemia, or represent the residua of ruptured blebs and bulla or post radiation therapy. Apical scars/cap have also been reported in patients with ankylosing spondylitis.
Histology	There is marked thickening of the visceral pleura and remodeling of the subpleural parenchyma architecture by a homogeneous mixture of dense collagen deposition and elastic tissue (fibroelastotic scarring) *(Figs. 20.1 and 20.2)*. Rare fibroblastic activity may be present at the leading edge of the fibroelastotic scarring. Mild chronic inflammation is commonly seen in the fibroelastotic zones, but the uninvolved lung parenchyma is characteristically free of significant inflammation or scarring. The margins between the fibroelastotic zones and the underlying normal lung are typically sharply defined. The uninvolved lung usually shows minimal abnormalities, mainly involving small airways, such as bronchiolectasis or bronchiolar fibrosis. Extensive pleural adhesions may be present, most likely secondary to common history of pneumothorax.	The morphology of apical cap is virtually identical to PPFE, showing subpleural fibroelastotic scarring *(Figs. 20.1–20.4)*.
Special studies	Pentachrome special stain decorates dense collagen deposition (yellow) admixed with elastic fibers (black) *(Figs. 20.3 and 20.4)*.	Same as PPFE.
Prognosis	Variable. Progressive disease with eventual death within several years has been reported.	The major difference between apical cap and PPFE is that the patients with PPFE are symptomatic and the disease is progressive, while patients with apical cap are asymptomatic. Apical cap has no clinical significance and requires no treatment.

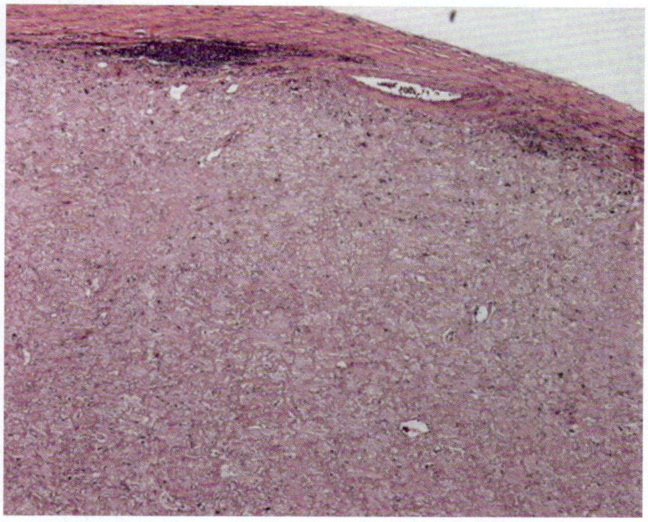

Figure 20.1 PPFE and apical cap: The morphology of apical cap is virtually identical to PPFE, showing thickening of the visceral pleura and remodeling of the subpleural parenchyma architecture by fibroelastotic scarring. Rare fibroblastic activity may be present at the leading edge of the fibroelastotic scarring in PPFE. The major difference between apical cap and PPFE is that the patients with PPFE are symptomatic and the disease is progressive.

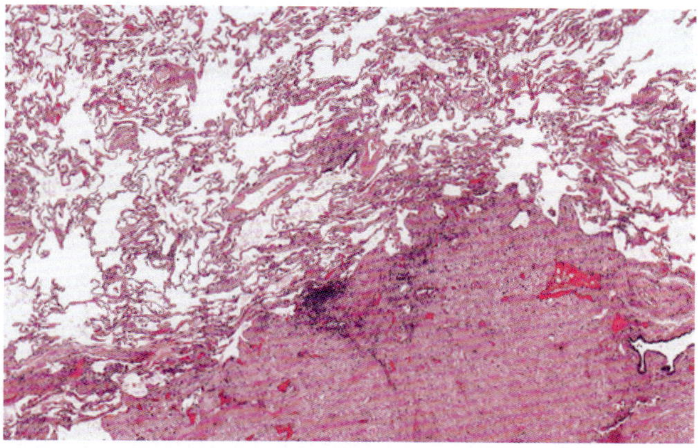

Figure 20.2 PPFE and apical cap: There is abrupt transition between fibroelastotic and normal lung parenchyma. The uninvolved lung parenchyma is characteristically free of significant inflammation or scarring. It affects characteristically upper lobes.

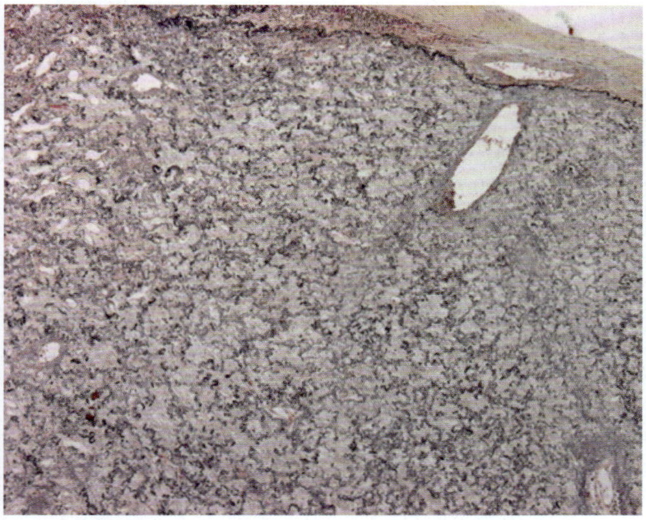

Figure 20.3 PPFE and apical cap: Pentachrome special stain demonstrates that the subpleural fibroelastotic scarring is composed of a homogeneous mixture of dense collagen deposition (*yellow*) and elastotic fibers (*black*).

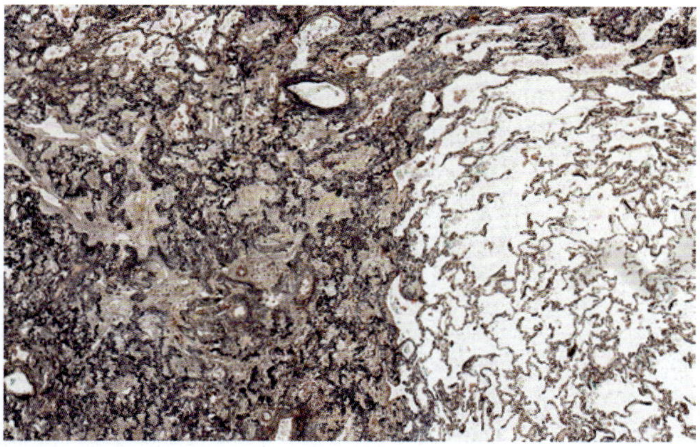

Figure 20.4 PPFE and apical cap: Pentachrome special stain demonstrates that fibroelastotic zones and underlying normal lung parenchyma have sharply defined margins.

21 CELLULAR NONSPECIFIC INTERSTITIAL PNEUMONIA VS. LYMPHOCYTIC INTERSTITIAL PNEUMONIA

	Cellular Nonspecific Interstitial Pneumonia (Cellular NSIP)	Lymphocytic Interstitial Pneumonia (LIP)
Age	The average age ranges from 40 to 57 y, but it can also be found in children. It is slightly more common in women.	The disease is most common in middle-aged women, but can be seen in both adults and children.
Location	It usually affects the lower lobes, spares subpleural spaces, and tends to be bilateral and symmetrical.	The disease can affect both lungs and typically involves the lung bases more severely. Cysts are often seen on HRCT of the chest.
Symptoms	The symptoms develop gradually. Shortness of breath, cough, fatigue, and weight loss are the most common symptoms. Fever and digital clubbing have been reported but are uncommon.	Cough, progressive dyspnea, and chest pain are common. Fever, fatigue, and weight loss are also commonly seen.
Signs	High-resolution computed tomography (HRCT) scans show bilateral lower-lobe predominant infiltrates and ground-glass attenuation. Pulmonary function tests usually reveal a restrictive pattern with decreased diffusing capacity of the lung carbon monoxide (DLCO).	HRCT scan shows ground-glass attenuation with thin-walled peribronchovascular cysts.
Etiology	Pulmonary manifestation of underlying autoimmune/collagen vascular disease (e.g., rheumatoid arthritis, Sjögren syndrome), immunodeficiency disorders (e.g., acquired immunodeficiency syndrome, common variable immunodeficiency), drug toxicity (e.g., Dilantin), or idiopathic.	The disease can be associated with viral infections such as Epstein–Barr virus (EBV) and human immunodeficiency virus (HIV) infections; be related to immune dysregulation in collagen vascular diseases, or may be the result of underlying immunodeficiency. Some consider LIP on the spectrum of lymphoproliferative disease and some cases have been reported to progress to mucosa-associated lymphoid tissue(MALT) and other forms of lymphoma.
Histology	There is diffuse and uniform interstitial (alveolar septal) expansion by mild-to-moderate chronic inflammatory cell infiltrate containing predominantly small mature lymphocytes and occasional plasma cells associated with alveolar pneumocyte prominence *(Figs. 21.1 and 21.2)*. The inflammatory process may be associated with scattered lymphoid aggregates (with or without germinal centers), chronic pleuritis, and increased perivascular collagen deposition, which although nonspecific, are features commonly associated with autoimmune disorder/collagen vascular disease manifesting in the lung. Scattered plugs of organizing pneumonia may be present within airspaces *(Fig. 21.3)*. Unlike many forms of interstitial lung disease that may be accentuated under the pleura, NSIP may show subpleural sparing *(Fig. 21.4)*.	There is marked and diffuse alveolar septal expansion by cellular infiltrate composed of small mature lymphocytes and variable amount of plasma cells and histiocytes. The infiltrate appears to be more prominent along the pleura, bronchovascular bundles and interlobular septa, following a lymphatic distribution. Lymphoid hyperplasia with germinal centers is frequently present *(Figs. 21.5–21.7)*. Small clusters of epithelioid histiocytes and loosely arranged poorly formed nonnecrotizing granulomas, often containing multinucleated giant cells, are commonly seen.

	Cellular Nonspecific Interstitial Pneumonia (Cellular NSIP)	Lymphocytic Interstitial Pneumonia (LIP)
Special studies	None suggested.	Epstein-Barr encoding region (EBER) in situ hybridization to exclude EBV associated infection. Immunoperoxidase stains show a mixture of B (CD20 positive) and T (CD 3 positive) cells, with the B cells present in germinal centers and T cells in intervening areas. IgH gene rearrangements can be helpful in excluding the possibility of lymphoma.
Prognosis	The prognosis of cellular NSIP is generally good. The 5-y survival rate for patients with cellular NSIP is close to 100%, with good response to corticosteroids therapy.	The prognosis is highly variable, with some patients spontaneously resolving and others resolving following immunosuppressive agents. A small percentage (5%) will progress to lymphoma.

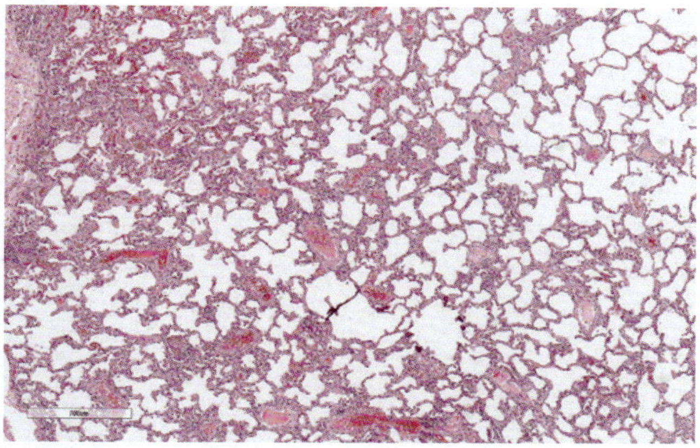

Figure 21.1 Cellular NSIP: A low-power view of cellular NSIP showing the diffuse and uniform expansion of the alveolar septa by chronic inflammatory cell infiltrate.

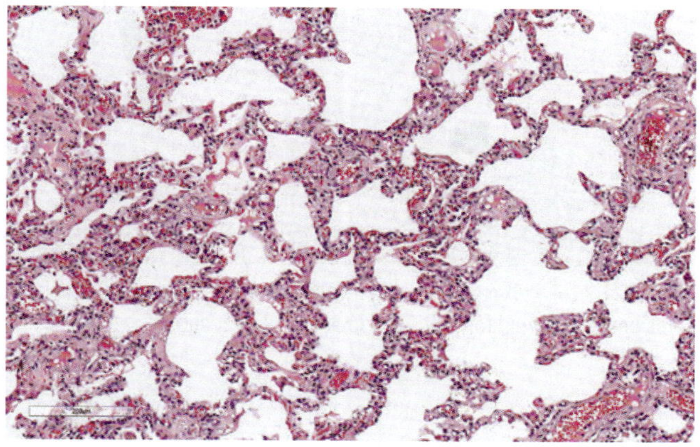

Figure 21.2 Cellular NSIP: There is mild uniform thickening of the alveolar septa by chronic inflammatory cells composed predominantly of small mature lymphocytes without significant fibrosis.

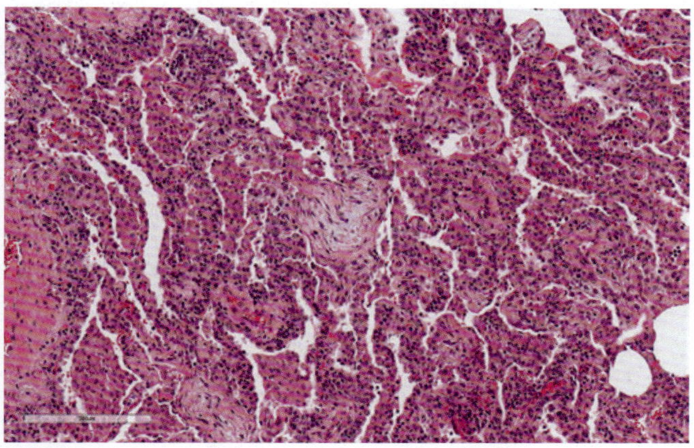

Figure 21.3 Cellular NSIP: In the center of the field there is a polypoid plug of loose myxoid fibroblastic tissue within an airspace (organizing pneumonia), which may be associated with cellular NSIP.

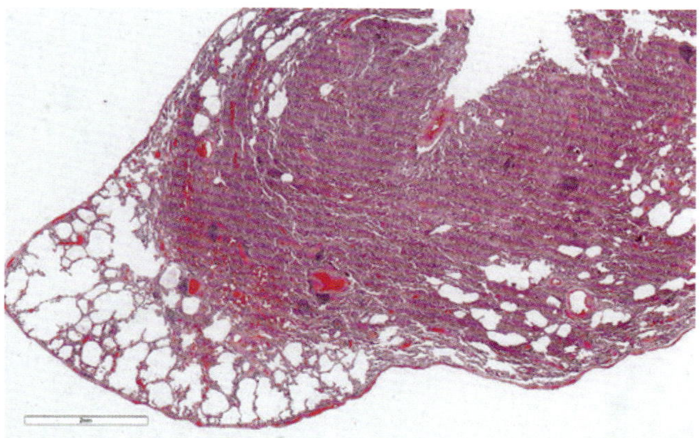

Figure 21.4 Cellular NSIP: Both radiographic and pathologic evidences of subpleural sparing are frequently seen.

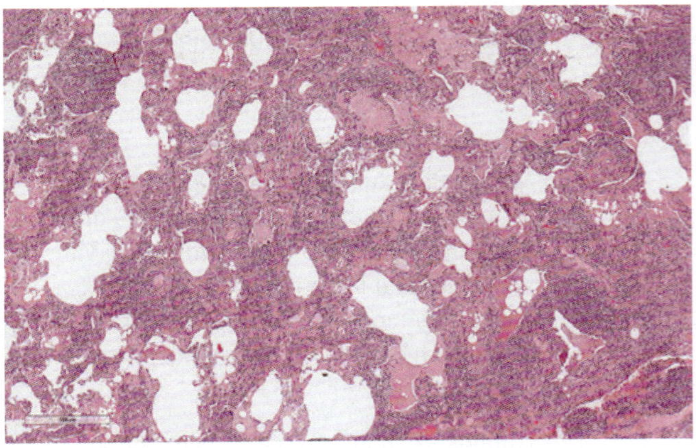

Figure 21.5 LIP: There is marked and diffuse alveolar septal expansion by lymphocytic inflammatory cell infiltrate.

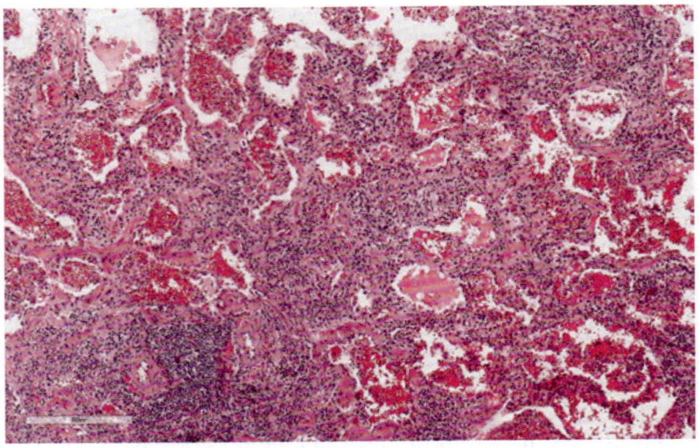

Figure 21.6 LIP: A higher power view with diffuse alveolar septal expansion by lymphocytic inflammatory cell infiltrate. Recent hemorrhage is present in this case and represents biopsy related hemorrhage.

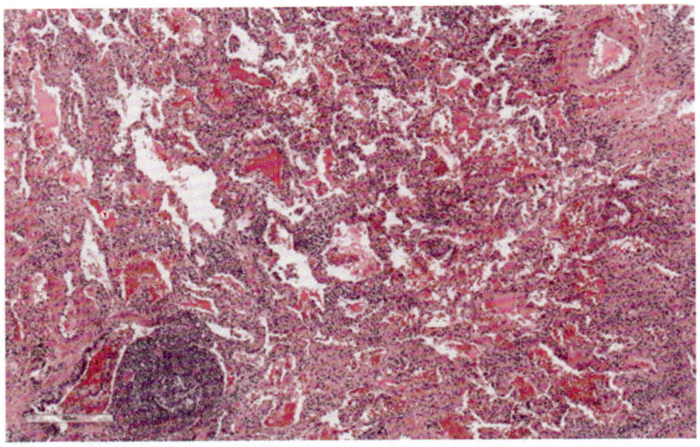

Figure 21.7 LIP: A case showing alveolar septal expansion by lymphocytes and a lymphoid follicle in the lower left lower corner.

22 LYMPHOCYTIC INTERSTITIAL PNEUMONIA VS. MALT LYMPHOMA

	Lymphocytic Interstitial Pneumonia (LIP)	MALT Lymphoma
Age	The disease is most common in middle-aged women, but can be seen in both adults and children.	Extranodal marginal zone lymphoma of mucosa-associated lymphoid tissue (MALT lymphoma) is the most common form of lymphoma involving the lung. It usually affects patients in their 60s with a slight female predominance.
Location	The disease can affect both lungs and typically involves the lung bases more severely. Cysts are often seen on high-resolution computed tomography (HRCT) of the chest.	Most pulmonary MALT lymphomas present bronchovascular consolidative masses and may also follow a lymphatic distribution. There is no clear lobar preference for disease.
Symptoms	Cough, progressive dyspnea, and chest pain are common. Fever, fatigue, and weight loss are also commonly seen.	Patients may be entirely asymptomatic or may present with B-symptoms such as fever, night sweats, and weight loss. Previous or synchronous MALT lymphomas at other extranodal sites are not uncommon.
Signs	HRCT scan shows ground-glass attenuation with thin-walled peribronchovascular cysts.	CT scan typically shows consolidating masses along the bronchovascular bundle. Many patients will also show splenomegaly and mediastinal lymphadenopathy.
Etiology	The disease can be associated with viral infections such as Epstein–Barr virus (EBV) and human immunodeficiency virus (HIV) infections; be related to immune dysregulation in collagen vascular diseases, or may be the result of underlying immunodeficiency. Some consider LIP on the spectrum of lymphoproliferative disease, and some cases have been reported to progress to MALT and other forms of lymphoma.	Lymphomas may be idiopathic, associated with collagen vascular diseases such as Sjögren syndrome, or may be immunodeficiency related (such as common variable immunodeficiency [CVID], HIV, or organ transplant). For lymphomas associated with immunodeficiency, EBER in situ hybridization may be helpful.

	Lymphocytic Interstitial Pneumonia (LIP)	MALT Lymphoma
Histology	The alveolar septa show widespread regions of alveolar septal expansion by cellular infiltrate composed of small mature lymphocytes and variable amount of plasma cells and histiocytes. The infiltrate may be more prominent along the pleura, bronchovascular bundles and interlobular and alveolar septa, following a lymphatic distribution. Lymphoid hyperplasia with germinal centers is frequently present *(Figs. 22.1–22.4)*. Small clusters of epithelioid histiocytes and loosely arranged poorly formed nonnecrotizing granulomas, often containing multinucleated giant cells, are commonly seen. Unlike a malignant lymphoproliferative process, LIP preserves the underlying structures of the lung and does not destroy epithelial structures.	In pulmonary MALT lymphoma, also known as bronchial-associated lymphoid tissue (BALT) lymphoma, there is diffuse infiltrate of lymphocytes with modest atypia associated with lymphoid follicles with germinal centers that track along lymphatics and cause effacement of the underlying lung parenchyma architecture. The malignant lymphocytes cause massive expansion of the alveolar septa and may form mass-like lesions and nodules *(Figs. 22.5 and 22.6)*. Infiltration of bronchial or bronchiolar wall, and alveolar epithelium (lymphoepithelial lesion) is characteristic, although not pathognomonic, since this lesion can also be seen in nonneoplastic pulmonary lymphoid infiltrates *(Figs. 22.7 and 22.8)*. Vascular infiltration and granuloma formation are not uncommon. It may also be associated with crystal-storing histiocytosis. MALT lymphomas are composed of monoclonal B cell population that show aberrant coexpression of CD20 and Bcl-2, associated with variable amount of reactive T cells (CD3 positive) in the background. Clonality of the B-cells may be inferred from IgH gene rearrangement studies; however, these may be rarely positive in patients responding to infections (particularly viral infections). Lack of Cyclin D1 expression help to exclude mantle cell lymphoma; and lack of CD10 and Bcl-6 expression help to exclude follicular lymphoma.
Special studies	Epstein-Barr virus encoded region (EBER) in situ hybridization to exclude EBV associated infection. Immunoperoxidase stains show a mixture of B (CD20 positive) and T (CD3 positive) cells, with the B cells present in germinal centers and T cells in intervening areas. IgH gene rearrangements can be helpful in excluding the possibility of lymphoma.	CD3, CD20, Bcl-2, CD10, EBER, and IgH gene rearrangements. Cytokeratin stains highlight lymphoepithelial lesions.
Prognosis	The prognosis is highly variable, with some patients spontaneously resolving and others resolving following immunosuppressive agents. A small percentage (5%) will progress to lymphoma.	The prognosis of stage I disease is good with up to 80% 5-y survival.

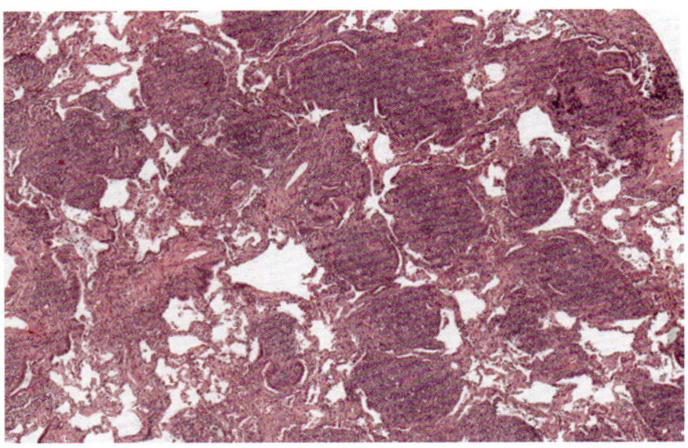

Figure 22.1 LIP: Bland lymphocytes expand the alveolar septa but may also form frequent lymphoid aggregates, some with prominent germinal centers.

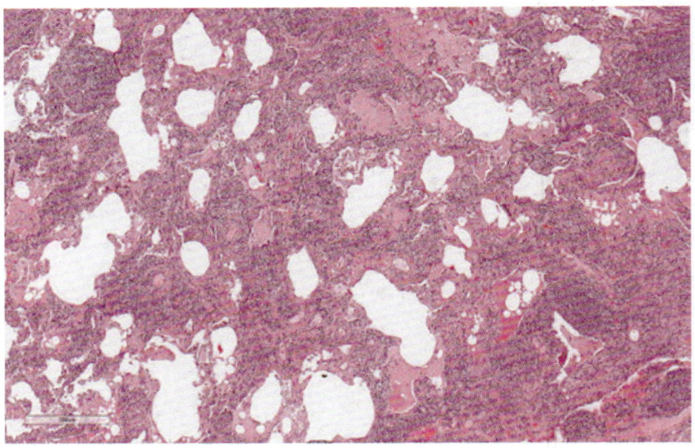

Figure 22.2 LIP: Another example showing marked diffuse alveolar septal expansion by lymphocytic inflammation.

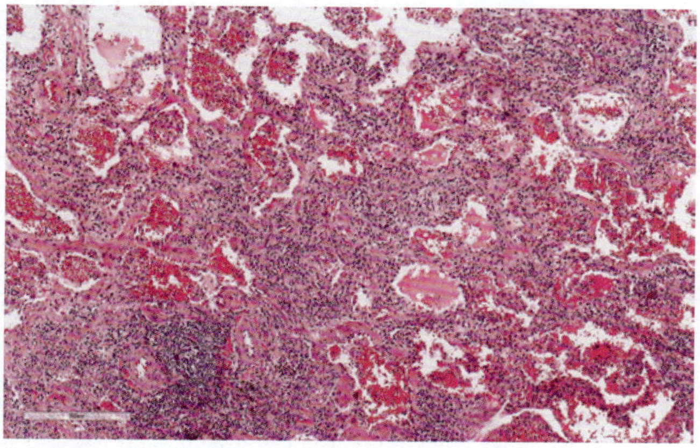

Figure 22.3 LIP: A higher-power view showing alveolar septal expansion by lymphocytes. Recent hemorrhage is present in this case and represents biopsy related hemorrhage.

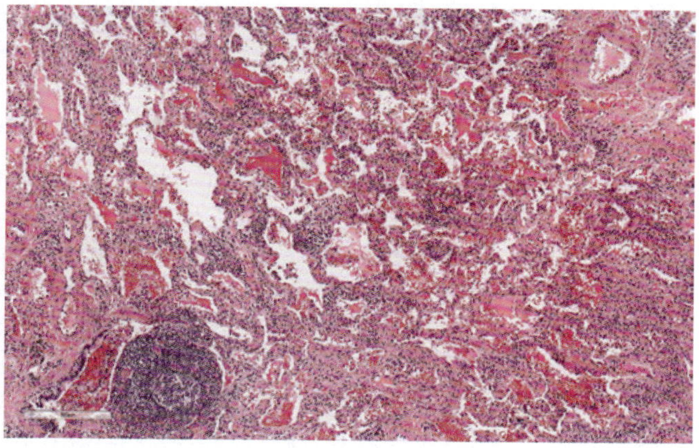

Figure 22.4 LIP: An example showing alveolar septal expansion by lymphocytes and a lymphoid follicle in the lower left-hand corner.

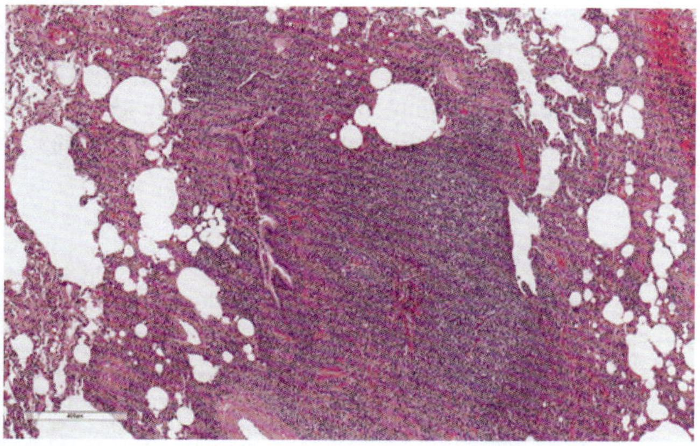

Figure 22.5 MALT lymphoma: An example showing mass-like region of lymphocytic infiltrate that effaces the normal architecture of the lung and contains small germinal centers.

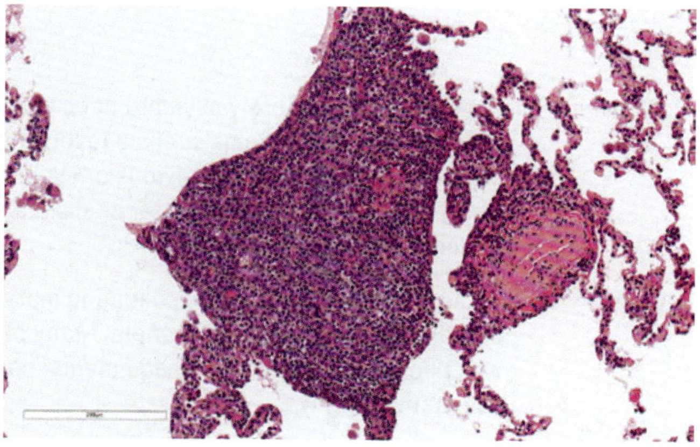

Figure 22.6 MALT lymphoma: A high-power view of malignant lymphocytes. Note that the cells appear small and it would be difficult to classify this case as lymphoma without additional studies such as molecular IgH gene rearrangement studies.

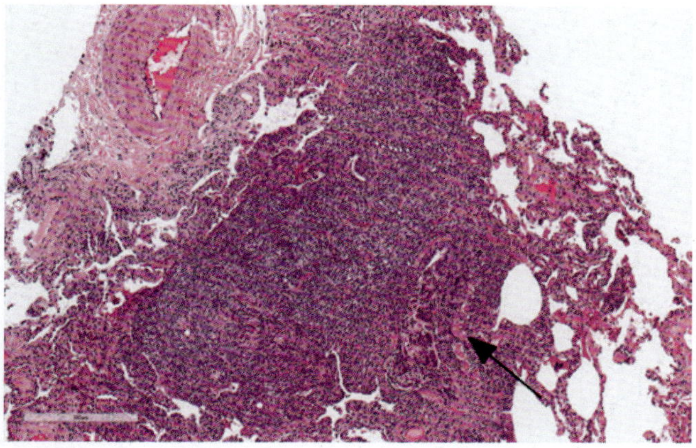

Figure 22.7 MALT lymphoma: Another example of MALT lymphoma showing infiltration and destruction of the epithelium and smooth muscle of the bronchiole (*arrow*).

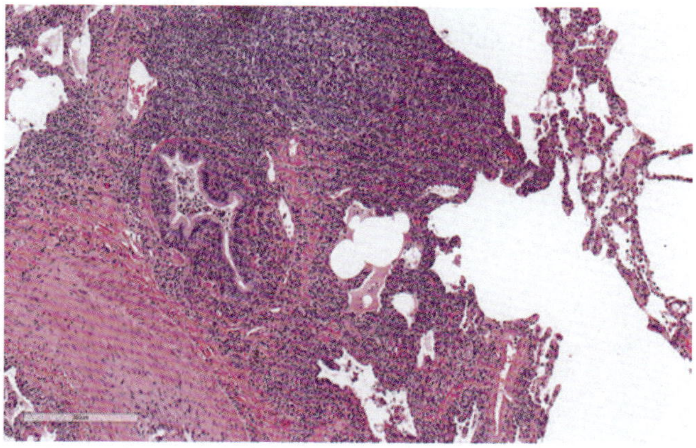

Figure 22.8 MALT lymphoma: The lymphocytes appear small, and there is a lymphoid follicle at the upper portion of the figure; however, the infiltration of the wall of the bronchiole and splaying of the collagen fibers of the bronchiolar adventitia suggest that this case is lymphoma.

23 MALT LYMPHOMA VS. LYMPHANGITIC CARCINOMA

	MALT Lymphoma	Lymphangitic Carcinoma
Age	Extranodal marginal zone lymphoma of mucosa-associated lymphoid tissue (MALT lymphoma) is the most common form of lymphoma involving the lung. It usually affects patients in their 60s with a slight female predominance.	Although lymphangitic spread of carcinoma may occur in any age group, the majority of these cases will be in adults with primary adenocarcinoma of the breast, lung, colon, stomach, prostate, cervix, or thyroid.
Location	Most pulmonary MALT lymphomas present bronchovascular consolidative masses and may also follow a lymphatic distribution. There is no clear lobar preference for disease.	Most cases show bilateral lung involvement, although some pulmonary primary carcinomas may show unilateral lymphangitic spread. Both the central lymphatic channels running along the bronchi/artery and the peripheral lymphatic channels in the pleura and intralobular septa may be involved with tumor.
Symptoms	Patients may be entirely asymptomatic or may present with B-symptoms such as fever, night sweats, and weight loss. Previous or synchronous MALT lymphomas at other extranodal sites are not uncommon.	In addition to symptoms from the primary tumor, many patients with lymphangitic carcinoma have dyspnea, cough, or hemoptysis.
Signs	CT scans typically show consolidating masses along the bronchovascular bundle. Many patients will also show splenomegaly and mediastinal lymphadenopathy.	CT scans typically show irregular thickened intralobular septa, bronchovascular thickening, and prominent centrilobular bundles. Lymphadenopathy and pleural effusions are frequently present.
Etiology	Lymphomas may be idiopathic, associated with collagen vascular diseases such as Sjögren syndrome, or may be immunodeficiency related (e.g., common variable immunodeficiency [CVID], HIV, or organ transplant). For lymphomas associated with immunodeficiency, Epstein–Barr virus encoding region (EBER) in situ hybridization may be helpful.	Diffuse metastasis of carcinoma through the lymphatic channels.

	MALT Lymphoma	**Lymphangitic Carcinoma**
Histology	In pulmonary MALT lymphoma, also known as bronchial-associated lymphoid tissue (BALT) lymphoma, there is diffuse infiltrate of lymphocytes with modest atypia associated with lymphoid follicles with germinal centers that track along lymphatics and cause effacement of the underlying lung parenchyma architecture. The malignant lymphocytes may form mass-like lesions and nodules *(Figs. 23-1 and 23-2)*. Infiltration of bronchial or bronchiolar wall, and alveolar epithelium (lymphoepithelial lesion) is characteristic, although not pathognomonic, since this lesion can also be seen in non-neoplastic pulmonary lymphoid infiltrates *(Figs. 23-3 and 23-4)*. Vascular infiltration and granuloma formation are not uncommon. It may also be associated with crystal-storing histiocytosis. MALT lymphomas are composed of monoclonal B cell population that show aberrant coexpression of CD20 and Bcl-2, associated with variable amount of reactive T cells (CD3 positive) in the background. Clonality of the B-cells may be inferred from IgH gene rearrangement studies; however, these may be rarely positive in patients responding to infections (particularly viral infections). Lack of Cyclin D1 expression help to exclude mantle cell lymphoma and lack of CD10 and Bcl-6 expression help to exclude follicular lymphoma.	Clusters of malignant epithelial cells may be found in the small lymphatic channels that are present in the adventitia of bronchi, in bronchioles, in arteries, within the interlobular septa, and in the lymphatic channels of the pleura *(Fig. 23.5)*.
Special studies	CD3, CD20, Bcl-2, CD10, EBER and IgH gene rearrangements. Cytokeratin stains highlight lymphoepithelial lesions.	In cases of patients with an unknown or undiscovered primary site of origin, the combination of pancytokeratin *(Fig. 23-6)* and the lymphatic marker D2-40 *(Fig. 23-7)* is useful in identifying lymphangitic tumor. For patients with a known primary tumor, lineage-specific immunostains may also be used; however, not all metastases continue to express the markers expressed within the primary tumor *(Fig. 23-8)*.
Prognosis	The prognosis of stage I disease is good, with up to 80% 5-y survival.	The prognosis is very poor with a mean survival of 3 mo.

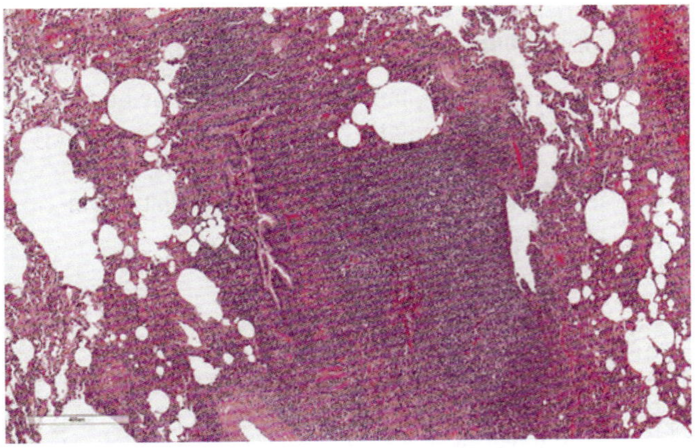

Figure 23.1 MALT lymphoma: An example of a pulmonary MALT lymphoma with mass-like region of lymphocytic infiltrate that effaces the normal architecture of the lung and contains small germinal centers.

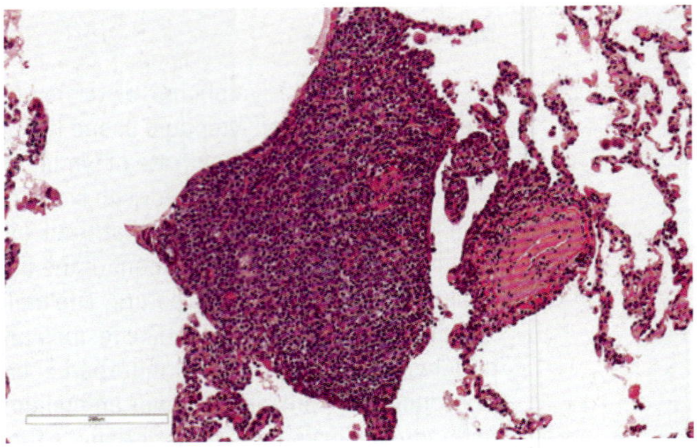

Figure 23.2 MALT lymphoma: A high-power view of malignant lymphocytes. Note that the cells appear small and it would be difficult to classify this case as lymphoma without additional studies such as molecular IgH gene rearrangement studies.

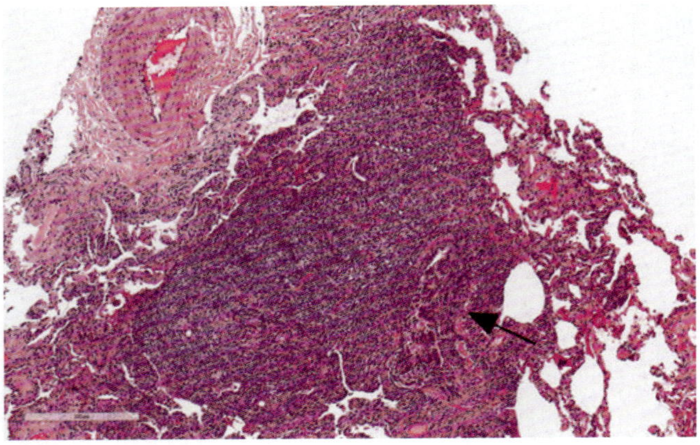

Figure 23.3 MALT lymphoma: Another example of MALT lymphoma showing infiltration and destruction of the epithelium and smooth muscle of the bronchiole (*arrow*).

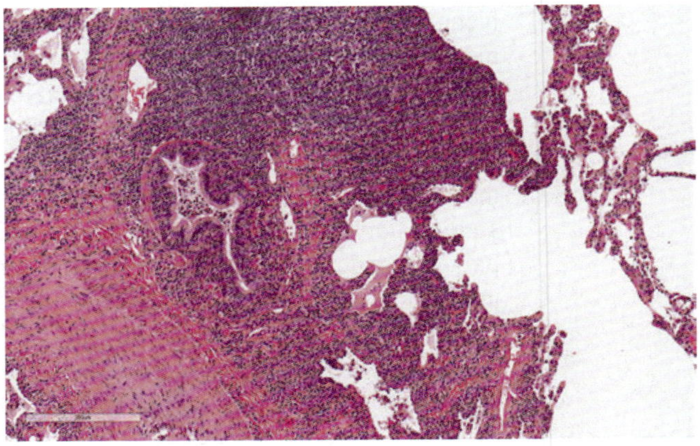

Figure 23.4 MALT lymphoma: The lymphocytes appear small, and there is a lymphoid follicle at the upper portion of the figure; however, the infiltration of the wall of the bronchiole and splaying of the collagen fibers of the bronchiolar adventitia suggest that this case is lymphoma.

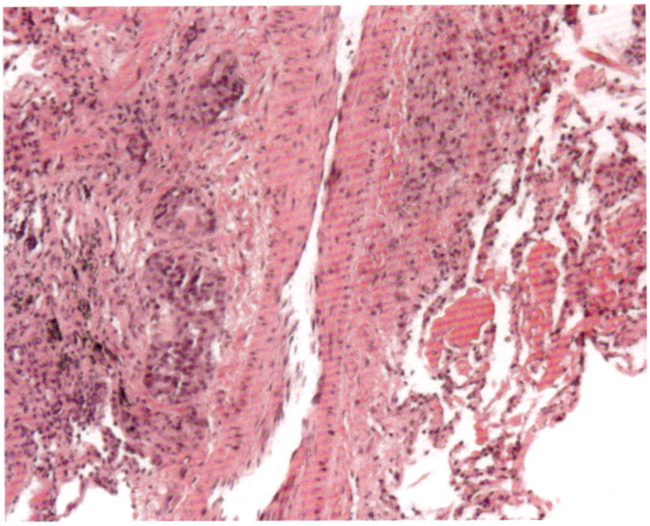

Figure 23.5 Lymphangitic carcinoma: To the left of the longitudinal blood vessel, there are clusters of epithelial cells sitting within distended perivascular lymphatic channels.

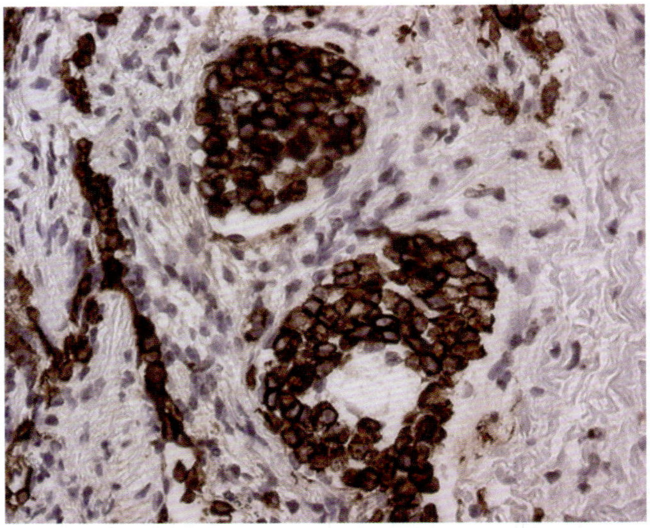

Figure 23.6 Lymphangitic carcinoma: Pancytokeratin stain (high power view of Figure 23.5) shows that the cell clusters seen within lymphatic channels are epithelial, confirming the diagnosis of lymphangitic spread of a carcinoma.

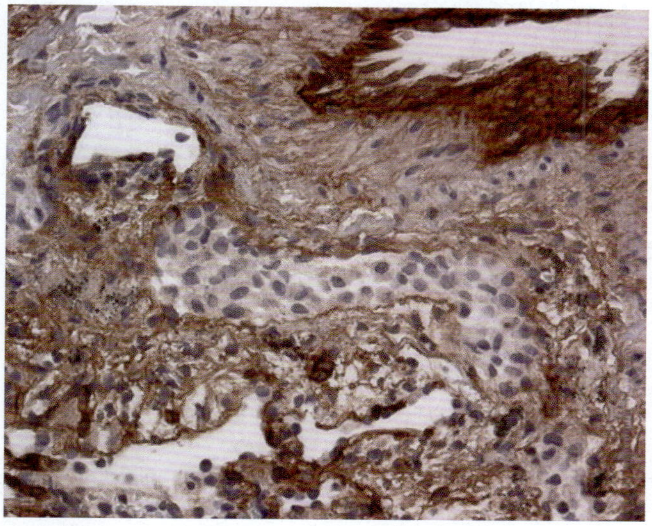

Figure 23.7 Lymphangitic carcinoma: In this example of lymphangitic carcinoma, vascular markers (CD31, CD34) or lymphatic-specific markers (D2-40) show that the previously shown (Fig 23.5 and 23.6) epithelial cells are sitting within endothelial-lined vessels and are not a retraction artifact of fixation.

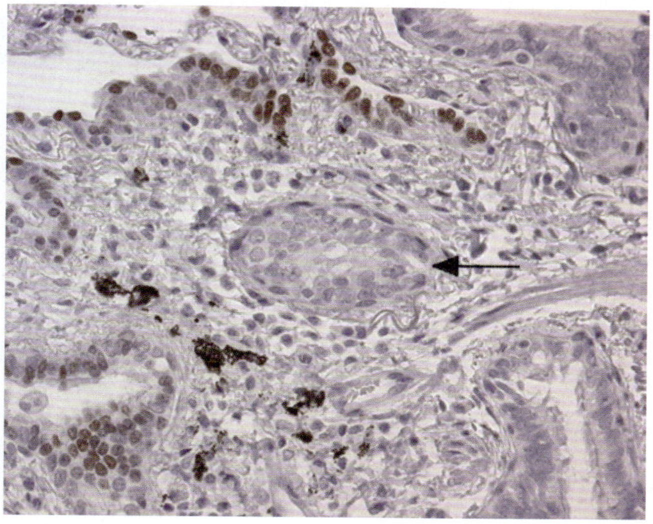

Figure 23.8 Lymphangitic carcinoma: A negative TTF-1 immunoexpression shows that the malignant cells (*arrow*), seen in this example of a lymphangitic carcinoma are likely not a primary adenocarcinoma of the lung. The normal pulmonary pneumocytes serve as a positive control.

24 NONSPECIFIC INTERSTITIAL PNEUMONIA VS. CHRONIC HYPERSENSITIVITY PNEUMONIA

	Nonspecific Interstitial Pneumonia (NSIP)	Chronic Hypersensitivity Pneumonia (HP)
Age	The average age ranges from 40 to 57 y, but it can also be found in children. It is slightly more common in women.	There is no gender or age predilection, although it is uncommon in children.
Location	It usually affects the lower lobes, spares subpleural zones, and tends to be bilateral and symmetrical.	It is usually a predominantly centrilobular/bronchiolocentric process involving the middle and upper lung zones.
Symptoms	The symptoms develop gradually. Shortness of breath, cough, fatigue, and weight loss are the most common symptoms. Fever and digital clubbing have been reported but are uncommon.	Insidious onset of dyspnea, often associated with dry cough, fatigue, and malaise.
Signs	High-resolution computed tomography (HRCT) scans show subpleural sparing, bilateral lower lobe predominant infiltrates, and ground glass attenuation. Pulmonary function tests usually reveal a restrictive pattern with decreased diffusing capacity of the lung carbon monoxide (DLCO).	Chest HRCT demonstrates mid-to-upper lobe predominant linear interstitial opacities and small nodules associated with traction bronchiectasis and honeycomb areas. If small airway obstruction is present, air trapping can be seen on expiratory HRCT manifesting as a mosaic attenuation pattern. Bronchoalveolar lavage marked lymphocytosis, although nonspecific, can further support the diagnosis of chronic HP.
Etiology	Pulmonary manifestation of underlying autoimmune/collagen vascular disease (e.g., rheumatoid arthritis, Sjögren syndrome), immunodeficiency disorders (e.g., acquired immunodeficiency syndrome, common variable immunodeficiency), drug toxicity (e.g., Dilantin), or idiopathic.	HP represents a combination of immune complex–mediated (type III) and T-cell–mediated, delayed (type IV) hypersensitivity reactions. Exposure to inhaled environmental antigens (e.g., mold, bacteria, animal proteins, avian proteins) or other allergen particles of small size (5 μm or smaller) triggers the disease. Sometimes the causal agent cannot be identified. The disease, which is also called extrinsic allergic alveolitis (EAA), may also be known by a great variety of names depending on the causal agent (farmer's lung, pigeon breeder's disease, ventilator pneumonitis). However, regardless of the pathologic responsible agent, the clinical presentation and pathologic findings are similar.

	Nonspecific Interstitial Pneumonia (NSIP)	Chronic Hypersensitivity Pneumonia (HP)
Histology	*Cellular variant:* There is diffuse and uniform interstitial (alveolar septal) expansion by mild-to-moderate chronic inflammatory cell infiltrate containing predominantly small mature lymphocytes and occasional plasma cells associated with alveolar pneumocyte prominence. The inflammatory process may be associated with lymphoid aggregates (with or without germinal centers), chronic pleuritis, and increase in perivascular collagen deposition, which although nonspecific, are features commonly associated with autoimmune disorder/collagen vascular disease manifesting in the lung *(Figs. 24.1–24.4)*. *Fibrosing variant:* There is diffuse and uniform interstitial expansion by dense collagen deposition (fibrosis), few fibroblasts, little amount of inflammation, and alveolar pneumocyte prominence *(Figs. 24.5–24.8)*. *Mixed cellular and fibrosing variant:* There is diffuse and uniform interstitial expansion by similar amount of inflammation and fibrosis. In all three forms of NSIP, the underlying lung architecture is preserved, with no honeycomb change. Fibroblastic foci may be present, but they are usually inconspicuous and never numerous. Few plugs of organizing pneumonia and variable amounts of peribronchiolar metaplasia may be present. Increased number of macrophages are frequently found within the alveolar spaces.	Chronic cellular interstitial pneumonia (typically showing bronchiolocentric accentuation), cellular chronic bronchiolitis, and small, predominantly interstitial, nonnecrotizing, poorly formed granulomas composed of loose clusters of epithelioid histiocytes, multinucleated giant cells, and lymphocytes *(Figs. 24.9–24.11)*. Peribronchiolar metaplasia, peribronchiolar fibrosis, and patchy foci of organizing pneumonia are frequently present *(Figs. 24.12 and 24.13)*. Constrictive bronchiolitis may occur, and foamy macrophages related to bronchiolar obstruction may be seen within the nearby alveolar spaces. In the advanced phase of chronic HP, interstitial scarring/fibrosis and honeycomb change may become prominent resembling UIP.
Special studies	None suggested.	Gomori methenamine silver (GMS) and acid-fast bacilli (AFB), special stains and tissue cultures should be performed to exclude infection.
Prognosis	The prognosis of cellular NSIP is better than that of fibrosing NSIP. The 5-y survival rate for patients with cellular NSIP is close to 100%, with good response to corticosteroids therapy. The 5- and 10-y survival rates for patients with fibrosing NSIP are 90% and 35%, respectively.	The prognosis is worse when associated with interstitial scarring. Some patients respond to removal of antigen exposure and corticosteroid therapy, but some cases become self-sustained and progress to fibrotic phase despite removal from the antigen exposure. How much fibrosis is required to move into the poor outcome group is unclear. Overall, once dense fibrosis develops with honeycomb change, the disease is irreversible.

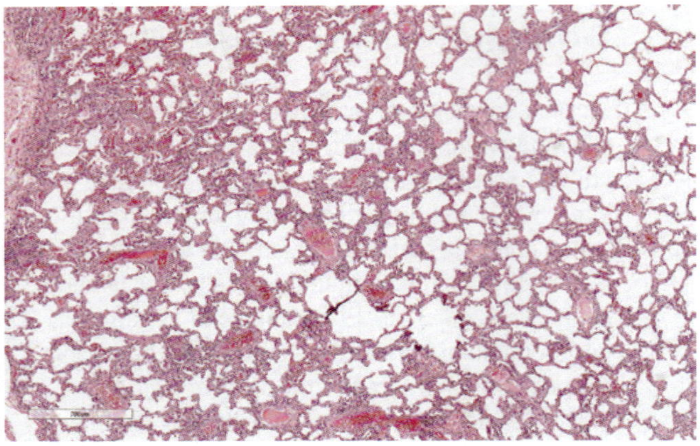

Figure 24.1 Cellular NSIP (low power): There is diffuse and uniform interstitial (alveolar septal) expansion.

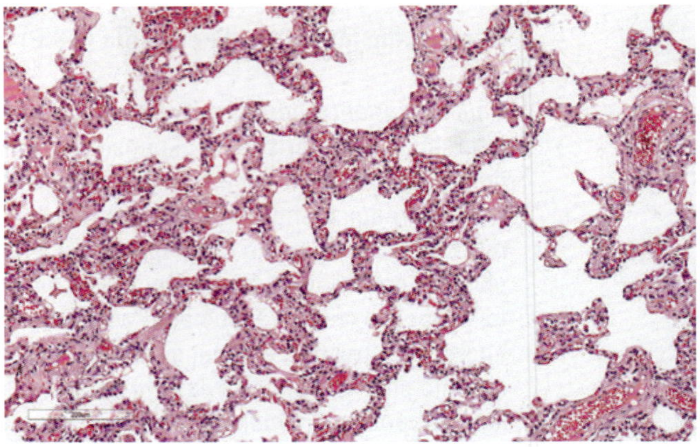

Figure 24.2 Cellular NSIP (high power view of Figure 24.1): The alveolar septal expansion is composed of mild-to-moderate inflammatory cell infiltrate containing predominantly small mature lymphocytes.

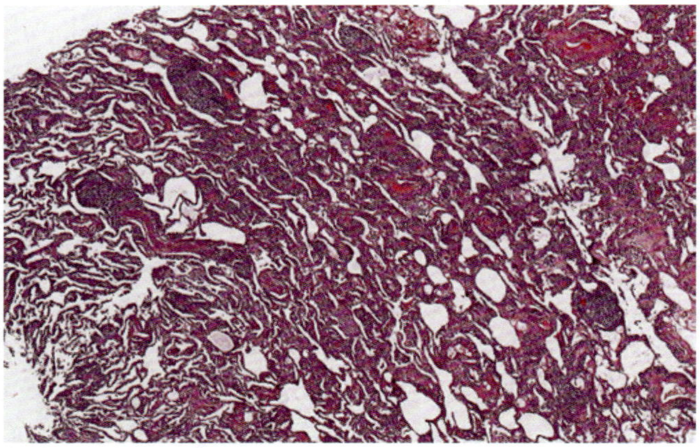

Figure 24.3 Cellular NSIP (low power): Cellular NSIP secondary to rheumatoid arthritis in a 62-year-old woman. Note diffuse and uniform alveolar septal cellular expansion associated with frequent lymphoid follicles.

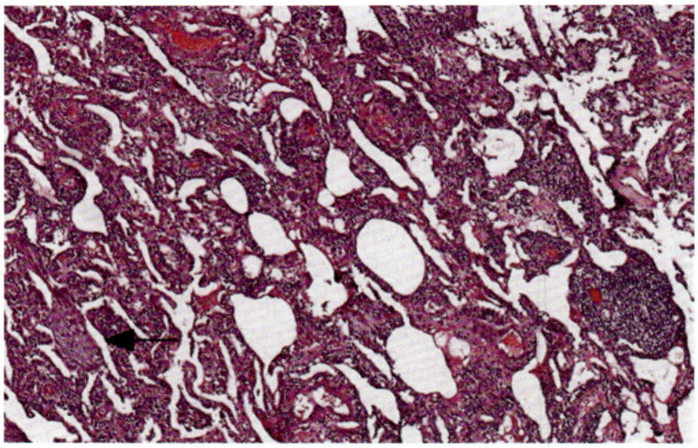

Figure 24.4 Cellular NSIP (high power of Figure 24.3): The cellular alveolar septal expansion is composed predominantly of lymphocytic inflammatory cell infiltrate. Note the rare plug of organizing pneumonia (*arrow*).

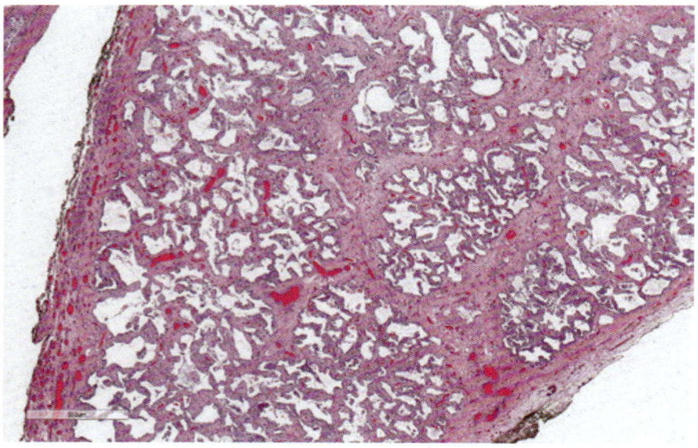

Figure 24.5 Fibrotic NSIP (low power): There is diffuse and uniform interstitial (alveolar septal) expansion by eosinophilic material.

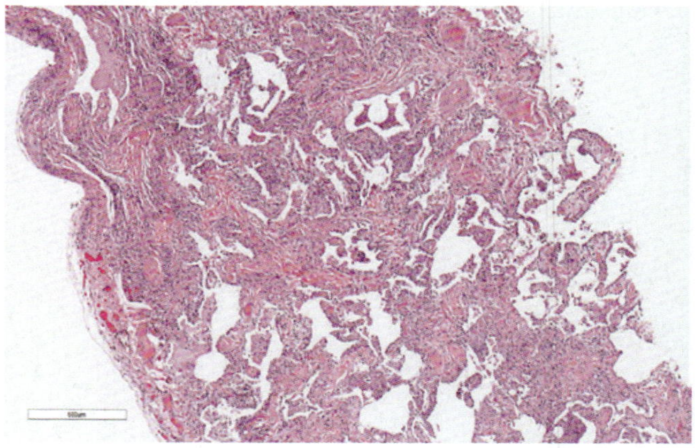

Figure 24.6 Fibrotic NSIP (high power): The interstitial eosinophilic material is composed of dense collagen deposition (fibrosis) and little inflammation.

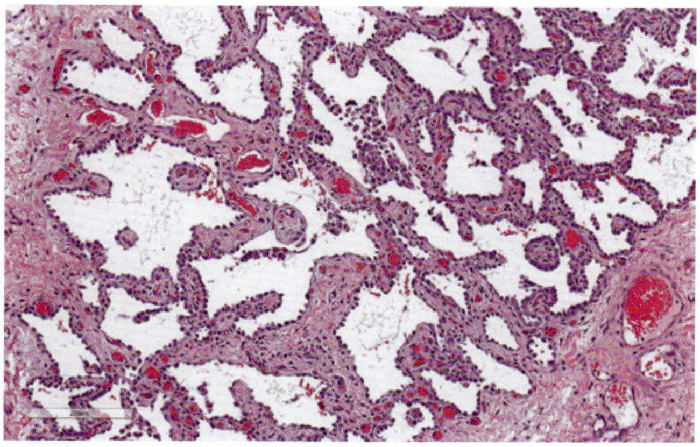

Figure 24.7 Fibrotic NSIP (low power): The alveolar septal scarring is frequently associated with alveolar pneumocyte prominence. Macrophages are frequently found within the alveolar spaces.

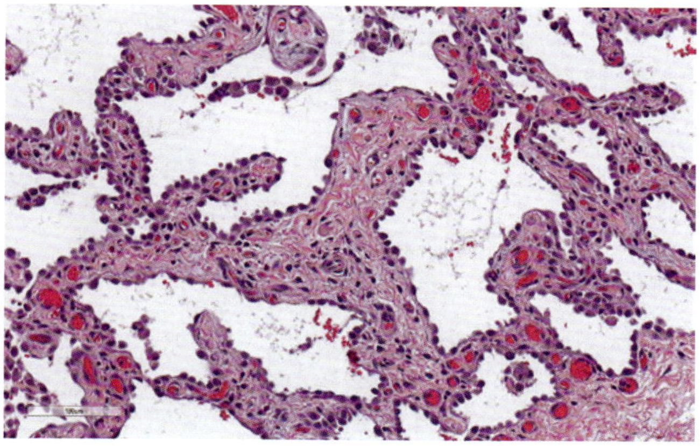

Figure 24.8 Fibrotic NSIP (high power view of Figure 24.7): Note alveolar pneumocyte prominence.

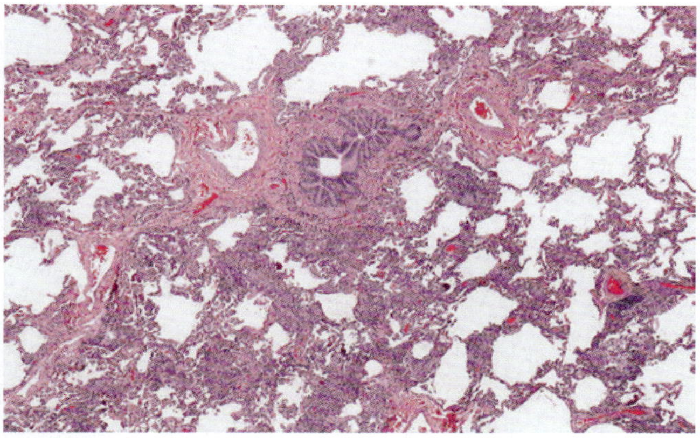

Figure 24.9 HP (low-power): There is diffuse expansion of the alveolar septa by chronic inflammatory cell infiltrate, which is more pronounced in peribronchiolar zones.

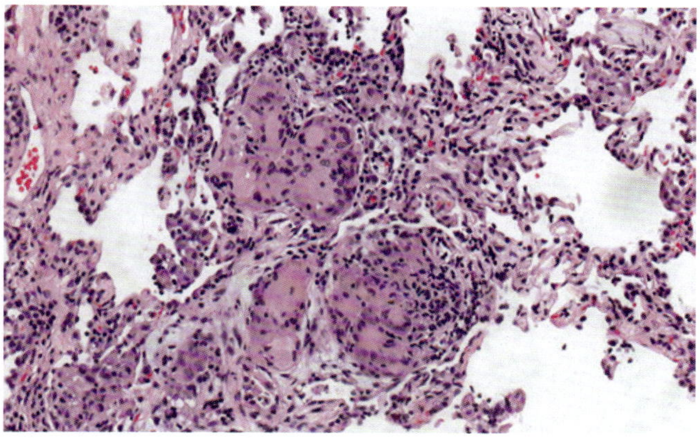

Figure 24.10 HP (high-power): The granulomas present in HP are not typically seen in alveolar spaces but in the interstitium (alveolar septa). They are poorly formed and may be composed of multinucleated giant cells and lymphocytes.

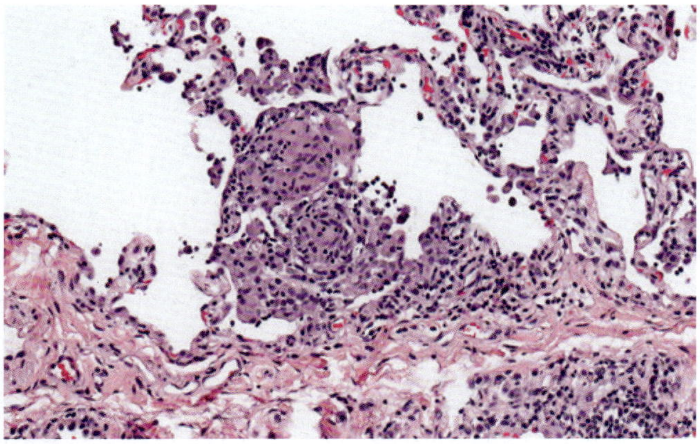

Figure 24.11 HP (high-power): Poorly formed nonnecrotizing granulomas composed of loosely arranged epithelioid histiocytes.

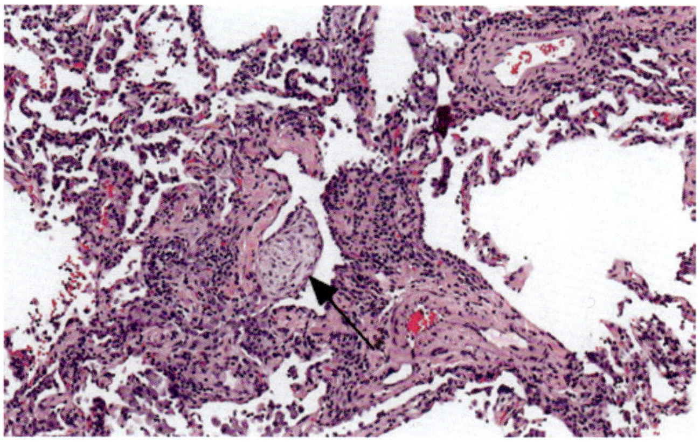

Figure 24.12 HP: Few foci of organizing pneumonia may be present (*arrow*), which do not represent the main pattern of injury in HP.

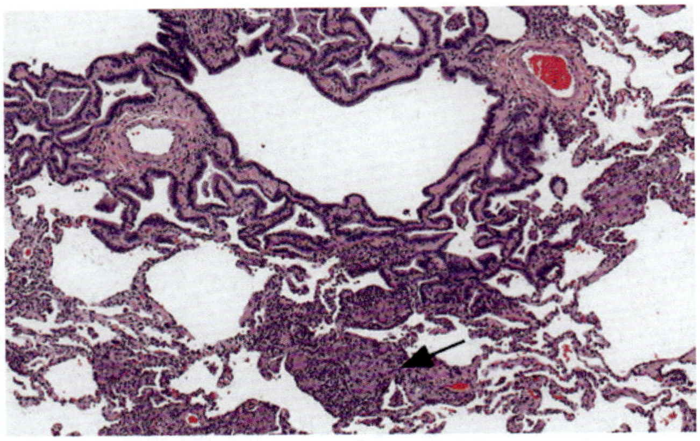

Figure 24.13 HP: Peribronchiolar metaplasia is another feature commonly seen in HP. Note the rare peribronchiolar granuloma (*arrow*).

25 CHRONIC HYPERSENSITIVITY PNEUMONIA VS. ASPIRATION PNEUMONIA

	Chronic Hypersensitivity Pneumonia (HP)	Aspiration Pneumonia
Age	There is no gender or age predilection, although it is uncommon in children.	Aspiration occurs in children and adult of both sexes.
Location	Usually, it is a predominantly centrilobular/bronchiolocentric process involving the middle and upper lung zones.	The process usually centers around bronchioles and most often affects basal segments of lower lobes, posterior segments of upper lobes, right middle lobe, and lingula.
Symptoms	Insidious onset of dyspnea, often associated with dry cough, fatigue, and malaise.	For many patients, aspiration is a silent event without symptoms. Other patients may experience shortness of breath, tachypnea, tachycardia, fever, purulent sputum, and marked leukocytosis.
Signs	Chest high-resolution computed tomography (HRCT) demonstrates mid-to-upper lobe predominant linear interstitial opacities and small nodules associated with traction bronchiectasis and honeycomb areas. If small airway obstruction is present, air trapping can be seen on expiratory HRCT manifesting as a mosaic attenuation pattern. Bronchoalveolar lavage marked lymphocytosis, although nonspecific, can further support the diagnosis of chronic HP.	Radiographic studies typically show infiltrates with or without cavities in a lobar or segmental distribution.
Etiology	HP represents a combination of immune complex-mediated (type III) and T-cell mediated, delayed (type IV) hypersensitivity reactions. Exposure to inhaled environmental antigens (e.g., mold, bacteria, animal proteins, avian proteins) or other allergen particles of small size (5 μm or smaller) triggers the disease. Sometimes the causal agent cannot be identified. The disease, which is also called extrinsic allergic alveolitis (EAA), may also be known by a great variety of names depending on the causal agent (farmer's lung, pigeon breeder's disease, ventilation pneumonitis). However, regardless of the pathologic responsible agent, the clinical presentation and pathologic findings are similar.	Aspiration events lead to injury through the introduction of acidic stomach fluid, proteolytic enzymes, and foreign material into the lung and airways. The acidic and enzymatic fluids of the stomach lead to direct injury to airways and pneumocytes, while the foreign material is typically processed by histiocytes and multinucleated giant cells. Bacterial organisms of the oropharynx may be inoculated into the lung and lead to a secondary bacterial infection. Risk factors for developing aspiration include loss of consciousness, impaired swallowing, abnormal esophageal motility, and gastroesophageal reflux.

	Chronic Hypersensitivity Pneumonia (HP)	Aspiration Pneumonia
Histology	Chronic cellular interstitial pneumonia (typically showing bronchiolocentric accentuation), cellular chronic bronchiolitis, and small, interstitial, nonnecrotizing, poorly formed granulomas composed of loose clusters of epithelioid histiocytes, multinucleated giant cells, and lymphocytes *(Figs. 25.1–25.3)*. Peribronchiolar metaplasia *(Fig. 25.4)*, peribronchiolar fibrosis, and patchy foci of organizing pneumonia are frequently present *(Fig. 25.5)*. Constrictive bronchiolitis may occur and foamy macrophages related to bronchiolar obstruction may be seen within the nearby alveolar spaces. In the advanced phase of chronic HP, interstitial scarring/fibrosis and honeycomb change may become prominent resembling UIP.	Patchy airway-centered foci of organizing pneumonia are commonly seen in aspiration pneumonia and may represent the main pattern of injury *(Figs. 25.6 and 25.7)*. The associated inflammation is a mixture of lymphocytes, histiocytes, and multinucleated giant cells. The presence of vegetable matter with cell walls *(Figs. 25.8 to 25.11)* is helpful in making the diagnosis, but is often not present in individual sections due to sampling. In addition to vegetable material, other foreign materials that may be seen associated with aspiration pneumonia include talk and microcrystalline cellulose, which are strongly polarizable; crospovidone *(Fig. 25.13)*, and kayexalate *(Fig. 25.14)*. Talc, microcrystalline cellulose, and crospovidone are components of various oral pharmaceutical tablets, and may represent accidental aspiration of these medications. Kayexalate is a polystyrene sulfonate used in the treatment of hyperkalemia. Acute bronchopneumonia with neutrophils and necrosis may develop as a consequence of inoculation of oropharyngeal bacteria *(Fig. 25.14)*. This is not a feature of chronic HP. Cases of massive aspiration may lead to acute lung injury with hyaline membranes.
Special studies	Gomori methenamine silver (GMS) and acid-fast bacilli (AFB) special stains and tissue cultures to exclude infection.	None.
Prognosis	The prognosis is worse when associated with interstitial scarring. Some patients respond to removal of antigen exposure and corticosteroid therapy but some cases become self-sustained and progress to fibrotic phase despite removal from the antigen exposure. How much fibrosis is required to move into the poor outcome group is unclear. Overall, once dense fibrosis develops with honeycomb change, the disease is irreversible.	The prognosis of aspiration is largely dependent on the severity of the aspiration event. Typical cases of silent or mildly symptomatic aspiration have good prognosis. Some pulmonologists believe that recurrent aspiration may lead to interstitial fibrosis, however, the contribution of aspiration to pulmonary fibrosis is not entirely understood. Cases of massive aspiration have a similar overall mortality to other etiologies for diffuse alveolar damage.

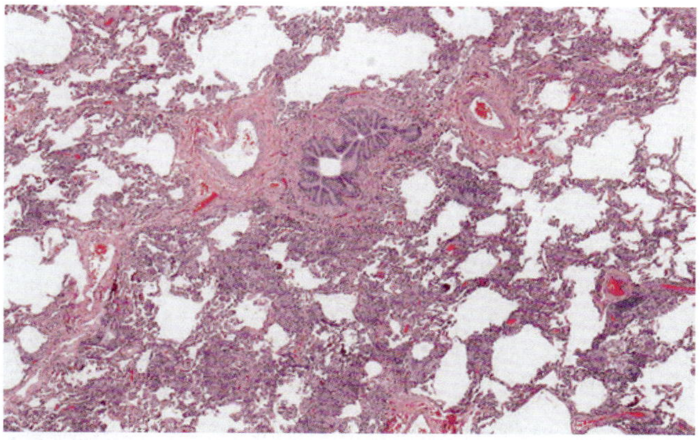

Figure 25.1 HP: There is diffuse expansion of the alveolar septa by chronic inflammatory cell infiltrate, which is more pronounced in the peribronchiolar zones.

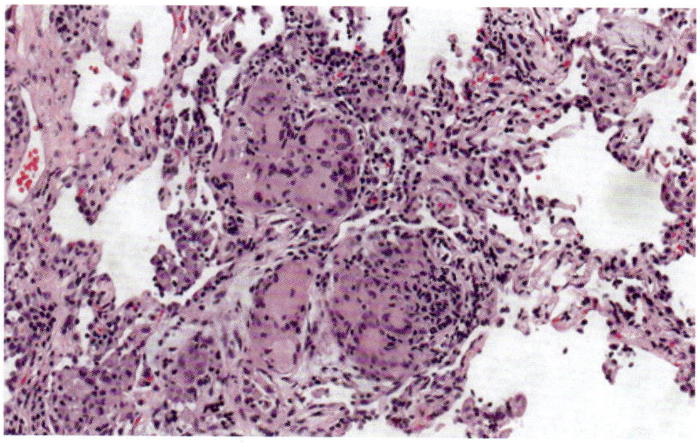

Figure 25.2 HP: The granulomas present in HP are not typically seen in alveolar spaces but in the interstitium (alveolar septa). They are poorly formed and may be composed of giant cells and lymphocytes. On contrary, in aspiration pneumonia there is foreign-body type of multinucleated giant cell reaction.

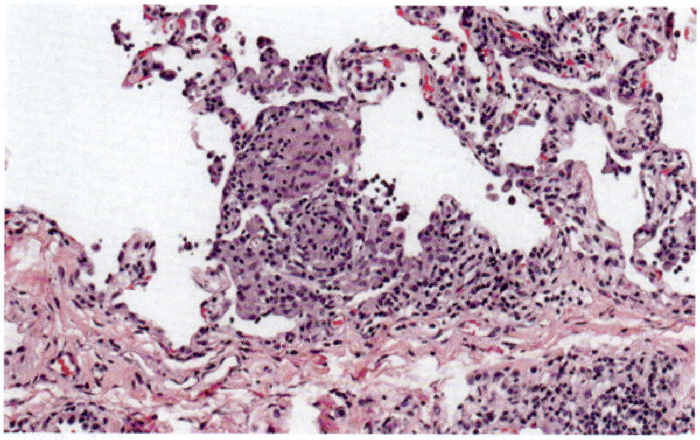

Figure 25.3 HP: High-power view showing nonnecrotizing poorly formed granuloma composed of loosely arranged epithelioid histiocytes is suggestive of chronic HP.

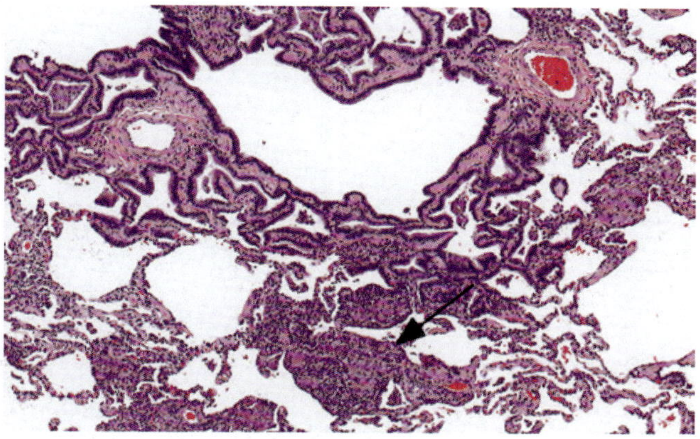

Figure 25.4 HP: Peribronchiolar metaplasia is another feature commonly seen in chronic HP. Note poorly formed peribronchiolar granuloma (*arrow*).

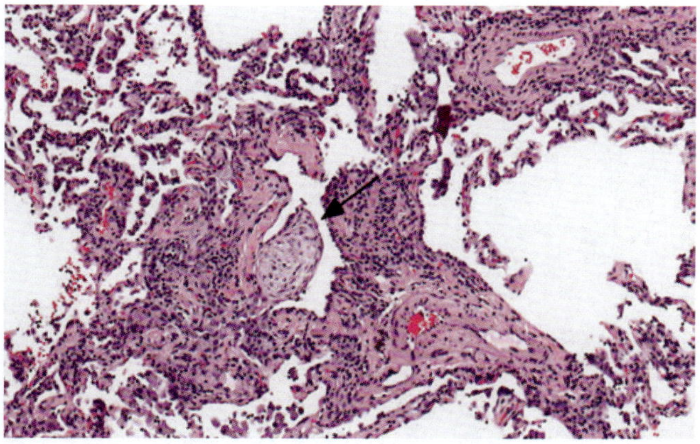

Figure 25.5 HP: Few foci of organizing pneumonia may be present (*arrow*), which do not represent the main pattern of injury in HP. Differently, in aspiration pneumonia the main patterns of injury are organizing pneumonia and acute bronchopneumonia associated with foreign-body type multinucleated giant cells.

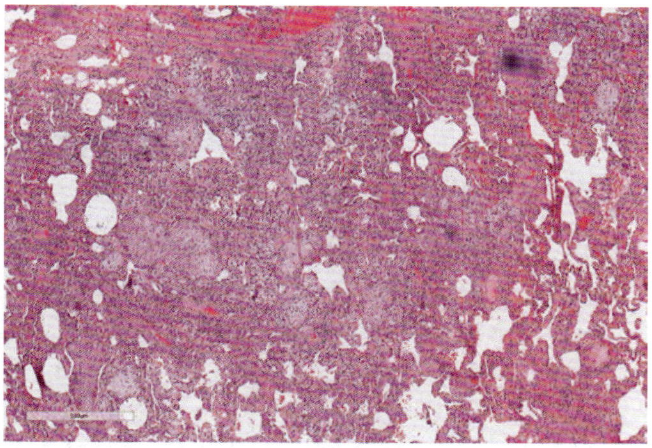

Figure 25.6 Aspiration pneumonia: Many cases of aspiration pneumonia show infiltrates in image studies that correspond to organizing pneumonia and mild chronic interstitial inflammation.

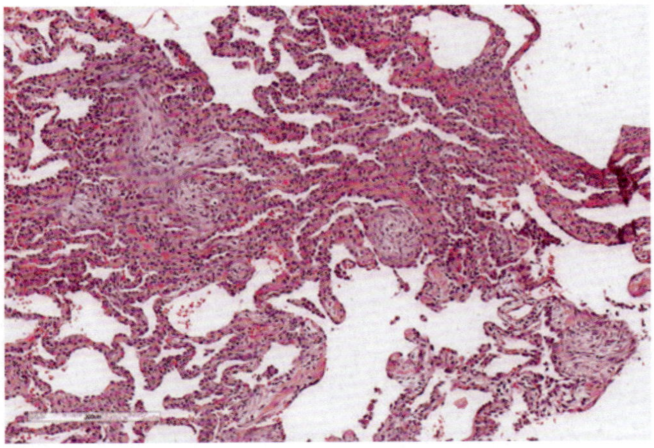

Figure 25.7 Aspiration pneumonia: A higher power view showing regions of fibroblastic tissue within airspaces (organizing pneumonia).

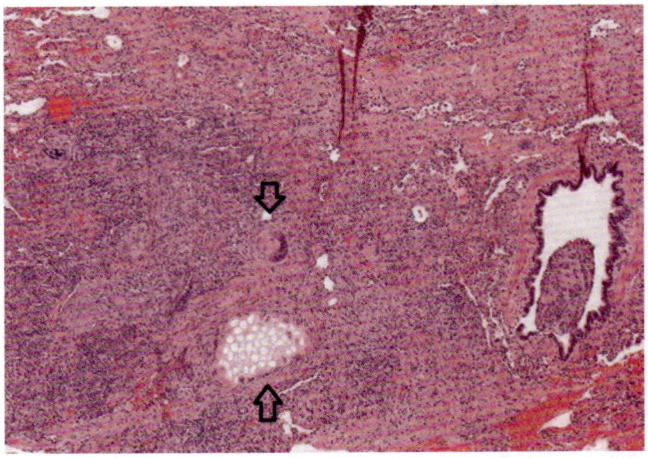

Figure 25.8 Aspiration pneumonia: There is dense acute and chronic inflammatory cell infiltrate around peribronchiolar zone associated with multinucleated giant cells processing vegetable material (*arrows*).

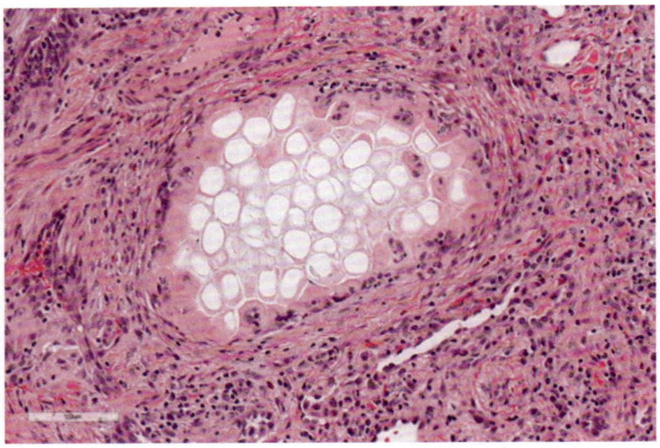

Figure 25.9 Aspiration pneumonia: A higher power view of aspirated plant/vegetable material seen in Figure 25.8 with the devitalized cell wall structure.

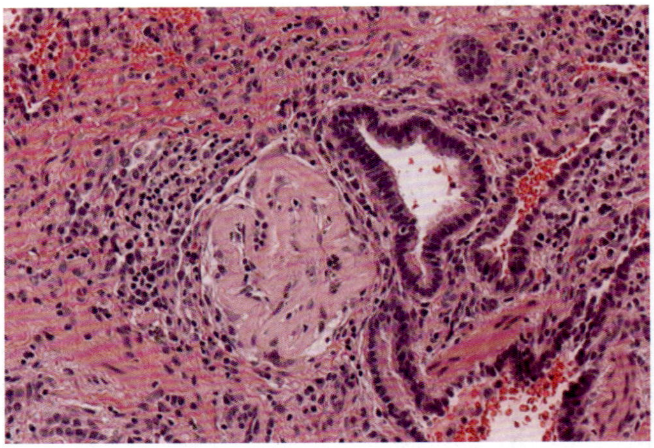

Figure 25.10 Aspiration pneumonia: In the early stage, vegetable matter is easily recognizable. Later on, the vegetable matter loses its structures and appears as eosinophilic amorphous cerebriform material.

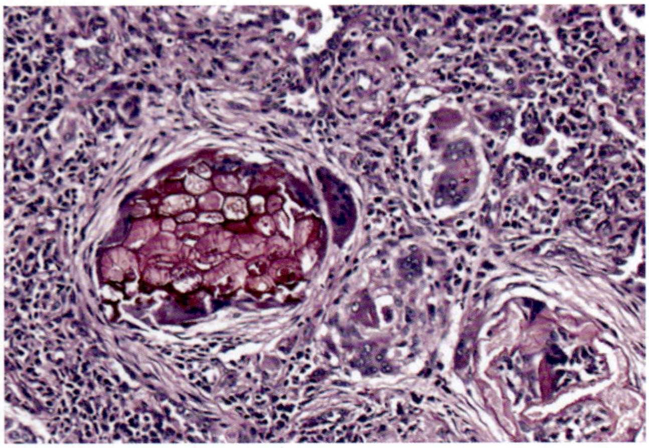

Figure 25.11 Aspiration pneumonia: Vegetable matter surrounded by foreign body type multinucleated giant cells.

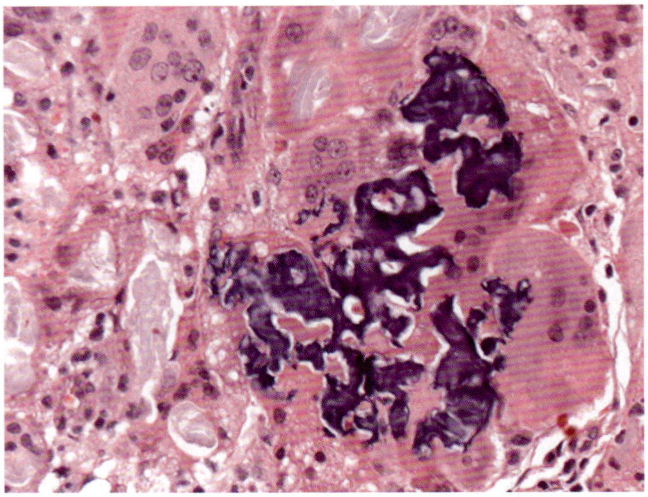

Figure 25.12 Aspiration pneumonia: Serpiginous coral-like dark basophilic particles of crospovidone may be seen associated with aspiration pneumonia. Note foreign body type multinucleated giant cells surrounding the crospovidone particles.

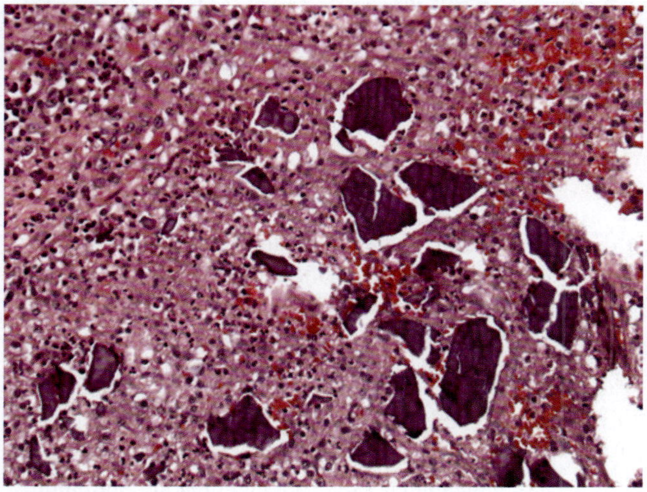

Figure 25.13 Aspiration pneumonia: Kayexalate, in this case within a background of acute inflammation, is another foreign material that may be seen associated with aspiration pneumonia.

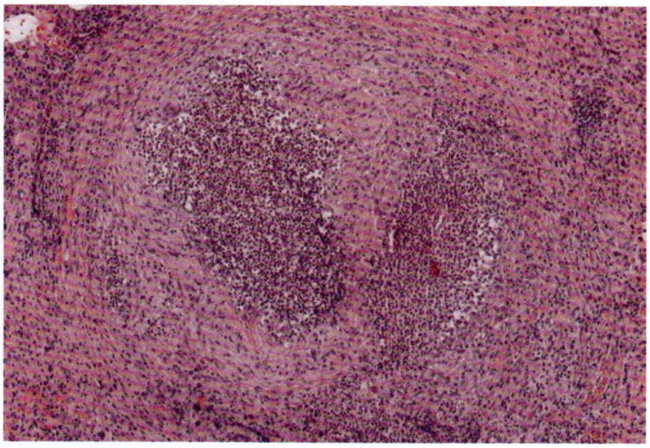

Figure 25.14 Aspiration pneumonia: Aspiration pneumonia may causes a bronchopneumonia pattern of injury with abundant neutrophils filling airways lumens and microabscess formation, both as a reaction to the acidic fluid of the stomach and secondary infection from the aspiration of bacterial flora from the oropharynx.

26 HYPERSENSITIVITY PNEUMONIA VS. HARD METAL PNEUMOCONIOSIS

	Hypersensitivity Pneumonia (HP)	Hard Metal Pneumoconiosis
Age	There is no gender or age predilection, although uncommon in children.	Hard metal pneumoconiosis is most common among adults of working age, with a mean age of 43 in small studies. The majority of cases have been associated with occupations involving the grinding and milling of hard-metal alloys that contain cobalt.
Location	Usually a predominantly centrilobular/ bronchiolocentric process involving the middle and upper lung zones.	The disease is generally diffuse in distribution, although some cases show modest accentuation in the lower lobes.
Symptoms	Insidious onset of dyspnea, often associated with dry cough, fatigue, and malaise.	Some patients show airway-related symptoms, with asthma being a common manifestation of the pneumoconiosis. For patients with interstitial disease and fibrosis, the symptoms are typical for fibrotic interstitial lung diseases and include dyspnea and a nonproductive cough.
Signs	Chest high-resolution computed tomography (HRCT) demonstrates mid-to-upper-lobe predominant linear interstitial opacities and small nodules associated with traction bronchiectasis and honeycomb areas. If small airway obstruction is present, air trapping can be seen on expiratory HRCT manifesting as a mosaic attenuation pattern. Although not entirely specific, a lymphocytosis in the bronchoalveolar lavage can further support the diagnosis of chronic HP.	The radiographic findings are not consistent, but often show small irregular opacities with some lower lobe predominance along with reticular changes and occasionally honeycombing.
Etiology	HP represents a combination of immune complex–mediated (type III) and T-cell–mediated, delayed (type IV) hypersensitivity reactions. Exposure to inhaled environmental antigens (e.g., mold, bacteria, animal proteins, avian proteins) or other allergen particles of small size (5 μm or smaller) triggers the disease. Sometimes the causal agent cannot be identified. The disease, which is also called extrinsic allergic alveolitis (EAA), may also be known by a great variety of names depending on the causal agent (farmer's lung, pigeon breeder's disease, ventilation pneumonitis). However, regardless of the pathologic responsible agent, the clinical presentation and pathologic findings are similar.	The disease is not well understood but appears to be an inflammatory disorder that can be initiated by cobalt and other hard metals. In the case of cobalt, the cobalt salts that form in the lung are excreted and typically no longer present by the time the patients present clinically. Interestingly, the disease once initiated does not require ongoing exposure to progress.

	Hypersensitivity Pneumonia (HP)	**Hard Metal Pneumoconiosis**
Histology	Chronic cellular interstitial pneumonia (typically showing bronchiolocentric accentuation), cellular chronic bronchiolitis, and small, interstitial and airspace, nonnecrotizing, poorly formed granulomas composed of loose clusters of epithelioid histiocytes and multinucleated giant cells *(Figs. 26.1–26.3)*. Peribronchiolar metaplasia *(Fig. 26.4)*, peribronchiolar fibrosis, and patchy foci of organizing pneumonia are frequently present *(Fig. 26.5)*. Constrictive bronchiolitis may occur, and foamy macrophages related to bronchiolar obstruction may be seen within the nearby alveolar spaces. In the advanced phase of chronic HP, interstitial scarring/fibrosis and honeycomb change may become prominent, resembling UIP.	Hard metal pneumoconiosis, also known as giant cell interstitial pneumonia, shows large number of multinucleated giant cells of histiocytic origin within the airspaces and clinging to the alveolar septa *(Figs. 26.6 and 26.7)*. There is alveolar type II pneumocyte prominence the pneumocytes may also appear multinucleated. Some giant cells show endocytosed inflammatory cells within their cytoplasm and are referred to as cannibalistic giant cells *(Fig. 26.8)*. DIP-like macrophages are also typically present within the airspaces. The alveolar septa show expansion by mild-to-moderate chronic inflammatory infiltrate and variable amounts of fibrosis *(Fig. 26.9)*. Occasionally, the fibrotic and inflammatory reaction may mimic UIP pattern of fibrosis with areas of honeycomb change.
Special studies	Gomori methenamine silver (GMS) and acid-fast bacilli (AFB) special stains and tissue cultures performed to exclude infection.	Analytic electron microscopy can be performed on transbronchial biopsy or bronchoalveolar lavage specimens and may demonstrate characteristic profile of metallic elements.
Prognosis	The prognosis is worse when associated with interstitial scarring. Some patients respond to removal of antigen exposure and corticosteroid therapy, but some cases become self-sustained and progress to fibrotic phase despite removal from the antigen exposure. How much fibrosis is required to move into the poor outcome group is unclear. Overall, once dense fibrosis develops with honeycomb change, the disease is irreversible.	The prognosis is highly variable with some patients responding well to immunosuppressive therapies, while others have died from the process or have required lung transplantation.

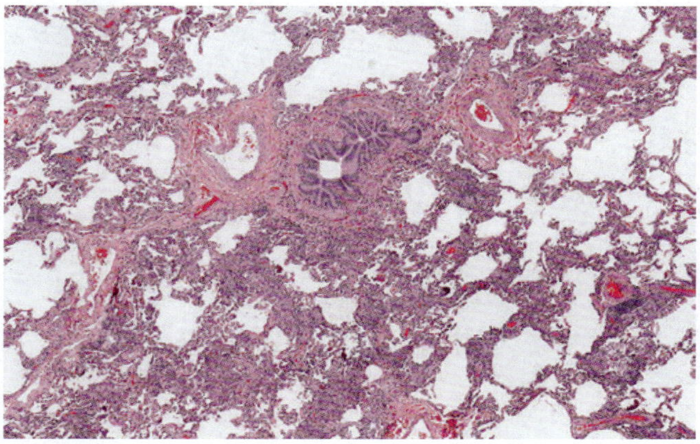

Figure 26.1 HP: A low-power view of a case of HP showing peribronchiolar chronic inflammation and nonnecrotizing granulomas.

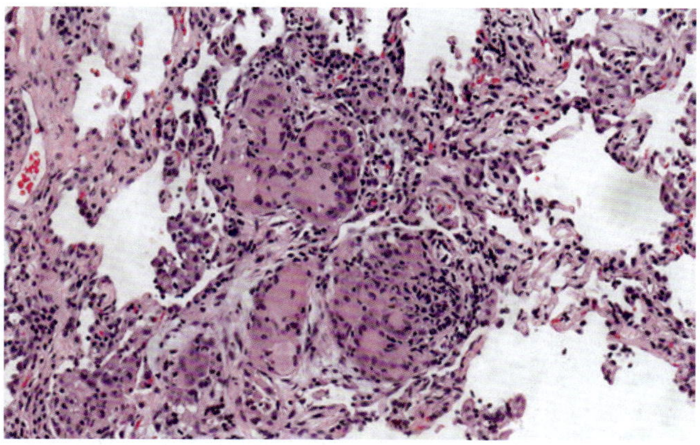

Figure 26.2 HP: A high-power view of the poorly formed nonnecrotizing granulomas and multinucleated giant cells in HP.

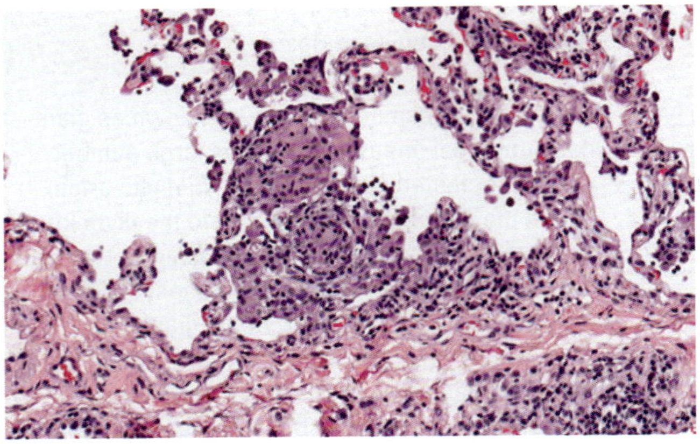

Figure 26.3 HP: A high-power view of the poorly formed nonnecrotizing granulomas composed of loosely arranged epithelioid histiocytes seen in airspaces and interstitium.

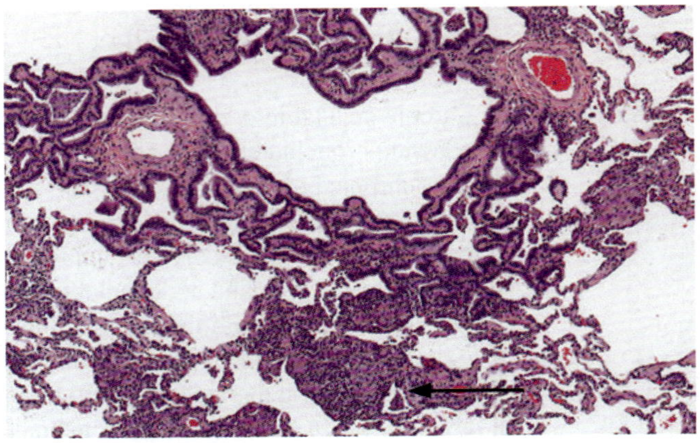

Figure 26.4 HP: Peribronchiolar metaplasia is another feature commonly seen in HP. Note the rare, poorly formed peribronchiolar granuloma (*arrow*).

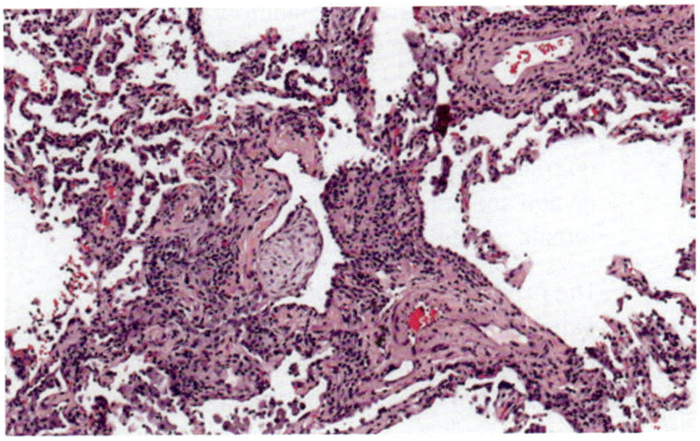

Figure 26.5 HP: Few foci of organizing pneumonia may be present, which do not represent the main pattern of injury in HP.

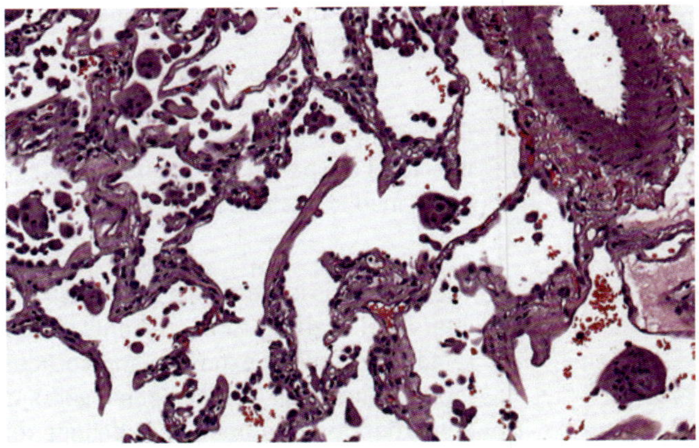

Figure 26.6 Hard metal pneumoconiosis: A case of hard metal pneumoconiosis/giant cell interstitial pneumonia showing mildly thickened alveolar septa with numerous multinucleated giant cells within the airspaces. Note that many of the multinucleated giant cells have engulfed inflammatory cells within them, also referred to as cannibalistic giant cells.

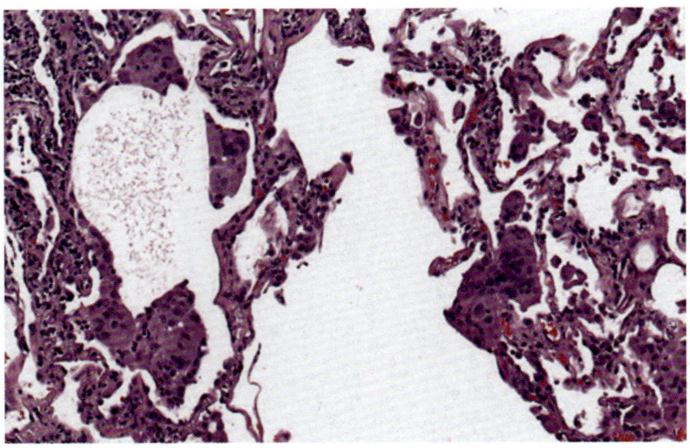

Figure 26.7 Hard metal pneumoconiosis: Another image demonstrating cannibalistic giant cells and the mild alveolar septal thickening typically seen in hard metal pneumoconiosis.

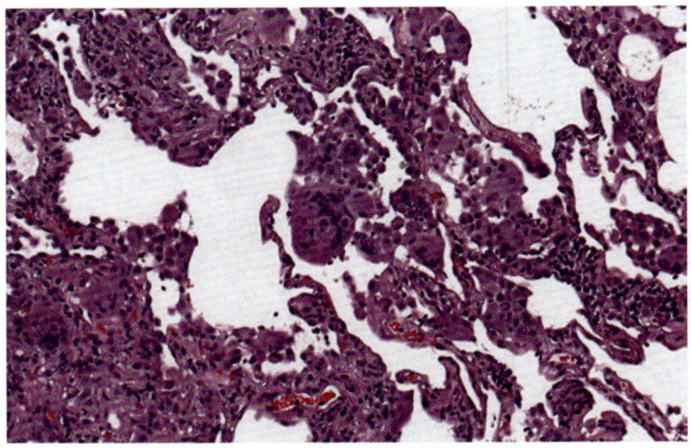

Figure 26.8 Hard metal pneumoconiosis: Cannibalistic giant cells of hard metal pneumoconiosis.

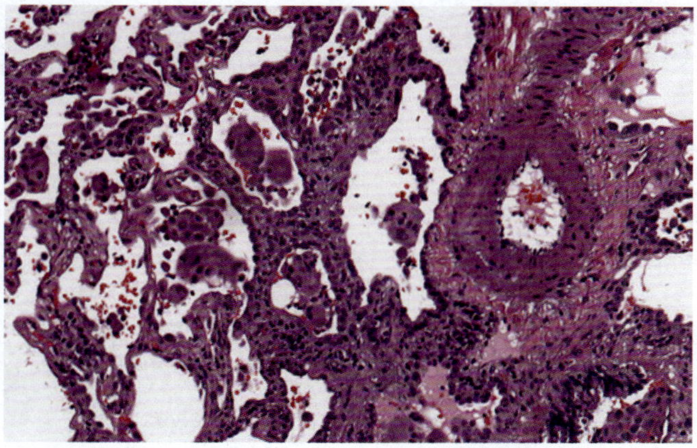

Figure 26.9 Hard metal pneumoconiosis: Thickened alveolar septa are lined by mildly hyperplastic pneumocytes. Numerous giant cells are in airspaces.

27 HYPERSENSITIVITY PNEUMONIA VS. SARCOIDOSIS

	Hypersensitivity Pneumonia (HP)	Sarcoidosis
Age	There is no gender or age predilection, although uncommon in children.	Sarcoidosis is most common in adults aged 20–30 and shows a modest female predominance. The disease is most common in African Americans, Irish, and Scandinavians, but can occur in any race.
Location	Usually a predominantly centrilobular/ bronchiolocentric process involving the middle and upper lung zones.	Pulmonary sarcoidosis typically involves both lungs and favors the upper and middle zones. Lymph node involvement of the hilum and mediastinum is common.
Symptoms	Insidious onset of dyspnea, often associated with dry cough, fatigue, and malaise.	Symptoms may either be acute or follow a slow and chronic course. The common presentation of sarcoidosis includes fatigue, anorexia, fever, weight loss, and cough. Skin and extrapulmonary organ involvement is common.
Signs	Chest high-resolution computed tomography (HRCT) demonstrates mid-to-upper-lobe predominant linear interstitial opacities and small nodules associated with traction bronchiectasis and honeycomb areas. If small airway obstruction is present, air trapping can be seen on expiratory HRCT manifesting as a mosaic attenuation pattern. Although not entirely specific, a lymphocytosis in the bronchoalveolar lavage can further support the diagnosis of chronic HP.	The disease typically follows a lymphatic pattern of distribution involving pleural and subpleural zones, interlobular septa, and coursing along bronchovascular bundles, associated with symmetric bilateral hilar and mediastinal lymphadenopathy. Pulmonary involvement typically shows nodular or reticulonodular changes in the middle and upper lung zones of both lobes equally.
Etiology	HP represents a combination of immune complex–mediated (type III) and T-cell–mediated, delayed (type IV) hypersensitivity reactions. Exposure to inhaled environmental antigens (e.g., mold, bacteria, animal proteins, avian proteins), or other allergen particles of small size (5 µm or smaller) triggers the disease. Sometimes, the causal agent cannot be identified. The disease, which is also called extrinsic allergic alveolitis (EAA), may also be known by a great variety of names depending on the causal agent (farmer's lung, pigeon breeder's disease, ventilation pneumonitis). However, regardless of the pathologic responsible agent, the clinical presentation and pathologic findings are similar.	Despite decades of research, little is understood about the mechanism of sarcoidosis. Current theories consider sarcoidosis to be a disease that causes an aberrant immune response driven by an unidentified antigen or antigens in genetically susceptible individuals. Multiple candidate etiologic agents including mycobacteria, propionibacteria, and environmental agents have been investigated with inconsistent results.

	Hypersensitivity Pneumonia (HP)	Sarcoidosis
Histology	Chronic cellular interstitial pneumonia (typically showing bronchiolocentric accentuation), cellular chronic bronchiolitis, and small, interstitial and airspace, nonnecrotizing, poorly formed granulomas composed of loose clusters of epithelioid histiocytes and multinucleated giant cells. *(Figs. 27.1–27.3).* Peribronchiolar metaplasia *(Fig. 27.4),* peribronchiolar fibrosis, and patchy foci of organizing pneumonia are frequently present *(Fig. 27.5).* Constrictive bronchiolitis may occur, and foamy macrophages related to bronchiolar obstruction may be seen within the nearby alveolar spaces. In the advanced phase of chronic HP, interstitial scarring/fibrosis and honeycomb changes may become prominent, resembling UIP.	Sarcoidosis typically shows coalescent well-formed nonnecrotizing granulomas following a lymphatic distribution, seen along pleural and subpleural zones, interlobular septa, and bronchovascular bundles *(Fig. 27.6).* The well-formed nature of the granulomas and the absence of airway-centered interstitial chronic inflammation distinguish sarcoidosis from HP. As sarcoidosis progresses, granulomas may become encased within concentric collagen and eventually become completely hyalinized *(Figs. 27.7 through 27.10).* Inclusion bodies, including polarizable endogenous calcium oxalate crystals, may be present within multinucleated giant cells. In large biopsies that sample numerous granulomas, it is not uncommon to find rare central necrosis. In necrotizing sarcoidosis, associated prominent vasculitis may be present, which may be granulomatous or may be characterized by transmural chronic inflammation. Multinucleated giant cells are prominent in some cases, but significant necrosis is usually not a feature. Widespread necrosis may indicate infection or granulomatosis with polyangiitis. Even in the absence of necrosis, sarcoidosis remains a diagnosis of exclusion that should only be considered if infectious entities, HP, and chronic beryllium disease have been excluded.
Special studies	Gomori methenamine silver (GMS) and acid-fast bacilli (AFB) special stains and tissue cultures should be performed to exclude infection.	Although there are no specific stains or markers for sarcoidosis, AFB and GMS stains, tissue cultures and appropriate molecular testing should be considered to exclude infection. Chronic beryllium disease is another condition that can mimic sarcoidosis and the possibility of beryllium exposure should be considered, which may be detected in the blood with the beryllium sensitization test (Blood lymphocyte proiferation test [BeBLPT]).
Prognosis	The prognosis is worse when associated with interstitial scarring. Some patients respond to removal of antigen exposure and corticosteroid therapy, but some cases become self-sustained and progress to fibrotic phase despite removal from the antigen exposure. How much fibrosis is required to move into the poor-outcome group is unclear. Overall, once dense fibrosis develops with honeycomb change, the disease is irreversible.	The overall prognosis for sarcoidosis is good, with an overall mortality of 1%–5%. Treatment is based on immunosuppression, and so infectious etiologies must be excluded prior to treatment.

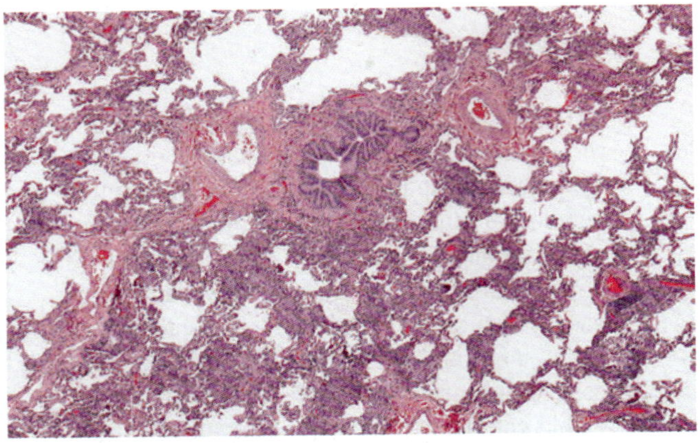

Figure 27.1 HP: A low-power view of a HP case showing characteristic airway centered chronic cellular interstitial pneumonia which is usually associated with poorly formed nonnecrotizing granulomas.

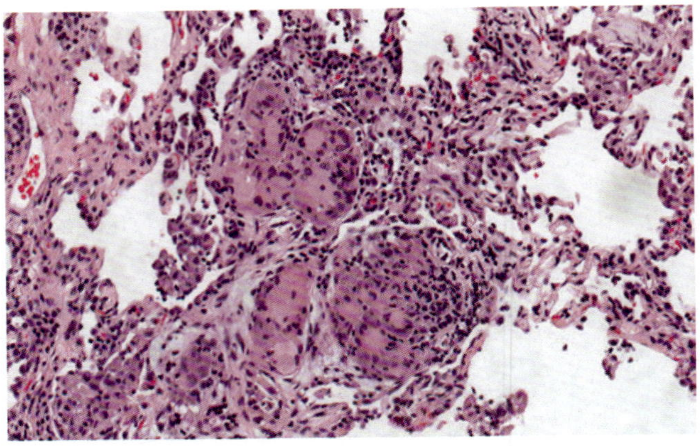

Figure 27.2 HP: A high-power view of the poorly formed nonnecrotizing granulomas and multinucleated giant cells in HP.

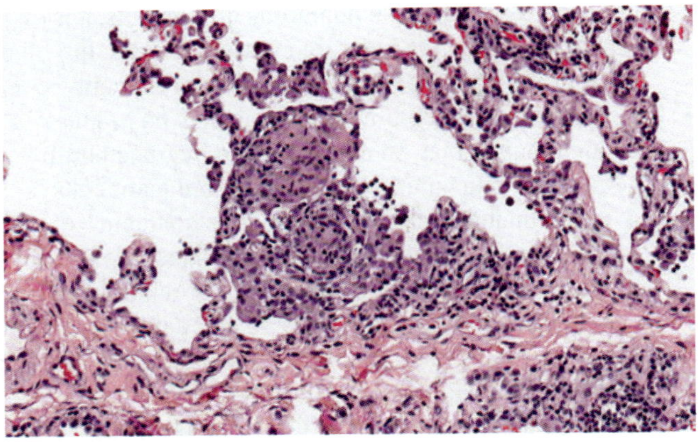

Figure 27.3 HP: A high-power view of the poorly formed nonnecrotizing granulomas composed of loosely arranged epithelioid histiocytes seen in airspace and interstitium.

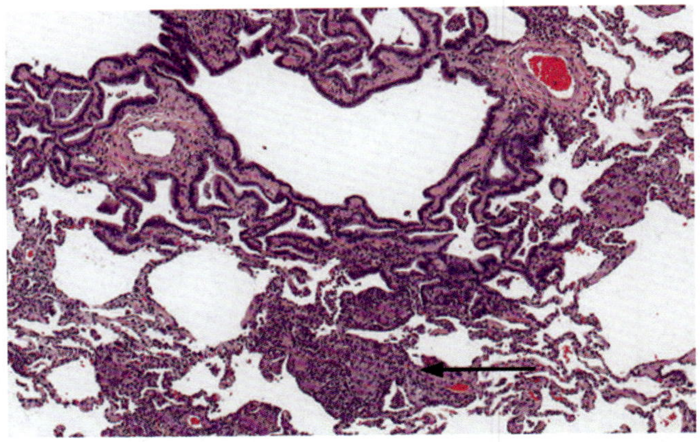

Figure 27.4 HP: Peribronchiolar metaplasia is another feature commonly seen in HP. Note the rare poorly formed peribronchiolar granuloma (*arrow*).

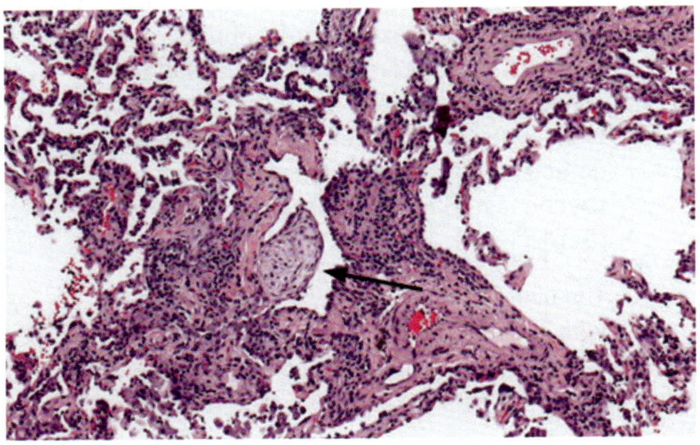

Figure 27.5 HP: Few foci of organizing pneumonia (*arrow*) may be present, which do not represent the main pattern of injury in HP.

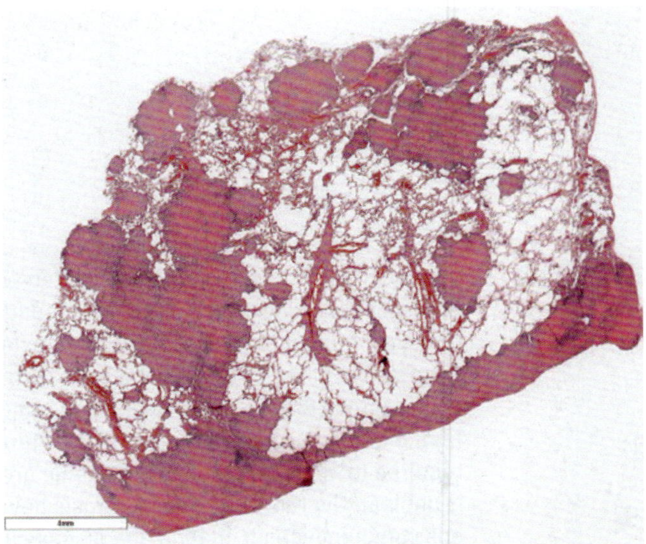

Figure 27.6 Sarcoidosis: A sarcoidosis case with mass-like nodules of dense collagen and nonnecrotizing granulomas at the junction with uninvolved lung. There is little associated interstitial chronic inflammation. Granulomas follow a lymphatic distribution with granulomas in the pleura, along the bronchovascular bundles and interlobular septa.

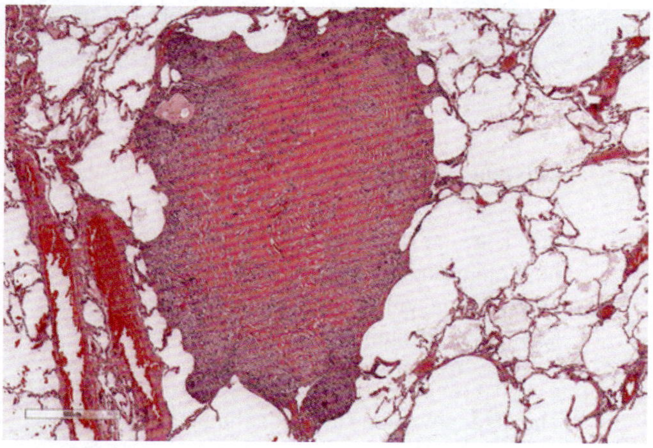

Figure 27.7 Sarcoidosis: Mass-like nodule of dense collagen and non-necrotizing granulomas at the junction with uninvolved lung. There is little associated interstitial chronic inflammation in the adjacent lung.

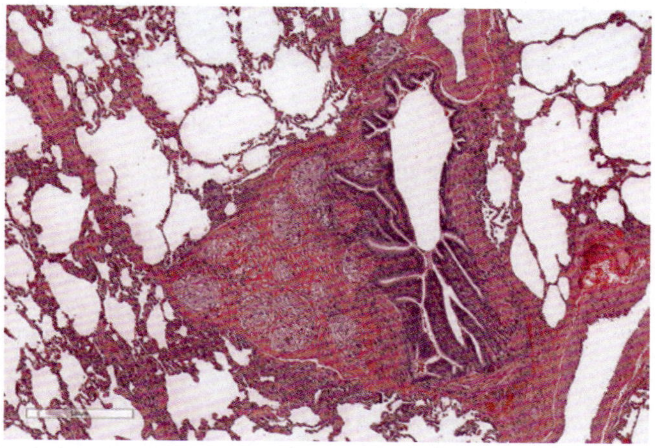

Figure 27.8 Sarcoidosis: A low-power view showing the peribronchiolar lymphatic distribution of granulomas in sarcoidosis.

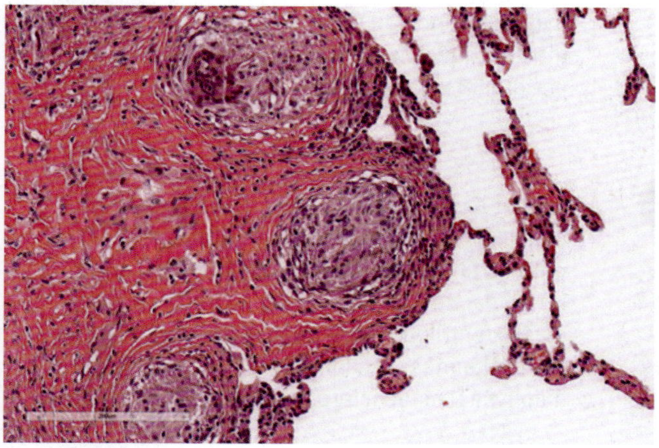

Figure 27.9 Sarcoidosis: A higher-power view of the dense concentric collagen surrounding well-formed granulomas.

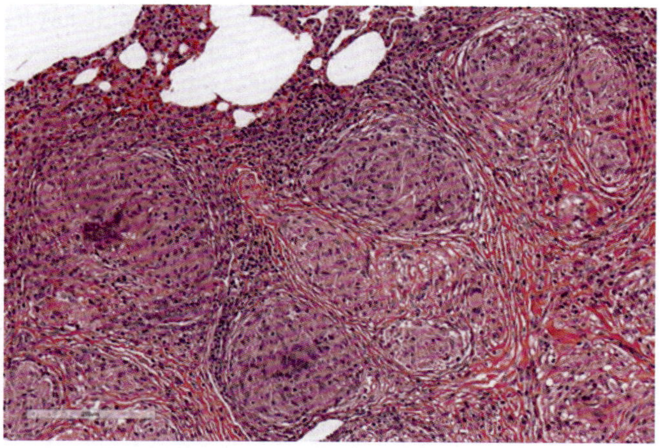

Figure 27.10 Sarcoidosis: Well-formed, coalescent nonnecrotizing granulomas showing typical concentric rings of dense collagen.

28 SARCOIDOSIS VS. ERDHEIM–CHESTER DISEASE

	Sarcoidosis	Erdheim–Chester Disease (ECD)
Age	Sarcoidosis is most common in adults aged 20–30 and shows a modest female predominance. The disease is most common in African Americans, Irish, and Scandinavians, but can occur in any race.	ECD is a very rare disease that can present in both children and adults, ranging from 4 to 87 years of age, with a mean age at diagnosis of 53 years, and slight male predominance.
Location	Pulmonary sarcoidosis typically involves both lungs and favors the upper and middle zones. Lymph node involvement of the hilum and mediastinum is common.	The disease usually involves the diaphyses of the long bones. However, more than 50% of cases have extraskeletal involvement. This can include lung, kidney, skin, brain, and orbit involvement, among other sites.
Symptoms	Symptoms may either be acute or follow a slow and chronic course. The common presentation of sarcoidosis includes fatigue, anorexia, fever, weight loss, and cough. Skin and extrapulmonary organ involvement is common.	Symptoms include dyspnea, pain in the bones of the legs, fever, weight loss, exophthalmos, and periorbital xanthomas.
Signs	The disease typically follows a lymphatic pattern of distribution involving pleural and subpleural zones, interlobular septa, and coursing along bronchovascular bundles, associated with symmetric bilateral hilar and mediastinal lymphadenopathy. Pulmonary involvement typically shows nodular or reticulonodular changes in the middle and upper lung zones of both lobes equally.	Similar to sarcoidosis, ECD also follows in the lung a lymphatic pattern of distribution. Radiographic findings in the lung include thickened interlobular septa, thickened lung fissures, ground glass, centrilobular nodularity, and reticular interstitial changes. The long bones show symmetric diaphyseal osteosclerosis.
Etiology	Despite decades of research, little is understood about the mechanism of sarcoidosis. Current theories consider sarcoidosis to be a disease that causes an aberrant immune response driven by an unidentified antigen or antigens in genetically susceptible individuals. Multiple candidate etiologic agents including mycobacteria, propionibacteria, and environmental agents have been investigated with inconsistent results.	ECD is a histiocytic disease of non–Langerhans cell histiocytes that derive from the monocyte lineage. The cause of the disease remains unknown. In some cases, BRAF V600E mutations and RAS mutations have been identified and are potential targets for treatment.

	Sarcoidosis	Erdheim–Chester Disease (ECD)
Histology	Sarcoidosis typically shows coalescent, well-formed, nonnecrotizing granulomas following a lymphatic distribution, seen along pleural and subpleural zones, interlobular septa, and bronchovascular bundles *(Fig. 28.1)*. As sarcoidosis progresses, granulomas may become encased within concentric collagen and eventually become completely hyalinized *(Figs. 28.2–28.5)*. Inclusion bodies, including polarizable endogenous calcium oxalate crystals, may be present within multinucleated giant cells. In large biopsies that sample numerous granulomas, it is not uncommon to find rare central necrosis. In necrotizing sarcoidosis, associated prominent vasculitis may be present, which may be granulomatous or may be characterized by transmural chronic inflammation. Multinucleated giant cells are prominent in some cases, but significant necrosis is usually not a feature. Widespread necrosis may indicate infection or granulomatosis with polyangiitis. Even in the absence of necrosis, sarcoidosis remains a diagnosis of exclusion that should only be considered if an infectious etiology could be rigorously clinically excluded. Chronic beryllium disease is another condition that can mimic sarcoidosis and the possibility of beryllium exposure should also be considered.	Biopsy shows foamy, lipid-laden histiocytes infiltrating the lung along the lymphatics with aggregates of histiocytes in the pleura *(Figs. 28.6–28.8)*, interlobular septa, and along the bronchovascular bundles *(Figs. 28.9 and 28.10)*. The lymphatic pattern of distribution is similar to sarcoidosis, but ECD has foamy lipid laden histiocytes, and not the epithelioid histiocytes of sarcoidosis. Histiocytes have round-to-oval nuclei and abundant eosinophilic foamy cytoplasm. The aggregates of histiocytes can be associated with variable amounts of fibrosis lymphocytes and plasma cells.
Special studies	Although there are no specific stains or markers for sarcoidosis, AFB and GMS stains, tissue cultures and appropriate molecular testing should be considered to exclude infection. Chronic beryllium disease is another condition that can mimic sarcoidosis and the possibility of beryllium exposure should be considered, which may be detected in the blood with the beryllium sensitization test (Blood lymphocyte proliferation test [BeBLPT]).	Unlike pulmonary Langerhans cell histiocytosis, the histiocytes of ECD are negative for CD1a, but express other histiocytic markers such as CD68 and S100. Oil red O in fresh tissue or bronchoalveolar lavage can highlight lipid droplets in the cytoplasm of the foamy histiocytes of ECD.
Prognosis	The overall prognosis for sarcoidosis is good, with an overall mortality of 1%–5%. Treatment is based on immunosuppression, and so infectious etiologies must be excluded prior to treatment.	The prognosis is poor with approximately 50% survival at 3 y. Treatment is aimed at immunosuppression/immune modulation, although cases associated with BRAF mutation have shown dramatic response to targeted therapy.

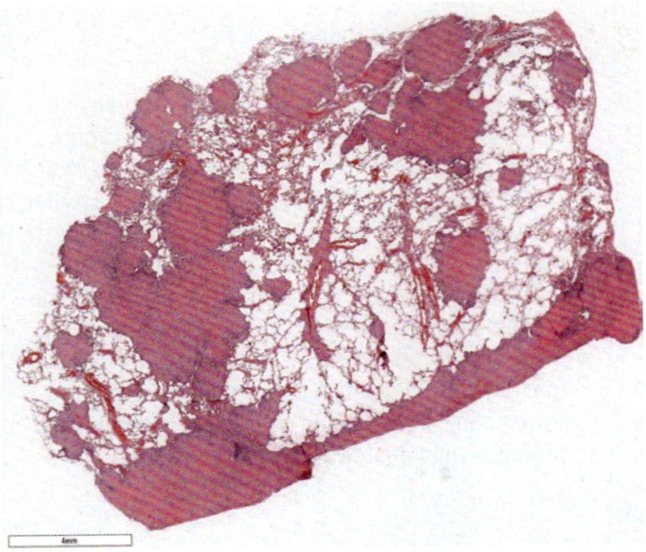

Figure 28.1 Sarcoidosis: A low-power view of sarcoidosis showing the mass-like collections of nonnecrotizing granulomas and dense collagen. The lymphatic distribution of sarcoidosis is similar to the lymphatic distribution of ECD.

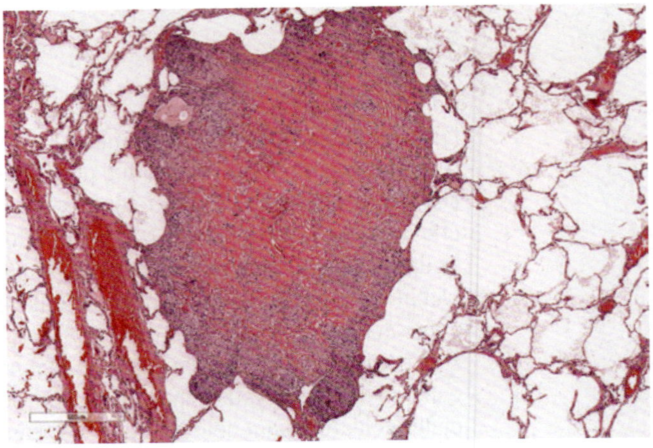

Figure 28.2 Sarcoidosis: A mass-like nodule composed of nonnecrotizing granulomas with central dense collagen deposition. This sarcoidosis case shows clear nonnecrotizing granulomas along the rim of the nodule, unlike ECD, which does not have granulomas.

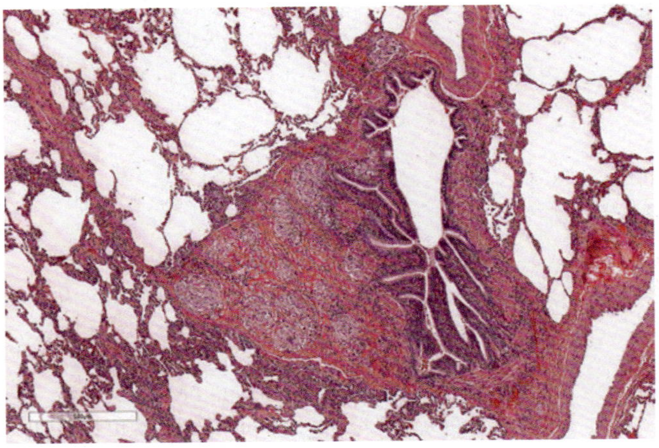

Figure 28.3 Sarcoidosis: A case of sarcoidosis showing granulomas along the lymphatic channels of the bronchiole and embedded in collagen. Although the lymphatic distribution of ECD is similar, ECD does not have well-formed granulomas.

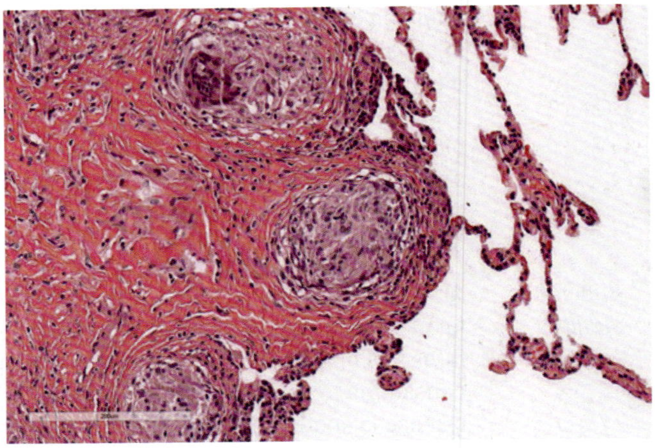

Figure 28.4 Sarcoidosis: A high-power view showing typical concentric collagen deposition around the well-formed nonnecrotizing granulomas.

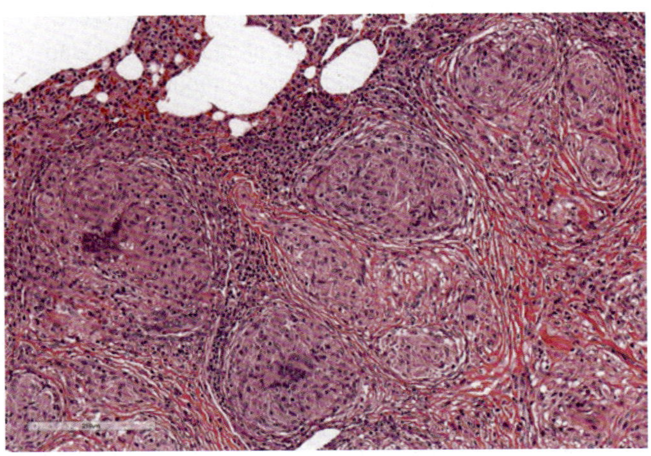

Figure 28.5 Sarcoidosis: A high-power view showing coalescent well-formed granulomas and typical concentric dense collagen deposition. Well-formed granulomas are not a feature of ECD.

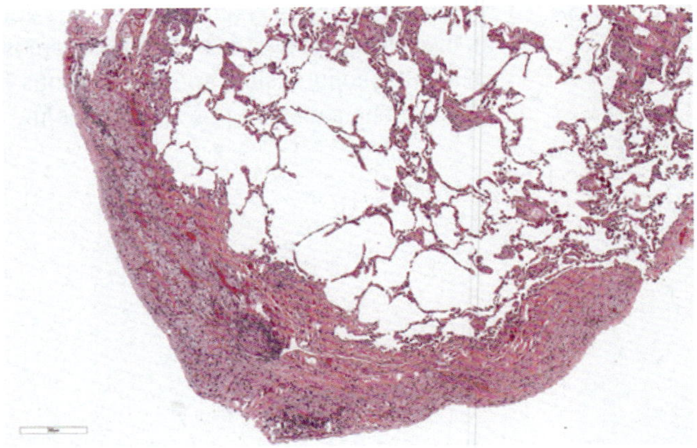

Figure 28.6 ECD: A low-power view of ECD showing collections of foamy histiocytes following a lymphatic distribution involving subpleural zone. Unlike sarcoidosis, which involves the pleura with granulomas, ECD has collections of foamy histiocytes.

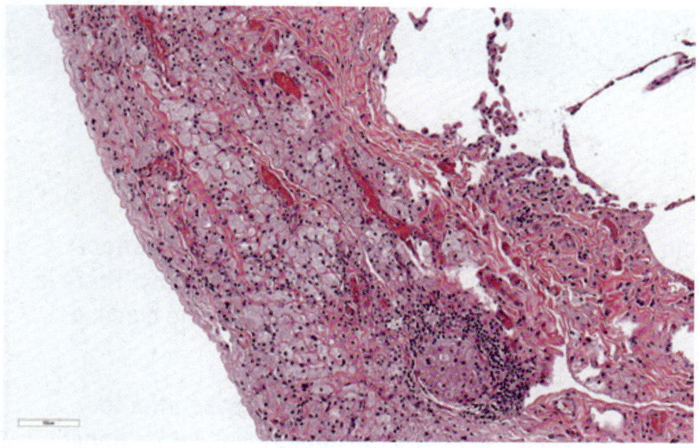

Figure 28.7 ECD: High-power view of Figure 28.6 showing foamy histiocytes of ECD involving the supleural zone. Foamy histiocytes are not a feature of sarcoidosis.

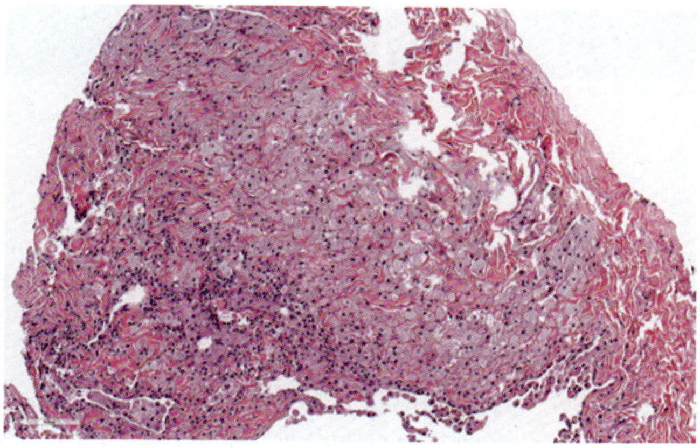

Figure 28.8 ECD: In this image, there are lipid-laden, foamy histiocytes embedded in the collagen of the pleura.

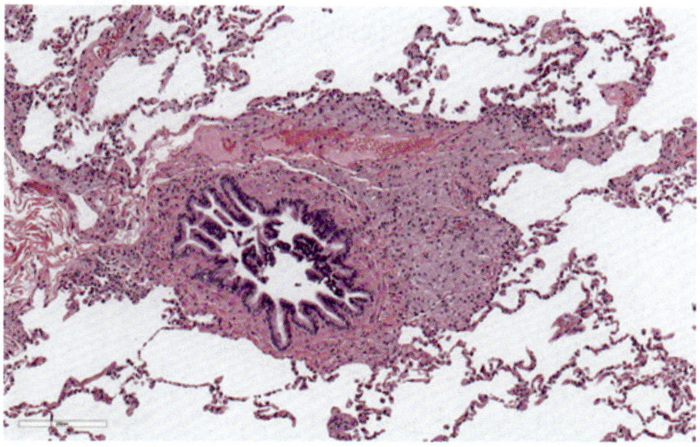

Figure 28.9 ECD: A case of ECD showing collections of foamy histiocytes along with lymphatic channels of the bronchovascular bundle. Although the lymphatic distribution of ECD is shared by sarcoidosis, ECD does not have granulomas.

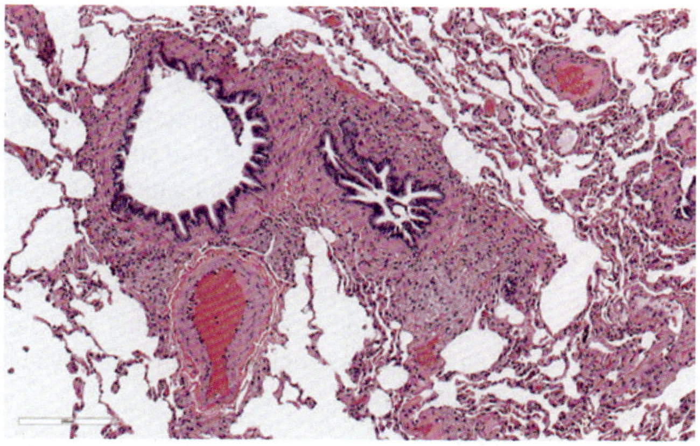

Figure 28.10 ECD: The foamy histiocytes of ECD are associated with the lymphatic channels of the bronchiole and pulmonary artery.

29 ERDHEIM–CHESTER DISEASE VS. MALAKOPLAKIA

	Erdheim–Chester Disease (ECD)	Malakoplakia
Age	ECD is a very rare disease that can present in both children and adults, ranging from 4 to 87 years of age, with a mean age at diagnosis of 53 years, and slight male predominance.	Malakoplakia is a rare disorder that can affect adults with underlying immunodeficiency. There is no known gender predominance to the disease.
Location	The disease usually involves the diaphyses of the long bones. However, more than 50% of cases have extraskeletal involvement. This can include lung, kidney, skin, brain, and orbit involvement, among other sites.	Although any part of the lung may be affected, this disease favors the upper lobes and is generally multifocal.
Symptoms	Symptoms include dyspnea, pain in the bones of the legs, fever, weight loss, exophthalmos, and periorbital xanthomas.	Patients often present with nonspecific signs of infections, including cough, fever, dyspnea, and chest pain.
Signs	EDC follows a lymphatic pattern of distribution in the lung involving pleural and subpleural zones, interlobular septa, and coursing along bronchovascular bundles. Radiographic findings in the lung include thickened interlobular septa, thickened lung fissures, ground glass, centrilobular nodularity, and reticular interstitial changes. The long bones show symmetric diaphyseal osteosclerosis.	Radiographic studies demonstrate upper-lobe predominant multifocal consolidation, often with cavitation. Bronchoalveolar lavage (BAL) and sputum cultures may be positive for *Rhodococcus equi, Acinetobacter, E. coli*, or other organisms that have been associated with malakoplakia.
Etiology	ECD is a histiocytic disease of non–Langerhans cell histiocytes that derive from the monocyte lineage. The cause of the disease remains unknown. In some cases, BRAF V600E mutations and RAS mutations have been identified and are potential targets for treatment.	Malakoplakia represents an infectious process that may develop in the setting of immunodeficiency. Organisms are present in the lung tissue and within the cytoplasmic endosomes of macrophages. The pathogenesis is related to a defect in the histiocyte function. There is inability to completely digest the microorganisms.
Histology	Biopsy shows foamy, lipid-laden histiocytes infiltrating the lung in a lymphatic pattern of distribution, with aggregates of histiocytes seen in the pleura and subpleural zones, *(Figs. 29.1–29.3)*, interlobular septa, and coursing along the bronchovascular bundles *(Figs. 29.4 and 29.5)*. Histiocytes have round-to-oval nuclei and abundant eosinophilic foamy cytoplasm *(Fig. 29.3)*. In contrast to malakoplakia, the histiocytes of ECD are lipid laden and do not have periodic acid–Schiff (PAS)-positive cytoplasmic material or calcified Michaelis–Gutmann bodies. The aggregates of histiocytes can be associated with variable amounts of fibrosis lymphocytes, and plasma cells, but is not associated with acute inflammation, abscess formation, or cavitation in contrast to malakoplakia.	Malakoplakia shows an acute inflammatory process with neutrophils and patchy necrosis. The lung tissue has abundant macrophages and histiocytes with eosinophilic cytoplasm *(Figs. 29.6 and 29.7)*. PAS-positive material is present within macrophages and can calcify to become Michaelis–Gutmann bodies *(Figs. 29.8 and 29.9 arrows)*. The bacterial organisms may be visualized on Gram stain and within the cytoplasmic endosomes of macrophages *(Fig. 29.8, arrowheads)*.

	Erdheim–Chester Disease (ECD)	Malakoplakia
Special studies	Unlike pulmonary Langerhans cell histiocytosis, the histiocytes of ECD are negative for CD1a, but express other histiocytic markers such as CD68 and S100. Oil red O in fresh tissue or bronchoalveolar lavage can highlight lipid droplets in the cytoplasm of foamy histiocytes of ECD.	Gram stain is useful in identifying the bacterial organisms. *R. equi* organisms are partially acid-fast and may show weak staining on Fite stain, but do not stain with Ziehl–Neelsen acid-fast stains. PAS stains can highlight accumulated cytoplasmic material. By electron microscopy, this PAS-positive material in the histiocytes cytoplasm has been shown to represent large phagolysosomes that contain broken-down organisms. This may calcify and form Michaelis–Gutmann bodies. Van Kossa and Prussian Blue special stains decorate the Michaelis–Gutmann bodies in malakoplakia *(Fig. 29.10* and *29.11)*.
Prognosis	The prognosis is poor, with approximately 50% survival at 3 y. Treatment is aimed at immunosuppression/immune modulation, although cases associated with BRAF mutation have shown dramatic response to targeted therapy.	Antibiotic treatment and multidrug regimens are often able to achieve a cure in infected patients. For patients with abscesses and extensive cavitation, surgical resection of the lesions may be required.

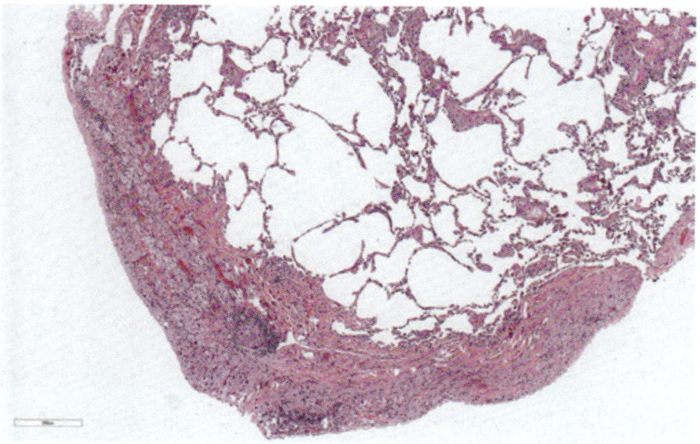

Figure 29.1 ECD: A low-power view of ECD showing the collections of foamy histiocytes, following a lymphatic distribution involving the pleura and subpleural zone. Unlike malakoplakia, ECD does not show acute inflammation, abscess formation, or necrosis/cavitary lesions.

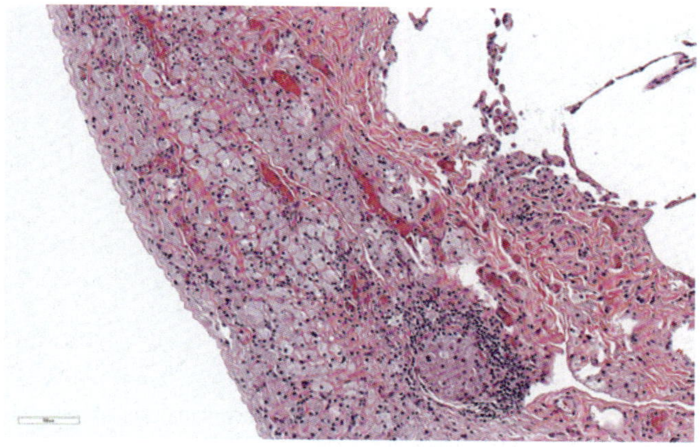

Figure 29.2 ECD: High-power view of Figure 29.1 showing foamy histiocytes of ECD involving the pleura and subpleural zone. The macrophages and histiocytes of ECD are lipid laden and do not have PAS-positive inclusions or Michaelis–Gutmann bodies like malakoplakia.

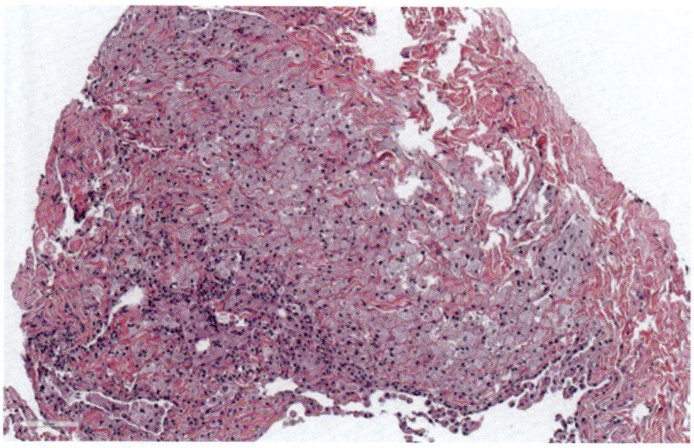

Figure 29.3 ECD: A high-power view showing the foamy histiocytes of ECD embedded in the collagen of the pleura.

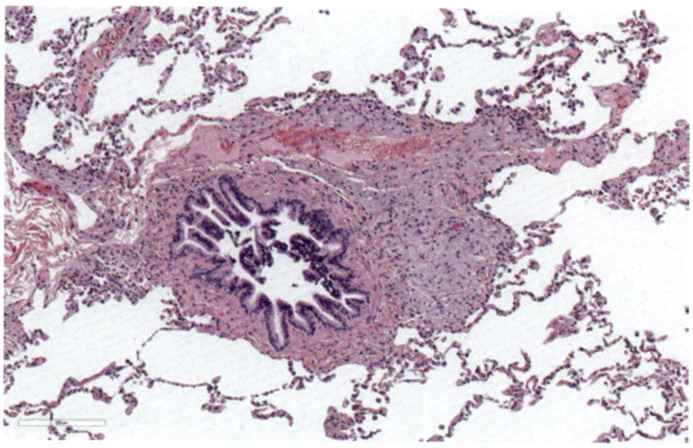

Figure 29.4 ECD: A case of ECD showing collections of foamy histiocytes along the lymphatic channels of the bronchovascular bundle.

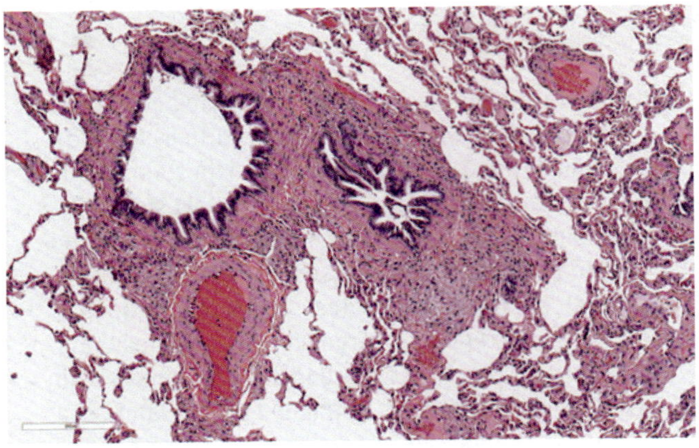

Figure 29.5 ECD: The foamy histiocytes are found in association with the lymphatic channels near the bronchiole and pulmonary artery.

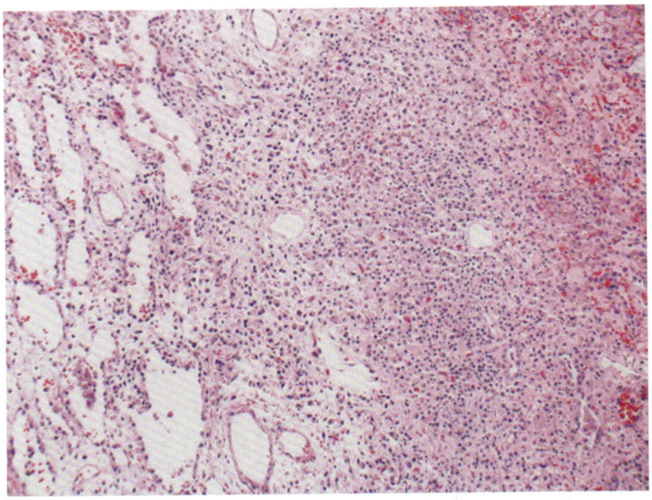

Figure 29.6 Malakoplakia: A low-power view of malakoplakia showing macrophages and mixed inflammatory cells (Courtesy of Dr. Yale Rosen).

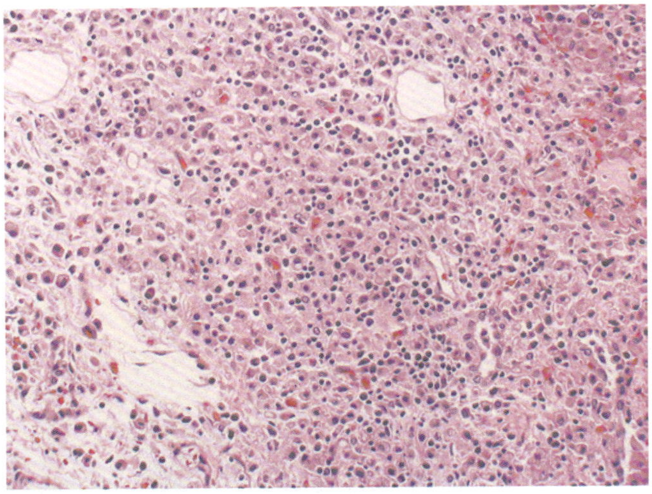

Figure 29.7 Malakoplakia: A higher-power view of malakoplakia showing macrophages with eosinophilic cytoplasm and mixed inflammatory cells. Unlike ECD, the macrophages of malakoplakia are not lipid laden. (Courtesy of Dr. Yale Rosen).

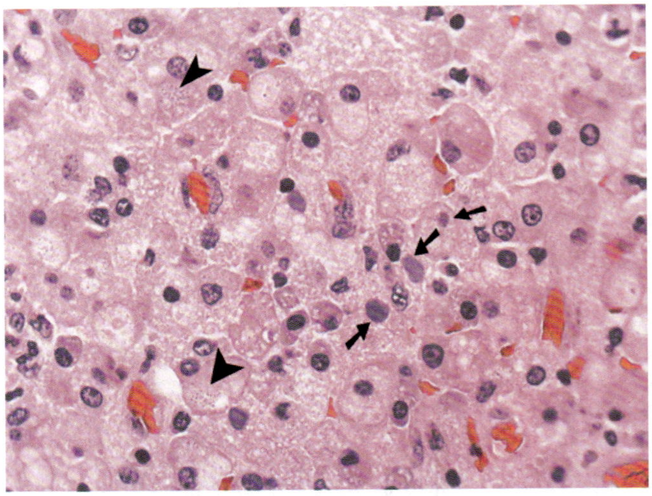

Figure 29.8 Malakoplakia: A high-power view of malakoplakia with bacterial organisms containing macrophage endosomes *(arrowheads)*, along with cytoplasmic calcified Michaelis–Gutmann bodies (*arrows*) (Courtesy of Dr. Yale Rosen).

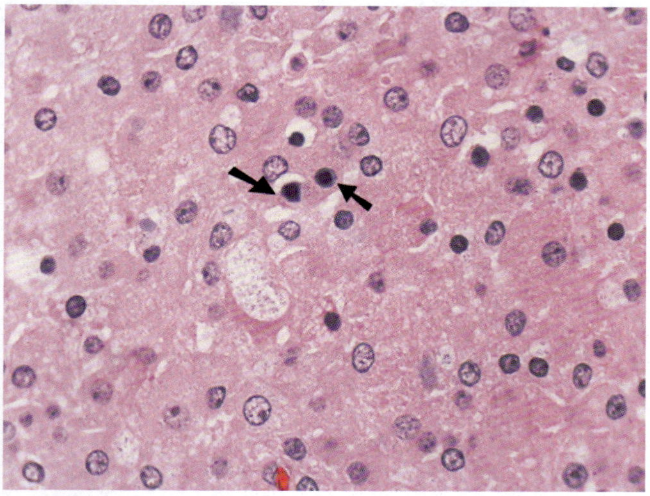

Figure 29.9 Malakoplakia: Michaelis-Gutmann bodies have a targetoid shape (*arrows*), and are pathognomonic of malakoplakia. They are composed of calcified debris of incompletely digested bacteria. (Courtesy of Dr. Yale Rosen).

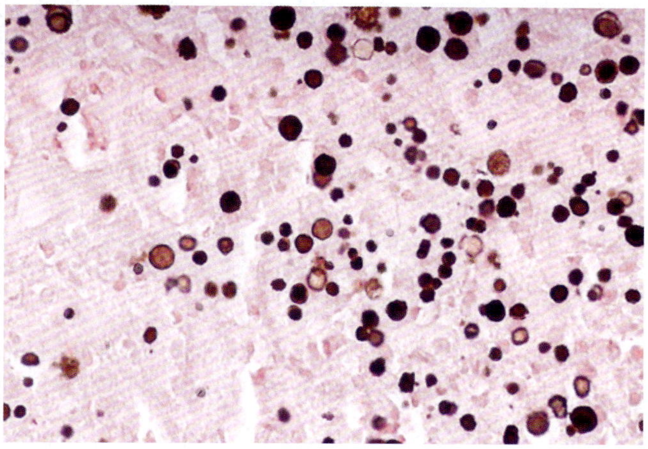

Figure 20.10 Malakoplakia: Von Kossa stain highlights the Michaelis–Gutmann (M–G) bodies. (Courtesy of Dr. Yale Rosen).

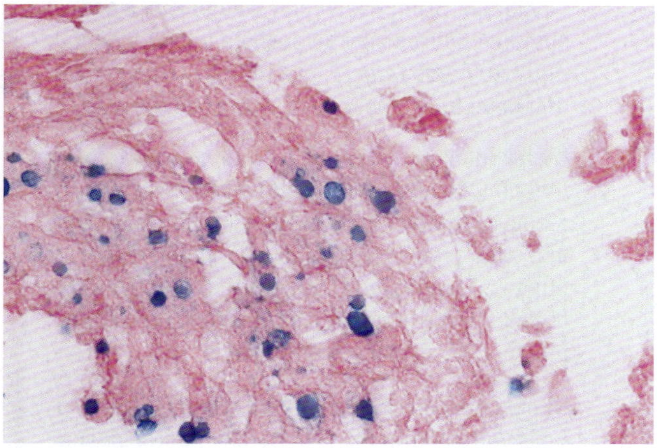

Figure 29.11 Malakoplakia: Iron stain decorates the M–G bodies (Courtesy of Dr. Yale Rosen).

30 CRYSTAL-STORING HISTIOCYTOSIS VS. MALAKOPLAKIA

	Crystal-Storing Histiocytosis (CSH)	Malakoplakia
Age	Pulmonary CSH is most commonly seen in patients 60 and older, with a similar incidence in men and women.	Malakoplakia is a rare disorder that can affect adults with underlying immunodeficiency. There is no known gender predominance to the disease.
Location	CSH may occur as a solitary mass or multiple masses anywhere in the lungs or pleura.	Although any part of the lung may be affected, this disease favors the upper lobes and is generally multifocal.
Symptoms	Since CSH is virtually always seen in the context of lymphoproliferative disease and multiple myeloma, the symptoms are largely those of the underlying hematologic condition.	Patients often present with nonspecific signs of infections, including cough, fever, dyspnea, and chest pain.
Signs	CSH may occur either as a solitary pulmonary nodule or as multiple nodules. The nodules may appear in either lung and do not show a clear lobar preference.	Radiographic studies demonstrate upper lobe predominant multifocal consolidation, often with cavitation. Bronchoalveolar lavage (BAL) and sputum cultures may be positive for *Rhodococcus equi*, *Acinetobacter*, *E. coli*, or other organisms that have been associated with malakoplakia.
Etiology	CSH results from intracytoplasmic deposition of crystalline immunoglobulins within nonneoplastic histiocytes and is usually associated with a lymphoplasmacytic/plasmacytic neoplasm. The intracytoplasmic crystalline immunoglobulins give the cells of CSH their granular cytoplasmic appearance.	Malakoplakia represents an infectious process that may develop in the setting of immunodeficiency. Organisms are present in the lung tissue and within the cytoplasmic endosomes of macrophages. The pathogenesis is related to a defect in the histiocyte function. There is inability to completely digest the microorganisms.
Histology	CSH presents as dense airspace filling by macrophages/histiocytes with eosinophilic crystalloid inclusions that are refractile on light microscopy *(Figs. 30.1–30.4)*. The histiocytes do not show cytologic atypia. The histiocytic lineage of the cells may be demonstrated on CD68 stain. The inclusions of CSH are PAS-positive and can easily be confused with the granular cytoplasm of malakoplakia. Immunostains for immunoglobulin light chains are helpful since most cases of CSH will show strong cytoplasmic staining for either the kappa or the lambda chains. Since kappa-restricted lymphoproliferative disease is more common than lambda-restricted disease, most cases of CSH are kappa restricted, which may be noted by differential immunostaining of the crystals. Gram stain will be negative for organisms on CSH unlike malakoplakia.	Malakoplakia shows an acute inflammatory process with neutrophils and patchy necrosis. The lung tissue has abundant macrophages and histiocytes with eosinophilic cytoplasm *(Figs. 30.5 and 30.6)*. Periodic acid–Schiff (PAS)-positive material is present within macrophages and can calcify to become Michaelis–Gutmann bodies *(Figs. 30.7 and 30.8 arrows)*. The bacterial organisms may be visualized on Gram stain and within the cytoplasmic endosomes of macrophages *(Fig. 30.7, arrowheads)*. Michaelis–Gutmann bodies have a targetoid shape and are pathognomonic of malakoplakia.

	Crystal-Storing Histiocytosis (CSH)	Malakoplakia
Special studies	Immunohistochemistry (IHC) is used for kappa and lambda light chains and CD68. Gram stain is used to rule out bacterial organisms. Electron microscopy shows rectangular, rhomboid, and needle-shaped intracytoplasmic crystals.	Gram stain is useful in identifying the bacterial organisms. *R. equi* organisms are partially acid-fast and may show weak staining on Fite stain, but do not stain with Ziehl–Neelsen acid-fast stains. PAS stain can highlight accumulated cytoplasmic material. By electron microscopy, this PAS-positive material in the histiocytes cytoplasm has been shown to represent large phagolysosomes that contain broken-down organisms. This may calcify and form Michaelis–Gutmann bodies. Van Kossa and Prussian Blue special stains decorate the Michaelis–Gutmann bodies in malakoplakia *(Fig.30.9 and 30.10)*.
Prognosis	The prognosis of patients with CSH is largely dominated by the prognosis of their underlying hematologic malignancy. As compared with patients who have the same underlying hematologic malignancy, patients with CSH typically have a worse prognosis than do patients without CSH.	Antibiotic treatment and multidrug regimens are often able to achieve a cure in infected patients. For patients with abscesses and extensive cavitation, surgical resection of the lesions may be required.

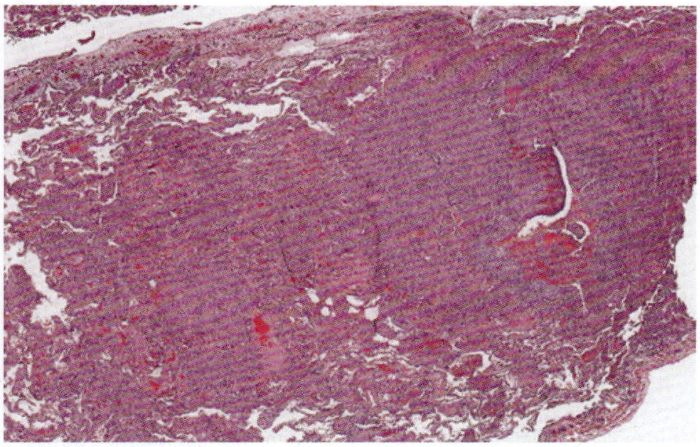

Figure 30.1 CSH: Low power view showing lung consolidation by dense mass-like lesion composed of histiocytes with eosinophilic cytoplasm.

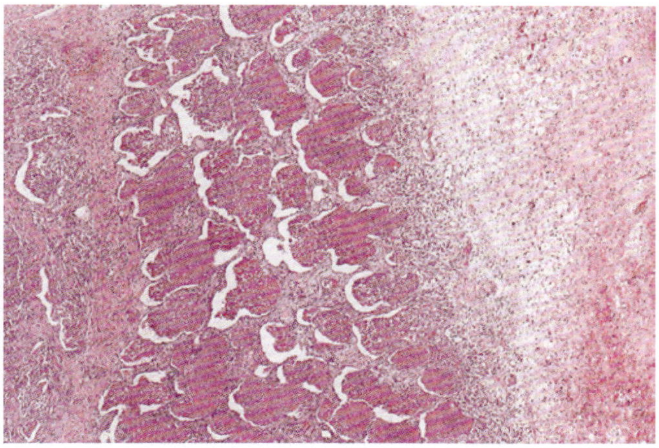

Figure 30.2 CSH: A low-power view showing dense airspace filling by macrophages with eosinophilic cytoplasm.

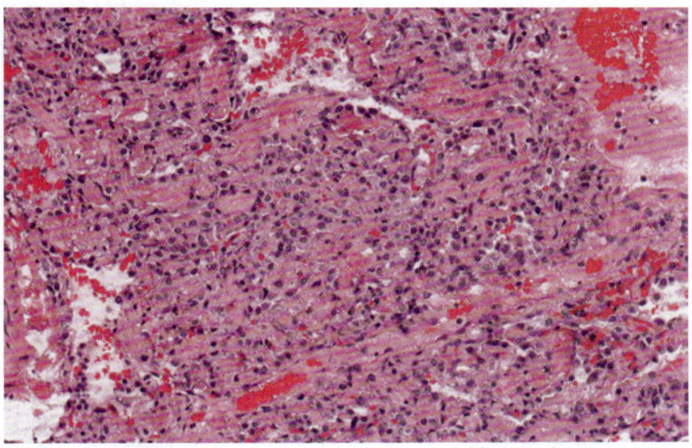

Figure 30.3 CSH: Higher-power view showing sheets of large polygonal histiocytes containing intracytoplasmic eosinophilic needle-like crystals. The crystals are PAS-positive and are composed immunoglobulin light chain.

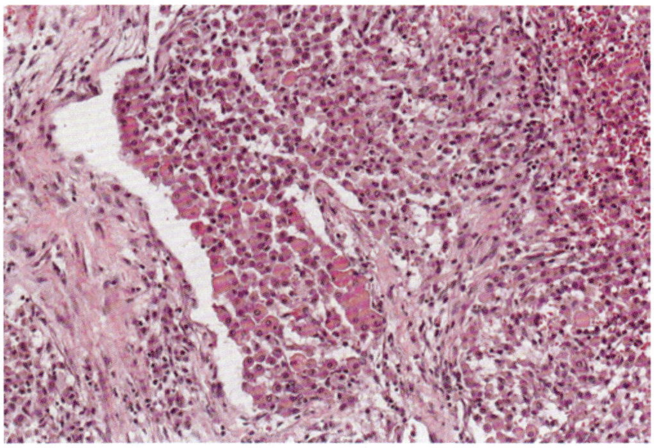

Figure 30.4 CSH: Airspaces consolidated by the crystal-laden eosinophilic macrophages.

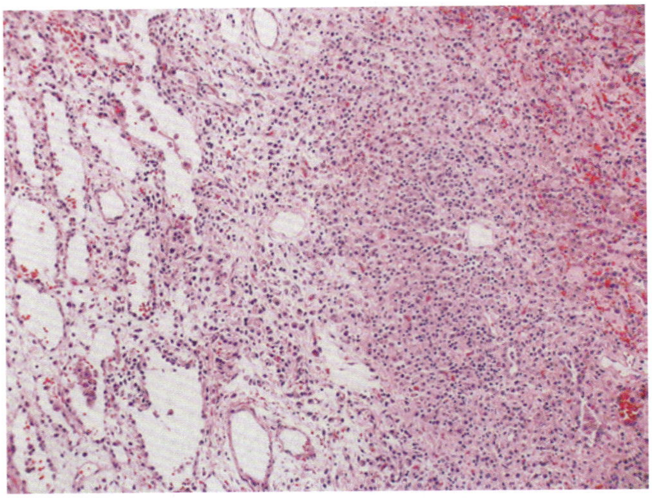

Figure 30.5 Malakoplakia: A low-power view showing macrophages and mixed inflammatory cells. (Courtesy of Dr. Yale Rosen.)

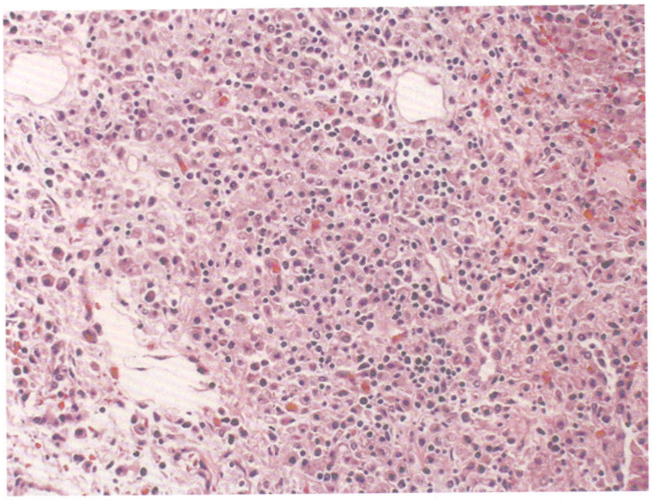

Figure 30.6 Malakoplakia: A high-power view showing macrophages with eosinophilic cytoplasm and mixed inflammatory cells. Unlike CSH, the macrophages of malakoplakia do not contain crystalloid cytoplasmic inclusions. (Courtesy of Dr. Yale Rosen.)

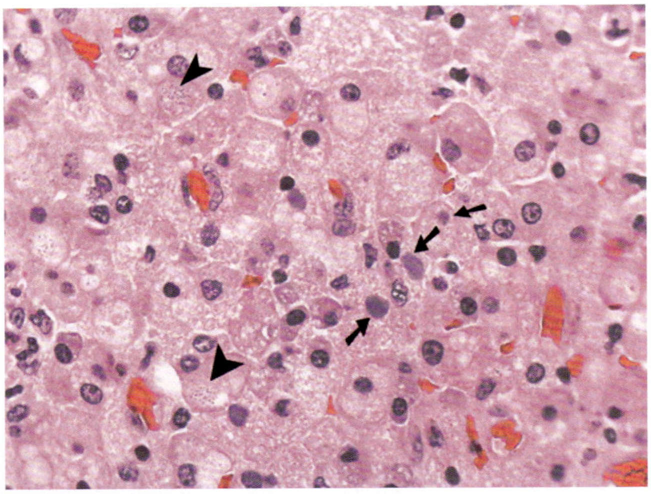

Figure 30.7 Malakoplakia: A high-power view showing bacterial organisms containing macrophage endosomes (*arrowheads*), along with cytoplasmic calcified Michaelis–Gutmann bodies (*arrows*). (Courtesy of Dr. Yale Rosen.)

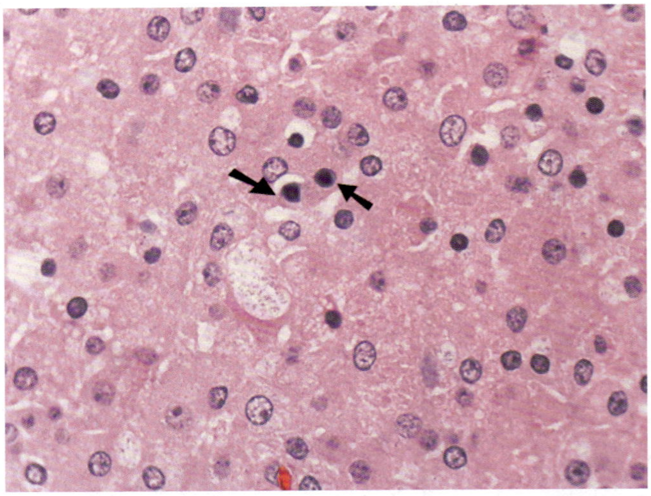

Figure 30.8 Malakoplakia: Michaelis–Gutmann bodies have a targetoid shape (*arrows*) and are pathognomonic of malakoplakia. They are composed of calcified debris of incompletely digested bacteria. (Courtesy of Dr. Yale Rosen.)

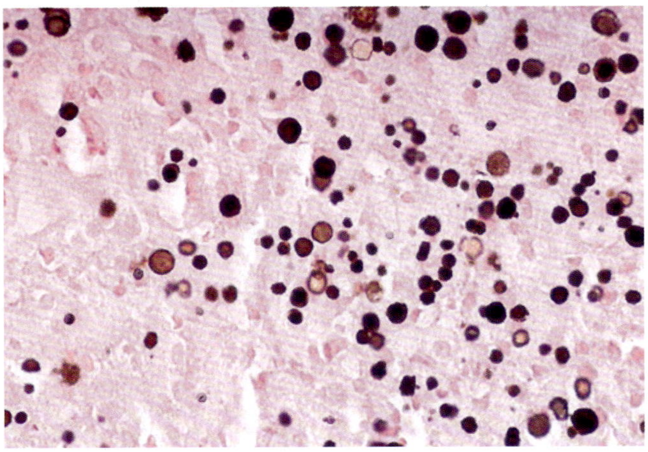

Figure 30.9 Malakoplakia: Von Kossa stain highlights the Michaelis–Gutmann bodies. (Courtesy of Dr. Yale Rosen.)

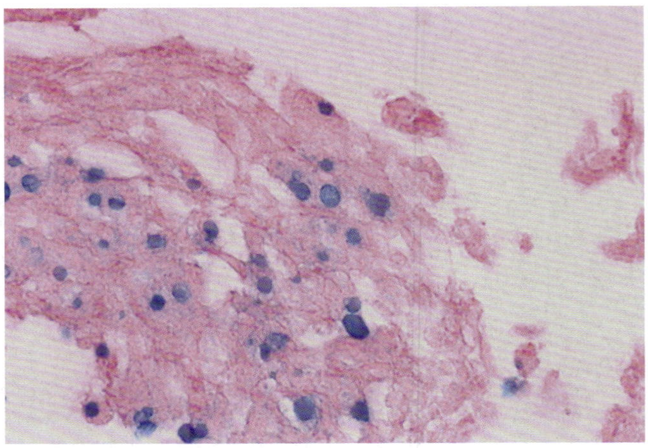

Figure 30.10 Malakoplakia: Iron stain decorates the Michaelis–Gutmann bodies. (Courtesy of Dr. Yale Rosen.)

31 ERDHEIM–CHESTER DISEASE VS. PULMONARY LANGERHANS CELL HISTIOCYTOSIS

	Erdheim–Chester Disease (ECD)	Pulmonary Langerhans Cell Histiocytosis (PLCH)
Age	ECD is a very rare disease that can present in both children and adults, ranging from 4 to 87 years of age, with a mean age at diagnosis of 53 years, and slight male predominance.	PLCH is a smoking-related disease of young adults, with most cases presenting in the second to fourth decades of life. Although the disease is more common in men, shifting smoking patterns are increasing the incidence in women.
Location	The disease usually involves the diaphyses of the long bones. However, more than 50% of cases have extraskeletal involvement. This can include lung, kidney, skin, brain, and orbit involvement, among other sites.	Like many of the inhalational and smoking-related diseases, PLCH affects the upper lobes more than the lower lobes and typically shows bilateral involvement.
Symptoms	Symptoms include dyspnea, pain in the bones of the legs, fever, weight loss, exophthalmos, and periorbital xanthomas.	Many cases of PLCH are asymptomatic, but others may present with dyspnea, nonproductive cough, and pleuritic pain. Patients with PLCH are at high risk for pneumothorax, and for some cases pneumothorax may be the initial presenting symptom.
Signs	EDC follows a lymphatic pattern of distribution in the lung involving pleural and subpleural zones, interlobular septa, and coursing along bronchovascular bundles. Radiographic findings in the lung include thickened interlobular septa, thickened lung fissures, ground glass, centrilobular nodularity, and reticular interstitial changes. The long bones show symmetric diaphyseal osteosclerosis.	On high-resolution CT scans of the chest, PLCH shows upper lobe predominant centrilobular nodules and thin-walled cysts.
Etiology	ECD is a histiocytic disease of non–Langerhans cell histiocytes that derive from the monocyte lineage. The cause of the disease remains unknown. In some cases, BRAF V600E mutations and RAS mutations have been identified and are potential targets for treatment.	Lung-limited PLCH is almost exclusively smoking related. Although tobacco appears to be the etiologic agent, the mechanism of disease is unknown.

	Erdheim–Chester Disease (ECD)	Pulmonary Langerhans Cell Histiocytosis (PLCH)
Histology	Biopsy shows foamy lipid-laden histiocytes infiltrating the lung in a lymphatic pattern of distribution with aggregates of histiocytes seen in the pleura and subpleural zones *(Figs. 31.1–31.3)*, interlobular septa, and coursing along the bronchovascular bundles *(Figs. 31.4 and 31.5)*. Histiocytes have round-to-oval nuclei and abundant eosinophilic foamy cytoplasm *(Fig. 31.3)*. In contrast, the histiocytes of PLCH are not foamy. The aggregates of histiocytes can be associated with variable amounts of fibrosis, but the scarring lacks the stellate character of PLCH.	*Proliferative* (*cellular*) *phase*: Airway-centered stellate to irregular cellular nodules composed of clusters of Langerhans cells *(Figs. 31.6 and 31.7)*, admixed with variable number of eosinophils, lymphocytes, plasma cells, neutrophils, and macrophages *(Fig. 31.8)*. Variable-sized cysts lacking cell lining are formed at the periphery of the nodules by traction of the adjacent alveolar septa or destructive dilation of bronchioles. *Fibrotic phase*: The nodules can be seen at different stages of cellularity and fibrosis. However, with the aging of the lesions, the Langerhans cells and other inflammatory cells become progressively decreased in number and overshadowed by fibrosis, eventually evolving into stellate-to-irregular scars *(Fig. 31.9)*. The airspaces adjacent to the fibrotic areas may become cystically dilated. In severe cases, interstitial fibrosis with honeycomb may develop. The bronchiolocentric fibrotic scars often maintain the stellate shape of the cellular lesions, which is a clue that suggests PLCH in cases where only fibrotic lesions are sampled in the biopsy.
Special studies	Unlike PLCH, the histiocytes of ECD are negative for CD1a, but express other histiocytic markers such as CD68 and S100. Oil red O in fresh tissue or bronchoalveolar lavage can highlight the lipid-laden histiocytes of ECD.	Immunoperoxidase stains CD1a *(Fig. 31.10)* and S100 decorate small clusters or sheets of Langerhans cells in the pulmonary interstitial nodular lesions as well as in adjacent alveoli. It should be noted that Langerhans cells can be found in other inflammatory (and neoplastic) lung diseases, where they occur *singly*. In PLCH, the Langerhans cells are *aggregated in clusters*, usually aggregates of more than 25 LCs. Cytoplasmic Birbeck granules and pentalaminar rod (or racket)-shaped organelles are identified by electron microscopic study. In contrast, the histiocytes of ECD are negative for CD1a. Some cases have a mutation in BRAF gene (V600E), although at this point relatively few of the tested cases were of lung origin.

	Erdheim–Chester Disease (ECD)	Pulmonary Langerhans Cell Histiocytosis (PLCH)
Prognosis	The prognosis is poor, with approximately 50% survival at 3 y. Treatment is aimed at immunosuppression/immune modulation, although cases associated with BRAF mutation have shown dramatic response to targeted therapy.	Variable and unpredictable. Clinical and radiologic stabilization or resolution of the disease occurs in 50% of patients, spontaneous regression in up to 25%, and progression to respiratory failure due to irreversible fibrosis in approximately 25%. In advanced cases, pulmonary hypertension and cor pulmonale may develop. Some patients develop and die of malignancies including lung cancer, lymphoma, and myeloproliferative disorders. The median survival is 12 y, with 5- and 10-y survival rates of 74% and 64%, respectively. Smoking cessation is recommended for all patients. Immunosuppression with corticosteroids, with or without the addition of chemotherapeutic agents, has been used to treat patients with variable results. Lung transplantation has been performed and has been successful in treating patients with advanced disease, although relapse of PLCH in the transplanted lung has been reported. BRAF target therapy might be useful.

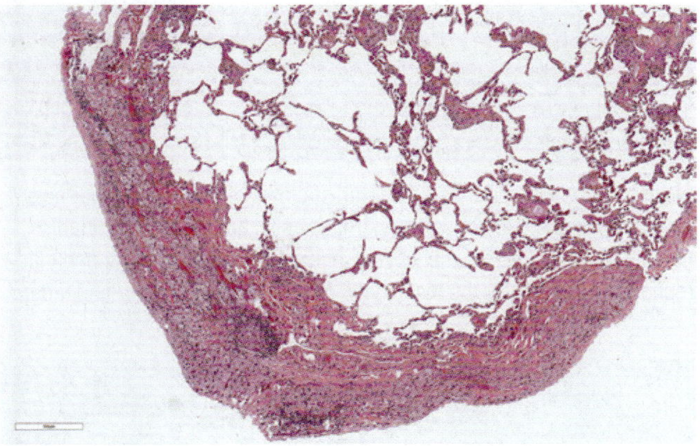

Figure 31.1 ECD: A low-power view showing collections of foamy histiocytes, following a lymphatic distribution involving the pleura and subpleural zone unlike PLCH, which follows an airway-centered distribution.

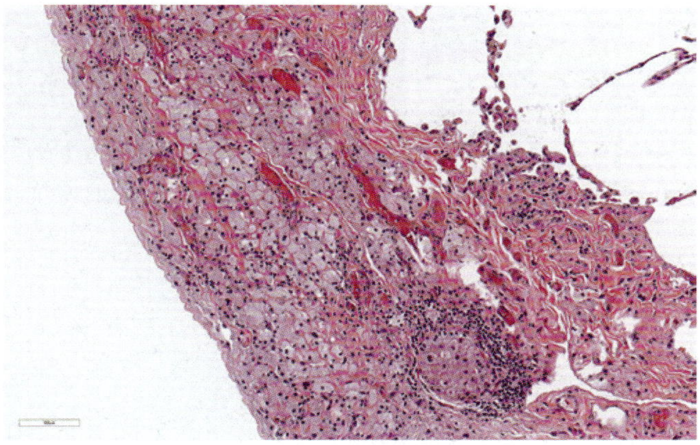

Figure 31.2 ECD: High-power view of Figure 31.1 showing foamy histiocytes of ECD involving the pleura and subpleural zone. Foamy histiocytes are not a feature of PLCH.

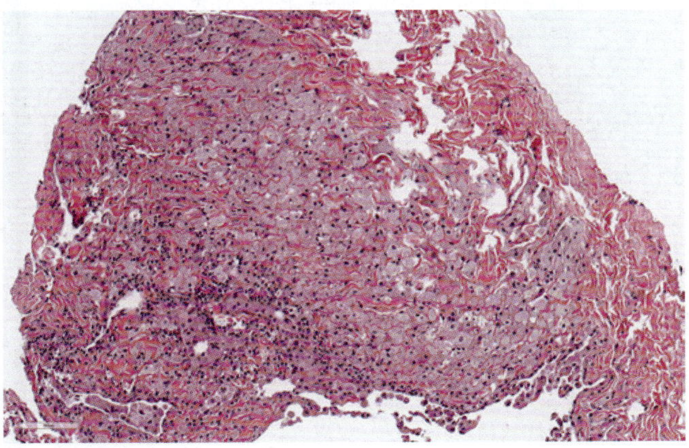

Figure 31.3 ECD: Foamy histiocytes are embedded in the collagen of the pleura.

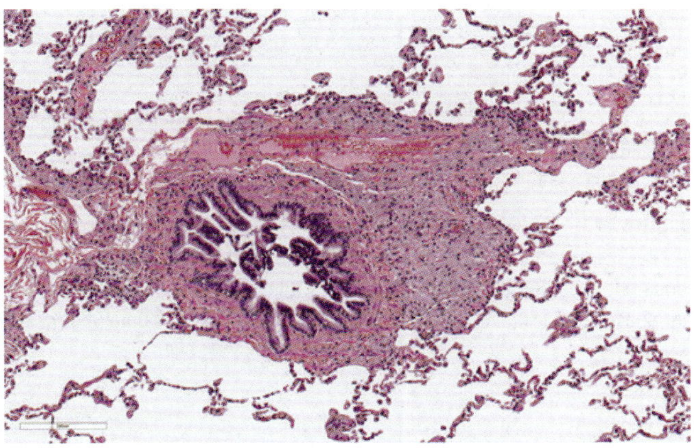

Figure 31.4 ECD: A case of ECD showing collections of foamy histiocytes along with lymphatic channels of the bronchovascular bundle. While PLCH may also involve the airway-centered parenchyma, the Langerhans cells are not foamy/lipid laden as seen in ECD.

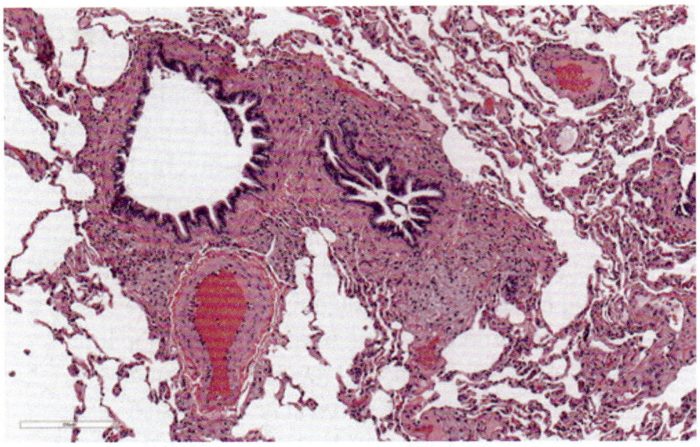

Figure 31.5 ECD: The foamy macrophages of ECD may be found along the lymphatic channels of the bronchioles and pulmonary arteries.

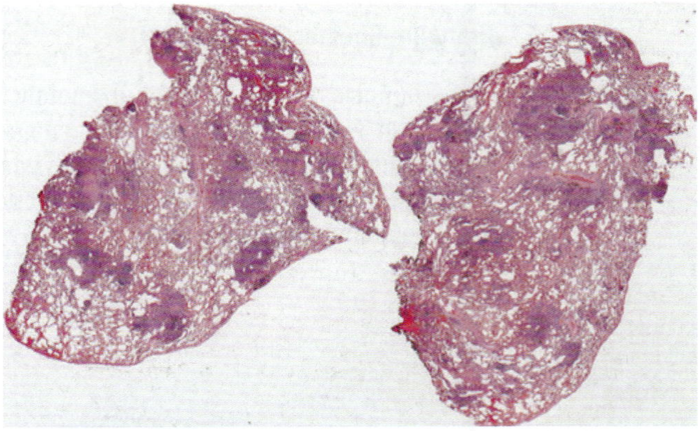

Figure 31.6 PLCH: Airway-centered stellate-to-irregular cellular nodules.

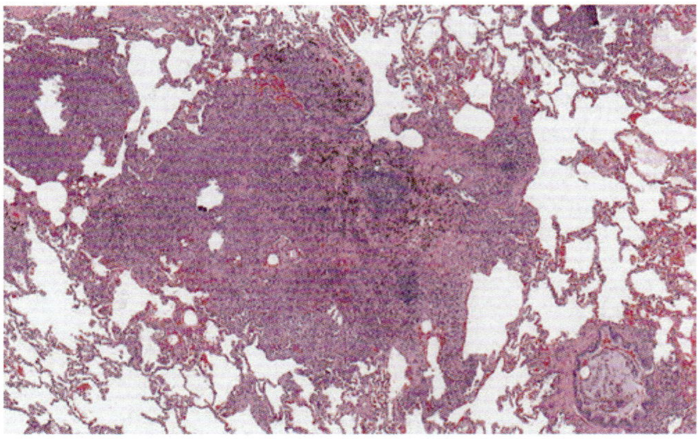

Figure 31.7 PLCH: PLCH cellular nodule. Note bronchiolectasis with mucostasis (*right lower corner*).

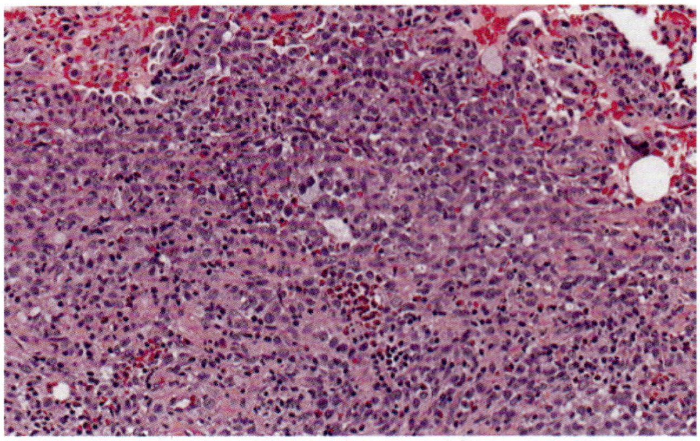

Figure 31.8 PLCH: Airway-centered stellate-to-irregular cellular nodules composed of clusters of Langerhans cells, admixed with variable number of eosinophils, lymphocytes, plasma cells, neutrophils, and macrophages. Unlike ECD, the histiocytes of PLCH are not foamy/lipid laden.

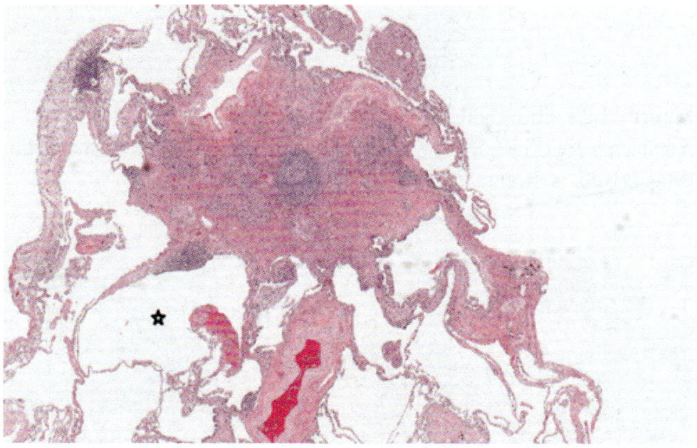

Figure 31.9 PLCH: As the lesions of PLCH age, they leave characteristic stellate scars encasing the bronchioles. In contrast, the fibrosis of ECD does not have a stellate airway-centered appearance. Note dilated alveolar space/peribronchiolar cyst adjacent to PLCH fibrotic nodule (*asterisk*).

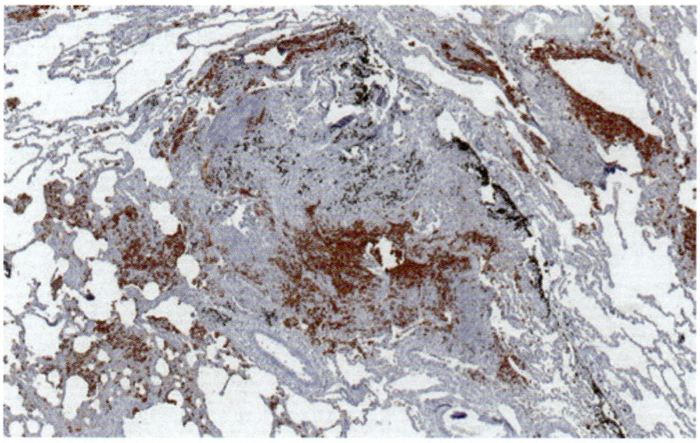

Figure 31.10 PLCH: Immunoperoxidase stain CD1a decorates clusters and sheets of Langerhans cells within the cellular nodule, confirming the diagnosis of PLCH. The histiocytes of ECD are lipid laden and negative for CD1a.

32 PULMONARY LANGERHANS CELL HISTIOCYTOSIS VS. LYMPHANGIOLEIOMYOMATOSIS

	Pulmonary Langerhans Cell Histiocytosis (PLCH)	**Lymphangioleiomyomatosis (LAM)**
Age	PLCH is a smoking-related disease of young adults with most cases presenting in the second to fourth decade. Although the disease is more common in males, shifting smoking patterns are increasing the incidence in women.	For sporadic cases, the disease is almost exclusively seen in women of reproductive age. In cases associated with tuberous sclerosis complex, men and children may rarely present with the disease.
Location	Like many of the inhalational and smoking-related diseases, PLCH affects the upper lobes more than the lower lobes and typically shows bilateral involvement.	The disease presents with cysts and small nodules randomly scattered throughout the lung, with no lobar preference.
Symptoms	Many cases of PLCH are asymptomatic, but others may present with dyspnea, nonproductive cough, and pleuritic pain. Patients with PLCH are at high risk for pneumothorax, and in some cases, pneumothorax may be the initial presenting symptom.	Spontaneous pneumothorax, dyspnea, and chylous effusions.
Signs	On high-resolution CT scans of the chest, PLCH shows upper lobe predominate centrilobular nodules and thin-walled cysts.	Scattered thin-walled cysts and small nodules found throughout the lung, with no preference for the upper lobes (as opposed to PLCH) or near the mediastinum (Birt–Hogg–Dube syndrome).
Etiology	Lung-limited PLCH is almost exclusively smoking related. Although tobacco appears to be the etiologic agent, the mechanism of disease is unknown.	The mechanism is thought to be a form of neoplasia with bundles of modified smooth muscle cells forming nodules or small masses associated with cystic dilation of airspaces.

	Pulmonary Langerhans Cell Histiocytosis (PLCH)	Lymphangioleiomyomatosis (LAM)
Histology	*Proliferative (cellular) phase*: Airway-centered stellate-to-irregular cellular nodules composed of clusters of Langerhans cells *(Figs. 32.1–32.3)*, admixed with variable number of eosinophils, lymphocytes, plasma cells, neutrophils, and macrophages *(Fig. 32.4)*. Variable-sized cysts lacking cell lining are formed at the periphery of the nodules by traction of the adjacent alveolar septa or destructive dilation of bronchioles. Patchy foci of airspace (organizing pneumonia, *Fig. 32.5*, *arrow*) and interstitial organization may be seen. Other smoking-related lung changes including desquamative interstitial pneumonia (DIP), respiratory bronchiolitis interstitial lung disease (RBILD), emphysematous change, small airway disease with mucostasis, and peribronchiolar metaplasia may be present. Vascular changes, such as intimal proliferation and medial thickening, are often present and may account for the clinical finding of pulmonary hypertension. The pleura may show reactive eosinophilic pleuritis if the patient had pneumothoraces. *Fibrotic phase*: The lung cellular nodules can be seen at different stages of cellularity and fibrosis. However, with the aging of the lesions, the Langerhans cells and other inflammatory cells become progressively decreased in number and overshadowed by fibrosis *(Figs. 32.6 and 32.7)*, eventually evolving into stellate-to-irregular scars. The airspaces adjacent to the fibrotic areas become cystically dilated (*Fig. 32.8*, *stars*). In severe cases, interstitial fibrosis with honeycomb change may develop. The bronchiolocentric fibrotic scars often maintain the stellate shape of the cellular lesions, which is a clue that suggests PLCH in cases where only fibrotic lesions are sampled in the biopsy.	LAM is characterized by proliferation of modified smooth muscle cells within the interstitium. The smooth muscle cells are usually spindle shaped with bland-appearing elongated nuclei *(Figs. 32.10 and 32.11)*. The distribution is quite random and nodules of smooth muscle can be found around bronchioles; in the alveolar septa; around arteries, veins, and lymphatic spaces; and in the pleura. Micronodular type 2 pneumocyte hyperplasia is frequently seen associated with the smooth muscle proliferation. Air-filled cysts that contain smooth muscle at least focally in their wall are commonly seen in LAM. *(Figs. 32.12 and 32.13)*.
Special studies	Immunoperoxidase stains CD1a *(Fig. 32.9)*, langerin, and S100 decorate small clusters or sheets of Langerhans cells in the pulmonary interstitial nodular lesions as well as in adjacent alveoli. It should be noted that Langerhans cells can be found in other inflammatory (and neoplastic) lung diseases, where they occur *singly*. In PLCH, the Langerhans cells *aggregate in clusters*, usually aggregates of more than 25 LCs. Cytoplasmic Birbeck granules and pentalaminar rod (or racket)-shaped organelles are identified by electron microscopic study. Some cases have a mutation in BRAF gene (V600E), although at this point relatively few of the tested cases were of lung origin.	HMB45 *(Fig. 32.14)*, and Melan A immunoperoxidase stains, even if expressed in rare cells, are supportive of a diagnosis of LAM. Desmin typically shows diffuse staining.

	Pulmonary Langerhans Cell Histiocytosis (PLCH)	Lymphangioleiomyomatosis (LAM)
Prognosis	Variable and unpredictable. Clinical and radiologic stabilization or resolution of the disease occurs in 50% of patients, spontaneous regression in up to 25%, and progression to respiratory failure due to irreversible fibrosis in approximately 25%. In advanced cases, pulmonary hypertension and cor pulmonale may develop. Some patients develop and die of malignancies including lung cancer, lymphoma, and myeloproliferative disorders. The median survival is 12 y, with 5-y and 10-y survival rates of 74% and 64%, respectively. Smoking cessation is recommended for all patients. Immunosuppression with corticosteroids, with or without the addition of chemotherapeutic agents, has been used to treat patients with variable results. Lung transplantation has been performed and has been successful in treating patients with advanced disease, although relapse of PLCH in the transplanted lung has been reported. BRAF target therapy might be useful.	Slow progression with poor long-term survival. Patients may undergo transplantation, although there are rare reported cases of recurrence within the transplanted lung.

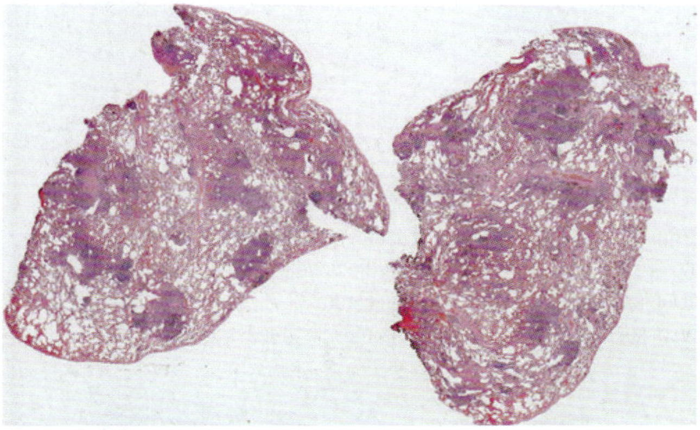

Figure 32.1 PLCH (cellular phase): Low-power view showing numerous airway-centered stellate-to-irregular cellular nodules.

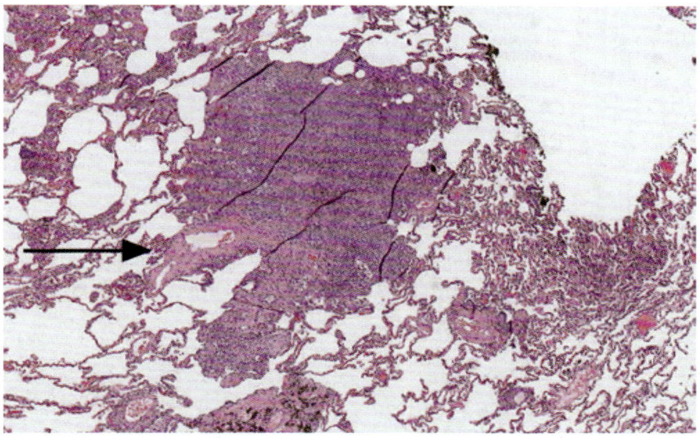

Figure 32.2 PLCH (cellular phase): High-power view of stellate-to-irregular airway-centered cellular nodule. Note pulmonary arteriole (*arrow*).

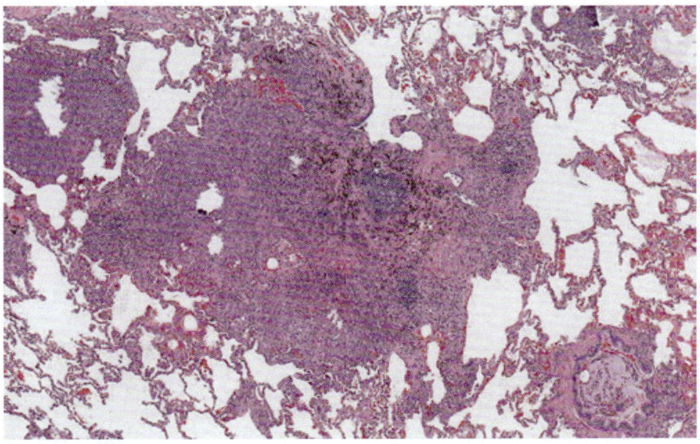

Figure 32.3 PLCH (cellular phase): Another example of PLCH cellular nodule. Note bronchiolectasis with mucostasis (*lower right corner*).

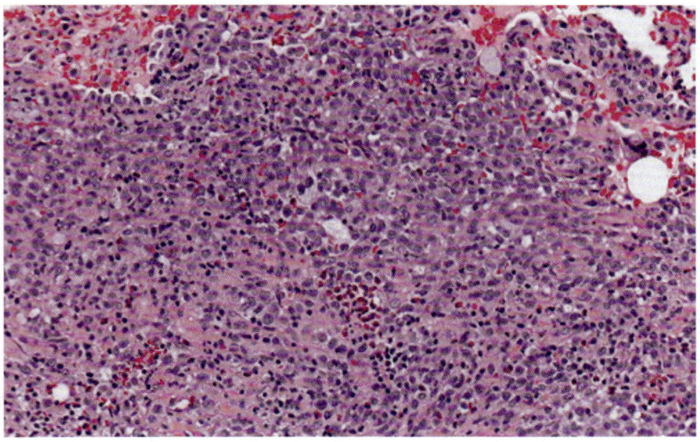

Figure 32.4 PLCH (cellular phase): The airway-centered stellate-to-irregular cellular nodules are composed of clusters of Langerhans cells, admixed with variable number of eosinophils, lymphocytes, plasma cells, neutrophils, and macrophages.

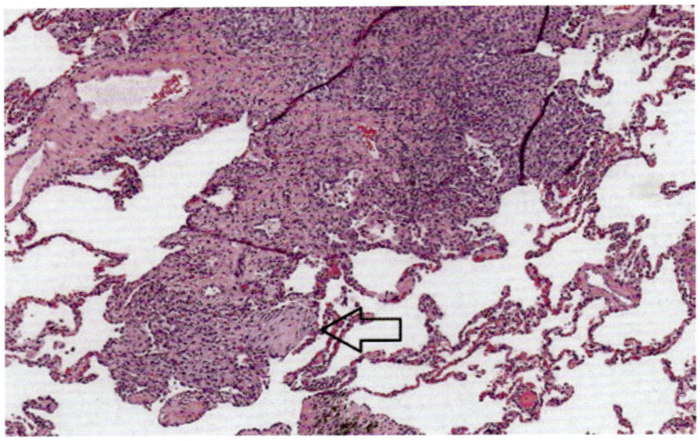

Figure 32.5 PLCH: Small foci of organizing pneumonia (*arrow*) may represent a small component of PLCH.

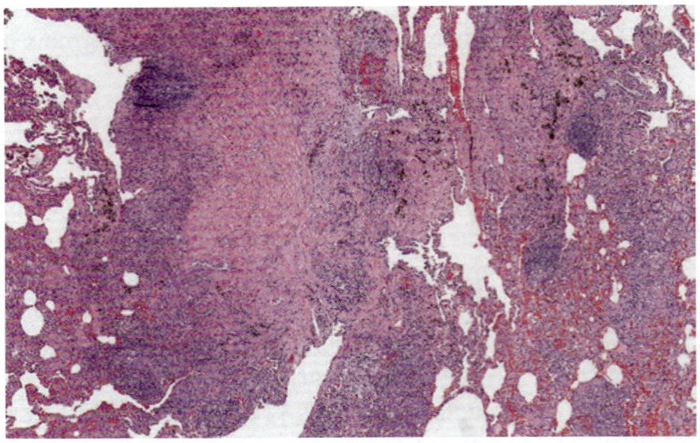

Figure 32.6 PLCH (fibrotic phase): With the aging of the lesions, the Langerhans cells and other inflammatory cells become progressively decreased in number and overshadowed by fibrosis, eventually evolving into stellate scars (see Fig. 32.7).

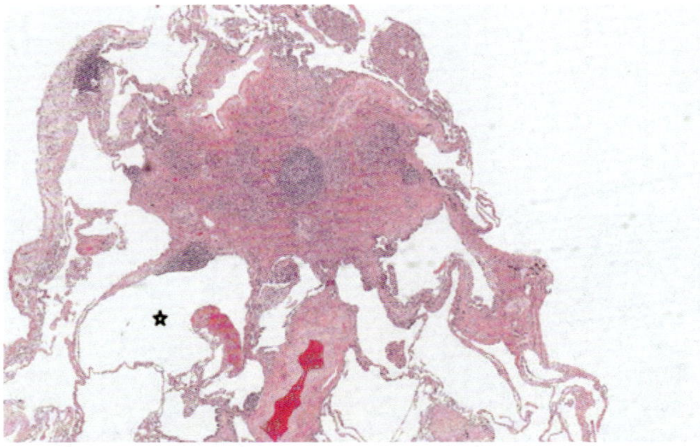

Figure 32.7 PLCH (fibrotic phase): The cellular nodules become progressively overshadowed by fibrosis, eventually evolving into stellate scars. *Star* indicates adjacent cyst.

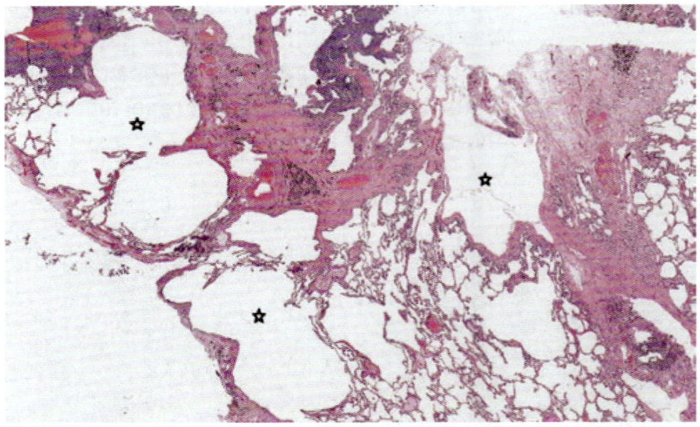

Figure 32.8 PLCH (fibrotic phase): Variable-sized cysts lacking cell lining are formed at the periphery of the nodules by traction of the adjacent alveolar septa (*stars*), also seen in Figure 32.7. Different from PLCH, the cysts seen in LAM contain smooth muscle at least focally in their walls.

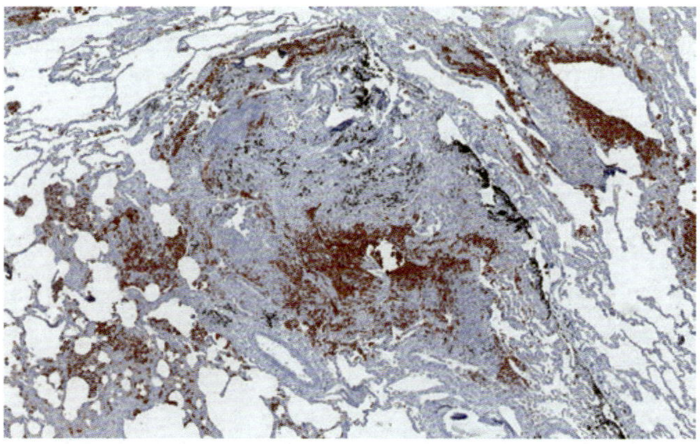

Figure 32.9 PLCH: Immunoperoxidase stain CD1a decorates clusters and sheets of Langerhans cells within the cellular nodule, confirming the diagnosis of PLCH. CD1a is negative in LAM.

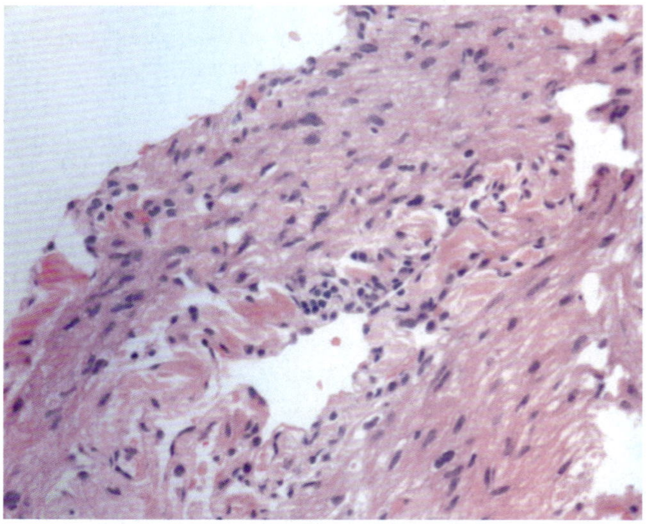

Figure 32.10 LAM: High-power view showing a proliferation of bland-appearing spindle-shaped smooth muscle cells with cigar-shaped nuclei and fibrillar eosinophilic cytoplasm.

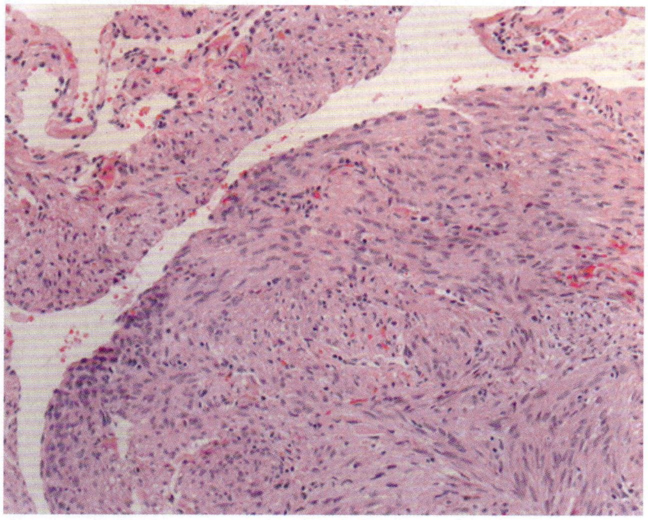

Figure 32.11 LAM: Another higher-power view of an LAM nodule showing a proliferation of modified smooth muscle cells.

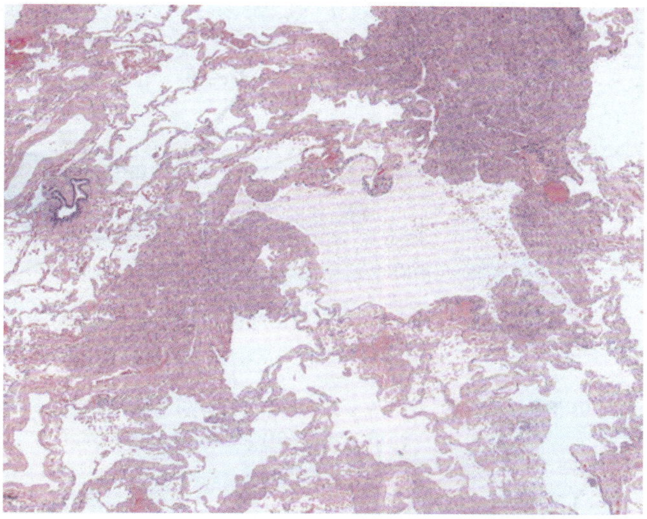

Figure 32.12 LAM: Multiple nodules of LAM cells with associated air-filled cysts seen in peribronchiolar zone (*note bronchiole in upper left*). While cysts seen in PLCH lack cell lining, the cysts seen in LAM contain smooth muscle at least focally in their walls.

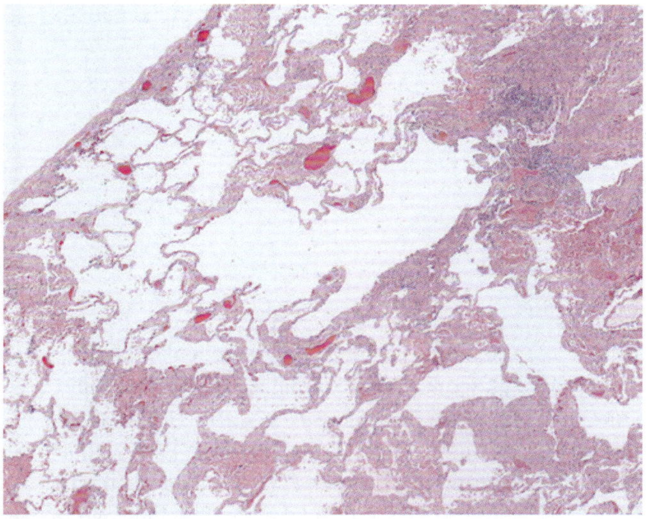

Figure 32.13 LAM: H&E stain showing a lower-power view of the nodules of smooth muscle cells associated with thin-walled air-filled cysts.

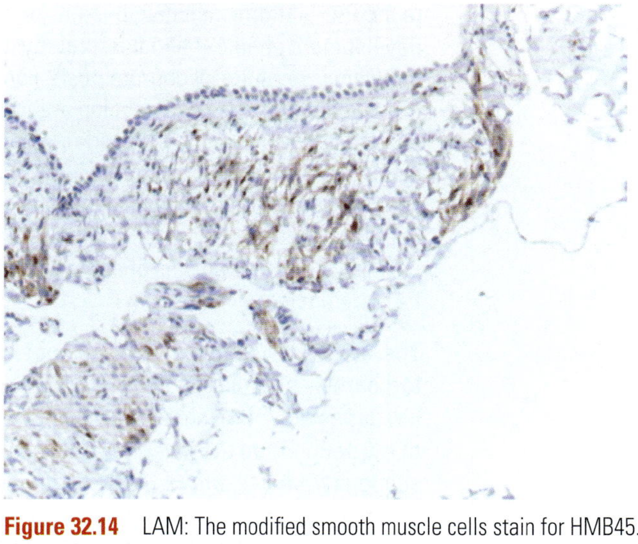

Figure 32.14 LAM: The modified smooth muscle cells stain for HMB45. HMB45 is negative in PLCH.

33 PULMONARY ALVEOLAR PROTEINOSIS VS. PULMONARY EDEMA

	Pulmonary Alveolar Proteinosis (PAP)	Pulmonary Edema
Age	PAP is typically seen in adults aged 30–50 and is more common in men than in women.	Any age.
Location	PAP is generally bilateral and symmetric in distribution.	Bilateral.
Symptoms	Many patients are asymptomatic but some develop cough and breathlessness.	If acute, breathlessness, anxiety, and feelings of drowning may develop. If more gradual, dyspnea on exertion, orthopnea, and cough. If severe, may have frothy sputum.
Signs	Radiographic studies show bilateral ground-glass opacities with interlobular septal thickening that is sometimes referred to as "crazy paving."	Classic chest x-ray shows bilateral infiltrates in a butterfly pattern with pleural effusions.
Etiology	There are several distinct mechanisms that can lead to the PAP pattern, including but not limited to the development of autoantibodies, underlying surfactant deficiency, or acute silicoproteinosis. For cases that are autoimmune, patients develop anti–GM-CSF antibodies that interfere with surfactant clearance, leading to the accumulation of fluid within the airspaces. Surfactant mutations can also cause impaired surfactant clearance and can result in PAP in children. The mechanisms of acute silicosis-induced PAP are unclear.	Cardiogenic (most common) and permeability (injury to capillary endothelial cells) causes.
Histology	There is accumulation of pink, homogeneous, fine-to-coarsely granular, protein-rich fluid within the airspaces that often shows "cracking" and a rim of retraction from the alveolar walls on permanent sections *(Figs. 33.1 and 33.2)*. The fluid may contain macrophages and needle-like acicular spaces resulting from cholesterol cleft deposition (acicular bodies). Amorphous solid eosinophilic globules are frequently seen inside the proteinaceous material. The alveolar septa remain thin, with nonreactive pneumocytes despite the fluid within the airspace. In some cases of PAP, mild septal thickening by chronic inflammation may be present *(Fig. 33.3)*. The process may appear patchy, with regions of dense fluid accumulation adjacent to uninvolved lung.	Pulmonary edema shows acellular, homogeneous pale eosinophilic material within alveolar spaces (*Figs. 33.4 and 33.5)*. The fluid of edema has less protein than PAP, with a lighter color. Unlike PAP, the fluid of edema does not have cracks within the fluid. No cholesterol clefts or globular material is present. The fluid is not associated with chronic interstitial pneumonia or type 2 cell hyperplasia.
Special studies	The periodic acid–Schiff (PAS) stain may be useful in demonstrating PAS and PAS diastase-resistant positive reactions of the PAP proteinaceous material. Electron microscopy shows abundant cellular debris and concentrically arranged laminated annular structures (lamellar bodies) within the alveolar spaces.	As pulmonary edema is a diagnosis of exclusion, PAS stain must be used to rule out alveolar proteinosis. Pneumocystis jiroveci pneumonia also enters in the differential diagnosis and GMS special stain should also be performed.

	Pulmonary Alveolar Proteinosis (PAP)	Pulmonary Edema
Prognosis	Overall prognosis is good. Some patients may spontaneously resolve while others may need lung lavage to clear the accumulated fluid. Immunosuppression has not been shown to be beneficial in most studies.	Prognosis is dependent on the cause.

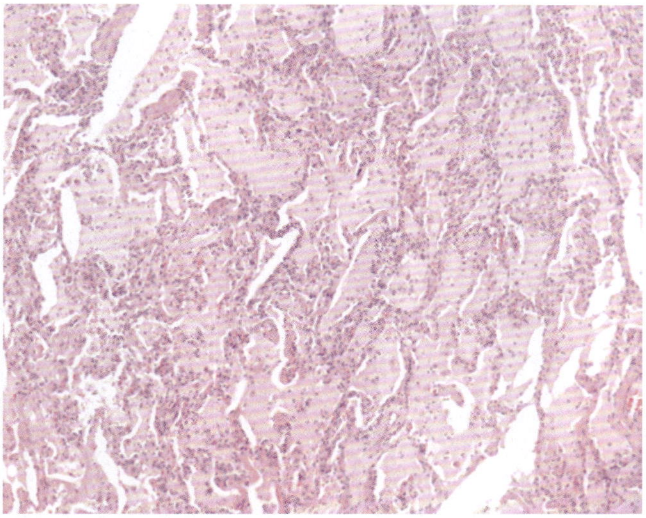

Figure 33.1 PAP: There is filling of the alveolar spaces by eosinophilic, homogeneous, fine-to-coarsely granular, amorphous material. The lung interstitial architecture is preserved.

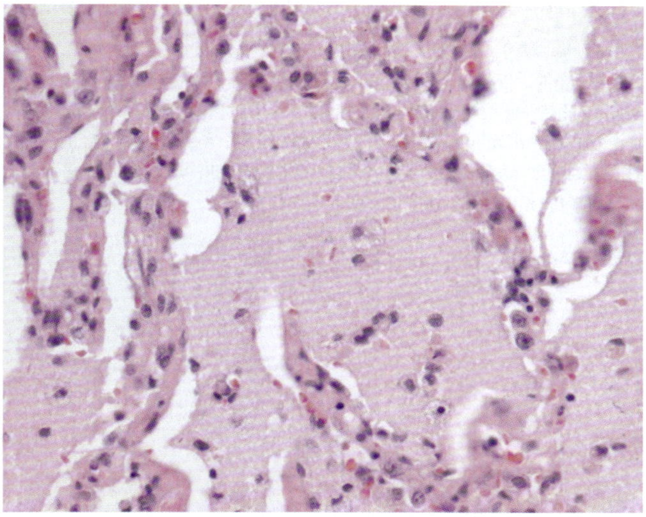

Figure 33.2 PAP: Note the granularity of the intra-alveolar material associated with a rim of retraction that separates the alveolar walls slightly from the exudates. Pulmonary edema is paler and lacks the granularity and retraction seen in PAP.

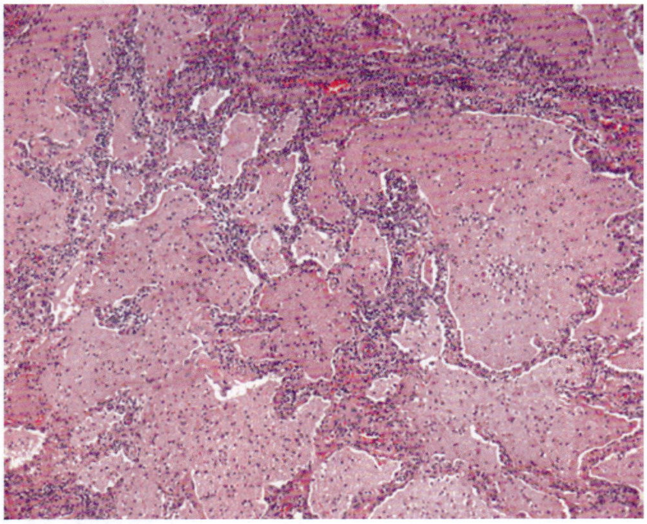

Figure 33.3 PAP: Note in this case the mild expansion of the alveolar septa by chronic inflammation. Significant inflammation and necrosis are not seen in uncomplicated cases, and their presence should suggest an associated infection.

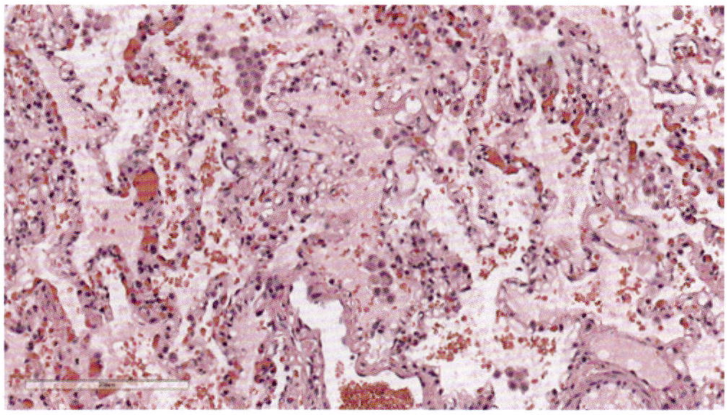

Figure 33.4 Pulmonary edema: A case of pulmonary edema showing the pale pink whispy fluid that has accumulated within the airspaces. The fluid has a low protein content, lacks granularity, and does not have the tendency to retract from the alveolar septa in the way that the fluid of PAP does.

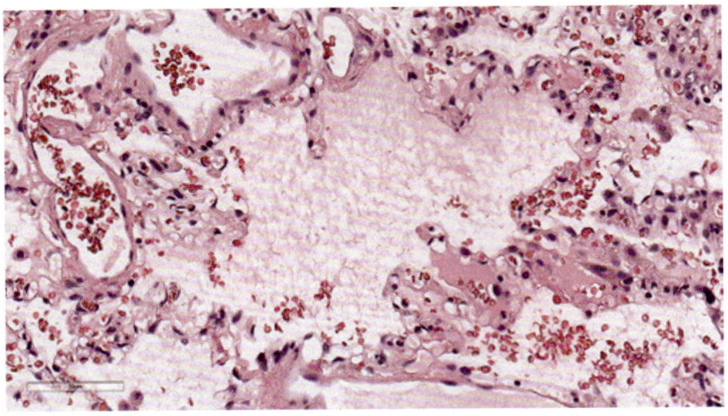

Figure 33.5 Pulmonary edema: A higher-power view of pulmonary edema showing pale homogeneous fluid and alveolar septa that are entirely free of inflammation. Some cases of PAP may show mild septal chronic inflammation, but pulmonary edema should not have any element of a chronic interstitial pneumonia.

34 CENTRILOBULAR EMPHYSEMA VS. PANACINAR EMPHYSEMA

	Centrilobular Emphysema	Panacinar Emphysema
Age	Centrilobular emphysema is generally diagnosed in adults between 50 and 75 y of age. Historically, men are more likely to develop centrilobular emphysema than are women.	Panacinar emphysema secondary to alpha-1–antitrypsin (A1AT) deficiency is often diagnosed in the third or fourth decade; however, concomitant smoking dramatically accelerates the emphysema, and smoking patients with A1AT deficiency may develop emphysema decades earlier. Both sexes are equally affected.
Location	As with many diseases associated with inhalational exposure, centrilobular emphysema is worse in the upper lobes. It involves the proximal/centriacinar aspect of the pulmonary lobule including respiratory bronchioles and surrounding airspaces.	In contrast with upper lobe predominance of centrilobular emphysema, panacinar emphysema is worse in the lung bases. It affects the whole pulmonary lobule uniformly.
Symptoms	Dyspnea is the most common presenting symptom with emphysema. While cough may be present, dyspnea is generally more debilitating.	The symptoms of panacinar emphysema are similar to centrilobular emphysema and consist predominantly of progressive dyspnea. In patients with panacinar emphysema secondary to A1AT deficiency, symptoms of liver disease may also be present.
Signs	Patients with emphysema show an obstructive pattern of pulmonary function tests with decreased FEV1 and increased total lung capacity (TLC) and residual volume (RV). CT scans show upper lobe predominant hyperinflation and lung destruction with flattening of the diaphragms. Cysts and bullae may be present.	The pulmonary function tests for panacinar emphysema are similar to centrilobular emphysema with an obstructive physiology. Chest CT scans, however, typically show basal predominant emphysema with loss of vascularity in the peripheral lungs.
Etiology	Centrilobular emphysema is highly associated with cigarette smoking. Although the mechanism of injury is not completely understood, it appears to represent a complex interplay of direct chemical damage, immunologic response to smoke exposure, and disorders in the injury repair mechanisms of the lung. The ultimate result is destruction of alveolar septa and dilation of the airspaces, leading to ineffective gas exchange and loss of elastic recoil.	For patients with emphysema secondary to A1AT deficiency, the mechanism is based on pulmonary parenchymal loss via the unregulated proteases activity (particularly elastase), in the absence of the protease inhibitor.

	Centrilobular Emphysema	Panacinar Emphysema
Histology	Centrilobular emphysema shows an airway-centered dilation of airspaces with breaking of the alveolar septa *(Figs. 34.1 and 34.2)*. The in vivo septal breakage and recoil of the broken ends may be seen as small "flags" or clubbing at the end of the broken septa *(Fig. 34.3)*. Respiratory bronchioles are enlarged or destroyed. The airspace dilation and septal damage decrease distal to the bronchioles at the center of the lobule, and this, along with the lobar distribution, is the primary difference between centrilobular and panacinar emphysema. Anthracotic pigment is frequently present in the peribronchiolar collagen as a result of smoke exposure *(Figs. 34.1 and 34.2)*. In severe cases, subpleural cysts and blebs may be present.	The distribution of alveolar airspace dilation and damage is the primary differentiator between centrilobular emphysema and panacinar emphysema. Whereas centrilobular emphysema is worse in the upper lobes and the parenchyma nearest to the bronchioles, panacinar emphysema is worse in the lower lobes and shows similar involvement of the entire lobule of the lung without the clear accentuation near bronchioles including distal alveolar sacs adjacent to the interlobular septa and pleura *(Figs. 34.4 and 34.5)*. In nonsmoking patients with panacinar emphysema, the deposition of anthracotic pigment is also less than smoking-related centrilobular emphysema.
Special studies	None.	The A1AT protease inhibitor (Pi) gene is located on the long arm of chromosome 14. There is a normal M allele and an abnormal Z allele. Analytical methods may be used to determine the A1AT phenotype. The PiMM phenotype is the most common phenotype occurring in 90% of the general population. Individuals homozygous for PiZ (PiZZ) have markedly reduced A1AT activity and are most commonly affected by symptomatic emphysema.
Prognosis	Centrilobular emphysema typically represents a progressive disease with increasing dyspnea. Patients may undergo periods of acute exacerbation of their disease with superimposed infections and respiratory failure. Medications offer modest improvements in function and quality of life. Lung transplant may be considered for patients in the appropriate age range.	The disease is characterized by slow progression of dyspnea and decline of pulmonary function. Transplant may be considered in severe cases.

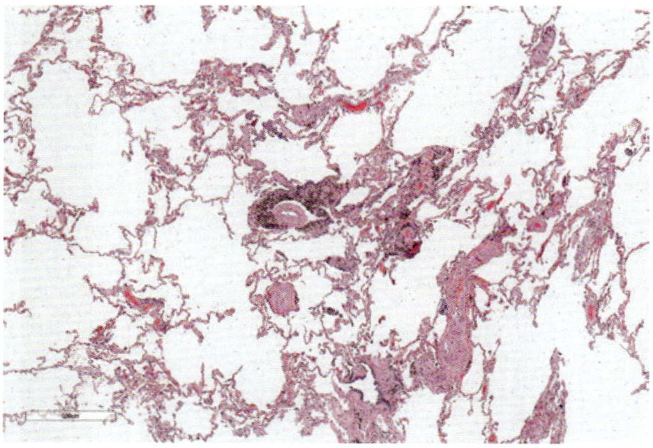

Figure 34.1 Centrilobular emphysema: An example of centrilobular emphysema with a bronchiole in the center of the image and anthracotic pigment in the adventitial collagen along with dilation of the surrounding airspaces.

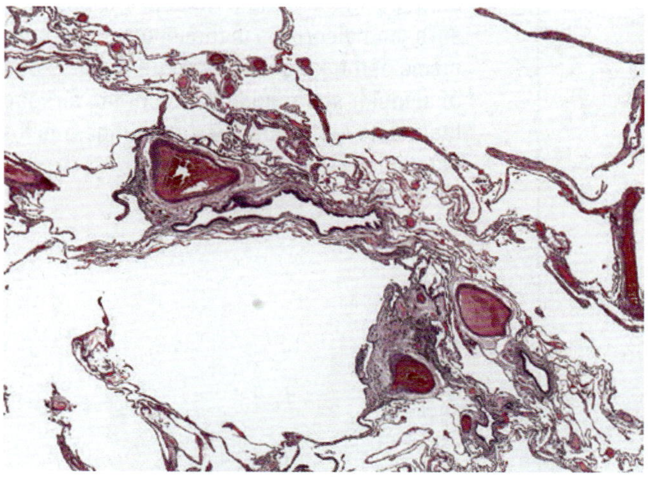

Figure 34.2 Centrilobular emphysema: Another example of centrilobular emphysema with enlargement of the air spaces surrounding the bronchiole.

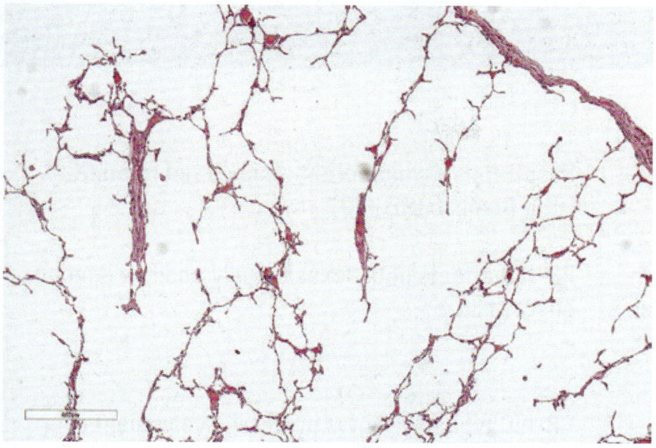

Figure 34.3 Centrilobular emphysema: A case of severe centrilobular emphysema with parenchymal loss and severe dilation of the airspaces. Note the clubbed ends, or "flags," on broken septa.

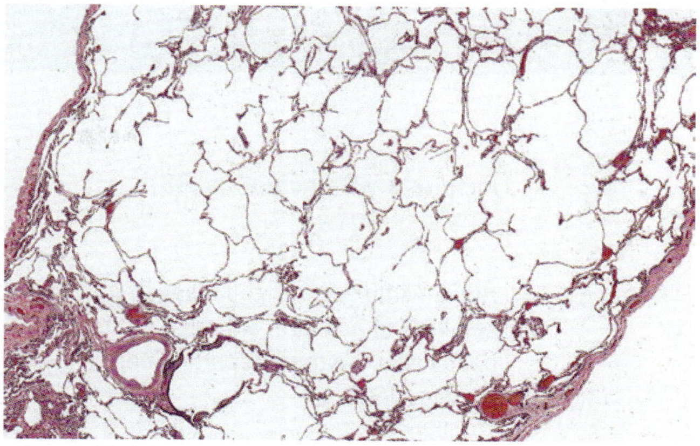

Figure 34.4 Panacinar emphysema: Panacinar emphysema showing the similar airspace dilation and parenchymal damage in both the parenchyma nearest the bronchiole and the remote parenchyma at the periphery of the lobule.

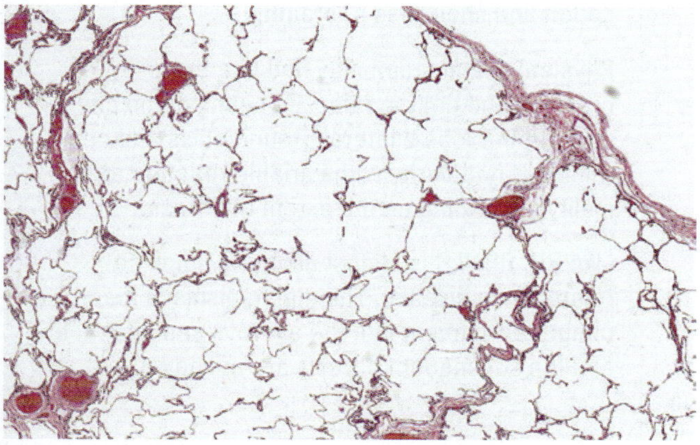

Figure 34.5 Panacinar emphysema: Another example of panacinar emphysema. Note the lack of anthracotic pigment in this nonsmoking case of A1AT-associated emphysema.

35 RESPIRATORY BRONCHIOLITIS VS. RESPIRATORY BRONCHIOLITIS–ASSOCIATED INTERSTITIAL LUNG DISEASE

	Respiratory Bronchiolitis (RB)	Respiratory Bronchiolitis–Associated Interstitial Lung Disease (RB-ILD)
Age	RB is a smoking-related disease that can occur in smokers of any age, although the mean for these cases is in the third decade. There is no clear sex predilection.	RB-ILD affects both sexes equally and has a mean onset of 36 y.
Location	As in many smoking-related and inhalational diseases, RB most commonly affects the upper lobes symmetrically.	RB-ILD typically shows bilateral involvement of the upper lobes with sparing of the lower lobes.
Symptoms	Patients with RB are by definition asymptomatic. It appears that nearly all smokers have some degree of RB on biopsy.	Patients with RB-ILD are by definition symptomatic and typically present with a nonproductive cough and shortness of breath.
Signs	CT scans of the chest typically show an upper lobe predominant process with hazy centrilobular ground glass and nodularity with bronchial wall thickening.	Physical examination may find fine bibasilar crackles and coarse rales. CT scans of the chest show upper lobe bilateral ground glass and centrilobular nodularity with variable reticular abnormality depending on the extent of fibrosis.
Etiology	RB is almost exclusively a smoking-related disease although some cases have been reported in association with other exposures to products of combustion. Macrophages engulf the pigmented particles and accumulate within the lumens of the smallest airways and adjacent airspaces.	Like RB, RB-ILD is almost always a smoking-related lung disease. The mechanisms of macrophage recruitment into the airways and airspaces and the subsequent fibrosis are unknown.
Histology	In cases of RB, light-brown–pigmented macrophages are seen within the lumens of bronchioles, often admixed with mucus *(Fig. 35.1)*. Additionally, there are collections of brown-pigmented macrophages within the airspaces adjacent to the bronchioles *(Figs. 35.2–35.4)*. The parenchyma furthest from the bronchiole is spared. In cases of RB as opposed to RB-ILD, there is no associated septal fibrosis or inflammation.	The histology of RB-ILD combines the features of RB with mild interstitial fibrosis. Like RB, there are brown-pigmented macrophages within the small airways and the airspaces nearest the airway *(Fig. 35.5)*. Additionally, there is often diffuse mild NSIP-like fibrosis, with septal expansion by collagen, which is usually seen in centrilobular zones. The fibrosis of RB-ILD is generally mild and upper lobe predominant *(Figs. 35.6–35.8)*. Fibroblastic foci and honeycombing are not typically seen.
Special studies	None.	None.
Prognosis	The prognosis of RB is good and will often resolve with smoking cessation.	The prognosis of RB-ILD is generally good, with most patients achieving either improvement or stabilization with smoking cessation. Steroids are sometimes used in this disease with modest response.

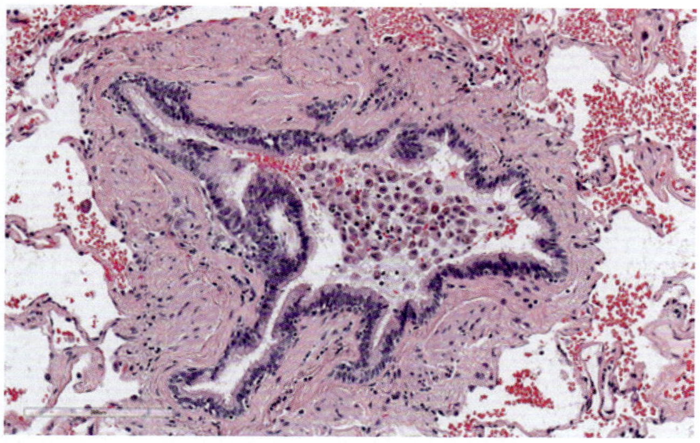

Figure 35.1 RB: A high-power view of a bronchiole with pigmented macrophages and mucus in the lumen. The bronchiole wall is essentially free of inflammation.

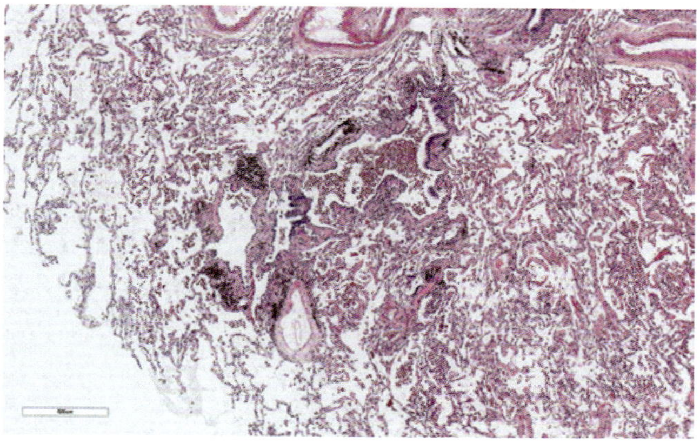

Figure 35.2 RB: A low-power image of RB in a smoker with clusters of macrophages sitting in the lumen of a bronchiole. Note the smoking-related anthracotic pigment in the peribronchiolar collagen. The alveolar septa remain thin and delicate.

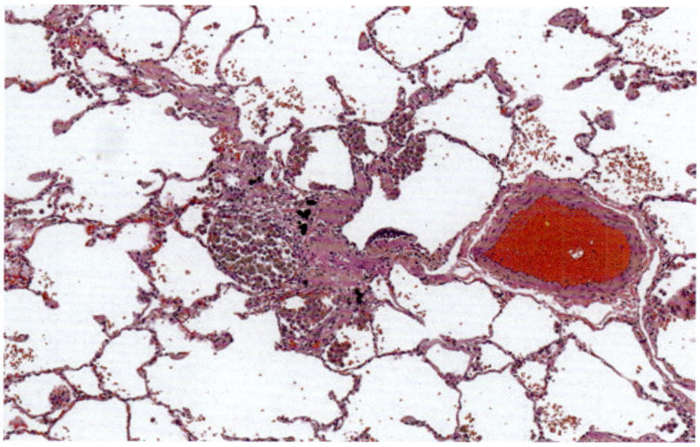

Figure 35.3 RB: A medium-power image of clustered pigmented macrophages within the lumen of a bronchiole and the adjacent alveolar airspaces.

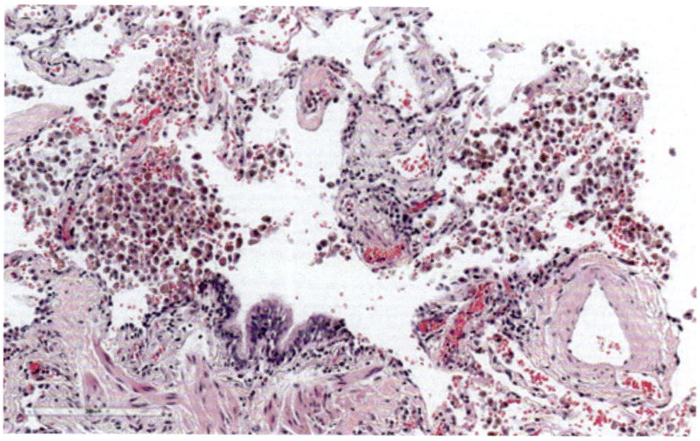

Figure 35.4 RB: A higher-power view of a bronchiole in RB showing the fine brown pigment in the cytoplasm of the macrophages.

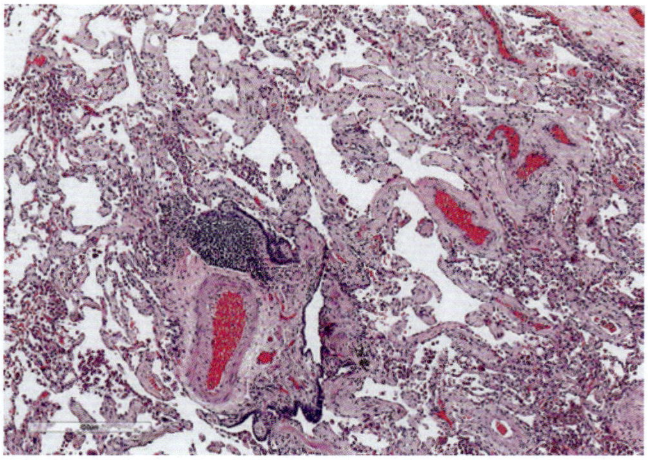

Figure 35.5 RB-ILD: A section of RB-ILD with a small bronchiole and surrounding airspaces containing light-brown–pigmented macrophages along with mild alveolar septal expansion by collagen deposition/fibrosis.

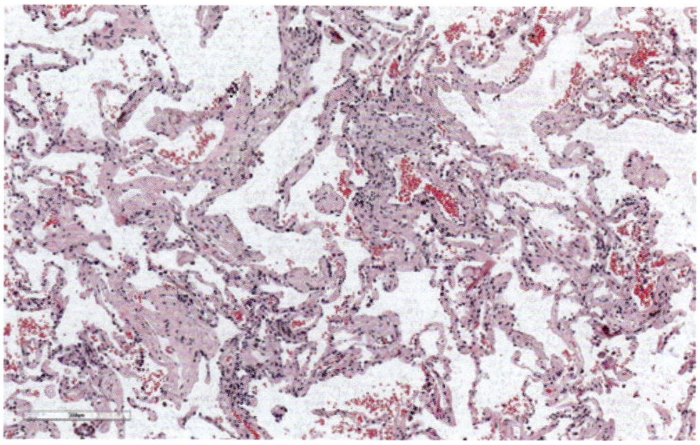

Figure 35.6 RB-ILD: A section of RB-ILD showing mild diffuse alveolar septal fibrosis along with scattered pigmented macrophages within the alveolar spaces.

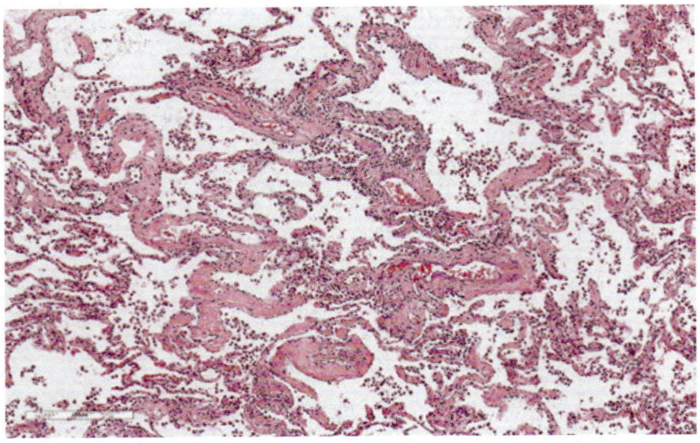

Figure 35.7 RB-ILD: Image of RB-ILD showing the combination of diffuse mild alveolar septal thickening by collagen and loosely clustered airspace macrophages.

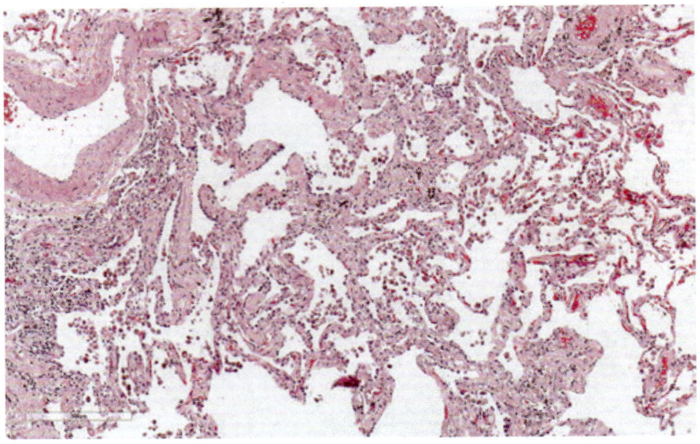

Figure 35.8 RB-ILD: Another example of RB-ILD in proximal acinar zone.

36 RESPIRATORY BRONCHIOLITIS VS. ALUMINUM PNEUMOCONIOSIS

	Respiratory Bronchiolitis (RB)	Aluminum Pneumoconiosis
Age	RB is a smoking-related disease that can occur in smokers of any age, although the mean for cases is in the third decade. There is no clear sex predilection.	As an occupational lung disease most commonly seen in metalworkers, aluminum smelting workers, and welders, aluminum pneumoconiosis is most commonly identified in men of working age.
Location	As in many smoking-related and inhalational diseases, RB most commonly affects the upper lobes symmetrically.	The disease diffusely involves the lungs bilaterally.
Symptoms	Patients with RB are by definition asymptomatic. It appears that nearly all smokers have some degree of RB on biopsy.	Most patients exhibit asthma-like symptoms with shortness of breath.
Signs	CT scans of the chest typically show an upper lobe predominant process with hazy centrilobular ground glass and nodularity with bronchial wall thickening.	The radiographic features are often nonspecific and are a mixture of reticular and nodular densities.
Etiology	RB is almost exclusively a smoking-related disease, although some cases have been reported in association with other exposures to products of combustion. Macrophages engulf the pigmented particles and accumulate within the lumens of the smallest airways and airway-adjacent airspaces.	As a foreign substance, aluminum particles are engulfed by macrophages, which then collect and migrate through the lymphatic system.
Histology	In cases of RB, light brown–pigmented macrophages are seen within the lumens of bronchioles, often admixed with mucus *(Fig. 36.1)*. Additionally, there are collections of brown-pigmented macrophages within the airspaces adjacent to the bronchioles *(Figs. 36.2–36.4)*. The parenchyma furthest from the bronchiole is spared. In cases of RB as opposed to RB-ILD, there is no associated septal fibrosis or inflammation.	In contrast to the brown macrophages of RB, or the golden inclusions of hemosiderin, the macrophages containing aluminum have a distinctive refractile gray-green appearance *(Fig. 36.5)*. The macrophages may be seen in the airspaces and form nodular aggregates within lymphatics adjacent to blood vessels and bronchioles *(Figs. 36.6–36.8)*. The tissue reaction to aluminum ranges from none to interstitial fibrosis to granulomatous inflammation. Cases with prominent granulomatous response may resemble sarcoidosis. Rare cases have been described with an alveolar proteinosis pattern, similar to that seen in acute silicoproteinosis.
Special studies	None.	Analytical electron microscopy shows electron-dense spherical particles composed of aluminum.
Prognosis	The prognosis of RB is good and often resolves with smoking cessation.	The prognosis is generally good, with few cases following a progressive fibrotic course. Treatment is largely centered on preventing or mitigating exposure.

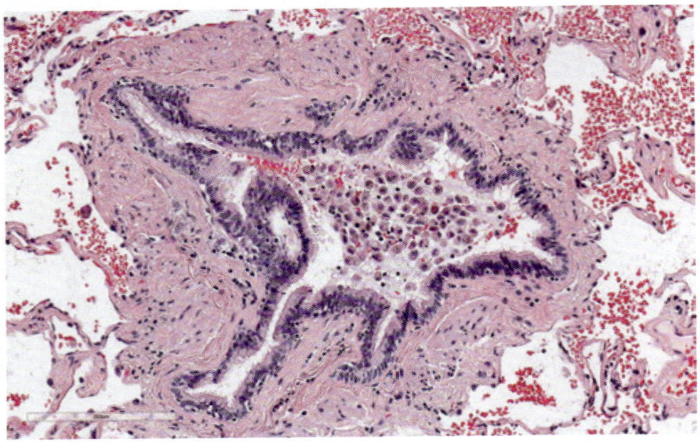

Figure 36.1 RB: A high-power view of a bronchiole with pigmented macrophages and mucus in the lumen. The bronchiole wall is essentially free of inflammation.

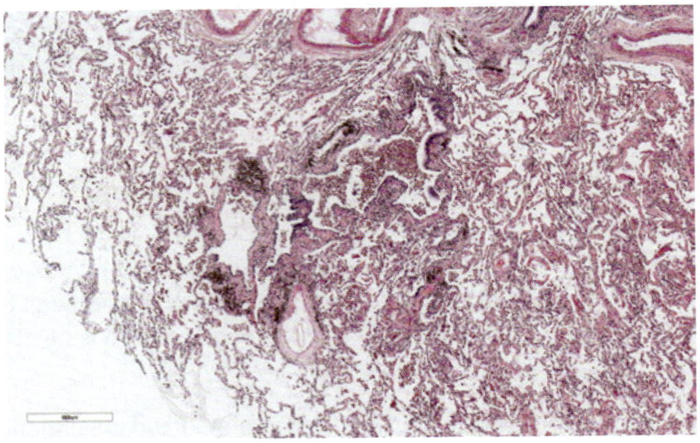

Figure 36.2 RB: A low-power image of RB in a smoker with clusters of macrophages sitting in the lumen of a bronchiole. Note the smoking-related anthracotic pigment in the peribronchiolar collagen. The alveolar septa remain thin and delicate.

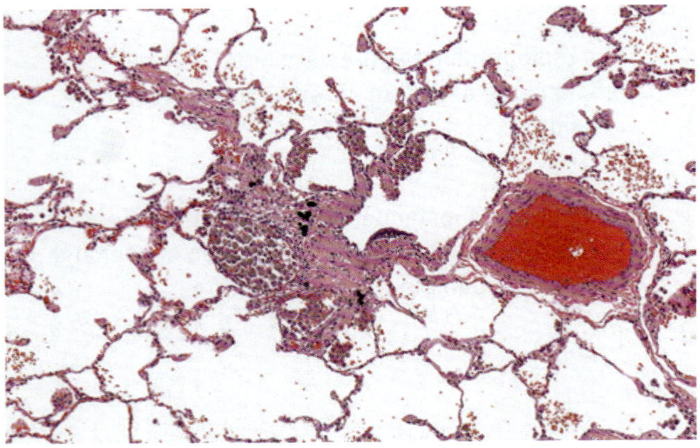

Figure 36.3 RB: A medium-power image of clustered pigmented macrophages within the lumen of a bronchiole and the adjacent alveolar airspaces.

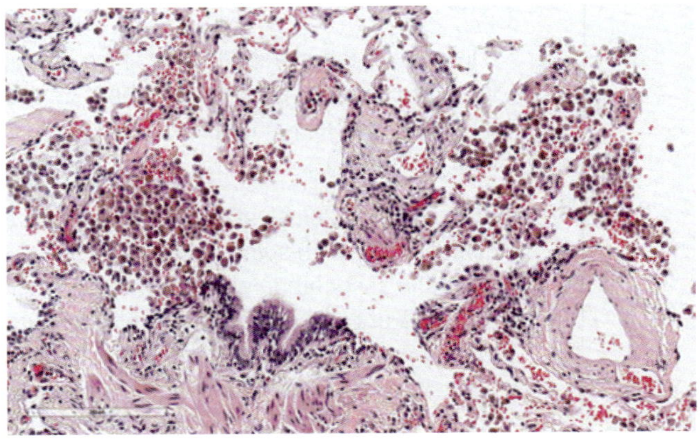

Figure 36.4 RB: A higher-power view of a bronchiole in RB showing the fine brown pigment in the cytoplasm of the macrophages.

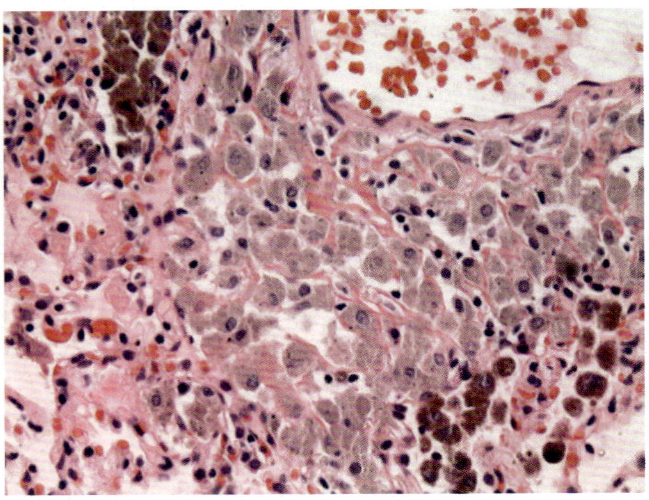

Figure 36.5 Aluminum pneumoconiosis: A high-power view of aluminum dust pneumoconiosis showing the aggregates of macrophages with gray-green refractile material. The case also includes some hemosiderin (iron)-laden macrophages at the upper left and lower right corners, showing the contrast between the dark golden-brown of iron and the light gray-green of aluminum.

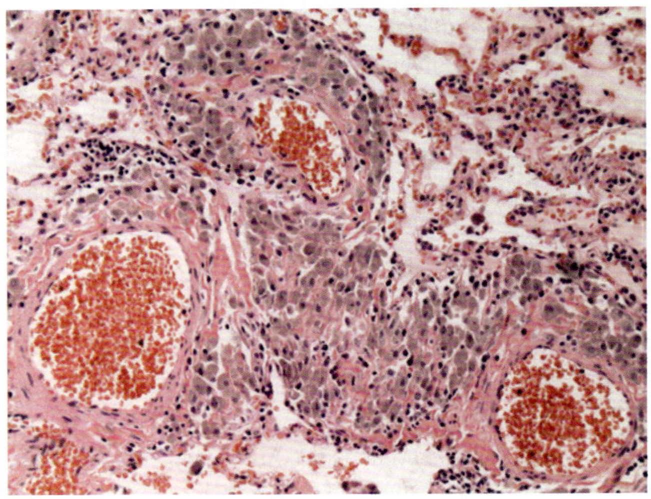

Figure 36.6 Aluminum pneumoconiosis: Aluminum dust containing macrophages in the airspaces and adventitial collagen around small blood vessels.

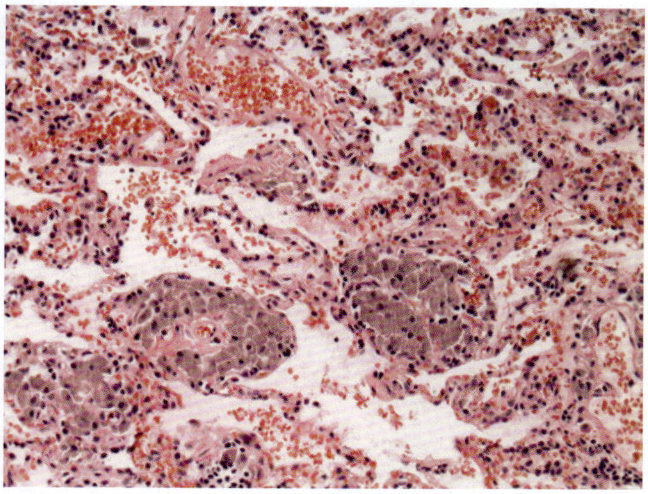

Figure 36.7 Aluminum pneumoconiosis: A medium-power view of aluminum dust containing macrophages in the interstitium and around small vessels. Note the absence of fibrosis in the alveolar septa.

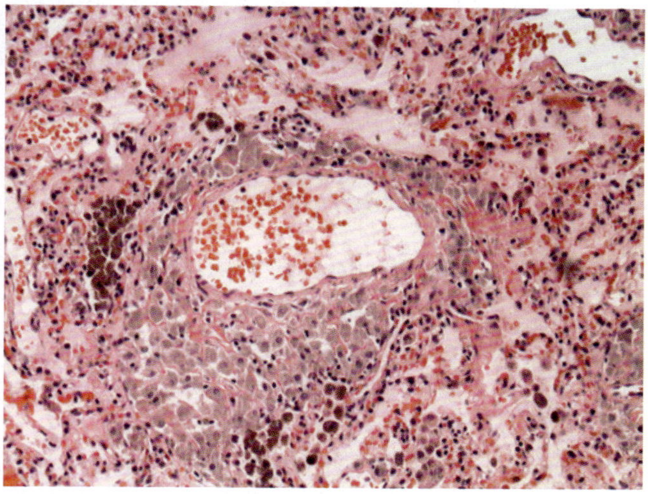

Figure 36.8 Aluminum pneumoconiosis: A blood vessel with dense collections of pigmented macrophages. The gray-green macrophages contain aluminum, while the dark-brown macrophages contain iron.

37 RESPIRATORY BRONCHIOLITIS–ASSOCIATED INTERSTITIAL LUNG DISEASE VS. SMOKING-RELATED INTERSTITIAL FIBROSIS

	Respiratory Bronchiolitis–Associated Interstitial Lung Disease (RB-ILD)	Smoking-Related Interstitial Fibrosis (SRIF)
Age	RB-ILD affects both sexes equally and has a mean onset of 36 y.	SRIF is most common in adults from the fifth to eighth decade, with an average age of 65.
Location	RB-ILD typically shows bilateral involvement of the upper lobes, with sparing of the lower lobes.	The disease involves both the subpleural and centrilobular parenchyma.
Symptoms	Patients with RB-ILD are by definition symptomatic and present with a nonproductive cough and shortness of breath.	SRIF is often either asymptomatic or minimally symptomatic. For many patients, the primary symptom is dyspnea from the underlying emphysema, rather than being symptomatic from the mild fibrosis.
Signs	Physical examination may find fine bibasilar crackles and coarse rales. CT scans of the chest show upper lobe bilateral ground glass and centrilobular nodularity with variable reticular abnormality, depending on the extent of fibrosis.	Pulmonary function tests typically show an obstructive, rather than restrictive, pattern. The presentation on chest CT includes bilateral ground glass and centrilobular densities.
Etiology	Like respiratory bronchiolitis (RB), RB-ILD is almost always a smoking-related lung disease. The mechanisms of macrophage recruitment into the airways and airspaces and the subsequent fibrosis are unknown.	Although the disease is associated with smoking, the mechanism of fibrosis is unclear.
Histology	The histology of RB-ILD combines the features of RB with mild interstitial fibrosis. Like RB, there are brown-pigmented macrophages within the small airways and the airspaces nearest the airway *(Fig. 37.1)*. Additionally, there is often diffuse mild nonspecific interstitial pneumonia (NSIP)–like fibrosis, with septal expansion by collagen, which is usually seen in centrilobular zones. Unlike SRIF that can have subpleural disease, the fibrosis of RB-ILD is accentuated near bronchioles. The fibrosis of RB-ILD is generally mild and upper lobe predominant *(Figs. 37.2–37.4)*. Fibroblastic foci and honeycombing are not typically seen.	SRIF shows mild subpleural and centrilobular fibrosis with minimal associated inflammation *(Figs. 37.5 and 37.6)*. The fibrosis has a dense eosinophilic hyalinized quality *(Fig. 37.7)*. SRIF is a relatively new classification, and there is significant histologic overlap between SRIF, RB-ILD, and desquamative interstitial pneumonia (DIP). Many cases that are currently diagnosed as SRIF may have been diagnosed as RB-ILD or DIP in the past. Although both RB-ILD and SRIF may share mild centrilobular fibrosis, subpleural fibrosis in RB-ILD is unusual. DIP, on the other hand, has a more diffuse NSIP-like fibrotic appearance without clear subpleural or centrilobular accentuation. Unlike usual interstitial pneumonia (UIP), the fibrosis of SRIF is temporally homogeneous and lacks both honeycombing and fibroblastic foci. SRIF has a background of smoking-related emphysema and may also have an element of RB if the patient is a current or recent smoker.
Special studies	None.	None.
Prognosis	The prognosis of RB-ILD is generally good, with most patients achieving either improvement or stabilization with smoking cessation. Steroids are sometimes used in this disease with modest response.	The prognosis of SRIF is good, and most patients who carry the diagnosis do not progress clinically.

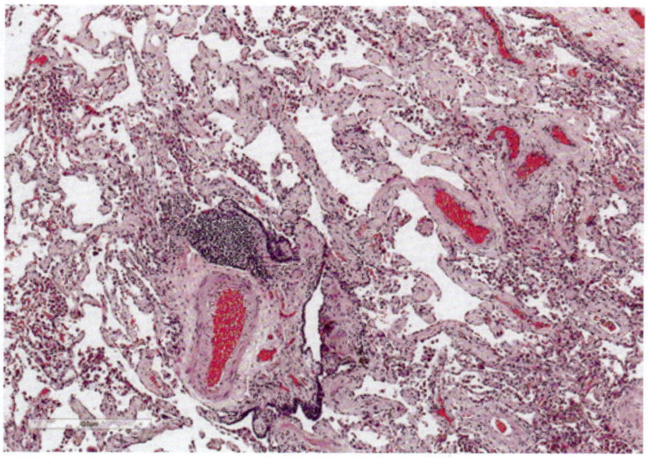

Figure 37.1 RB-ILD: A section of RB-ILD showing a bronchovascular bundle (*lower center*), and surrounding airspaces containing light-brown–pigmented macrophages along with mild alveolar septal expansion by collagen deposition/fibrosis.

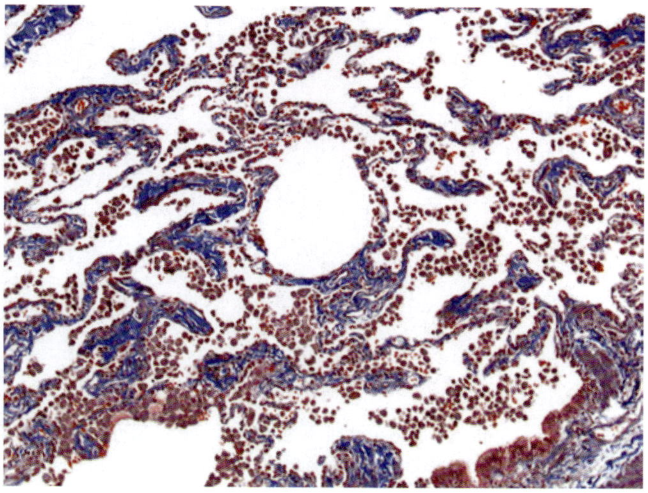

Figure 37.2 RB-ILD: An image showing mild peribronchiolar alveolar septal fibrosis (decorated by trichrome special stain/blue), along with scattered pigmented macrophages. Note bronchiole (*right lower corner*).

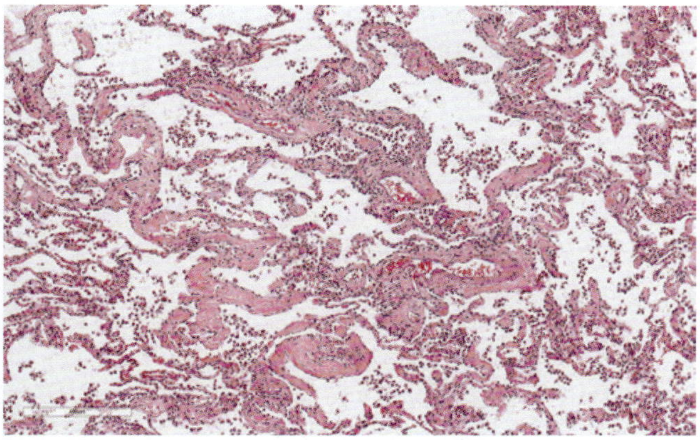

Figure 37.3 RB-ILD: An image showing the combination of diffuse mild alveolar septal thickening by collagen and loose-clustered airspace macrophages.

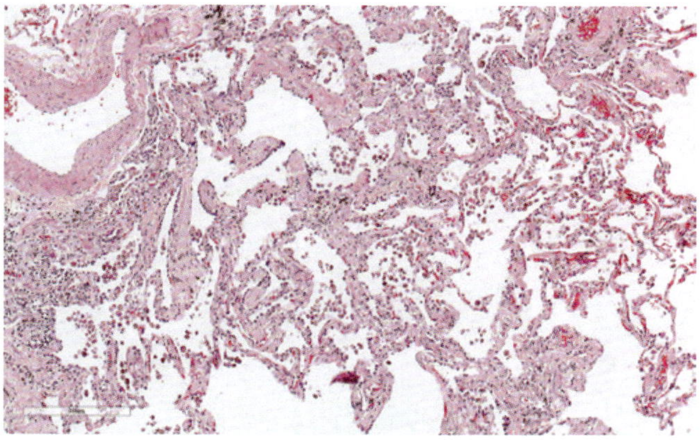

Figure 37.4 RB-ILD: Another example of RB-ILD with mild centrilobular alveolar septal thickening by fibrosis.

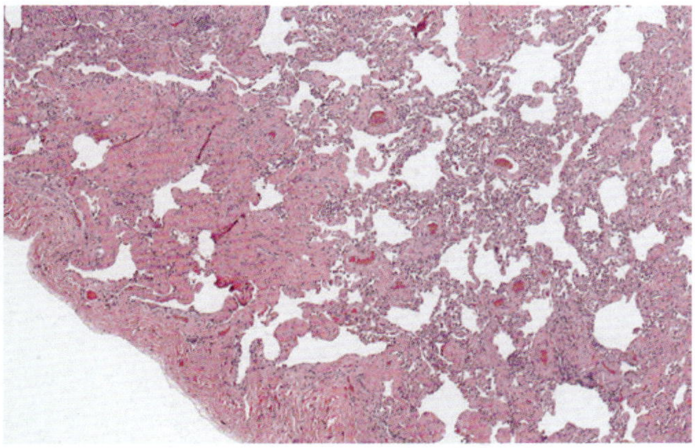

Figure 37.5 SRIF: A case of SRIF with mild subpleural alveolar septal fibrosis without significant inflammation. No fibroblastic foci or honeycombing is present. Airspaces show pigmented macrophages.

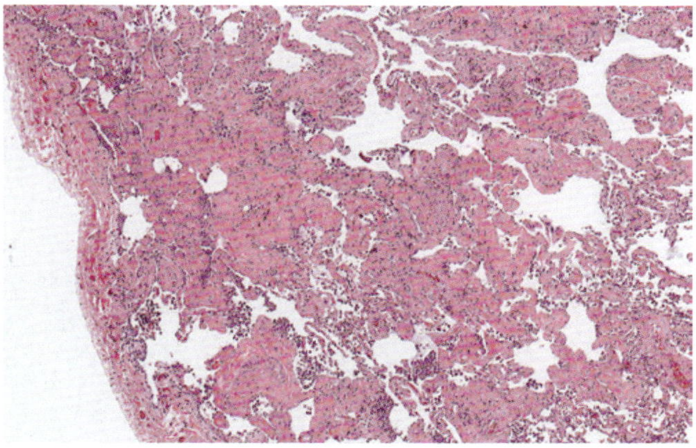

Figure 37.6 SRIF: Another case of SRIF showing subpleural alveolar septal thickening by hyalinized collagen deposition.

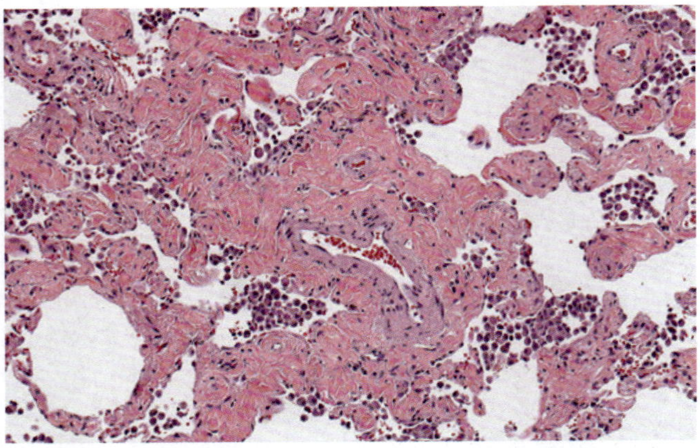

Figure 37.7 SRIF: A high-power view of the fibrosis of SRIF showing the densely hyalinized ropy collagen bundles and near-absence of inflammation.

38 RESPIRATORY BRONCHIOLITIS–ASSOCIATED INTERSTITIAL LUNG DISEASE VS. DESQUAMATIVE INTERSTITIAL PNEUMONIA

	Respiratory Bronchiolitis–Associated Interstitial Lung Disease (RB-ILD)	Desquamative Interstitial Pneumonia (DIP)
Age	RB-ILD affects both sexes equally and has a mean onset of 36 y.	DIP most commonly presents in the fourth to fifth decade and is more common in men.
Location	RB-ILD typically shows bilateral involvement of the upper lobes, with sparing of the lower lobes.	Typically, cases show bilateral involvement of all lobes of the lung.
Symptoms	Patients with RB-ILD are by definition symptomatic and present with a nonproductive cough and shortness of breath.	Most patients present with dyspnea and cough. Digital clubbing may be found in some patients with DIP.
Signs	Physical examination may find fine bibasilar crackles and coarse rales. CT scans of the chest show upper lobe bilateral ground glass and centrilobular nodularity with variable reticular abnormality, depending on the extent of fibrosis.	CT scans show diffuse bilateral ground glass opacities.
Etiology	Like respiratory bronchiolitis (RB), RB-ILD is almost always a smoking-related lung disease. The mechanisms of macrophage recruitment into the airways and airspaces and the subsequent fibrosis are unknown.	Similar to RB and RB-ILD, DIP represents a smoking-related macrophage-driven disease. The mechanisms of macrophage recruitment and interstitial damage remain unknown.
Histology	The histology of RB-ILD combines the features of RB with mild interstitial fibrosis. Like RB, there are brown-pigmented macrophages within the small airways and the airspaces nearest the airway *(Fig. 38.1)*. Additionally, there is often diffuse, mild nonspecific interstitial pneumonia (NSIP)–like fibrosis, with alveolar septal expansion by collagen, which is usually seen in centrilobular zones. The fibrosis of RB-ILD is generally mild and upper lobe predominant *(Figs. 38.2–38.4)*. Fibroblastic foci and honeycombing are not typically seen.	DIP shows diffuse accumulation of brown-pigmented macrophages throughout the biopsy *(Fig. 38.5)*. Although the pigment in the macrophages is identical to RB, the distribution of DIP is diffuse without being accentuated near the airways *(Fig. 38.6)*. Additionally, the process in DIP affects all the lobes similarly rather than having a clear preference for the upper lobe. Many cases of DIP will show an element of lymphoid hyperplasia with germinal centers present *(Fig. 38.7)*. Fibrosis is not uncommon in DIP, with many cases showing a diffuse, mild NSIP-like alveolar septal fibrosis that lacks chronic inflammation *(Figs. 38.7–38.9)*.
Special studies	None.	None.
Prognosis	The prognosis of RB-ILD is generally good, with most patients achieving either improvement or stabilization with smoking cessation. Steroids are sometimes used in this disease with modest response.	The 5- and 10-y survival rates for DIP are 95% and 70%, respectively. Smoking cessation is the main treatment strategy, although immunosuppression may also be used.

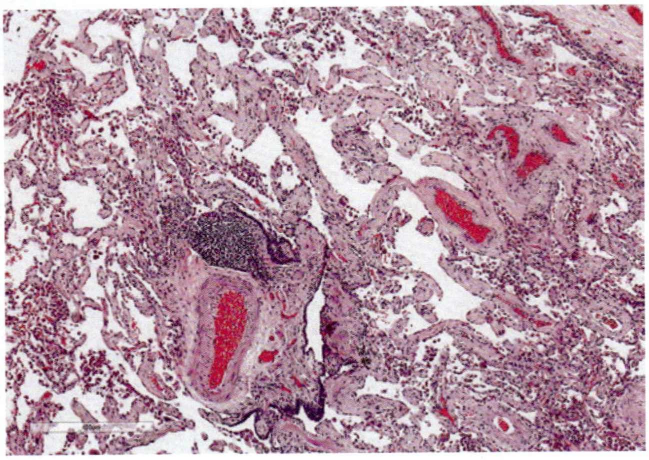

Figure 38.1 RB-ILD: A section of RB-ILD showing a bronchovascular bundle (*lower center*), and surrounding airspaces containing light-brown–pigmented macrophages along with mild alveolar septal expansion by collagen deposition/fibrosis.

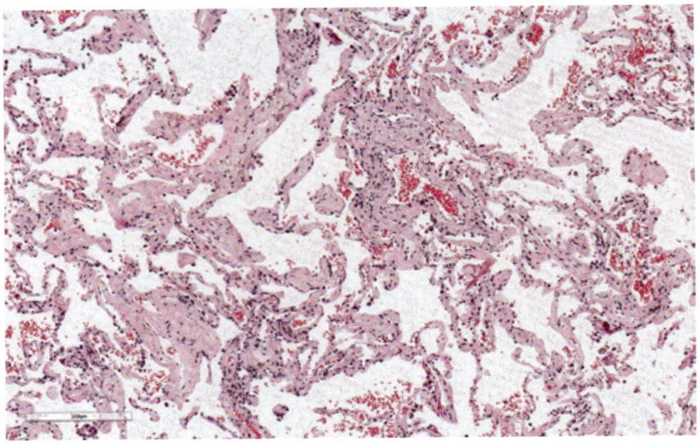

Figure 38.2 RB-ILD: H&E section showing mild alveolar septal fibrosis along with scattered pigmented macrophages in the alveolar spaces.

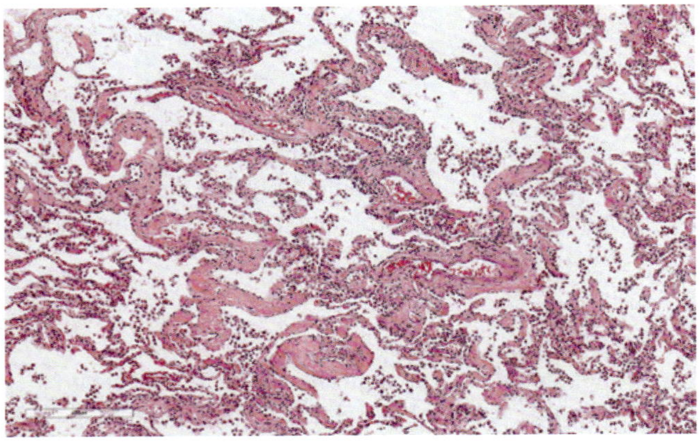

Figure 38.3 RB-ILD: Image showing the combination of mild alveolar septal thickening by collagen and loosely-clustered airspace macrophages.

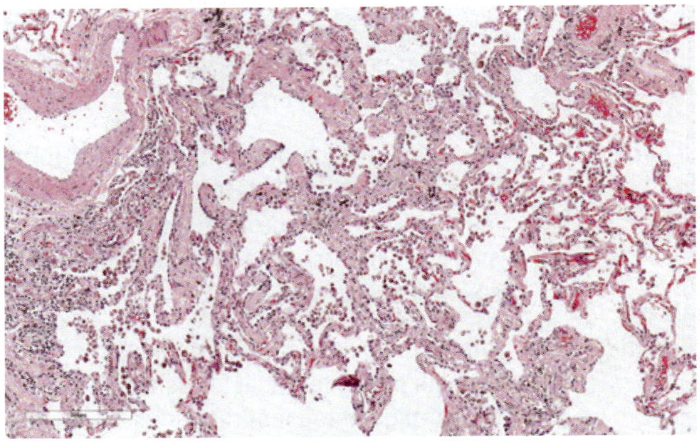

Figure 38.4 RB-ILD: Scattered pigmented airspace macrophages along with mild alveolar septal fibrosis.

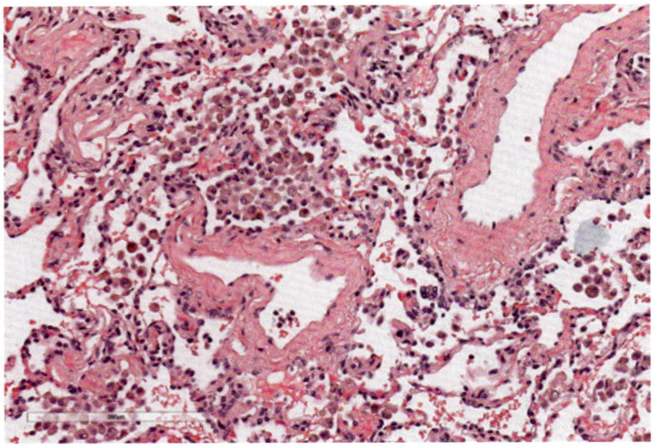

Figure 38.5 DIP: An image of a case of DIP showing that the pigmented macrophages are identical to those seen in the airspaces of RB or RB-ILD.

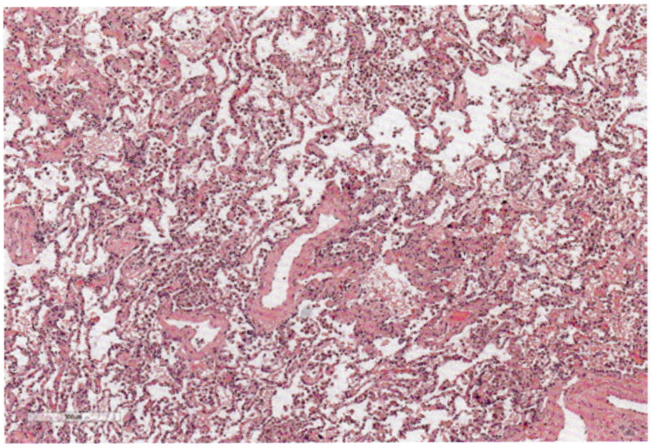

Figure 38.6 DIP: A low-power view of DIP showing the diffuse airspace filling by pigmented macrophages. This particular case did not have associated alveolar septal fibrosis.

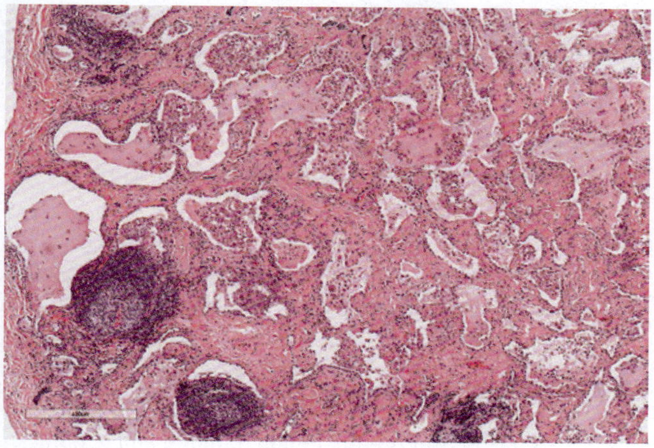

Figure 38.7 DIP: H&E showing lymphoid hyperplasia with prominent germinal centers along with mild-to-moderate amounts of diffuse alveolar septal fibrosis.

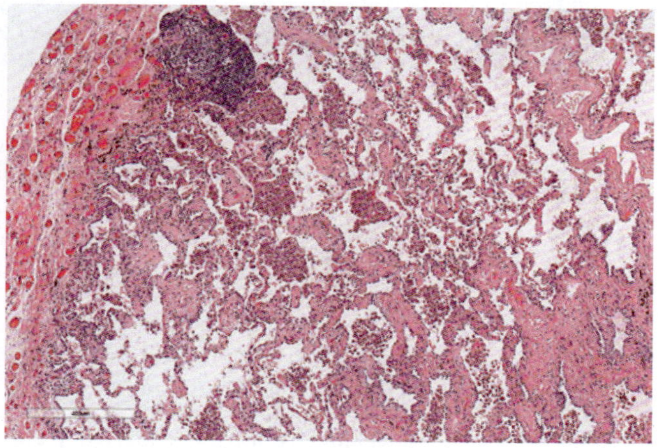

Figure 38.8 DIP: Section showing pigmented airspace macrophages, a single lymphoid follicle and mild alveolar septal fibrosis.

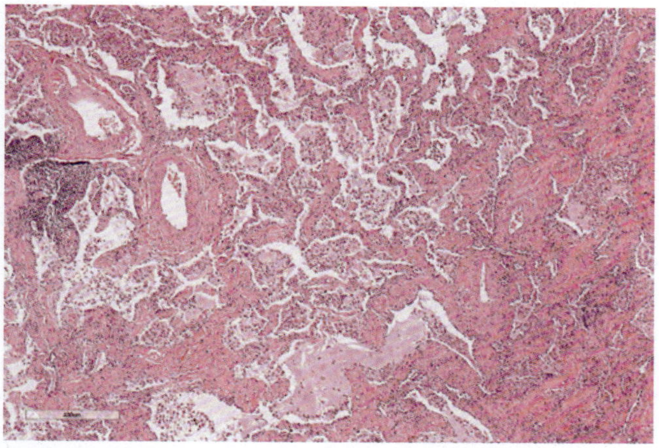

Figure 38.9 DIP: A case showing diffuse airspace filling by macrophages along with diffuse alveolar septal expansion by collagen. As there was similar involvement of all lobes of the biopsy, this case fits best with DIP rather than RB-ILD.

39 DESQUAMATIVE INTERSTITIAL PNEUMONIA VS. NONSPECIFIC INTERSTITIAL PNEUMONIA

	Desquamative Interstitial Pneumonia (DIP)	Nonspecific Interstitial Pneumonia (NSIP)
Age	DIP most commonly presents in the fourth to fifth decade and is more common in men.	The average age ranges from 40 to 57, but it can also be found in children. It is slightly more common in women.
Location	Typically, cases show bilateral involvement of all lobes of the lung.	It usually affects the lower lobes of the lung and tends to be bilateral and symmetrical.
Symptoms	Most patients present with dyspnea and cough. Digital clubbing may be found in some patients with DIP.	Shortness of breath, cough, fatigue, and weight loss are the most common symptoms. Fever and digital clubbing have been reported but are uncommon.
Signs	CT scans show diffuse bilateral ground glass opacities.	Pulmonary function tests demonstrate a restrictive pattern. High-resolution computed tomography (HRCT) scans show bilateral lower lobe predominant ground glass opacities that evolve into traction bronchiectasis as the disease becomes fibrotic. Honeycombing is generally not present.
Etiology	Similar to respiratory bronchiolitis (RB) and respiratory bronchiolitis–associated interstitial lung disease (RB-ILD), DIP represents a smoking-related macrophage-driven disease. The mechanisms of macrophage recruitment and interstitial damage remain unknown.	Pulmonary manifestation of underlying collagen vascular disease is the most common associated finding (e.g., rheumatoid arthritis, Sjögren syndrome). Other etiologies include immunodeficiency disorders (e.g., acquired immunodeficiency syndrome, common variable immunodeficiency), drug toxicity (e.g., Dilantin), or idiopathic disease.

	Desquamative Interstitial Pneumonia (DIP)	Nonspecific Interstitial Pneumonia (NSIP)
Histology	DIP shows diffuse accumulation of brown-pigmented macrophages throughout the biopsy *(Figs. 39.1 and 39.2)*. Although the pigment in the macrophages is identical to RB, the distribution of DIP is diffuse without being accentuated near the airways. Many cases of DIP will show an element of lymphoid hyperplasia with germinal centers present *(Fig. 39.3)*. Fibrosis is not uncommon in DIP, with many cases showing a diffuse mild NSIP-like alveolar septal fibrosis that lacks chronic inflammation *(Figs. 39.3–39.5)*.	*Cellular variant*: There is diffuse and uniform interstitial (alveolar septal) expansion by mild-to-moderate chronic inflammatory cell infiltrates containing predominantly small mature lymphocytes and occasional plasma cells associated with alveolar pneumocyte prominence. The inflammatory process may be associated with lymphoid aggregates (with or without germinal centers), chronic pleuritis, and increase in perivascular collagen deposition, which although nonspecific, are features commonly associated with autoimmune disorder/collagen vascular disease manifesting in the lung *(Figs. 39.6–39.9)*. *Fibrosing variant*: There is diffuse temporally homogeneous alveolar septal fibrosis, little amount of inflammation and alveolar pneumocyte prominence *(Figs. 39.10–39.13)*. *Mixed cellular and fibrosing*: There is diffuse and uniform interstitial expansion by similar amounts of inflammation and fibrosis. In all three forms of NSIP, the underlying lung architecture is preserved, with no honeycomb change. Fibroblastic foci may be present, but they are usually inconspicuous and never numerous. Few plugs of organizing pneumonia and variable amounts of peribronchiolar metaplasia may be present. Increased numbers of macrophages are frequently found within the alveolar spaces; however, unlike DIP, these macrophages are not pigmented unless the patient is a smoker.
Special studies	None.	None.
Prognosis	The 5- and 10-y survival rates for DIP are 95% and 70%, respectively. Smoking cessation is the main treatment strategy, although immunosuppression may also be used.	The prognosis of cellular NSIP is better than that of fibrosing NSIP. The 5-y survival rate for patients with cellular NSIP is close to 100%, with good response to corticosteroid therapy. The 5- and 10-y survival rates for patients with fibrosing NSIP are 90% and 35%, respectively.

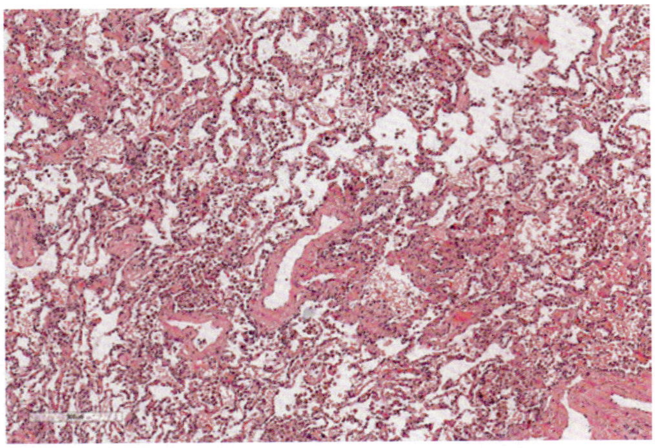

Figure 39.1 DIP: A low-power image of DIP showing the diffuse airspace filling by loose clusters of brown-pigmented macrophages.

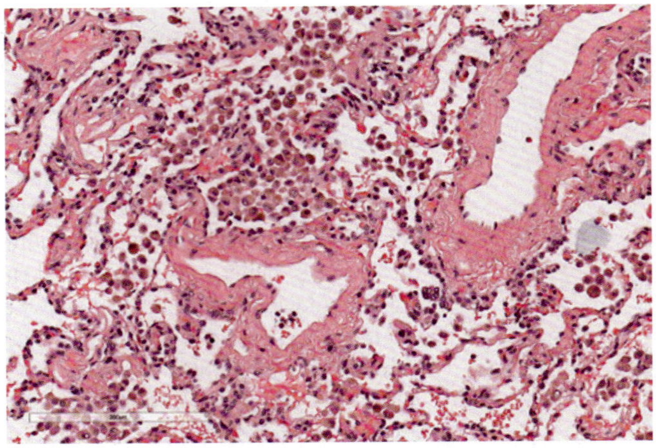

Figure 39.2 DIP: A higher-power of Figure 39.1 showing brown-pigmented macrophages within the airspaces.

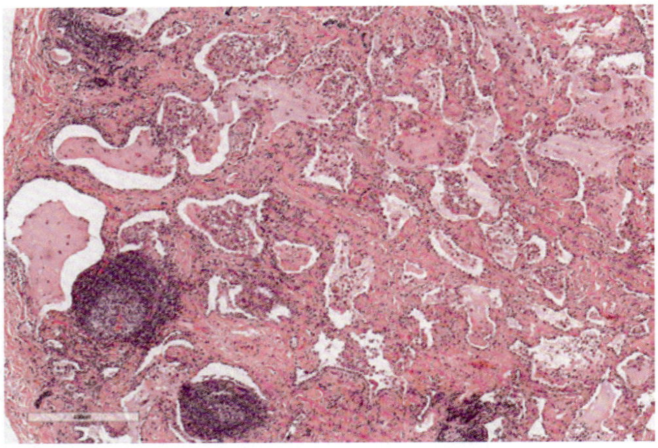

Figure 39.3 DIP: A case showing numerous lymphoid follicles containing germinal centers along with diffuse, moderate alveolar septal fibrosis without honeycombing.

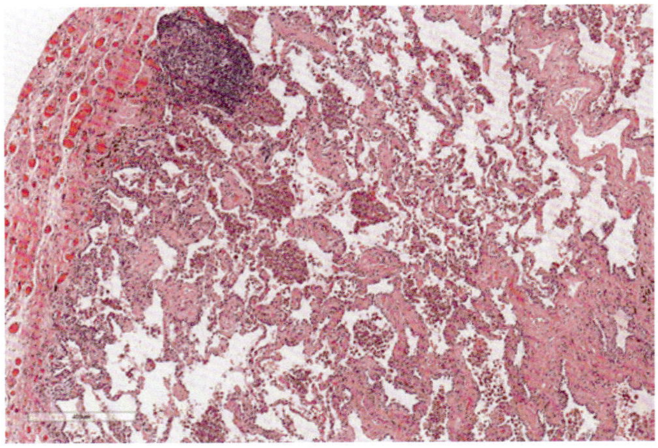

Figure 39.4 DIP: Section showing a subpleural lymphoid follicle, pigmented airspace macrophages, and mild alveolar septal fibrosis developing in the lower right corner.

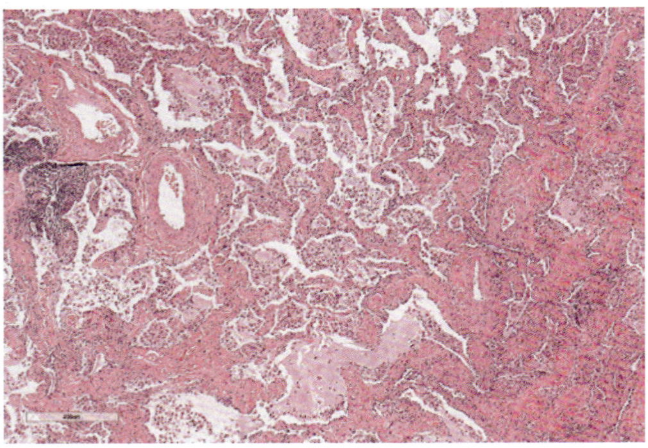

Figure 39.5 DIP: H&E stain with pigmented airspace macrophages and diffuse fibrotic alveolar septa without honeycombing.

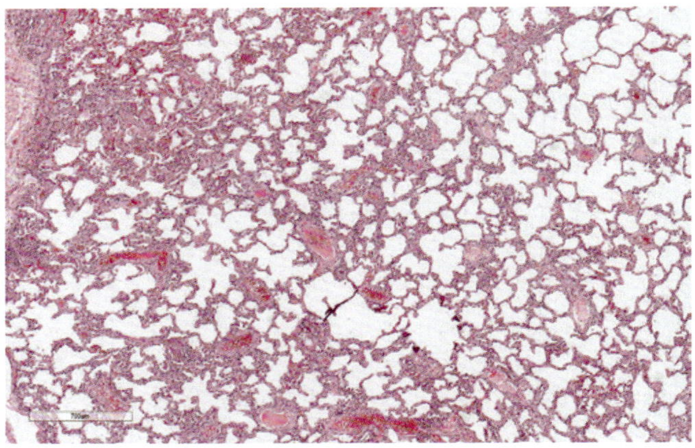

Figure 39.6 Cellular NSIP: There is diffuse and uniform interstitial (alveolar septal) expansion by chronic inflammatory cells.

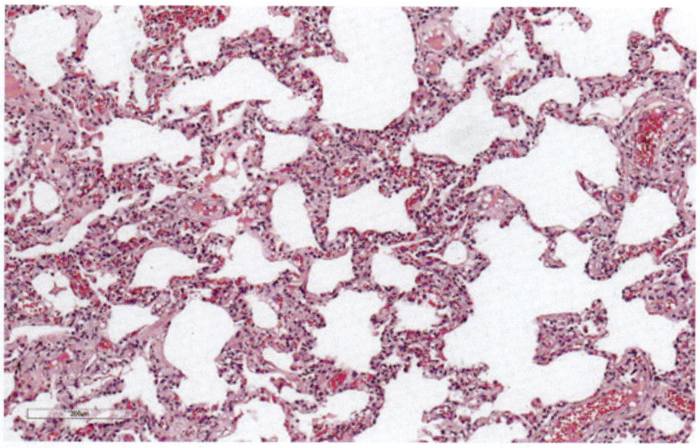

Figure 39.7 Cellular NSIP (high power): The alveolar septal expansion is composed of mild-to-moderate chronic inflammatory cell infiltrate consisting predominantly of lymphocytes.

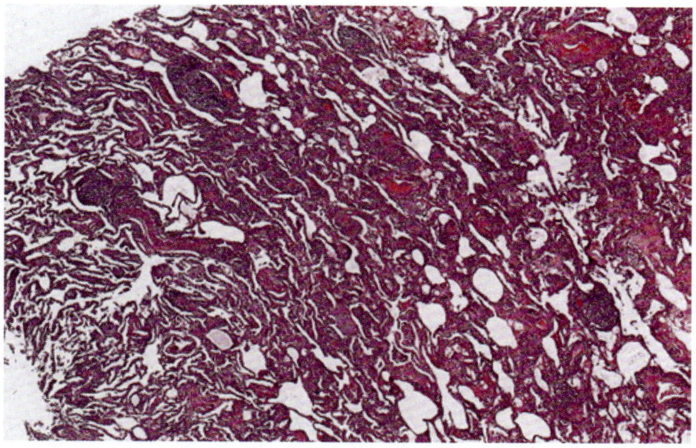

Figure 39.8 Cellular NSIP: A case secondary to rheumatoid arthritis in a 62-year-old woman. Note diffuse and uniform alveolar septal expansion associated with scattered lymphoid follicles.

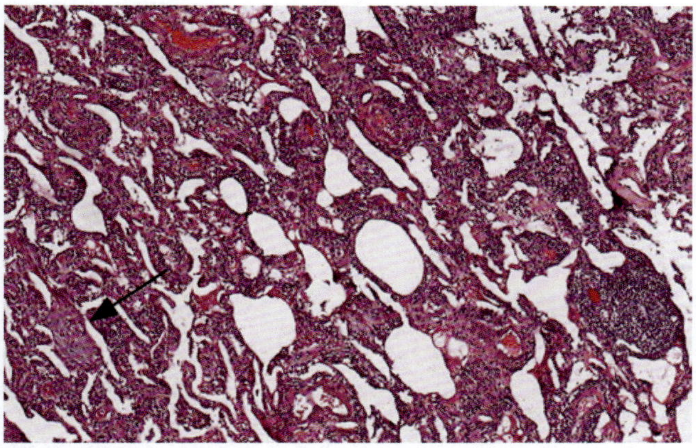

Figure 39.9 Cellular NSIP (high power): Same patient from Figure 39.8. The alveolar septal expansion is composed mainly of lymphocytes. Note small focus of organizing pneumonia (*lower left/arrow*).

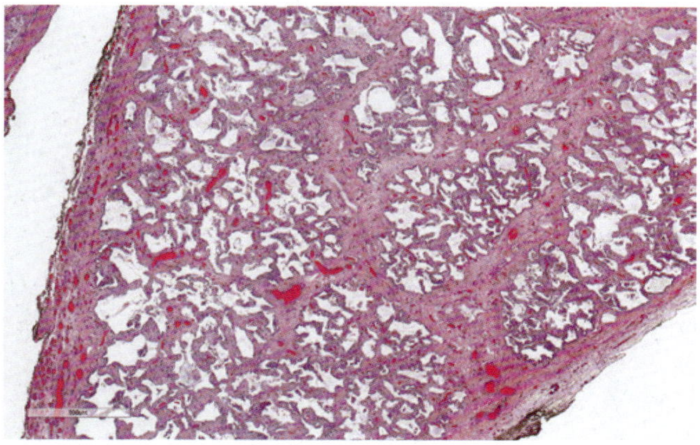

Figure 39.10 Fibrotic NSIP: There is diffuse and uniform interstitial (alveolar septal) expansion by eosinophilic acellular material.

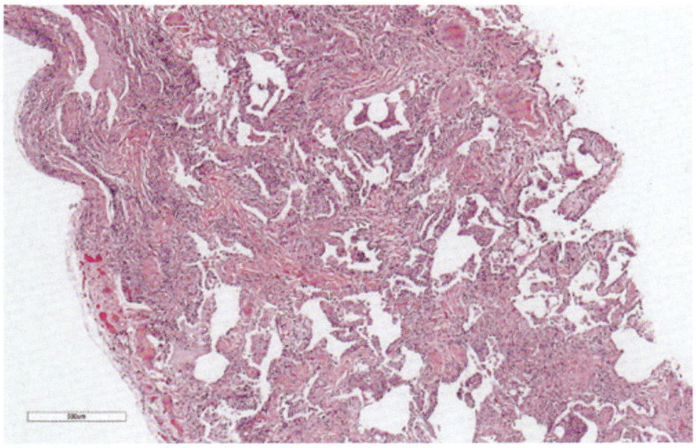

Figure 39.11 Fibrotic NSIP: The interstitial expansion is composed of dense collagen deposition (fibrosis) and little inflammation.

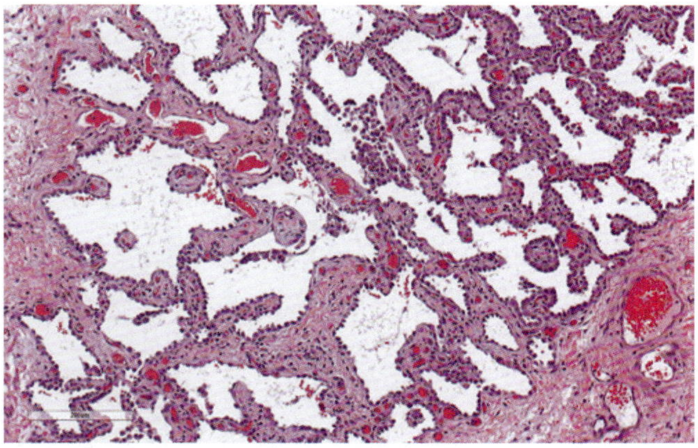

Figure 39.12 Fibrotic NSIP: The alveolar septal scarring is frequently associated with alveolar pneumocyte prominence. Macrophages are found in the alveolar spaces but they do not represent the main pattern of injury.

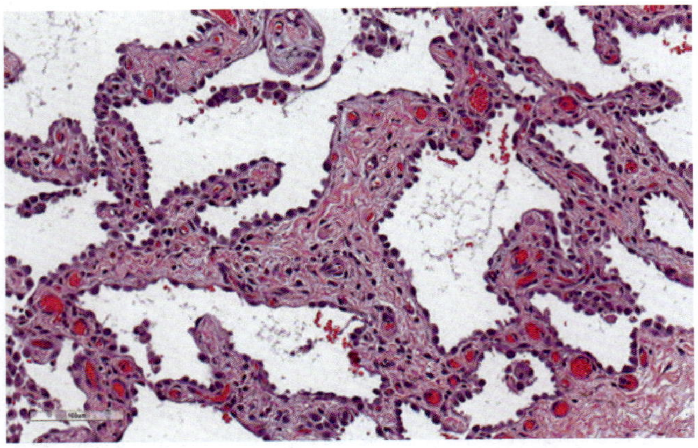

Figure 39.13 Fibrotic NSIP (high power): Note the alveolar pneumocyte prominence along the thickened/fibrotic alveolar septa.

40 DESQUAMATIVE INTERSTITIAL PNEUMONIA VS. EOSINOPHILIC PNEUMONIA

	Desquamative Interstitial Pneumonia (DIP)	Eosinophilic Pneumonia (EP)
Age	DIP most commonly presents in the fourth to fifth decade of life and is more common in men.	Can develop at any age, with mean age of 45 at diagnosis. Women are more affected than men.
Location	Typically, cases show bilateral involvement of all lobes of the lung.	Airspace-filling process that usually involves periphery of middle and upper lung zones.
Symptoms	Most patients present with dyspnea and cough. Digital clubbing may be found in some patients with DIP.	Chronic disease characterized by relapsing subacute episodes of dyspnea, cough, and chest pain, which is often associated with fatigue, malaise, fever, chills, and weight loss that may last for several weeks or months. Clinical history of chronic asthma, chronic rhinitis, or chronic sinusitis is common.
Signs	CT scans show diffuse bilateral ground glass opacities.	Physical examination may reveal wheezes or crackles. Peripheral blood, sputum, and bronchoalveolar lavage (BAL) containing markedly increased eosinophils and elevated IgE are usually present. Chest CT demonstrates patchy, bilateral, often peripheral (subpleural), poorly defined "migratory" infiltrates, which are transient infiltrates that tend to resolve and reappear in the same location or elsewhere. Migration of the infiltrates over time is strongly suggestive of the diagnosis. The predominant dense peripheral distribution of the infiltrates is often referred to as reverse pulmonary edema pattern.
Etiology	Similar to respiratory bronchiolitis (RB) and respiratory bronchiolitis–associated interstitial lung disease (RB-ILD), DIP represents a smoking-related macrophage-driven disease. The mechanisms of macrophage recruitment and interstitial damage remain unknown.	Potential etiologies include but are not limited to drug toxicity (e.g., ampicillin, bleomycin, cromoglycate, glafenine, hydralazine, naproxen, nitrofurantoin, para-aminosalicylic acid, penicillin, streptomycin, sulfasalazine, sulfonamides, tetracycline, L-tryptophan, etc.), fungal organisms, particularly *Aspergillus* sp., *Coccidioides* sp, parasites, bacteria, viruses, inhalants (e.g., cocaine, nickel, carbonyl vapor), and other allergens. Some cases have been associated with the initiation of smoking, or changes in smoking habits. Rare cases of EP may be an initial manifestation of autoimmune disease, and therefore a rheumatologic panel is indicated. In the absence of known etiologies, the case falls into the cryptogenic EP category.

	Desquamative Interstitial Pneumonia (DIP)	Eosinophilic Pneumonia (EP)
Histology	DIP shows diffuse accumulation of brown-pigmented macrophages throughout the biopsy *(Fig. 40.1)*. While the pigment in the macrophages is identical to RB, the distribution of DIP is diffuse without being accentuated near the airways *(Fig. 40.2)*. Additionally, the process in DIP affects all the lobes of the biopsy similarly rather than having a clear preference for the upper lobe. Many cases of DIP will show an element of lymphoid hyperplasia with germinal centers present *(Fig. 40.3)*. Fibrosis is not uncommon in DIP, with many cases showing a diffuse, mild nonspecific interstitial pneumonia (NSIP)–like alveolar septal fibrosis that lacks chronic inflammation *(Figs. 40.3–40.5)*.	Alveolar spaces filled by eosinophils admixed with variable number of macrophages, proteinaceous-to-fibrinous exudates, and frequent foci of organizing pneumonia. Granulomatous formation may be seen, characterized by dense accumulation of macrophages, sometimes accompanied by multinucleated giant cells. Eosinophilic abscesses may be seen, characterized by the presence of a central area of necrosis surrounded by palisading histiocytes mixed with eosinophils. The predominantly airspace-filling process is usually accompanied by mild-to-moderate interstitial pneumonia characterized by expansion of the alveolar septa by a mixture of eosinophils, lymphocytes, and plasma cells with associated alveolar pneumocyte type II prominence *(Figs. 40.6–40.9)*. Necrosis of the intra-alveolar cellular infiltrate is common, but septal (interstitial) necrosis does not occur. Mild perivascular and transmural infiltration by non-necrotizing, eosinophil-rich, chronic inflammatory cell infiltrate involving small arteries and venules is often seen *(Fig. 40.10)*. However, this finding does not indicate Churg–Strauss syndrome since necrotizing vasculitis should not be present. Chronicity may be suggested by the presence of variable interstitial fibrosis. Of note, if the patient has received steroids prior to the biopsy, the tissue eosinophilia may be inconspicuous or absent, and the alveolar spaces may be filled with macrophages only, resembling DIP and requiring correlation with clinical history and laboratory findings of peripheral eosinophilia to support the diagnosis.
Special studies	None.	GMS special stains and tissue cultures to exclude infection.
Prognosis	The 5- and 10-y survival rates for DIP are 95% and 70%, respectively. Smoking cessation is the main treatment strategy, although immunosuppression may also be used.	The clinical course depends on the underlying causal agent, but overall most patients respond favorably to corticosteroid therapy, although recurrences are common and prolonged therapy may be necessary.

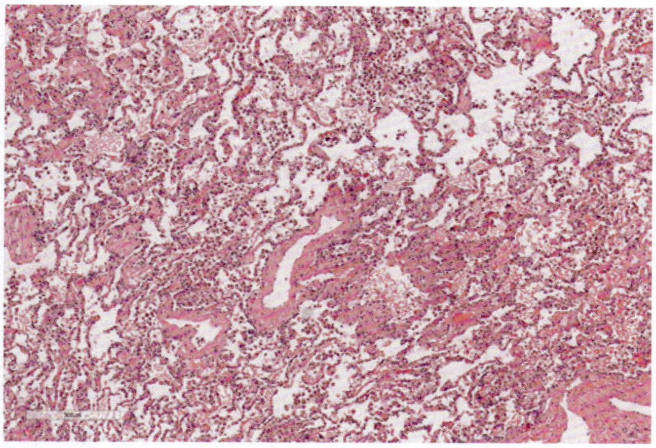

Figure 40.1 DIP: A low-power view of DIP showing the diffuse involvement of all airspaces by pigmented macrophages. This particular case did not have associated fibrosis.

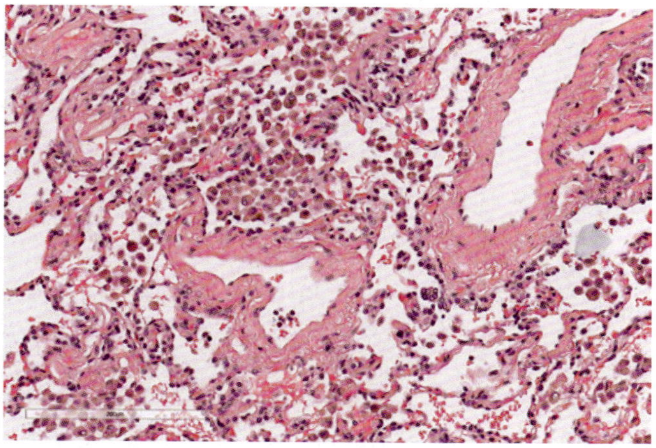

Figure 40.2 DIP: High power view of Figure 40.1 showing that the pigmented macrophages are identical to those seen in the airspaces of RB or RB-ILD. Note lack of eosinophils or fibrin typically seen in alveolar spaces of EP.

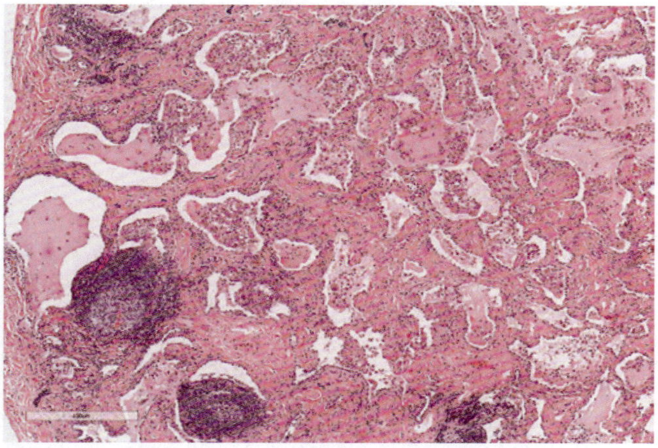

Figure 40.3 DIP: A case showing lymphoid hyperplasia with prominent germinal centers along with moderate alveolar septal fibrosis

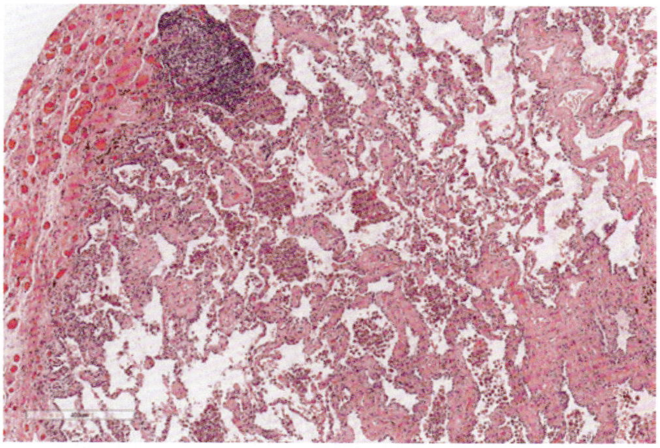

Figure 40.4 DIP: Image showing pigmented airspace macrophages, a single lymphoid follicle, and mild alveolar septal fibrosis.

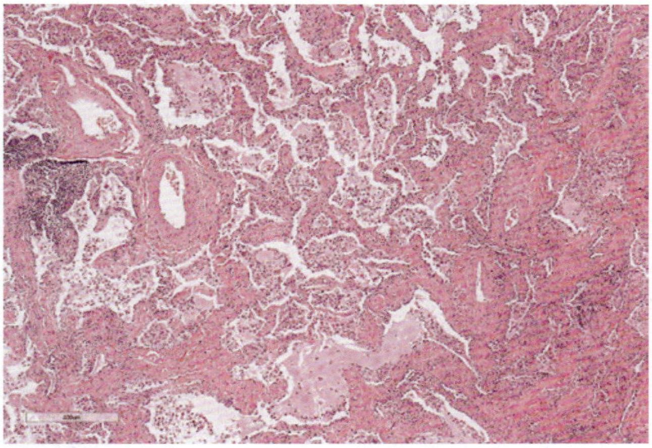

Figure 40.5 DIP: A case of DIP showing diffuse airspace macrophages along with diffuse alveolar septal expansion by collagen deposition/fibrosis.

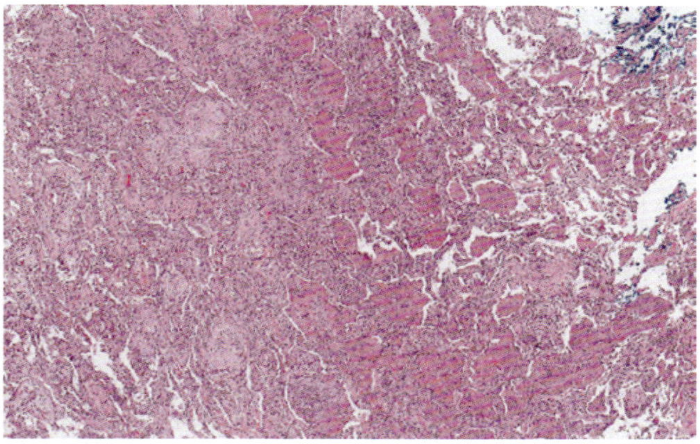

Figure 40.6 EP: There is dense lung parenchyma consolidation with filling of the alveolar spaces by proteinaceous-to-fibrinous exudates, (*dark pink material, middle right*), and polypoid-to-elongated plugs of organizing pneumonia (*middle left*).

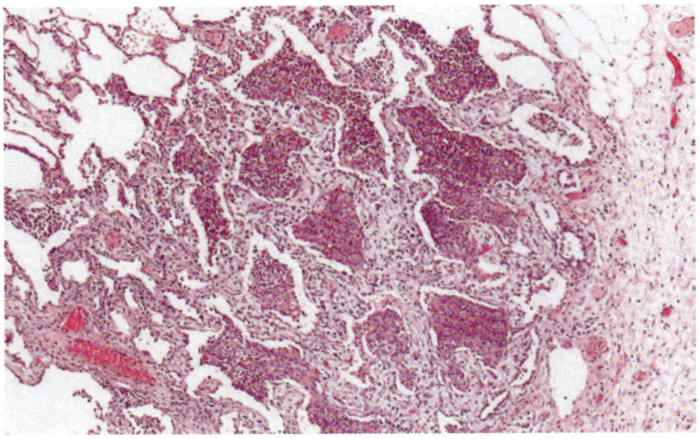

Figure 40.7 EP: Another example of EP with airspaces filling by fibrin, eosinophils and macrophages.

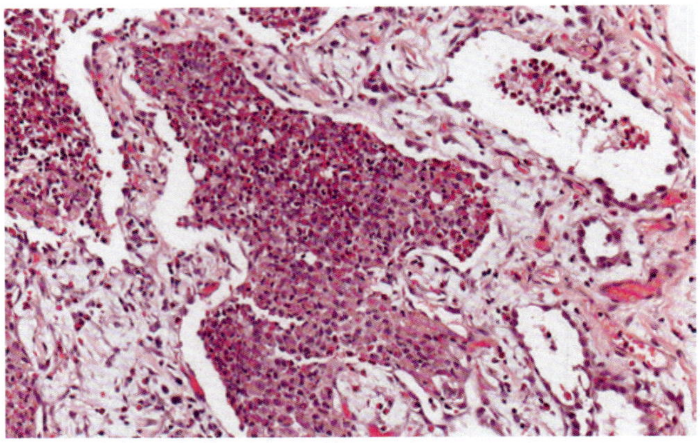

Figure 40.8 EP: High-power view of Figure 40.7 showing airspace filling by fibrin eosinophils and macrophages.

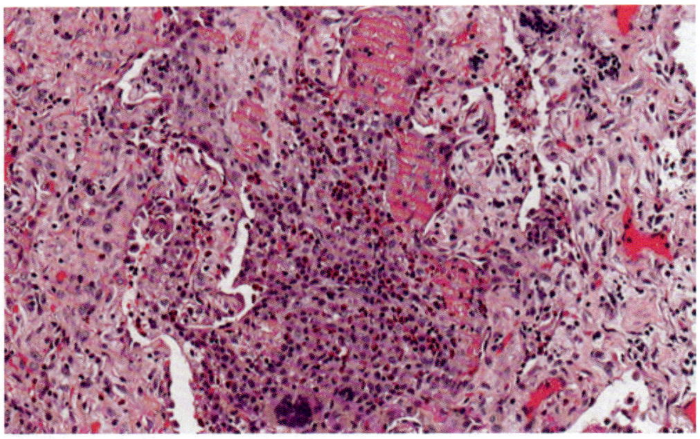

Figure 40.9 EP: High-power image showing airspace filling by fibrinous exudate (*dark-pink, middle right*) and inflammatory cell infiltrate composed of macrophages and numerous eosinophils (*middle left*). Fibrin exudation and eosinophilia are not features of DIP. However, if the patient has received steroids prior to the biopsy, the tissue eosinophilia may be inconspicuous or absent, and the alveolar spaces may be filled with macrophages only, resembling DIP and requiring correlation with clinical history and laboratory findings of peripheral eosinophilia to support the diagnosis.

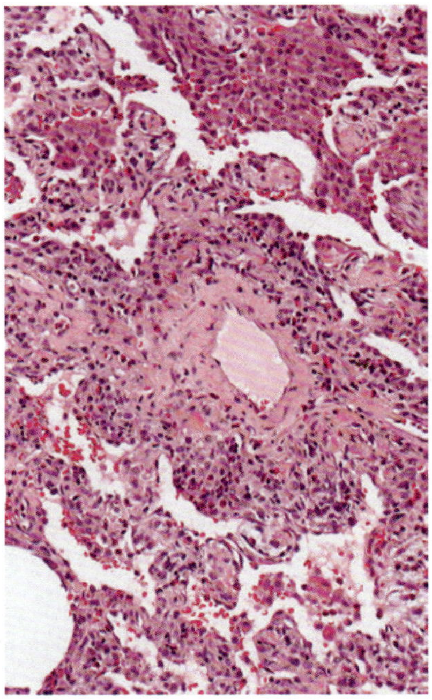

Figure 40.10 EP: Mild perivascular and transmural infiltration by eosinophils is often seen involving small arteries and venules.

41 DESQUAMATIVE INTERSTITIAL PNEUMONIA VS. PULMONARY ALVEOLAR HEMOSIDEROSIS

	Desquamative Interstitial Pneumonia (DIP)	Pulmonary Alveolar Hemosiderosis (PAH)
Age	DIP most commonly presents in the fourth to fifth decade of life and is more common in men.	PAH may occur at any age in both adult and children; however, it is most common in children aged 1–7. There appears to be no sex predilection.
Location	Typically shows bilateral involvement of all lobes of the lung.	Bilateral involvement of lungs.
Symptoms	Most patients present with dyspnea and cough. Digital clubbing may be found in some patients with DIP.	Hemoptysis, dyspnea, and shortness of breath. Not all cases have a history of hemoptysis.
Signs	CT scans show diffuse bilateral ground glass opacities.	Chest x-ray shows patchy or diffuse opacities. Chest CT shows patchy to diffuse, bilateral or unilateral, ground glass or consolidative opacities. Often more central than peripheral.
Etiology	Similar to respiratory bronchiolitis (RB) and respiratory bronchiolitis–associated interstitial lung disease (RB-ILD), DIP represents a smoking-related, macrophage-driven disease. The mechanisms of macrophage recruitment and interstitial damage remain unknown.	Most cases of PAH are thought to result from chronic alveolar hemorrhage. Potential etiologies include congestive and valvular heart disease, vasculitis, capillaritis, coagulopathies, antiphospholipid syndrome, sleep apnea, and drug reactions, or may be idiopathic.
Histology	There is diffuse alveolar spaces accumulation of pigmented macrophages with fine granular light golden-brown cytoplasm, throughout the biopsy *(Fig. 41.1–Fig. 41.2)*. Many cases of DIP will show an element of lymphoid hyperplasia with germinal centers *(Fig. 41.3)*. Fibrosis is not uncommon in DIP, with many cases showing a diffuse, mild nonspecific interstitial pneumonia (NSIP)–like alveolar septal fibrosis *(Fig. 41.3–Fig. 41.5)*.	There is alveolar space accumulation of pigmented hemosiderin-laden macrophages with chunky, coarsely granular, and dark brown cytoplasm *(Figs. 41.6 and 41.7)*. Additionally, hemosiderin-laden macrophages and extracellular hemosiderin may be found within the interstitium or in the adventitial collagen of vessels and airways. In chronic cases, calcium and hemosiderin-laden salts may encrust the elastic lamina of vessels or airways (also known as endogenous pneumoconiosis) *(Figs. 41.8 and 41.10)*. Some cases may show considerable fibrosis. It is important to exclude vasculitis and capillaritis in a biopsy showing alveolar hemosiderosis.
Special studies	Prussian blue stain demonstrates faint, uneven, light blue pattern of staining in macrophages.	Prussian blue demonstrates coarse granules in the cytoplasm of macrophages with uniform and dark blue pattern of staining *(Figs. 41.9 and 41.10)*.
Prognosis	The 5- and 10-y survival rates for DIP are 95% and 70%, respectively. Smoking cessation is the main treatment strategy, although immunosuppression may also be used.	The overall prognosis is quite variable and often related to the etiology of the hemorrhage. In idiopathic cases, 86% survive beyond 5 y. Treatment is largely based on immunosuppression with steroids and treating the underlying cause of the hemorrhage, if known.

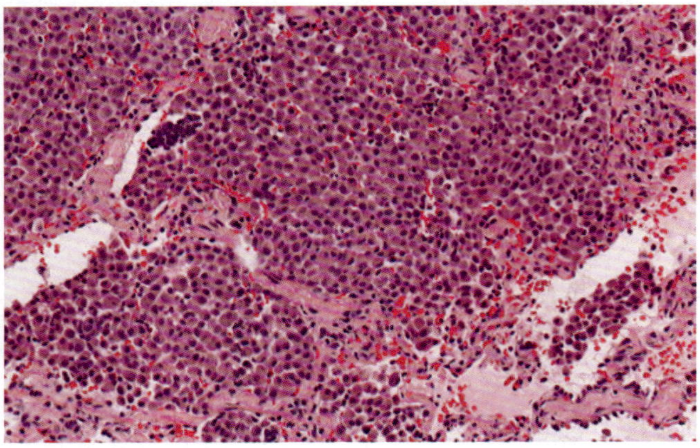

Figure 41.1 DIP (high-power view): There is diffuse alveolar spaces accumulation of pigmented macrophages with fine granular light golden-brown cytoplasm.

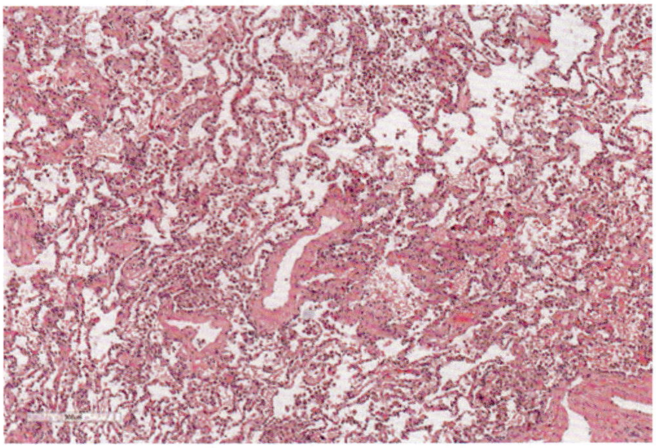

Figure 41.2 DIP: A low-power view of DIP showing the diffuse involvement of all airspaces by pigmented macrophages. This particular case did not have associated alveolar septal fibrosis.

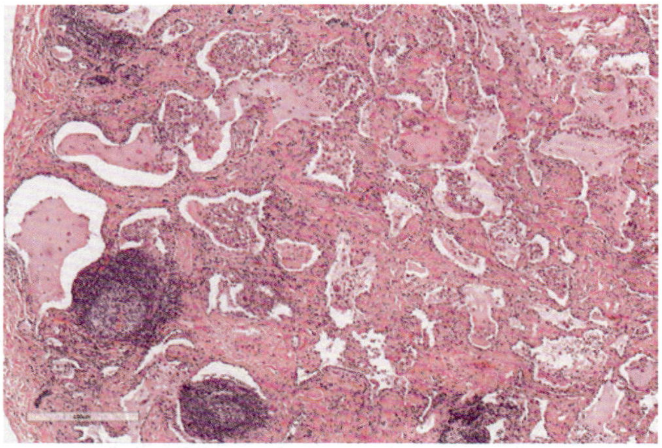

Figure 41.3 DIP: An image showing lymphoid hyperplasia with prominent germinal centers along with moderate amount of diffuse septal fibrosis.

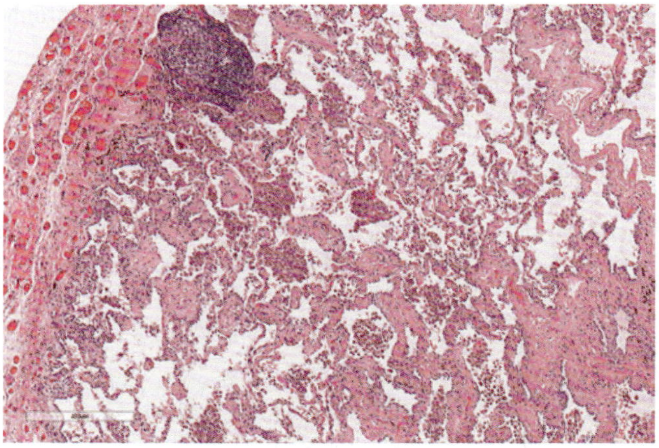

Figure 41.4 DIP: Histologic section showing pigmented airspace macrophages, a single lymphoid follicle, and mild septal fibrosis in the lower left corner.

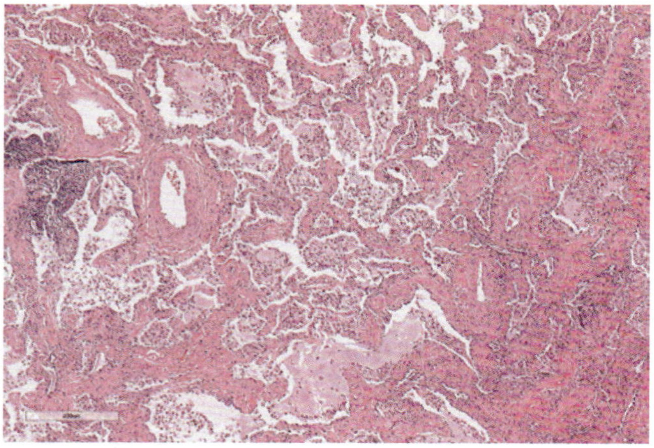

Figure 41.5 DIP: H&E stain showing diffuse airspace macrophages along with diffuse alveolar septal expansion by collagen.

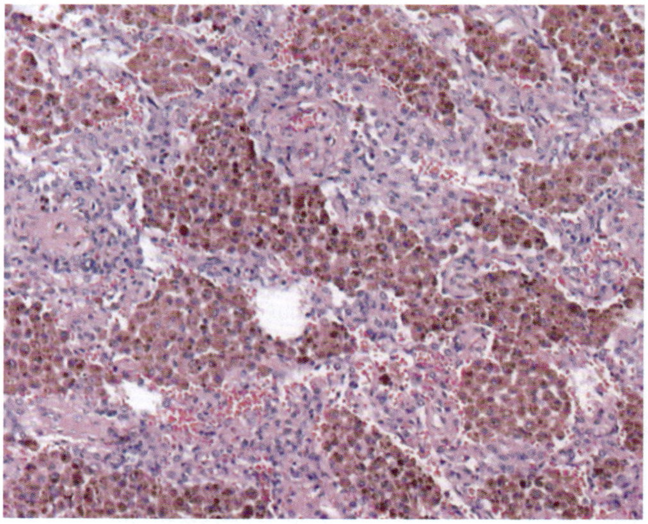

Figure 41.6 PAH: An image with dense airspace clusters of macrophages containing hemosiderin. Unlike smoking pigment, the hemosiderin inclusions may be large and coalesce to form spherical golden-brown inclusions within macrophages. The alveolar septa are expanded by inflammation.

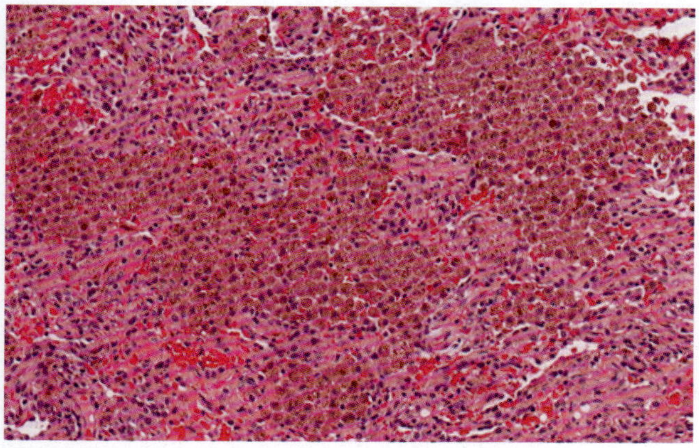

Figure 41.7 PAH (high-power view): There is alveolar space accumulation of pigmented hemosiderin-laden macrophages with chunky, coarsely granular, and dark golden brown cytoplasm.

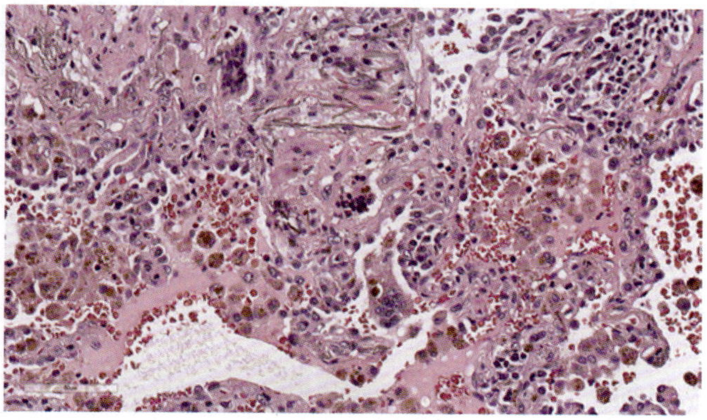

Figure 41.8 PAH (H&E stain): A case with coarse golden-brown macrophage inclusions and "endogenous pneumoconiosis" with elastic fibers encrusted with iron and calcium (upper middle portion of the image).

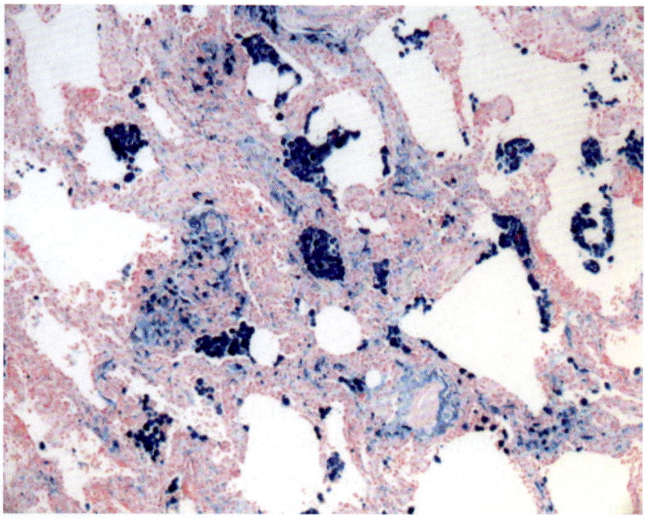

Figure 41.9 PAH: Prussian blue stain demonstrates chunky cytoplasmic granules with uniform dark blue pattern of staining.

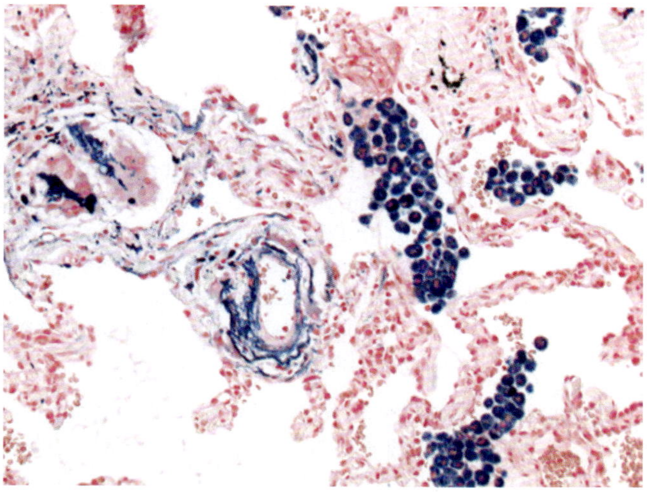

Figure 41.10 PAH: Prussian blue (iron stain) showing hemosiderin-laden macrophages within airspaces and endogenous pneumoconiosis, characterized by the presence of iron and calcium encrustation of vascular elastic tissue. Note foreign body multinucleated giant cell reaction (*upper left*). This lesion may be seen in any type of chronic alveolar hemorrhage.

42 DIFFUSE ALVEOLAR HEMORRHAGE VS. PROCEDURE-RELATED HEMORRHAGE

	Diffuse Alveolar Hemorrhage (DAH)	Procedure-Related Hemorrhage
Age	Age varies depending on cause.	Procedure-related hemorrhage may occur in children and adult populations with a wide range of age.
Location	Alveolar spaces. Hemorrhage may also be found in larger airways.	Alveolar spaces.
Symptoms	Symptoms vary and range from absent/minimal to frank hemoptysis. Onset is usually less than 7 d. Typical symptoms include cough, hemoptysis (variable), fever, and dyspnea. Symptoms associated with anemia.	No hemoptysis. In general, no symptoms related to the histologic findings.
Signs	Inspiratory crackles, tachypnea, and bronchial breath sounds on physical examination. Pulmonary function tests may show an increase in diffusing capacity of the lungs for carbon monoxide (DLCO) above 100% predicted because of the increased availability of hemoglobin within the alveoli. As DLCO is a sensitive marker for DAH, it is often used to monitor recurrences. Chest x-ray shows patchy or diffuse opacities. Chest CT shows patchy to diffuse, bilateral or unilateral, ground-glass or consolidative opacities. Often more central than peripheral.	No clinical signs of disease related to procedure-related hemorrhage.
Etiology	DAH may occur in a variety of situations. Most common causes are the small vessel vasculitic, pauci-immune disorders, including granulomatosis with polyangiitis (GPA) (previously referred to as Wegener granulomatosis), microscopic polyangiitis (MPA), and Churg–Strauss angiitis/granulomatosis (eosinophilic granulomatosis with polyangiitis). These diseases are associated with concomitant capillaritis or vasculitis on biopsy. Additional etiologies for DAH include immune complex vasculitic diseases such as Goodpasture syndrome (anti–glomerular basement membrane antibody disease), connective tissue–associated and immune complex–associated glomerulonephritis, and others. Idiopathic pulmonary alveolar hemosiderosis is a rare disease that is localized to the lungs (unlike many of the others that have an associated glomerulonephritis). Other causes of DAH include drug reactions, inhalants (such as cocaine), bone marrow transplantation, and coagulopathies (such as thrombocytopenia).	Bleeding occurs secondary to disruption of capillaries and small blood vessels during the process of the biopsy or other procedures. Common in transbronchial biopsies. The importance in recognizing lies in not overdiagnosing true alveolar hemorrhage.
Histology	Extensive intra-alveolar hemorrhage characterized by evidence of recent and ongoing hemorrhage. Thus, there should be a mix of fresh blood (intact and "smeared out" red blood cells), fibrin, alveolar hemosiderosis, and erythrophagocytosis by macrophages. Hemosiderin implies chronicity as it takes 2 d to form after hemorrhage and up to 4 wk to clear *(Figs. 42.1–42.3)*.	Like DAH, there are red blood cells within alveolar spaces; however, there is no fibrin, alveolar hemosiderosis, or erythrophagocytosis. Usually distinct red blood cells without any disintegration of red cell membranes are seen *(Figs. 42.10–42.12)*.

	Diffuse Alveolar Hemorrhage (DAH)	Procedure-Related Hemorrhage
	If concurrent vasculitis, then disruption of vessel elastic laminae by inflammatory cells with associated fibrinoid necrosis. Or, if capillaritis, then alveolar septa destroyed by neutrophilic infiltrates *(Fig. 42.4)*. Nonspecific thickening of alveolar septa and alveolar pneumocyte hyperplasia *(Fig. 42.5)*. If longstanding, may have disruption and encrustation of vascular elastic tissue by iron and calcium, imparting a particular blue-black hue to the elastic fibers. Associated engulfment by foreign body type giant cells may be seen (thus the term *endogenous pneumoconiosis*) *(Figs. 42.6 and 42.7)*.	No disruption of vascular elastic laminae. Often patchy with areas of unaffected lung readily identified.
Special studies	Elastic tissue stains or pentachrome (Movat) stain are necessary to evaluate destruction and disruption of the vascular elastic laminae. Additionally, immunofluorescence stains can be helpful in Goodpasture syndrome (anti–glomerular basement antibody disease) *(Fig. 42.8)* as well as in hemorrhage associated with systemic lupus erythematosus (SLE). Iron stains may be necessary to differentiate between smoker's pigment (faint uneven dusky blue to no staining) and hemosiderin (bright blue and coarsely granular) *(Fig. 42.9)*.	May perform iron stain to rule out hemosiderin deposition. Elastic tissue stains to evaluate vascular elastic laminae.
Prognosis	Prognosis depends on the etiology of the DAH. The most important step is to identify the underlying cause and begin treatment based on specific etiology.	No clinical sequelae to artefactual hemorrhage.

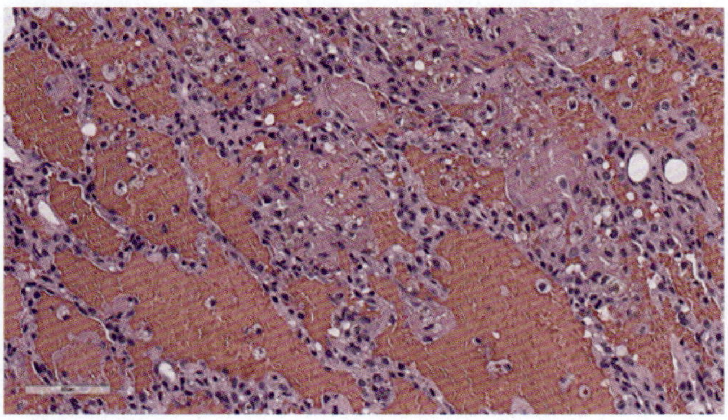

Figure 42.1 DAH: Real hemorrhage shows a mix of fibrin, hemosiderin-laden macrophages, and red blood cells that show indistinct borders.

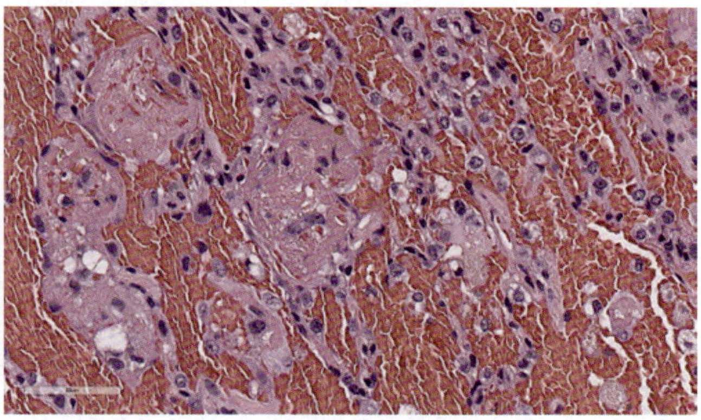

Figure 42.2 DAH: Fibrin mixed with red blood cells in real hemorrhage.

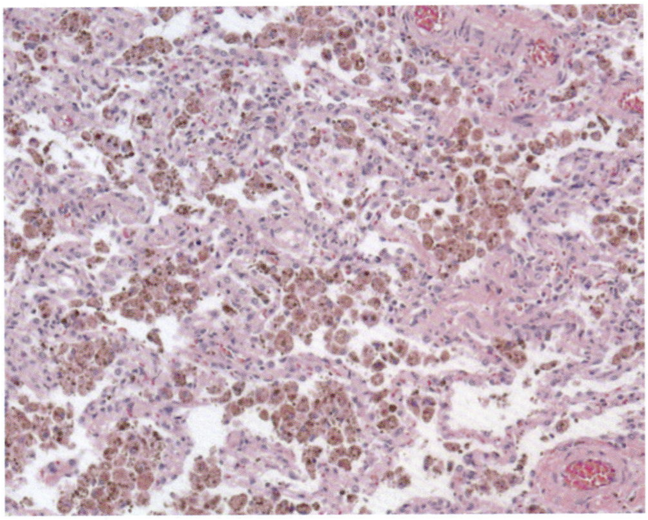

Figure 42.3 DAH: Hemosiderin-laden macrophages appear as chunky, coarse, golden-brown refractile cytoplasmic granules.

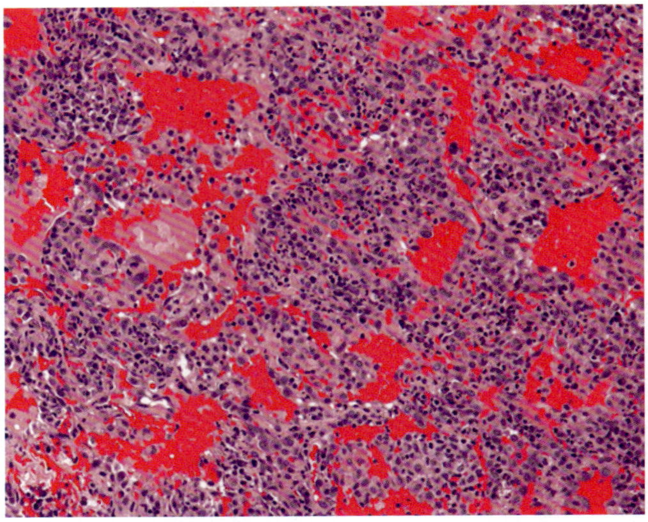

Figure 42.4 DAH: In this image of real hemorrhage, there is capillaritis, characterized by alveolar septal expansion by clusters of neutrophils demonstrating karyorrhectic debris. The adjacent airspaces contain coalescent red blood cells—no distinct borders are identified. Reactive pneumocytes line alveolar septa.

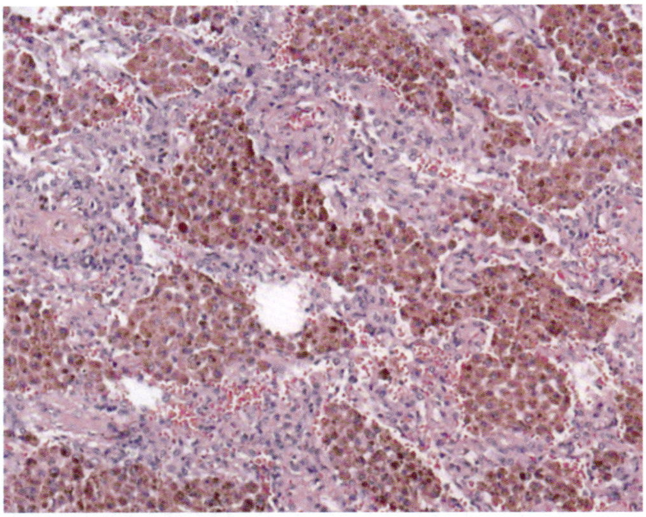

Figure 42.5 DAH: The alveolar septa may become thickened and the lining pneumocytes hyperplastic, imparting a low-power image of interstitial lung disease. In this image, note the coarse golden-brown hemosiderin pigment within the alveolar macrophages.

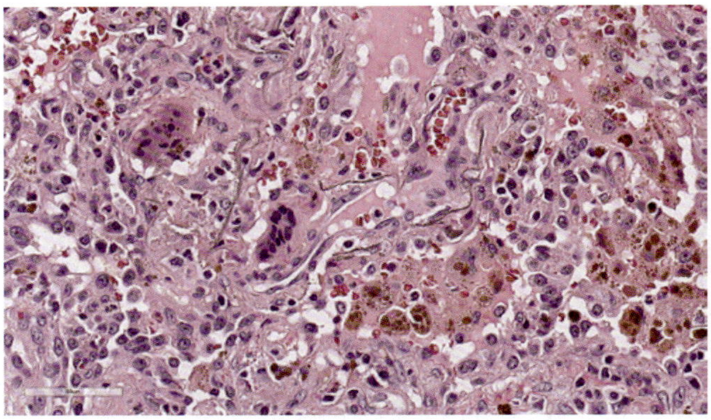

Figure 42.6 DAH: Encrustation of disrupted elastic tissue fibers occurs with longstanding bleeding from any cause. The fibers become disrupted and are visible on hematoxylin and eosin stain by their gray-black appearance, which is caused by iron and calcium deposition. Giant cells engulf these fibers, thus the term *endogenous pneumoconiosis*. Also note the extensive hemosiderin-laden macrophages in the background. The alveolar septa are nonspecifically thickened and show pneumocyte hyperplasia.

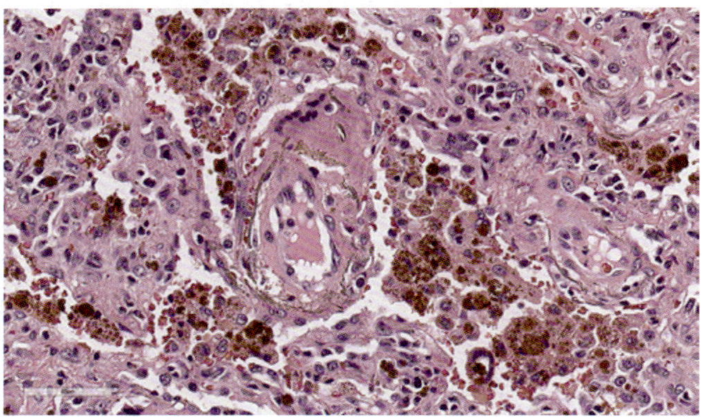

Figure 42.7 DAH: Higher-power view of gray-black elastic fibers engulfed by giant cell.

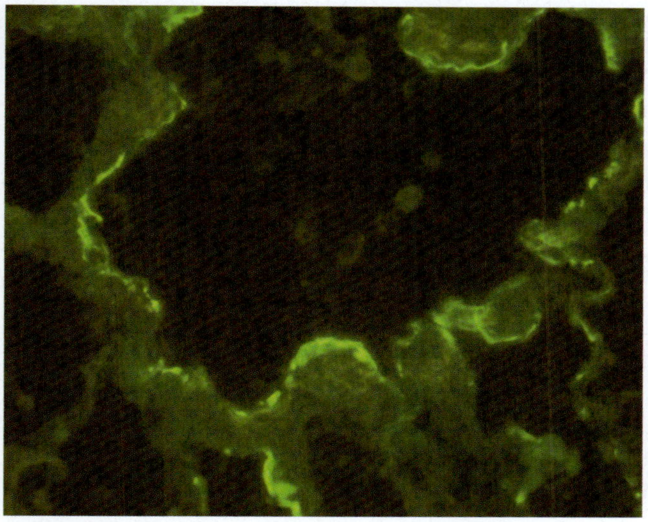

Figure 42.8 DAH: In a case of Goodpasture syndrome, an IgG immunofluorescence stain shows linear deposits along alveolar basement membrane. SLE typically shows granular staining of capillary basement membranes for immunoglobulins and complement.

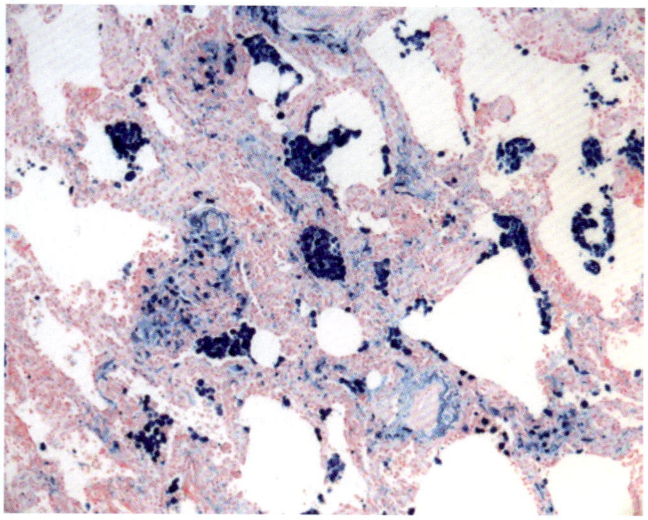

Figure 42.9 DAH: Iron stain shows bright-to-deep blue staining of hemosiderin within macrophages. In this image, the iron stain is also highlighting the vascular encrustation of elastic fibers (the so-called endogenous pneumoconiosis).

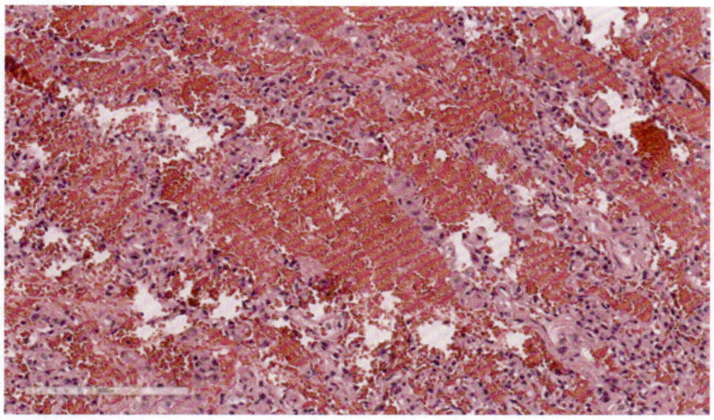

Figure 42.10 Procedure-related hemorrhage: Contrast this image of artifactual hemorrhage with that of real hemorrhage (Fig. 42.1). In artifactual hemorrhage, the majority of the red blood cells show distinct cell borders. No hemosiderin or fibrin is admixed with the blood. No pneumocyte hyperplasia is noted.

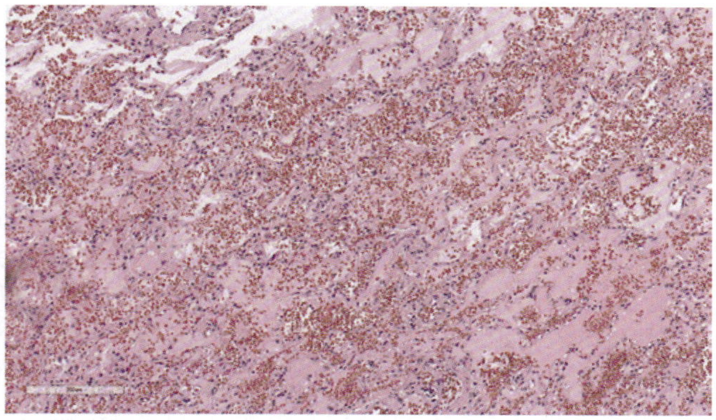

Figure 42.11 Procedure-related hemorrhage: Artifactual hemorrhage with focal airspace edema, which should not be mistaken for fibrin. Edema fluid lacks the density and the admixed macrophages and disintegrating red blood cells that are more characteristic of fibrin.

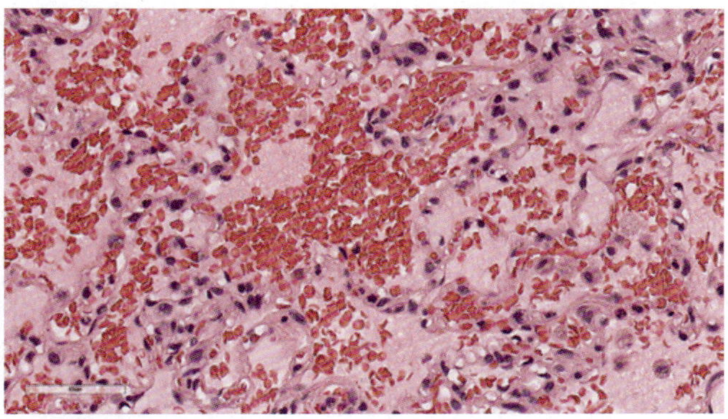

Figure 42.12 Procedure-related hemorrhage: Higher-power view showing distinct red blood cell borders and edema.

43 GRANULOMATOSIS WITH POLYANGIITIS VS. EOSINOPHILIC GRANULOMATOSIS WITH POLYANGIITIS (CHURG–STRAUSS SYNDROME)

	Granulomatosis with Polyangiitis (GPA; Wegener Granulomatosis)	Eosinophilic Granulomatosis with Polyangiitis (Churg–Strauss Syndrome)
Age	Adults, mean age 40, but can affect adolescents and, rarely, children.	Mean age of vasculitis onset approximately 40–50, but can affect adults of all ages.
Location	Systemic necrotizing vasculitis with a classic triad of upper airways (sinusitis/otitis, upper airway ulceration), lower respiratory tract, and kidney (glomerulonephritis) involvement. May also affect other organs, including eye, middle ear, nervous system, joints, and skin. May solely involve the lung (limited or localized GPA). Involves small to medium-sized arteries and veins, as well as capillaries.	Upper airway, lungs, skin, and peripheral nerves are main sites of involvement. May involve heart and kidneys (less commonly). Vascular involvement includes small arteries, veins, and capillaries. Airspace involvement.
Symptoms	Constitutional: fever, weight loss, malaise, fatigue. Pulmonary: cough, chest pain, shortness of breath, hemoptysis. Other symptoms depend on organ system involved.	Asthma (often severe, steroid-requiring, and longstanding) or allergies. Chronic rhinitis and sinusitis (with or without nasal polyposis). Weight loss, fever, arthralgias, and myalgias with development of vasculitis. Symptoms may overlap with other eosinophilic lung diseases.
Signs	Nonspecific lung findings with inspiratory crackles most common. If acute with hemorrhage, may have increased diffusing capacity of the lungs for carbon monoxide (DLCO); if chronic, may have restriction and gas exchange abnormalities. Chest x-ray may show multiple bilateral opacities. High-resolution computed tomography (HRCT) often shows bilateral ground-glass opacities or patchy consolidation; occasionally, centrilobular nodules are noted. Cavitation of nodules, diffuse ground-glass opacities (especially with diffuse alveolar hemorrhage [DAH]), atelectasis, and airway complications such as stenosis and ulcerations may also be seen. Bronchoalveolar lavage (BAL) is useful as there are increased red blood cell counts in subsequent aliquots, even in patients without clinical hemoptysis. Laboratory findings usually include anemia and leukocytosis. Positive c-ANCA and anti-proteinase 3 (PR3) autoantibodies are usually present in active disease, but are not present in nearly one-third of patients with limited disease.	Classic triad of (1) asthma, (2) peripheral blood eosinophilia, and (3) necrotizing vasculitis. Chest CT shows waxing and waning parenchymal opacities that may change location, often with peripheral or random distribution of air space consolidation. Unlike GPA, cavitary lesions are unusual. Peripheral blood eosinophilia is the major feature (generally between 5 and 20×10^9). BAL and pleural fluid eosinophilia seen, often greater than 60%. Perinuclear anti-neutrophil cytoplasmic antibody (p-ANCA) with myeloperoxidase (MPO) specificity is positive in 40%. Anemia common. Classification criteria of the American College of Rheumatology based on four or more of the following six criteria in a patient with a proven systemic vasculitis: asthma; blood eosinophilia $>10\%$; mononeuritis or polyneuropathy; fluctuating opacities on chest imaging; bilateral maxillary sinus abnormalities; eosinophils on biopsy.
Etiology	The cause is unknown; however, it is clearly mediated by the immune system, resulting in cytoplasmic antineutrophil cytoplasmic antibodies (c-ANCA) directed against specific proteins in white blood cells—proteinase 3 (PR3) in the case of GPA. Another name for ANCA-associated disease is ANCA-associated vasculitis (AAV).	Autoimmune process involving T cells, endothelial cells, and eosinophils. Possible relationship to leukotriene antagonists in a small proportion of cases.

	Granulomatosis with Polyangiitis (GPA; Wegener Granulomatosis)	**Eosinophilic Granulomatosis with Polyangiitis (Churg–Strauss Syndrome)**
Histology	Characteristically, the major histologic features include (1) lung parenchymal necrosis *(Fig. 43.1)*, (2) vasculitis (generally involving small to medium-sized arteries, and occasionally veins and capillaries) *(Fig. 43.2)*, and (3) granulomatous inflammation *(Fig. 43.3)*. Often large serpiginous necrotic zones replace lung parenchyma, resulting in the so-called geographic necrosis (deeply basophilic areas with irregular jagged borders) *(Fig. 43.4)*. May have smaller microscopic foci of microabscesses with irregular-to-round borders. Palisading histiocytes and scattered multinucleated giant cells can be found associated with areas of abscess. The giant cells do not form sarcoid-like granulomas and have a pyknotic quality *(Fig. 43.5)*. Necrotizing vasculitis, which can involve both arteries and veins, characterized by foci of necrosis and granulomatous inflammation. May see partial involvement of vessel walls by microabscesses. Fibrinoid necrosis is usually present *(Fig. 43.6)*. Variant cases may show capillaritis with DAH as the sole histologic abnormalities. Capillaritis is inferred if there are neutrophils with nuclear debris (indicative of apoptosis) within the alveolar septa and there is some evidence of injury—fibrin exudates, pneumocyte reactivity, organization *(Fig. 43.7)*. Although eosinophils are usually inconspicuous, occasionally may have eosinophil-rich variants. Must differentiate from polyangiitis with eosinophils (Churg–Strauss syndrome). Rarely (1%), bronchocentric variant is present. Differentiation from bronchocentric granulomatosis is based on the presence or absence of necrotizing vasculitis.	Necrotizing small-vessel (arteries, veins, capillaries) vasculitis with eosinophils, lymphocytes, and occasionally giant cells/granulomas *(Figs. 43.9 and 43.10)*. Eosinophilic pneumonia with airspace eosinophils and pink macrophages (absent in GPA) *(Fig. 43.11)*. Parenchymal granulomatous necrosis characterized by central areas of necrosis containing abundant necrotic eosinophils, surrounded by palisading histiocytes and multinucleated giant cells *(Fig. 43.12)*. Changes of chronic asthma in bronchi and bronchioles. Pulmonary hemorrhage not common (in contrast to GPA). Histologic diagnostic issues arise when a patient is treated with steroids prior to biopsy, as eosinophils are exquisitely sensitive to corticosteroids and disappear rapidly.
Special studies	Elastic tissue stains or pentachrome (Movat) stain may be used to evaluate vessel walls *(Fig. 43.8)*.	Elastic tissue stains to evaluate vascular elastic laminae.
Prognosis	5-y survival of 75% with appropriately treated disease.	Overall 5-y survival rates between 70% and 100% with appropriate treatment.

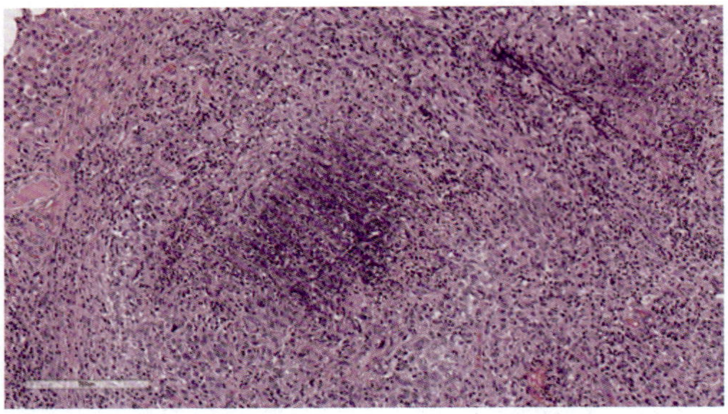

Figure 43.1 GPA: Focus of parenchymal necrosis characterized by basophilic central necrosis surrounded by histiocytes and other inflammatory cells.

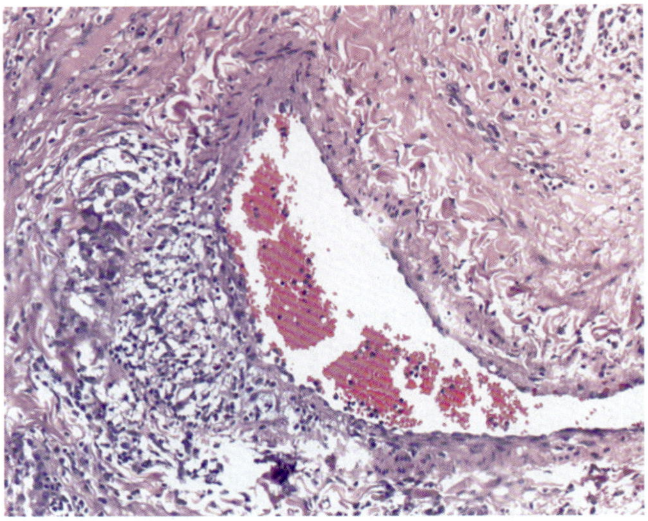

Figure 43.2 GPA: Granulomatous vasculitis in which there is disruption of the left side of artery wall by an inflammatory infiltrate composed of histiocytes, lymphocytes, eosinophils, and, at the outer aspect, multinucleated giant cells. GPA may partially or circumferentially destroy the vessel wall.

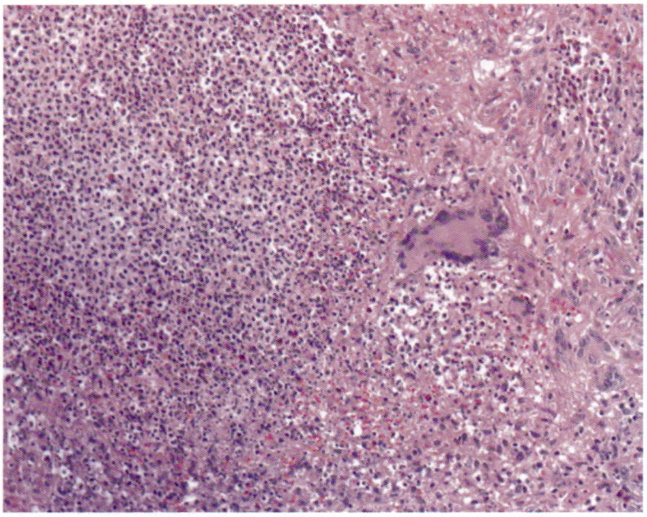

Figure 43.3 GPA: Classic giant cell of GPA, which is an isolated giant cell easily visible at low power.

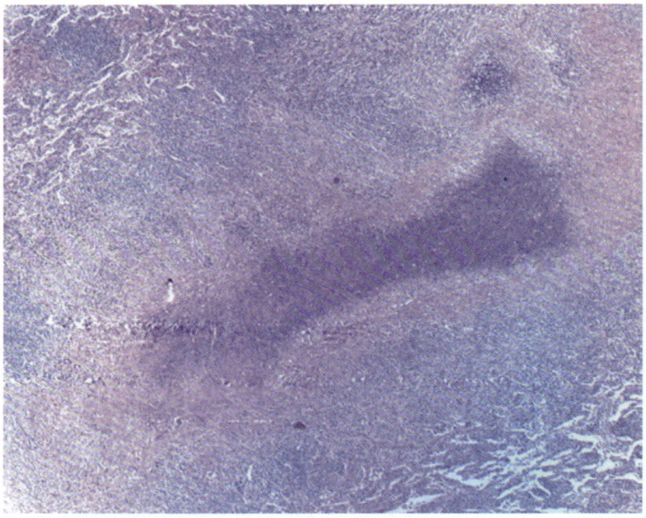

Figure 43.4 GPA: Geographic necrosis is characterized by irregularly bordered basophilic necrotic zones, which are usually surrounded by epithelioid histiocytes. The necrosis has a "dirty," granular-to-basophilic appearance due to pyknotic nuclei and abundant cellular debris.

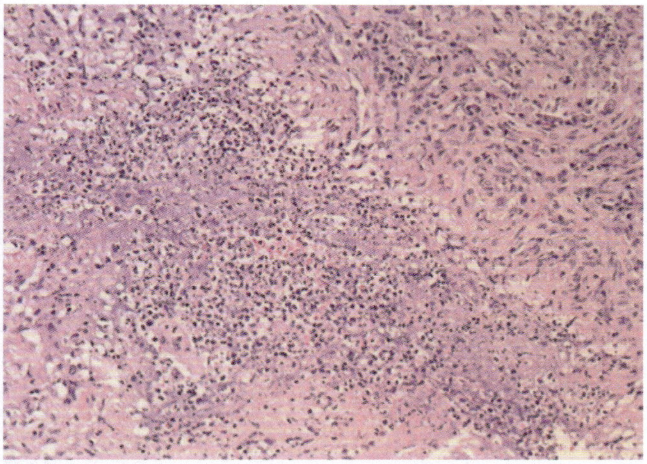

Figure 43.5 GPA: Microabscess surrounded by palisading histiocytes.

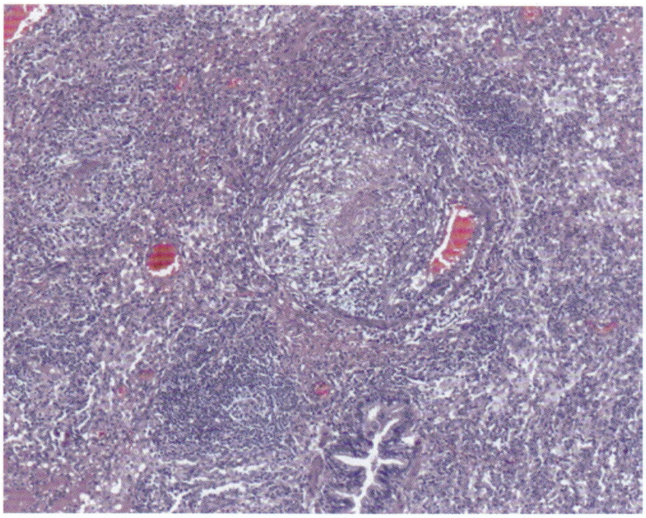

Figure 43.6 GPA: Here, an artery is partially destroyed by an eccentric infiltrate. Fibrinoid necrosis is present. An intact small airway (bronchiole) can be seen at the bottom of the image.

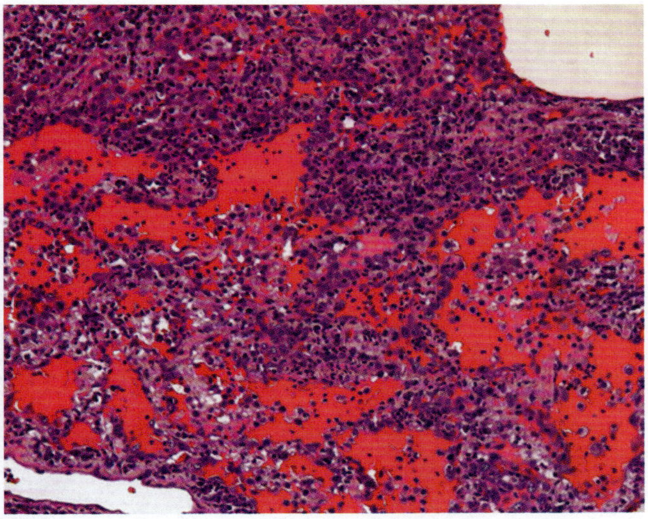

Figure 43.7 GPA: In this case of GPA, the only histologic feature is capillaritis with associated alveolar hemorrhage. The capillaritis is characterized by expansion of the alveolar septa by clustered neutrophils and associated nuclear debris. Airspaces show hemorrhage. Some of the neutrophils spill over into the airspaces, but the septal neutrophils are much more prominent than the airspace neutrophils.

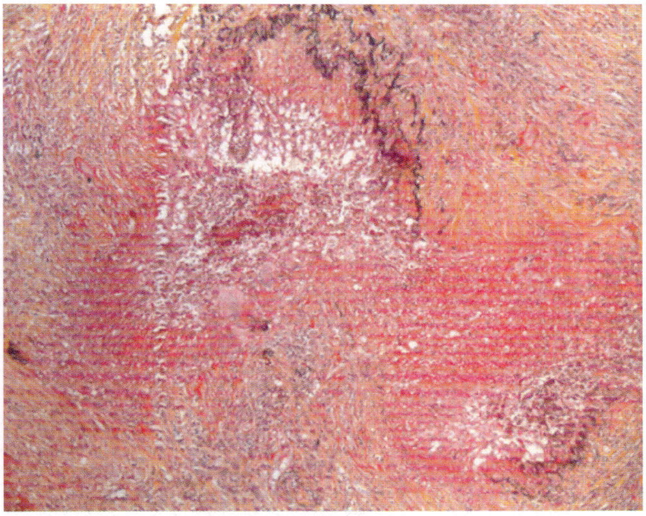

Figure 43.8 GPA: The pentachrome (Movat) stain shows a nearly circumferentially destroyed vessel wall as illustrated by the remnant double elastic laminae of the pulmonary artery.

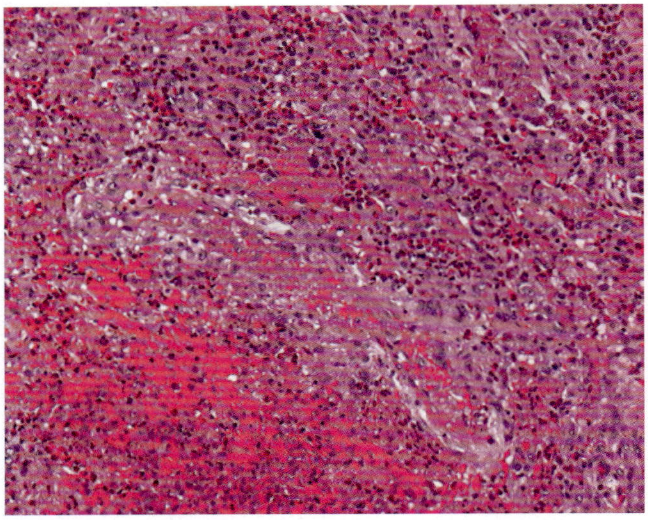

Figure 43.9 Eosinophilic granulomatosis with polyangiitis: Small vessel infiltrated by numerous eosinophils. There is fibrinoid necrosis of the wall. Alveolar red blood cells and fibrin fill adjacent airspaces.

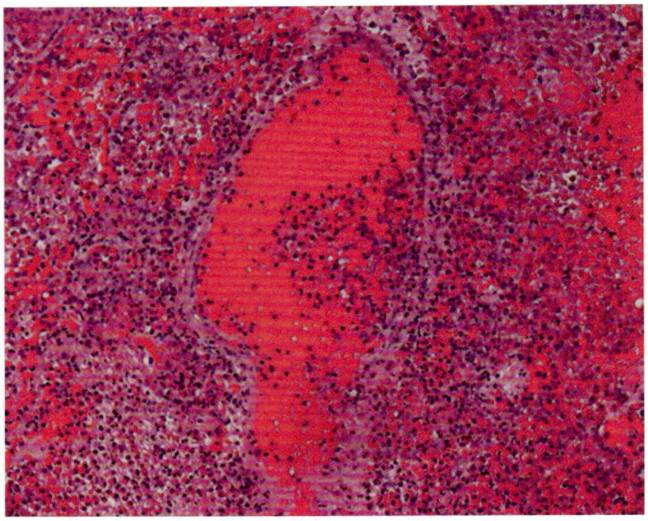

Figure 43.10 Eosinophilic granulomatosis with polyangiitis: Destruction of a vein by eosinophilic infiltrate and hemorrhage in adjacent airspaces.

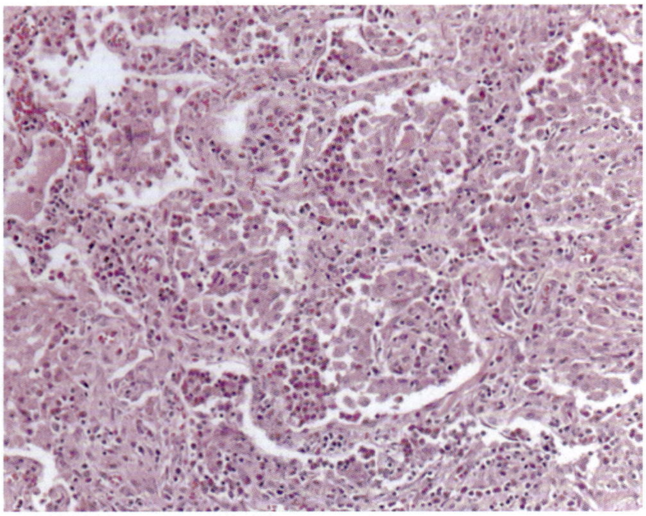

Figure 43.11 Eosinophilic granulomatosis with polyangiitis: Eosinophilic pneumonia component of Churg–Strauss syndrome is characterized by airspace collections of eosinophils admixed with pink macrophages. The adjacent septa are also infiltrated by eosinophils and chronic inflammatory cells.

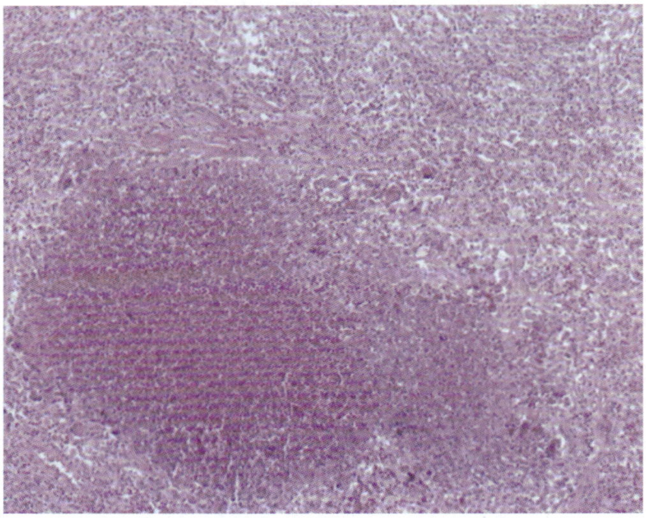

Figure 43.12 Eosinophilic granulomatosis with polyangiitis: Central eosinophilic abscess surrounded by a zone of chronic inflammation, eosinophils, and multinucleated giant cells.

44 GRANULOMATOSIS WITH POLYANGIITIS VS. MICROSCOPIC POLYANGIITIS

	Granulomatosis with Polyangiitis (GPA; Wegener Granulomatosis)	Microscopic Polyangiitis (MPA)
Age	Adults, mean age 40, but can affect adolescents and, rarely, children.	Adults, mean age 50.
Location	Systemic necrotizing vasculitis with a classic triad of upper airways (sinusitis/otitis, upper airway ulceration), lower respiratory tract, and kidney (glomerulonephritis) involvement. May also affect other organs, including eye, middle ear, nervous system, joints, and skin. May solely involve the lung (limited or localized GPA). Involves small- to medium-sized arteries and veins, as well as capillaries.	Lungs (up to 30% of patients) and kidney (nearly universal). MPA is the most common cause of pulmonary–renal syndrome. Also can involve ear, upper respiratory tract, and skin. Involves lung capillaries.
Symptoms	Constitutional: fever, weight loss, malaise, fatigue. Pulmonary: cough, chest pain, shortness of breath, hemoptysis. Other symptoms depend on organ system involved.	Fever, asthenia, fatigue, malaise, myalgias, and arthralgias, followed by symptoms of renal disease.
Signs	Nonspecific lung findings with inspiratory crackles most common. If acute, may have increased diffusing capacity of the lungs for carbon monoxide (DLCO); if chronic, may have restriction and gas exchange abnormalities. Chest x-ray may show multiple bilateral opacities. High-resolution computed tomography (HRCT) often shows bilateral ground-glass opacities or patchy consolidation; occasionally, centrilobular nodules are noted. Cavitation of nodules, diffuse ground-glass opacities (especially with diffuse alveolar hemorrhage [DAH]), atelectasis, and airway complications such as stenosis and ulcerations may also be seen. Bronchoalveolar lavage (BAL) is useful as there are increased red blood cell counts in subsequent aliquots, even in patients without clinical hemoptysis. Laboratory findings usually include anemia and leukocytosis. Positive c-ANCA and anti-proteinase 3 (PR3) autoantibodies are usually present in active disease, but are not present in nearly one-third of patients with limited disease.	Chest CT demonstrates bilateral alveolar opacities without pulmonary nodules, predominantly involving lower lobes. BAL with acute hemorrhage and/or hemosiderin-laden macrophages. p-ANCAs with myeloperoxidase (MPO) specificity in $>80\%$.
Etiology	The cause is unknown; however, it is clearly mediated by the immune system, resulting in cytoplasmic antineutrophil cytoplasmic antibodies (c-ANCA) directed against specific proteins in white blood cells—proteinase 3 (PR3) in the case of GPA. Another name for ANCA-associated disease is ANCA-associated vasculitis (AAV).	Etiology unknown. Considered a small vessel variant of polyarteritis nodosa. Autoimmune process. One of the ANCA-associated vasculitides with p-ANCAs directed against MPO.
Histology	Characteristically, the major histologic features include (1) lung parenchymal necrosis, (2) vasculitis (generally involving small- to medium-sized arteries, and occasionally veins and capillaries), and (3) granulomatous inflammation. Often large serpiginous necrotic zones replace lung parenchyma, resulting in the so-called geographic necrosis (deeply basophilic areas with irregular jagged borders) *(Fig. 44.1)*.	Capillaritis characterized by neutrophilic infiltrate of septal walls with karyorrhectic debris *(Figs. 44.4 and 44.5)*. Alveolar hemorrhage with fibrin and hemosiderin *(Figs. 44.6–44.8)*.

	Granulomatosis with Polyangiitis (GPA; Wegener Granulomatosis)	Microscopic Polyangiitis (MPA)
	May have smaller microscopic foci of microabscesses with irregular-to-round borders *(Fig. 44.2)*. Palisading histiocytes and scattered multinucleated giant cells can be found associated with areas of abscess. The giant cells do not form sarcoid-like granulomas and have a pyknotic quality. Necrotizing vasculitis, which can involve both arteries and veins, characterized by foci of necrosis and granulomatous inflammation. Partial involvement of vessel walls by microabscesses may be seen. Fibrinoid necrosis is usually present. Variant cases may show capillaritis with DAH as the sole histologic abnormalities. Capillaritis is inferred if there are neutrophils with nuclear debris (indicative of apoptosis) within the alveolar septa and there is some evidence of injury—fibrin exudates, pneumocyte reactivity, organization *(Fig. 44.3)*. Although eosinophils are usually inconspicuous, occasionally may have eosinophil-rich variants. Must differentiate from polyangiitis with eosinophils (Churg–Strauss syndrome). Rarely (1%), bronchocentric variant is present. Differentiation from bronchocentric granulomatosis is based on the presence or absence of necrotizing vasculitis.	Secondary changes of organizing pneumonia and reactive pneumocytes *(Fig. 44.9)*. Rarely, fibrotic interstitial lung disease occurs after recurrent DAH. No granulomas.
Special studies	Elastic tissue stains or pentachrome (Movat) stain may be used to evaluate vessel walls.	Iron stains may be helpful in differentiating smoker's pigment from hemosiderin.
Prognosis	5-y survival of 75% with appropriately treated disease.	5-y survival of 65% with treatment. Early mortality rate of 25% with DAH.

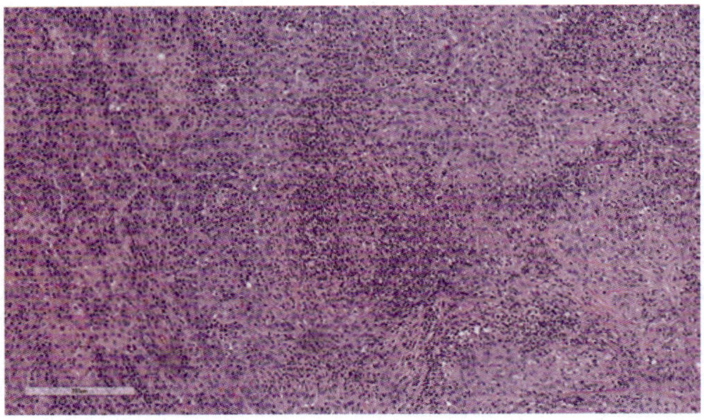

Figure 44.1 GPA: Necrosis and abscess characterized by basophilic necrosis and collections of neutrophils surrounded by histiocytes and other inflammatory cells.

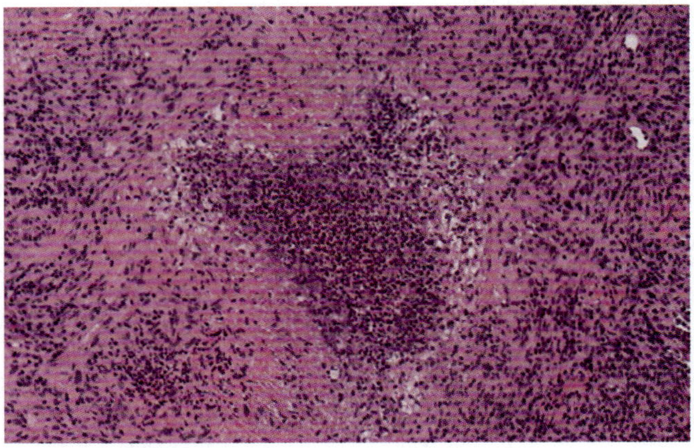

Figure 44.2 GPA: Microabscess surrounded by palisading histiocytes.

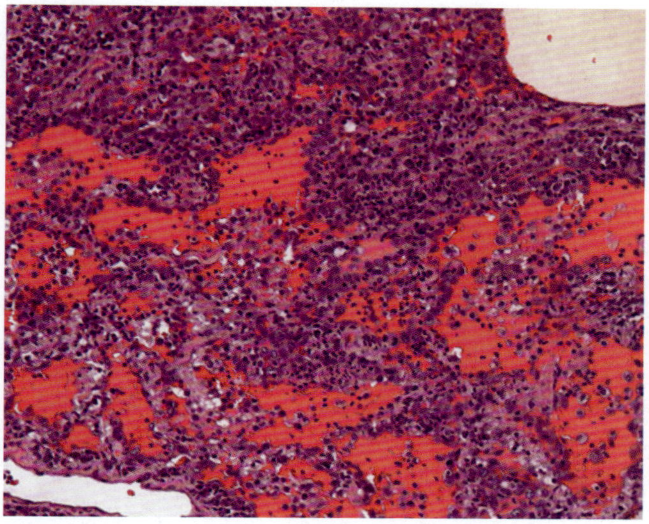

Figure 44.3 GPA: Capillaritis in GPA (note that the appearance is identical to capillaritis in MPA). Need additional features of granulomatous inflammation and parenchymal necrosis, or serologic studies, to help establish GPA.

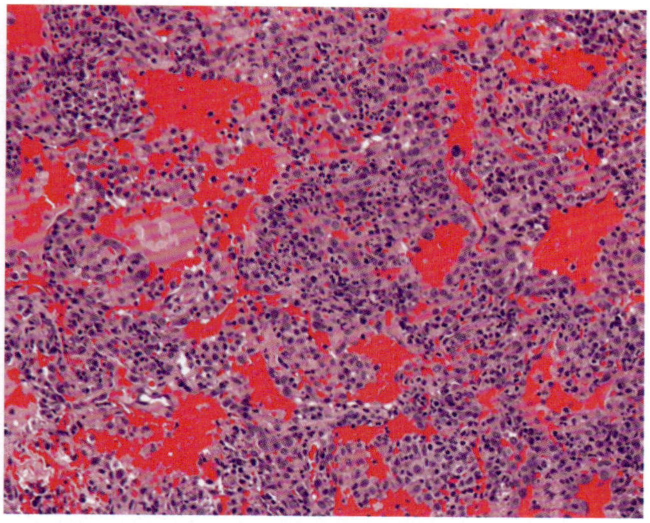

Figure 44.4 MPA: Capillaritis characterized by infiltration of septal walls with neutrophils. Red blood cells are present in adjacent airspaces. These histologic findings are indistinguishable from those of the rare capillaritis variant of GPA. However, most cases of GPA will also have areas of more typical granulomatous inflammation. Distinguishing the two diseases can be problematic, though, especially on small needle core biopsies. Correlation with serologic studies is helpful.

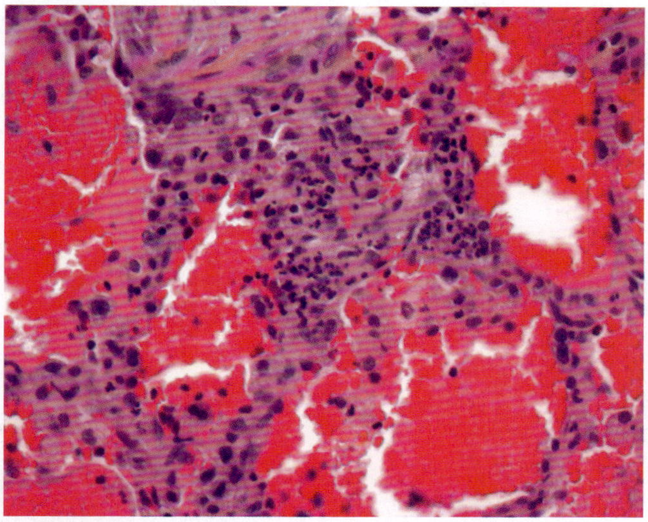

Figure 44.5 MPA: Higher-power image of expansion and destruction of alveolar walls by neutrophilic infiltrates. There is karyorrhectic debris. Some spillover of neutrophils into the adjacent airspaces is noted. Disintegrating red blood cells and fibrin are present in adjacent airspaces.

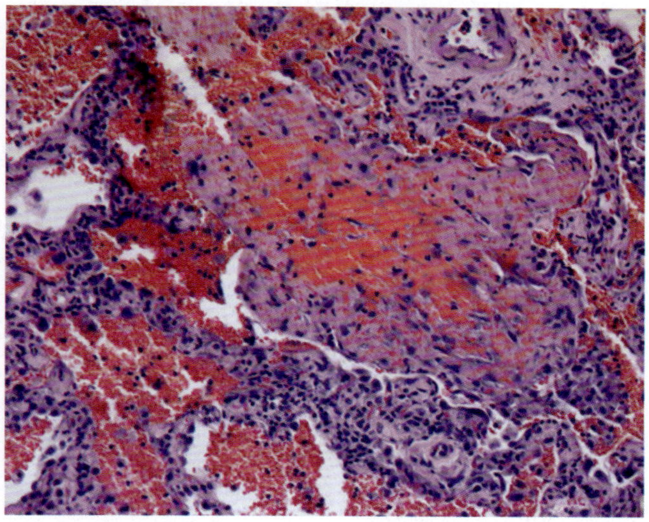

Figure 44.6 MPA: The histology of alveolar hemorrhage in this disease is similar to all other forms of pulmonary alveolar hemorrhage—there is airspace fibrin, red blood cells, and hemosiderin-laden macrophages.

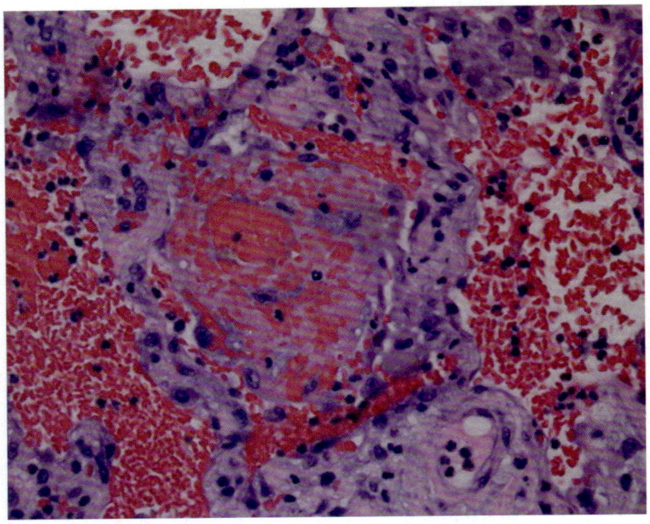

Figure 44.7 MPA: Airspaces with recent hemorrhage are indicated by the intact red blood cells; the area of true hemorrhage (*center*) shows the more typical indistinct appearance of the red blood cells. Additionally, true hemorrhage also demonstrates fibrin and hemosiderin-laden macrophages.

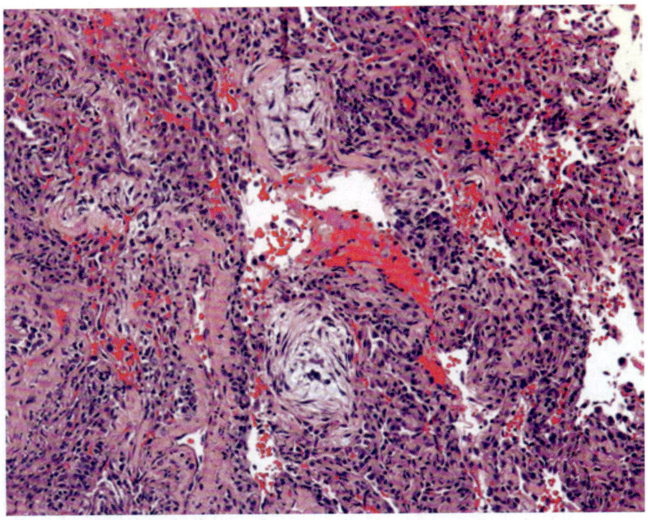

Figure 44.9 MPA: The nonspecific finding of organizing pneumonia is common to many lung injuries.

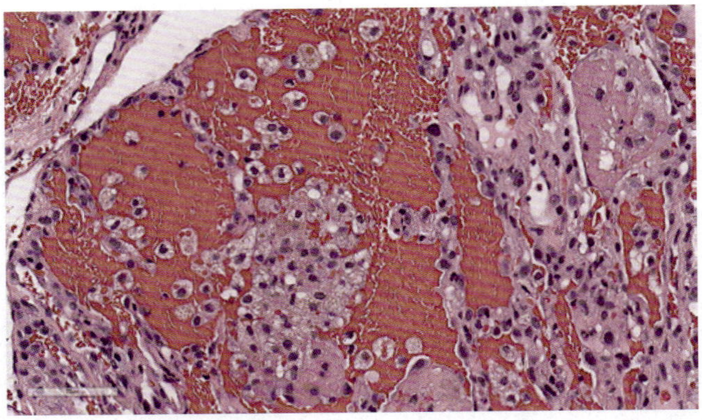

Figure 44.8 MPA: Hemorrhage consisting of hemosiderin-laden macrophages, fibrin, and disrupted red blood cells.

45 GRANULOMATOSIS WITH POLYANGIITIS VS. LYMPHOMATOID GRANULOMATOSIS

	Granulomatosis with Polyangiitis (GPA; Wegener Granulomatosis)	Lymphomatoid Granulomatosis (LYG)
Age	Adults, mean age 40, but can affect adolescents and, rarely, children.	Can develop at any age; median age at diagnosis is 60.
Location	Systemic necrotizing vasculitis with a classic triad of upper airways (sinusitis/otitis, upper airway ulceration), lower respiratory tract, and kidney (glomerulonephritis) involvement. May also affect other organs, including eye, middle ear, nervous system, joints, and skin. May solely involve the lung (limited or localized GPA). Involves small- to medium-sized arteries and veins, as well as capillaries.	Lung, central nervous system, skin, liver and kidneys. Vasculitis involves small- to medium-sized pulmonary vessels.
Symptoms	Constitutional: fever, weight loss, malaise, fatigue. Pulmonary: cough, chest pain, shortness of breath, hemoptysis. Other symptoms depend on the organ system involved.	Cough, chest pain, dyspnea, fever, weight loss, and hemoptysis.
Signs	Nonspecific lung findings with inspiratory crackles most common. If acute, may have increased diffusing capacity of the lungs for carbon monoxide (DLCO); if chronic, may have restriction and gas exchange abnormalities. Chest x-ray may show multiple bilateral opacities. High-resolution computed tomography (HRCT) often shows bilateral ground-glass opacities or patchy consolidation; occasionally, centrilobular nodules are noted. Cavitation of nodules, diffuse ground-glass opacities (especially with diffuse alveolar hemorrhage [DAH]), atelectasis, and airway complications such as stenosis and ulcerations may also be seen. Bronchoalveolar lavage (BAL) is useful as there are increased red blood cell counts in subsequent aliquots, even in patients without clinical hemoptysis. Laboratory findings usually include anemia and leukocytosis. Positive c-ANCA and anti-proteinase 3 (PR3) autoantibodies are usually present in active disease, but are not present in nearly one-third of patients with limited disease.	Chest CT demonstrates bilateral peripheral smooth lung nodules, ranging from 2 to 10 cm, which wax and wane. May also present as solitary mass or diffuse infiltrate. Ground-glass opacities may be present. No peripheral or mediastinal lymphadenopathy.
Etiology	The cause is unknown; however, it is clearly mediated by the immune system, resulting in cytoplasmic antineutrophil cytoplasmic antibodies (c-ANCA) directed against specific proteins in white blood cells—proteinase 3 (PR3) in the case of GPA. Another name for ANCA-associated disease is ANCA-associated vasculitis (AAV).	T-cell rich, Epstein–Barr virus (EBV)–associated B-cell lymphoproliferative disorder. LYG- and EBV-related posttransplant lymphoproliferative diseases are likely closely related, with both arising in a background of latent EBV infection. Prolonged immunosuppression or immune deficiency are frequent underlying conditions in LYG.

	Granulomatosis with Polyangiitis (GPA; Wegener Granulomatosis)	Lymphomatoid Granulomatosis (LYG)
Histology	Characteristically, the major histologic features include (1) lung parenchymal necrosis, (2) vasculitis (generally involving small- to medium-sized arteries, and occasionally veins and capillaries), and (3) granulomatous inflammation. Often large serpiginous necrotic zones replace lung parenchyma, resulting in the so-called geographic necrosis (deeply basophilic areas with irregular jagged borders) *(Fig. 45.1)*. May have smaller microscopic foci of microabscesses with irregular-to-round borders. Palisading histiocytes and scattered multinucleated giant cells can be found associated with areas of abscess. The giant cells do not form sarcoid-like granulomas and have a pyknotic quality. Necrotizing vasculitis, which can involve both arteries and veins, characterized by foci of necrosis and granulomatous inflammation. Partial involvement of vessel walls by microabscesses may be seen. Fibrinoid necrosis is usually present *(Figs. 45.2 and 45.3)*. Variant cases may show capillaritis with DAH as the sole histologic abnormalities. Capillaritis is inferred if there are neutrophils with nuclear debris (indicative of apoptosis) within the alveolar septa and there is some evidence of injury—fibrin exudates, pneumocyte reactivity, organization. Although eosinophils are usually inconspicuous, occasionally may have eosinophil-rich variants. Must differentiate from polyangiitis with eosinophils (Churg–Strauss syndrome). Rarely (1%), bronchocentric variant is present. Differentiation from bronchocentric granulomatosis is based on the presence or absence of necrotizing vasculitis.	Nodules with central necrosis and atypical polymorphous lymphoid infiltrates *(Fig. 45.4)*. Angiocentric infiltrates of small- to medium-sized vessel walls by atypical lymphoid cells with associated necrosis in high-grade lesions *(Figs. 45.5–45.7)*. Although the name implies a granulomatous process, in fact, granulomas are not typical, and their presence implies another diagnosis such as infection or GPA. The name is a misnomer as the original description by Liebow (more than 40 y ago) noted overlapping features with Wegener granulomatosis and lymphoma, thus "lymphomatoid granulomatosis."
Special studies	Elastic tissue stains or pentachrome (Movat) stain may be used to evaluate vessel walls.	CD20 to highlight atypical B cells *(Fig. 45.8)*, CD3 to confirm background reactive lymphocytes, and EBV in situ hybridization (ISH) to quantify EBV-positive B cells *(Fig. 45.9)*. LYG may be divided into three grades according to number of EBV-infected cells (Grade 1, $<$5 EBV+ cells/hpf; Grade 2, 5–20 EBV+ cells/hpf; Grade 3, $>$20 EBV+ cells/hpf). Immunoglobulin heavy chain gene rearrangements.
Prognosis	5-y survival of 75% with appropriately treated disease.	Clinical course varies. Nearly 70% of patients die of the disease. A minority undergo spontaneous regression. Higher grade lesions correlate with worse prognosis. Newer treatments (e.g., anti-CD20 therapy) may afford better prognoses.

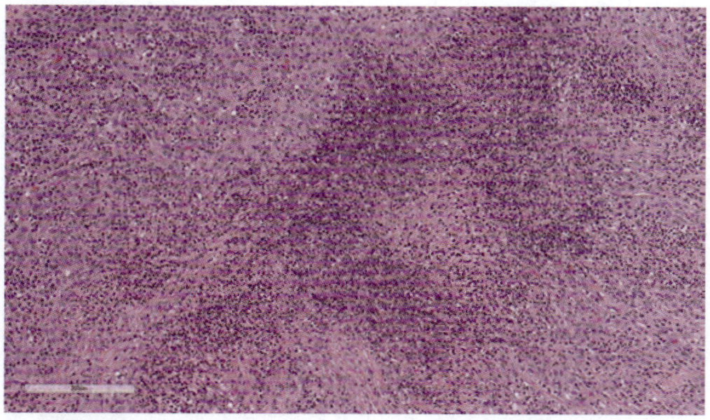

Figure 45.1 GPA: Geographic necrosis demonstrating irregularly bordered outlines with central basophilic necrosis. Note the prominent neutrophilic component in the surrounding tissue.

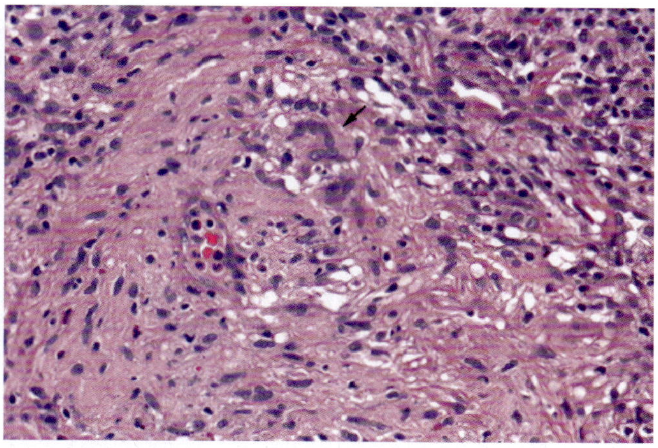

Figure 45.2 GPA: Vasculitis characterized by infiltration of vessel wall by giant cells (*arrow*).

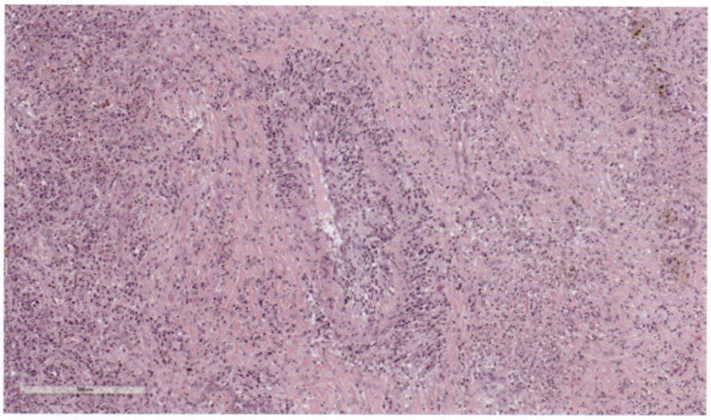

Figure 45.3 GPA: Eccentric infiltration of a vessel wall by lymphocytes, histiocytes, and plasma cells. No atypical lymphoid cells are present.

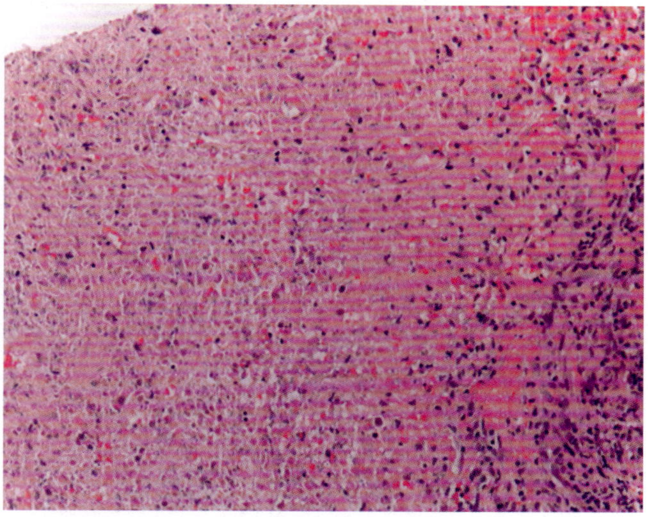

Figure 45.4 LYG: This image demonstrates the typical necrosis surrounded by lymphocytes and chronic inflammatory cells. Pyknotic large nuclei are evident in the area of necrosis, likely indicating necrotic tumor cells.

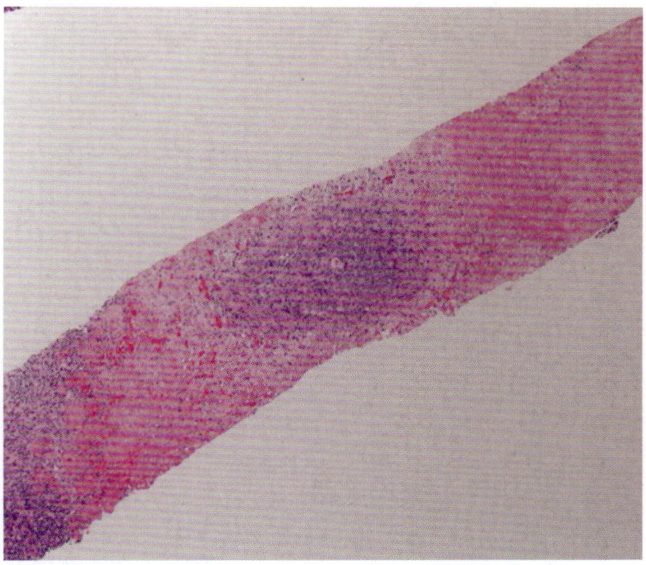

Figure 45.5 LYG: A needle core biopsy of a patient with Grade 3 disease. At the center of the image, there is a small vessel surrounded by chronic inflammatory cells, which in turn are surrounded by areas of necrosis.

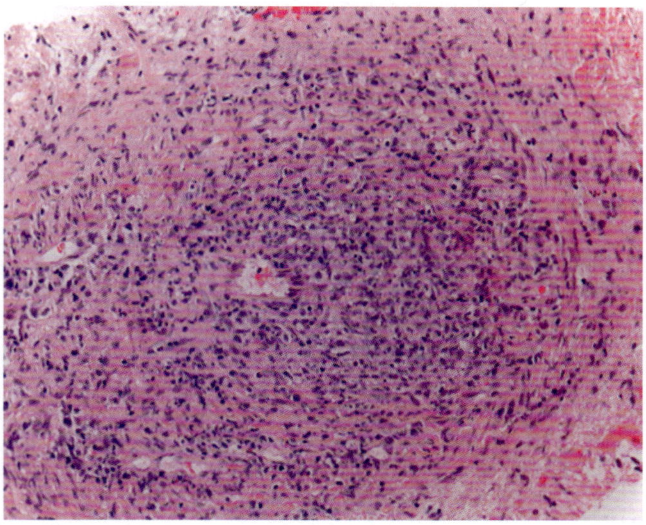

Figure 45.6 LYG: Higher magnification of the same vessel as in Figure 45.5. The atypical lymphoid cells are readily identified.

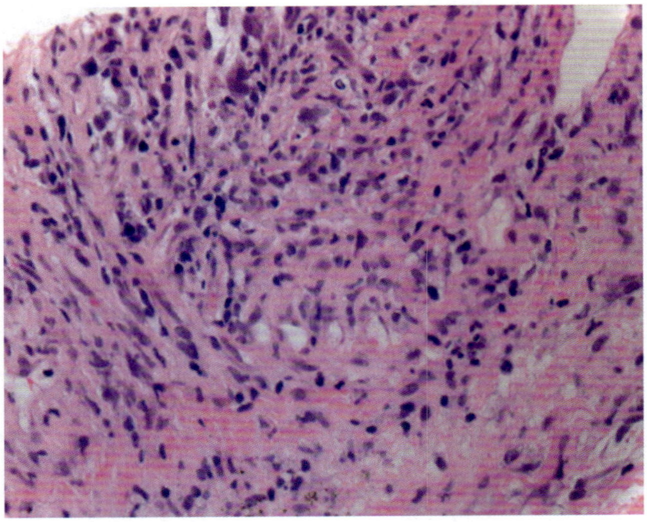

Figure 45.7 LYG: A higher magnification of the atypical lymphoid cells. The cells show varying degrees of atypia, with enlarged nuclei and amphophilic cytoplasm. Unlike many of the other vasculitides, including GPA, the infiltrates typically lack multinucleated giant cells, eosinophils, and neutrophils.

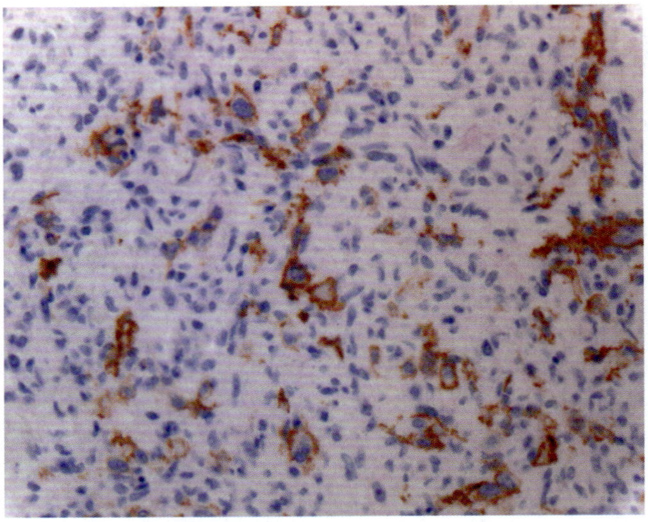

Figure 45.8 LYG: CD20 immunostain highlights the large atypical B cells found in LYG. The normal background lymphocytes are CD3-positive T cells. Although originally thought to be a T-cell lymphoproliferative process, the majority of LYG cases in the lung are now known to be B-cell lymphoproliferative lesions.

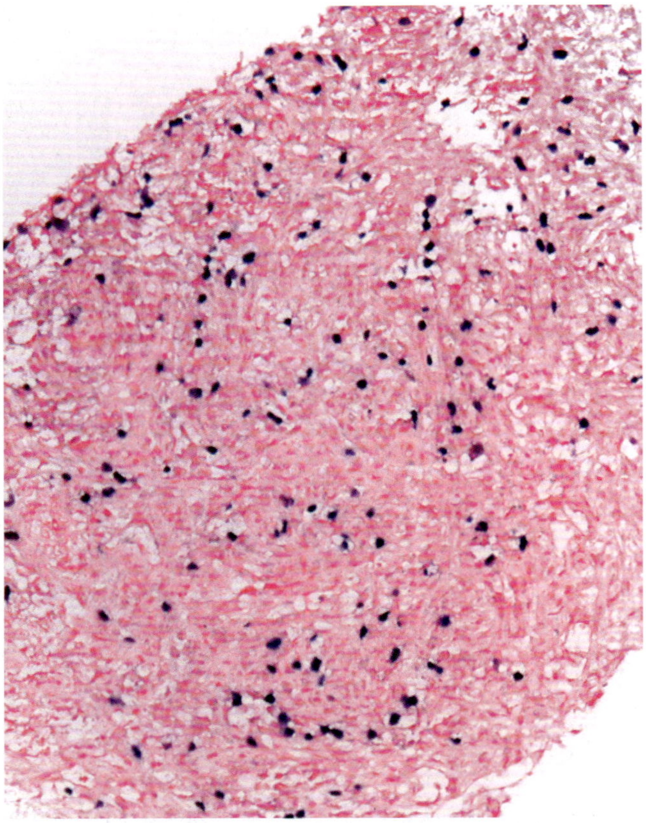

Figure 45.9 LYG: This Epstein–Barr-encoded RNA (EBER) in situ hybridization stain demonstrates EBV expression in the atypical B cells.

46 GRANULOMATOSIS WITH POLYANGIITIS VS. NECROTIZING SARCOID GRANULOMATOSIS

	Granulomatosis with Polyangiitis (GPA; Wegener Granulomatosis)	Necrotizing Sarcoid Granulomatosis (NSG)
Age	Adults, mean age 40, but can affect adolescents and, rarely, children.	Can develop at all ages; mean age 50.
Location	Systemic necrotizing vasculitis with a classic triad of upper airways (sinusitis/otitis, upper airway ulceration), lower respiratory tract, and kidney (glomerulonephritis) involvement. May also affect other organs, including eye, middle ear, nervous system, joints, and skin. May solely involve the lung (limited or localized GPA). Involves small- to medium-sized arteries and veins, as well as capillaries.	Lung; rarely involves extrapulmonary organs. Lymphangitic distribution. Vasculitis affects arteries and veins.
Symptoms	Constitutional: fever, weight loss, malaise, fatigue. Pulmonary: cough, chest pain, shortness of breath, hemoptysis. Other symptoms depend on the organ system involved.	Cough, chest pain, fever, and shortness of breath. About 20% are asymptomatic.
Signs	Nonspecific lung findings with inspiratory crackles are most common. If acute, may have increased diffusing capacity of the lungs for carbon monoxide (DLCO); if chronic, may have restriction and gas exchange abnormalities. Chest x-ray may show multiple bilateral opacities. High-resolution computed tomography (HRCT) often shows bilateral ground-glass opacities or patchy consolidation; occasionally, centrilobular nodules are noted. Cavitation of nodules, diffuse ground-glass opacities (especially with diffuse alveolar hemorrhage [DAH]), atelectasis, and airway complications such as stenosis and ulcerations may also be seen. Bronchoalveolar lavage (BAL) is useful as there are increased red blood cell counts in subsequent aliquots, even in patients without clinical hemoptysis. Laboratory findings usually include anemia and leukocytosis. Positive c-ANCA and anti-proteinase 3 (PR3) autoantibodies are usually present in active disease, but are not present in nearly one-third of patients with limited disease.	PFTs may show decreased forced vital capacity and decreased O_2 saturation. Chest CT shows unilateral, localized disease with nodules, often in lower lobes; bilateral lung involvement can occur. Unlike sarcoidosis, hilar adenopathy is rare (<10% of patients). Laboratory findings are nonspecific, but often show elevated erythrocyte sedimentation rate (ESR). Angiotensin converting enzyme (ACE) levels are not elevated (in contrast to sarcoidosis).
Etiology	The cause is unknown; however, it is clearly mediated by the immune system, resulting in cytoplasmic antineutrophil cytoplasmic antibodies (c-ANCA) directed against specific proteins in white blood cells—proteinase 3 (PR3) in the case of GPA. Another name for ANCA-associated disease is ANCA-associated vasculitis (AAV).	Generally considered a vasculitis and most likely a variant of systemic sarcoidosis. Etiology unknown.

	Granulomatosis with Polyangiitis (GPA; Wegener Granulomatosis)	**Necrotizing Sarcoid Granulomatosis (NSG)**
Histology	Characteristically, the major histologic features include (1) lung parenchymal necrosis, (2) vasculitis (generally involving small- to medium-sized arteries, and occasionally veins and capillaries), and (3) granulomatous inflammation. Often large serpiginous necrotic zones replace lung parenchyma, resulting in the so-called geographic necrosis (deeply basophilic areas with irregular jagged borders). May have smaller microscopic foci of microabscesses with irregular-to-round borders. Palisading histiocytes and scattered multinucleated giant cells can be found associated with areas of abscess. The giant cells do not form sarcoid-like granulomas and have a pyknotic quality *(Figs. 46.1 and 46.2).* Necrotizing vasculitis, which can involve both arteries and veins, characterized by foci of necrosis and granulomatous inflammation. Partial involvement of vessel walls by microabscesses may be seen. Fibrinoid necrosis is usually present *(Fig. 46.3).* Variant cases may show capillaritis with DAH as the sole histologic abnormalities. Capillaritis is inferred if there are neutrophils with nuclear debris (indicative of apoptosis) within the alveolar septa and there is some evidence of injury—fibrin exudates, pneumocyte reactivity, organization. Although eosinophils are usually inconspicuous, occasionally may have eosinophil-rich variants. Must differentiate from polyangiitis with eosinophils (Churg–Strauss syndrome). Rarely (1%), bronchocentric variant is present. Differentiation from bronchocentric granulomatosis is based on the presence or absence of necrotizing vasculitis.	Like sarcoidosis, has lymphangitic distribution of granulomas with subpleural, paraseptal, and bronchovascular distribution. Granulomas may coalesce *(Fig. 46.4)* and show small areas of central necrosis *(Fig. 46.5).* Unlike sarcoidosis, NSG also has large zones of infarct-like necrosis *(Fig. 46.6).* Unlike GPA, granulomas in NSG are well formed (contrast with *Figs. 46.1 and 46.2*). Lymphocytic and/or giant cell/granulomatous vasculitis affect both veins and arteries *(Figs. 46.7 and 46.8).* Organizing pneumonia may be present.
Special studies	Elastic tissue stains or pentachrome (Movat) stain may be used to evaluate vessel walls.	Elastic tissue stains may help clarify vascular destruction *(Fig. 46.9).*
Prognosis	5-y survival of 75% with appropriately treated disease.	Excellent prognosis. No deaths due to disease. Surgical resection is curative.

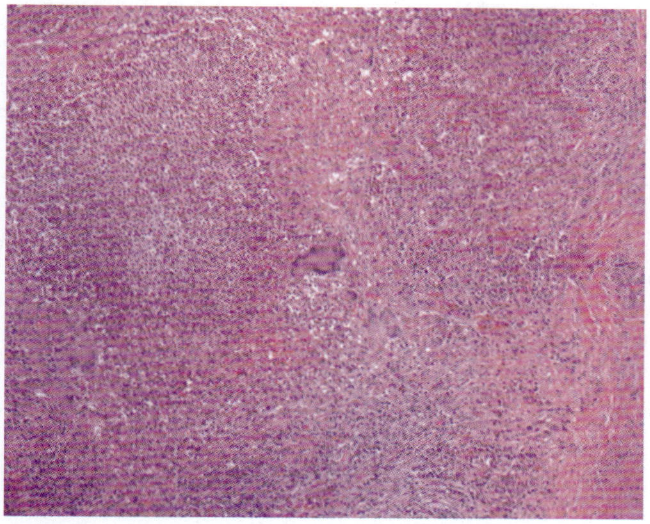

Figure 46.1 GPA: Large area of basophilic necrosis and an isolated giant cell is seen in this condition.

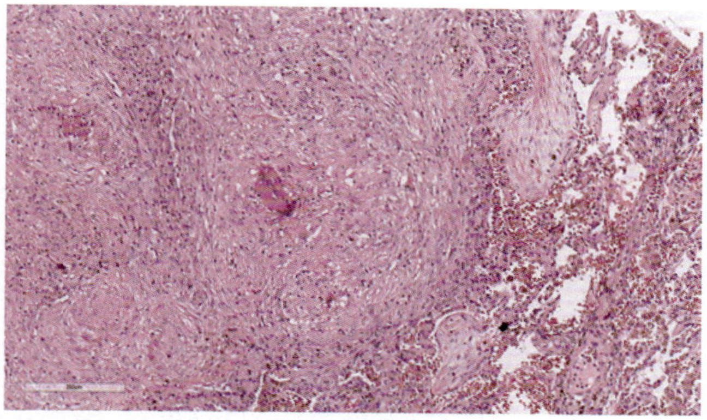

Figure 46.2 GPA: Single giant cell surrounded by epithelioid histiocytes and fibroblastic tissue. Foci of organizing pneumonia surround the poorly formed granuloma.

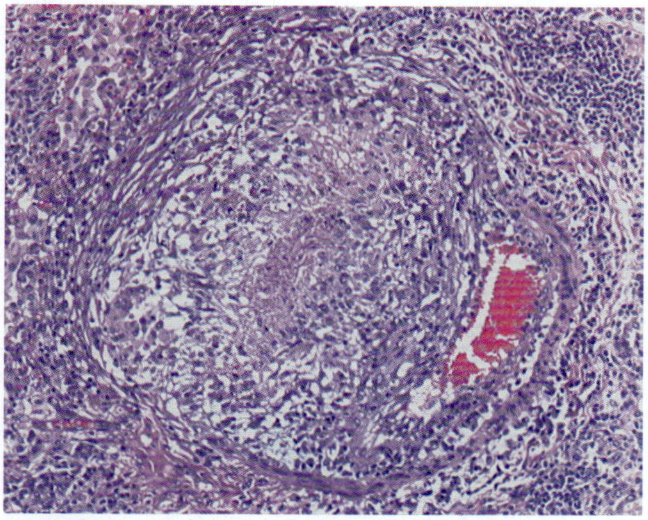

Figure 46.3 GPA: Partial destruction of vessel wall with concomitant fibrinoid necrosis.

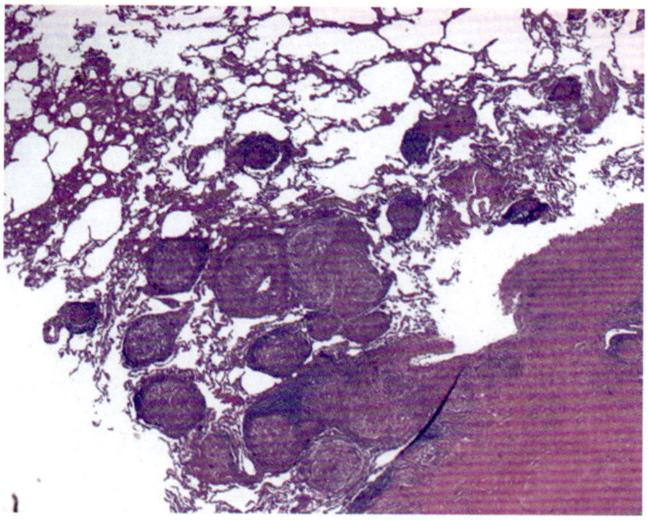

Figure 46.4 NSG: Well-formed granulomas characterize sarcoidosis. Classically, the granulomas follow a lymphangitic distribution. In this image, there are multiple well-formed granulomas demonstrating a coalescing pattern, with an area of dense fibrosis at the lower right.

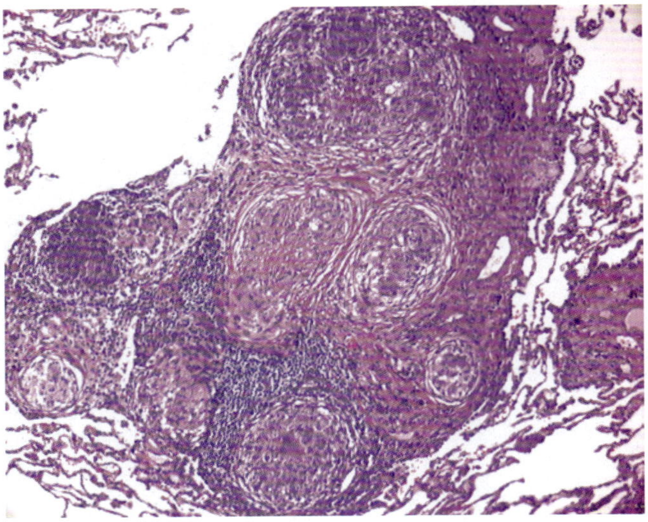

Figure 46.5 NSG: Higher-power image of confluent well-formed granulomas. The granulomas at the top and center of the image show small areas of central necrosis.

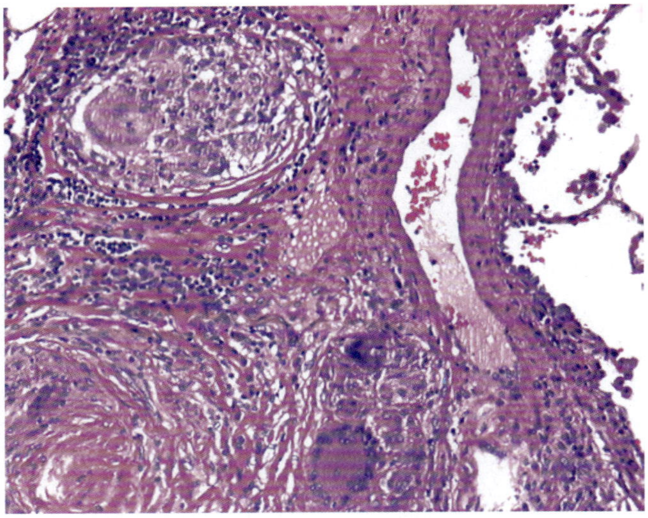

Figure 46.7 NSG: Infiltration of small vessel by granulomas and giant cells. Note the well-formed granuloma at the upper left.

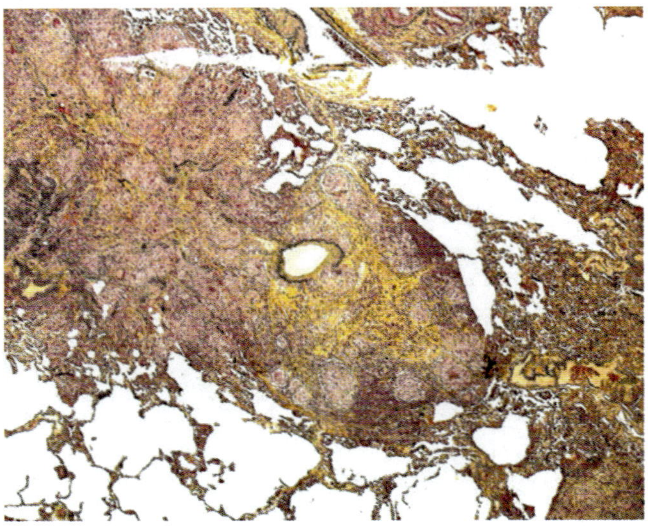

Figure 46.9 NSG: The pentachrome (Movat) stain shows infiltration and partial destruction of the elastic lamina in this small vein. The granulomas are clearly visible as coalescing, rounded nodules surrounding the vascular structure.

Figure 46.6 NSG: In this case, there is a zone of infarct-like necrosis on the right surrounded by chronic (predominantly lymphocytic) inflammation and myofibroblastic tissue. Like GPA, the borders of the necrosis are irregular, but the necrosis is eosinophilic and infarct-like, unlike the "dirty," basophilic necrosis of GPA (compare with Fig. 46.1).

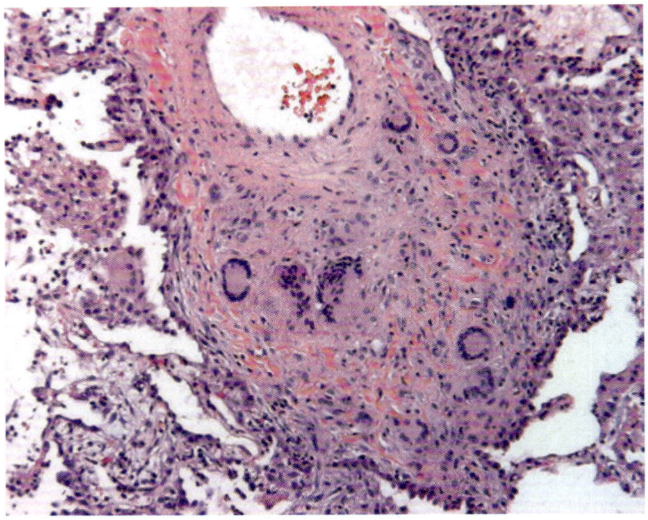

Figure 46.8 NSG: Granulomas infiltrate small pulmonary artery.

47 GRANULOMATOSIS WITH POLYANGIITIS WITH BRONCHOCENTRIC PATTERN VS. BRONCHOCENTRIC GRANULOMATOSIS

	Granulomatosis with Polyangiitis (GPA; Wegener Granulomatosis)	Bronchocentric Granulomatosis (BCG)
Age	Adults, mean age 40, but can affect adolescents and, rarely, children.	Can develop at any age. If asthma-related, onset can be in childhood, but remains occult for years to decades.
Location	Systemic necrotizing vasculitis with a classic triad of upper airways (sinusitis/otitis, upper airway ulceration), lower respiratory tract, and kidney (glomerulonephritis) involvement. May also affect other organs, including eye, middle ear, nervous system, joints, and skin. May solely involve the lung (limited or localized GPA). Involves small- to medium-sized arteries and veins, as well as capillaries.	Bronchiolocentric with extension into surrounding lung parenchyma.
Symptoms	Constitutional: fever, weight loss, malaise, fatigue. Pulmonary: cough, chest pain, shortness of breath, hemoptysis. Other symptoms depend on organ system involved.	Fever, cough, severe wheezing (if asthmatic).
Signs	Nonspecific lung findings with inspiratory crackles are the most common. If acute, may have increased diffusing capacity of the lungs for carbon monoxide (DLCO); if chronic, may have restriction and gas exchange abnormalities. Chest x-ray may show multiple bilateral opacities. High-resolution computed tomography (HRCT) often shows bilateral ground-glass opacities or patchy consolidation; occasionally, centrilobular nodules are noted. Cavitation of nodules, diffuse ground-glass opacities (especially with diffuse alveolar hemorrhage [DAH]), atelectasis, and airway complications such as stenosis and ulcerations may also be seen. Bronchoalveolar lavage (BAL) is useful as there are increased red blood cell counts in subsequent aliquots, even in patients without clinical hemoptysis. Laboratory findings usually include anemia and leukocytosis. Positive c-ANCA and anti-proteinase 3 (PR3) autoantibodies are usually present in active disease, but are not present in nearly one-third of patients with limited disease.	Half the patients have a history of chronic asthma and show obstructive pulmonary function tests consistent with asthma; nonasthmatic patients are heterogeneous with variable presentations. CT imaging may show masses, alveolar opacities, or reticulonodular opacities, predominantly in the upper lobes. Unilateral in a majority of patients. Eosinophilia is present in patients with untreated asthma; nonasthmatics generally have no eosinophilia.
Etiology	The cause is unknown; however, it is clearly mediated by the immune system, resulting in cytoplasmic antineutrophil cytoplasmic antibodies (c-ANCA) directed against specific proteins in white blood cells—proteinase 3 (PR3) in the case of GPA. Another name for ANCA-associated disease is ANCA-associated vasculitis (AAV).	Infections, including mycobacteria and fungi; allergic, including allergic bronchopulmonary fungal disease and especially in association with allergic aspergillosis with mucoid impaction of bronchi.

	Granulomatosis with Polyangiitis (GPA; Wegener Granulomatosis)	Bronchocentric Granulomatosis (BCG)
Histology	Characteristically, the major histologic features include (1) lung parenchymal necrosis, (2) vasculitis (generally involving small- to medium-sized arteries, and occasionally veins and capillaries), and (3) granulomatous inflammation. Often large serpiginous necrotic zones replace lung parenchyma, resulting in the so-called geographic necrosis (deeply basophilic areas with irregular jagged borders) *(Fig. 47.1)*. May have smaller microscopic foci of microabscesses with irregular-to-round borders. Palisading histiocytes and scattered multinucleated giant cells can be found associated with areas of abscess. The giant cells do not form sarcoid-like granulomas and have a pyknotic quality. Necrotizing vasculitis, which can involve both arteries and veins, characterized by foci of necrosis and granulomatous inflammation. Partial involvement of vessel walls by microabscesses may be seen. Fibrinoid necrosis is usually present. Variant cases may show capillaritis with DAH as the sole histologic abnormalities. Capillaritis is inferred if there are neutrophils with nuclear debris (indicative of apoptosis) within the alveolar septa and there is some evidence of injury—fibrin exudates, pneumocyte reactivity, organization. Although eosinophils are usually inconspicuous, occasionally may have eosinophil-rich variants *(Fig. 47.2)*. Must differentiate from polyangiitis with eosinophils (Churg–Strauss syndrome) and, occasionally, bronchocentric granulomatosis if an allergic component is present. Rarely (1%), bronchocentric variant is present. Differentiation from bronchocentric granulomatosis is based on the presence or absence of necrotizing vasculitis *(Fig. 47.3)*.	Necrotizing granulomatous inflammation of the small bronchi and bronchiolar walls characterized by palisading histiocytes with luminal necrosis, and complete-to-partial destruction of the bronchiolar wall *(Figs. 47.5–47.9)*. Eosinophils may be prominent in allergic forms *(Figs. 47.10 and 47.11)*. May see fungal hyphae if associated with allergic bronchopulmonary fungal disease *(Fig. 47.12)*. Differentiated from GPA by lack of vasculitis *(compare Fig. 47.4 with 47.8 and 47.9)*.
Special studies	Elastic tissue stains or pentachrome (Movat) stain may be used to evaluate vessel walls *(Fig. 47.4)*.	Mycobacterial and fungal stains, tissue cultures, and appropriate molecular testing are necessary to rule out infectious etiologies. Elastic tissue stains will highlight the partial-to-complete destruction of the airway elastic laminae. Elastic tissue stains will also help in ruling out a necrotizing vasculitis *(Fig. 47.13)*.
Prognosis	5-y survival of 75% with appropriately treated disease.	Excellent prognosis with steroid treatment for both allergic and nonallergic BCG. Refractory lesions may require resection.

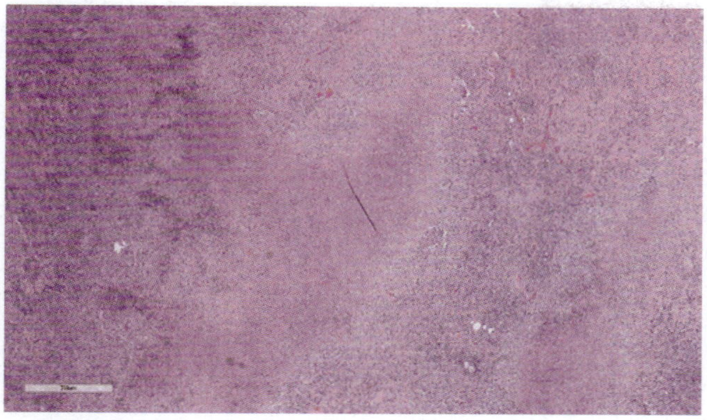

Figure 47.1 GPA: "Dirty," basophilic necrosis.

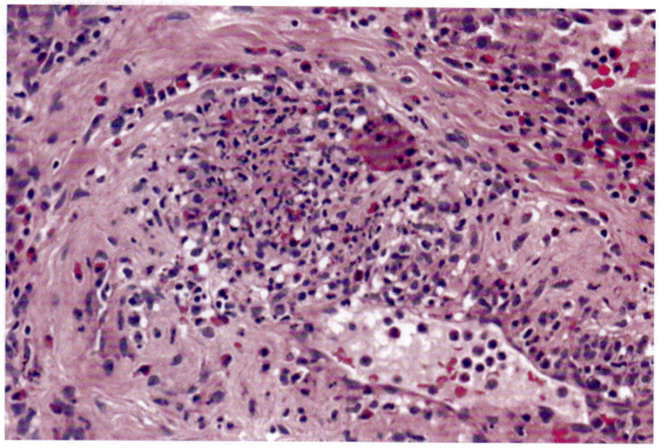

Figure 47.2 GPA: Early infiltrative, transmural chronic inflammatory infiltrate. Focal fibrinoid necrosis is present. Eosinophils are prominent in this case.

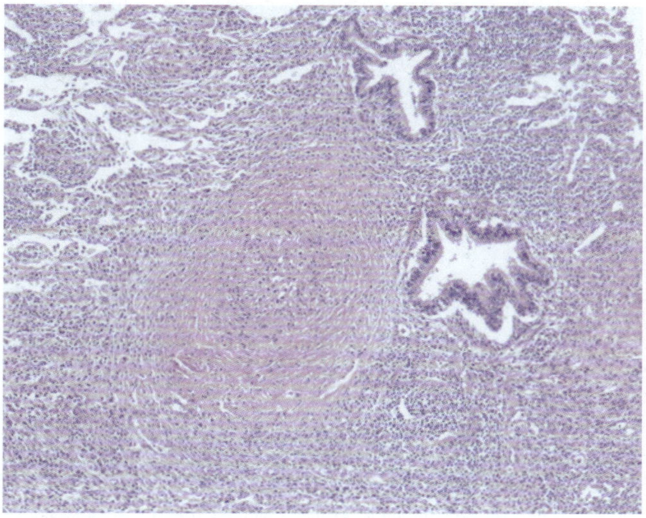

Figure 47.3 GPA: Necrotizing vasculitis. Note the intact bronchiolar wall on the right.

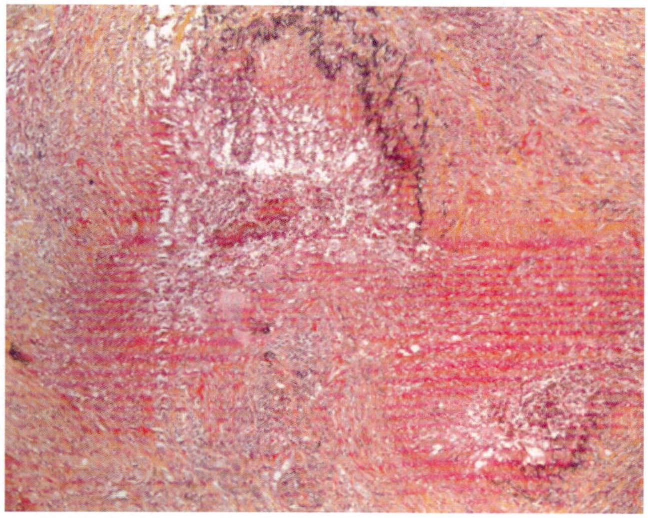

Figure 47.4 GPA: Pentachrome (Movat) stain is helpful in delineating vascular destruction (as in this case) from bronchiolar wall destruction.

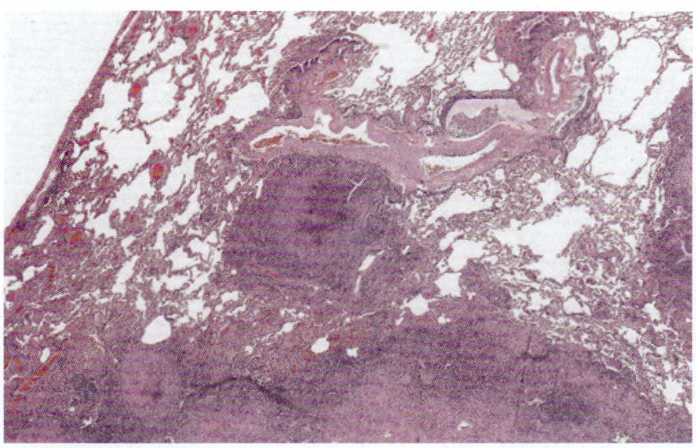

Figure 47.5 BCG: Below the pulmonary artery is a partially destroyed bronchiole with purulent material in the center of the lesion. The artery is unaffected by the inflammatory process.

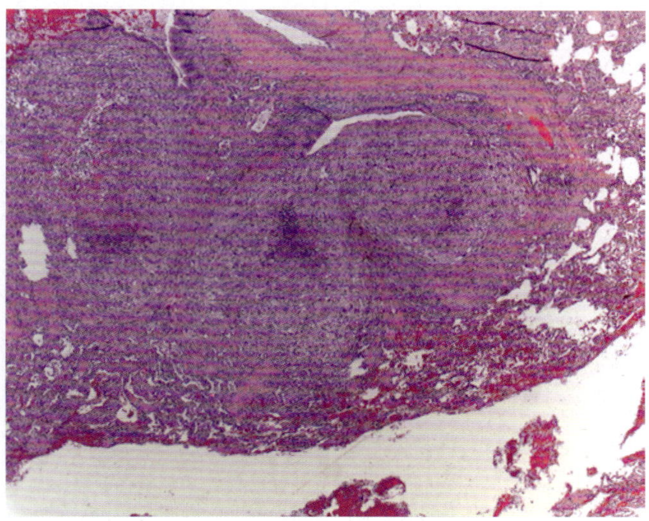

Figure 47.6 BCG: Higher-power image of a partially destroyed bronchiolar wall. Again, note the unaffected adjacent pulmonary artery.

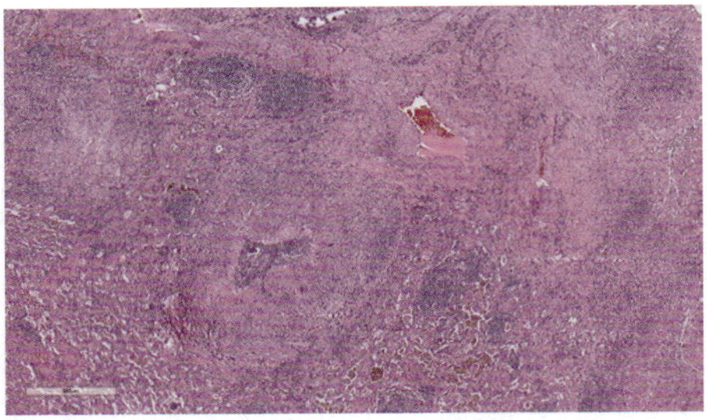

Figure 47.7 BCG: In this image, the bronchiolar wall is circumferentially replaced by palisading histiocytes and purulent material in the lumen.

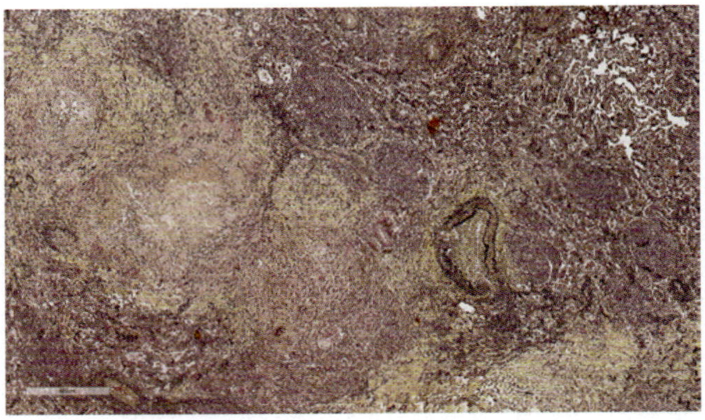

Figure 47.8 BCG: Same image as 47.7, stained with the pentachrome (Movat) stain. This stain highlights the destroyed elastic tissue of the bronchiolar wall and the relatively intact elastic laminae of the accompanying pulmonary artery on the right.

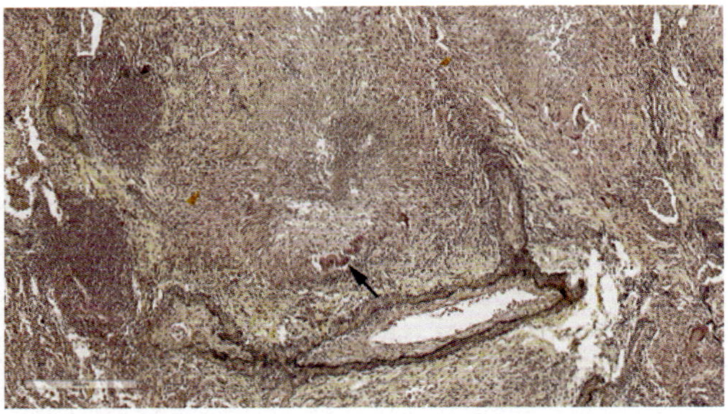

Figure 47.9 BCG: Another pentachrome (Movat) stain of a nearly totally destroyed airway wall. A small amount of residual bronchiolar-type epithelium is noted at the bottom of the airway (*arrow*). The pulmonary artery, located beneath the destroyed airway, is intact, without evidence of necrosis.

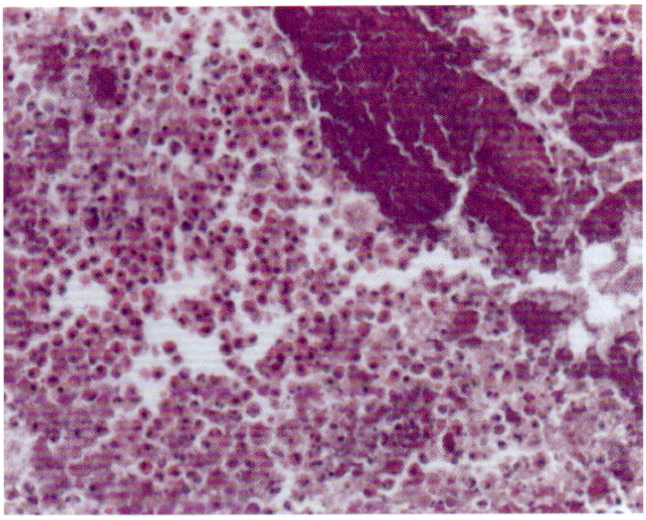

Figure 47.10 BCG: Eosinophilic abscess with necrosis.

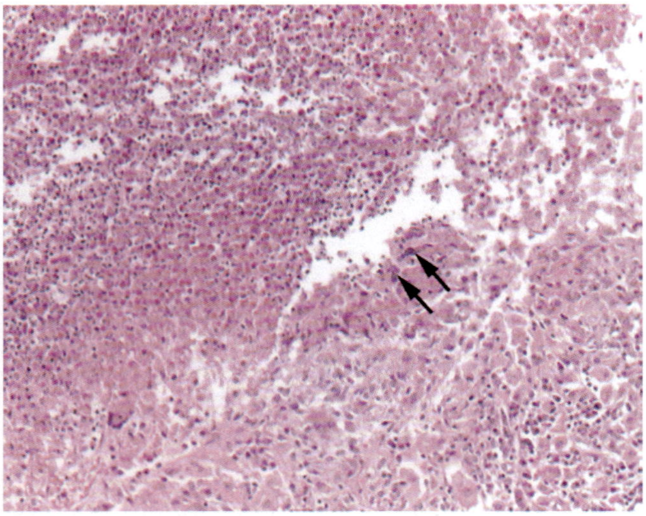

Figure 47.11 BCG: Necrotic eosinophils are surrounded by palisading histiocytes and giant cells. Fungal hyphae are evident in the necrotic region (*arrows*).

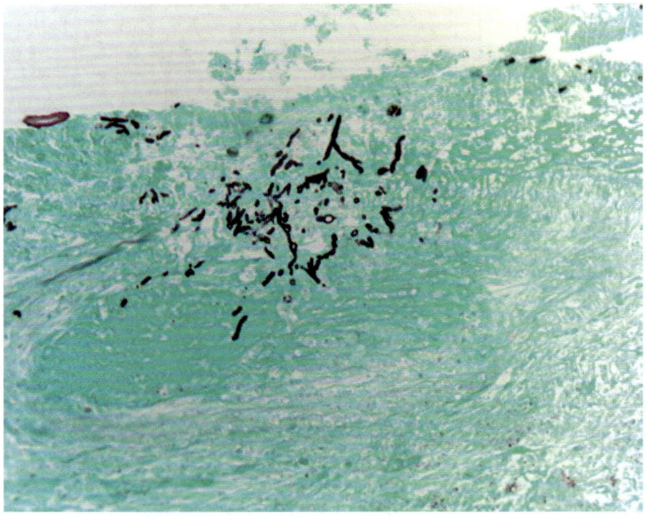

Figure 47.12 BCG: GMS stain highlights the branching hyphal forms of *Aspergillus*. The fungi are usually found within the luminal material, but may be difficult to locate due to small numbers and fragmented forms.

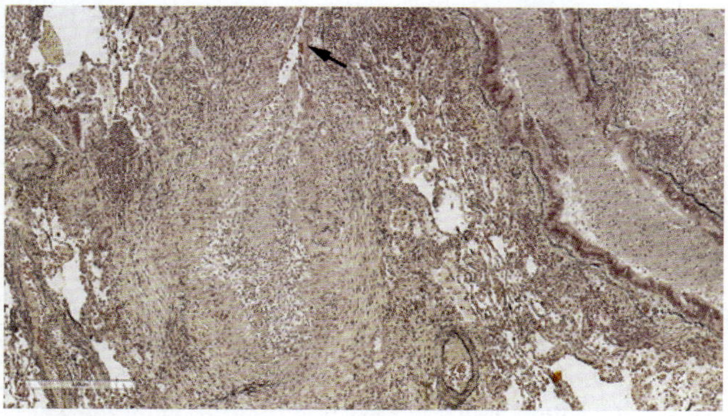

Figure 47.13 BCG: Elastic stains are useful in differentiating airways from pulmonary arteries. In this case, the structure on the left mimics a vessel; however, there is intact airway epithelium (*arrow*) and a single elastic lamina, compatible with an airway, not a vessel.

48 GRANULOMATOSIS WITH POLYANGIITIS VS. MYCOBACTERIA INFECTION

	Granulomatosis with Polyangiitis (GPA; Wegener Granulomatosis)	Mycobacteria Infection
Age	Adults, mean age 40, but can affect adolescents and, rarely, children.	Any age. *Mycobacterium tuberculosis* (MTB) is the most common infectious cause of death in adults worldwide. MTB more common in young adults in the United States. Nontuberculous mycobacteria (NTM) disease more common in the middle-aged and elderly.
Location	Systemic necrotizing vasculitis with a classic triad of upper airways (sinusitis/otitis, upper airway ulceration), lower respiratory tract, and kidney (glomerulonephritis) involvement. May also affect other organs, including eye, middle ear, nervous system, joints, and skin. May solely involve the lung (limited or localized GPA). Involves small- to medium-sized arteries and veins, as well as capillaries.	Patchy, random distribution. Upper lobe disease more common in reactivated disease.
Symptoms	Constitutional: fever, weight loss, malaise, fatigue. Pulmonary: cough, chest pain, shortness of breath, hemoptysis. Other symptoms depend on organ system involved.	Cough, weight loss, fatigue, low-grade fever, night sweats. Some patients are asymptomatic.
Signs	Nonspecific lung findings with inspiratory crackles most common. If acute, may have increased diffusing capacity of the lungs for carbon monoxide (DLCO); if chronic, may have restriction and gas exchange abnormalities. Chest x-ray may show multiple bilateral opacities. High-resolution computed tomography (HRCT) often shows bilateral ground-glass opacities or patchy consolidation; occasionally, centrilobular nodules are noted. May also see cavitation of nodules, diffuse ground-glass opacities (especially with diffuse alveolar hemorrhage [DAH]), atelectasis, and airway complications such as stenosis and ulcerations. Bronchoalveolar lavage (BAL) is useful as there are increased red blood cell counts in subsequent aliquots, even in patients without clinical hemoptysis. Laboratory findings usually include anemia and leukocytosis. Positive c-ANCA and anti-proteinase 3 (PR3) autoantibodies are usually present in active disease, but are not present in nearly one-third of patients with limited disease.	Varied. Radiographically, lesions can be nodular, multinodular cavitary, or diffusely infiltrative. Bronchiectasis is often present. May have hilar and mediastinal lymphadenopathy. Pleural effusions may be present. Cultures necessary to differentiate MTB from NTM and to distinguish between the various environmental mycobacteria that cause disease.
Etiology	The cause is unknown; however, it is clearly mediated by the immune system, resulting in cytoplasmic antineutrophil cytoplasmic antibodies (c-ANCA) directed against specific proteins in white blood cells—proteinase 3 (PR3) in the case of GPA. Another name for ANCA-associated disease is ANCA-associated vasculitis (AAV).	Infectious.

	Granulomatosis with Polyangiitis (GPA; Wegener Granulomatosis)	Mycobacteria Infection
Histology	Characteristically, the major histologic features include (1) lung parenchymal necrosis, (2) vasculitis (generally involving small- to medium-sized arteries, and occasionally veins and capillaries), and (3) granulomatous inflammation. Often large serpiginous necrotic zones replace lung parenchyma, resulting in the so-called geographic necrosis (deeply basophilic areas with irregular jagged borders). May have smaller microscopic foci of microabscesses with irregular to round borders *(Fig. 48.1)*. Palisading histiocytes and scattered multinucleated giant cells can be found associated with areas of abscess. The giant cells do not form sarcoid-like granulomas and have a pyknotic quality *(Figs. 48.2 and 48.3)*. Necrotizing vasculitis, which can involve both arteries and veins, characterized by foci of necrosis and granulomatous inflammation. Partial involvement of vessel walls by microabscesses may be seen. Fibrinoid necrosis is usually present *(Fig. 48.4)*. Variant cases may show capillaritis with DAH as the sole histologic abnormalities. Capillaritis is inferred if there are neutrophils with nuclear debris (indicative of apoptosis) within the alveolar septa and there is some evidence of injury—fibrin exudates, pneumocyte reactivity, organization. Although eosinophils are usually inconspicuous, occasionally may have eosinophil-rich variants. Must differentiate from polyangiitis with eosinophils (Churg–Strauss syndrome). Rarely (1%), bronchocentric variant is present. Differentiation from bronchocentric granulomatosis is based on the presence or absence of necrotizing vasculitis.	Necrotizing (caseating) and nonnecrotizing granulomas *(Figs. 48.5–48.7)*. Necrosis is usually less basophilic and more rounded than that seen in GPA. Granulomas may fibrose and calcify over time *(Fig. 48.8)*. Bronchiectasis often present. Incidental vascular involvement may be seen, but true necrotizing vasculitis is uncommon *(Fig. 48.9)*. Mycobacteria may be demonstrated with an acid-fast stain *(Figs. 48.10 and 48.11)*; negative stain does NOT rule out mycobacterial disease. Must correlate with cultures and appropriate molecular testing.
Special studies	Elastic tissue stains or pentachrome (Movat) stain may be used to evaluate vessel walls.	Mycobacterial stains (immunohistochemical, immunofluorescent, histochemical) and molecular testing are all used to evaluate tissue. Fungal stains should also be performed to rule out a fungal organism. Elastic tissue stains can help with assessing the presence or absence of necrotizing vasculitis.
Prognosis	5-y survival of 75% with appropriately treated disease.	Without treatment, mortality approaches 50% in 5 y. With treatment, most patients can be cured. Those with multidrug-resistant strains of TB have higher relapse rates and may require surgical resection.

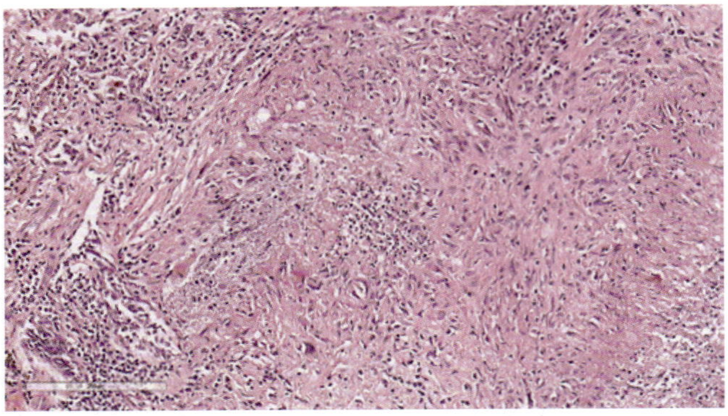

Figure 48.1 GPA: Microabscess surrounded by palisading histiocytes and rare giant cells.

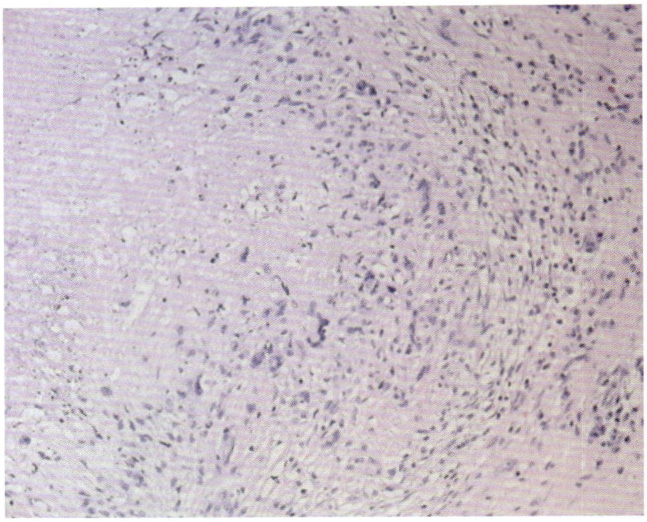

Figure 48.2 GPA: Zone of necrosis surrounded by multinucleated giant cells, epithelioid type histiocytes, and other chronic inflammatory cells.

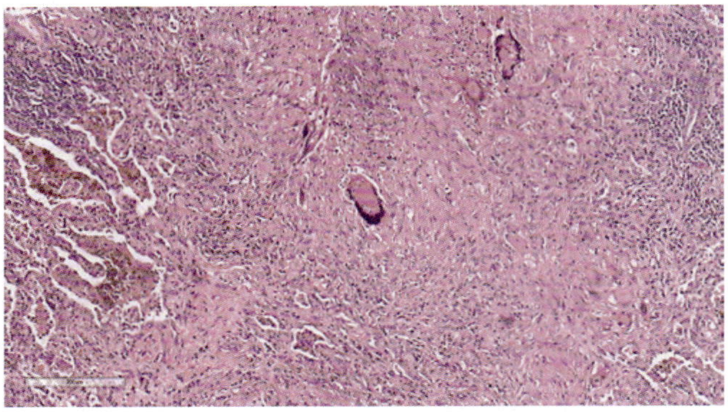

Figure 48.3 GPA: Isolated giant cells, epithelioid histiocytes, and other chronic inflammatory cells form an area of granulomatous inflammation. Note the hemosiderin-laden macrophages to the left.

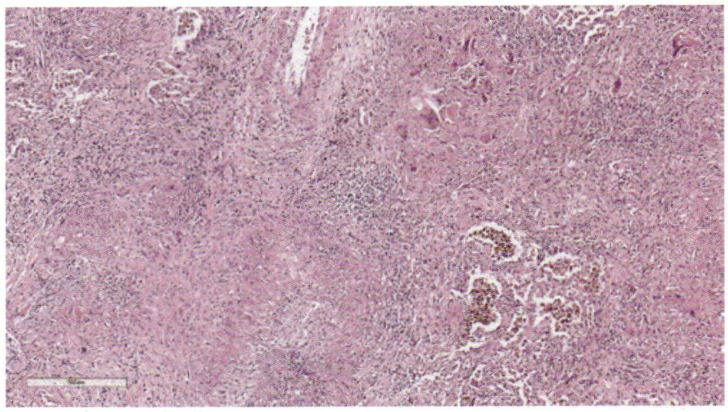

Figure 48.4 GPA: Necrotizing vasculitis affecting an artery. Also note the isolated giant cells, foci of neutrophils, and airspace hemosiderin-laden macrophages.

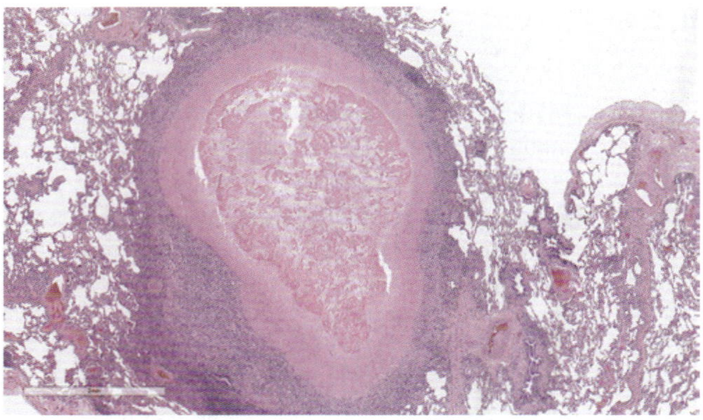

Figure 48.5 Mycobacteria infection: Low-power image of a nodular necrotizing granuloma with central necrosis surrounded by granulomatous and chronic inflammation. Organisms are usually best identified with acid-fast stains in the central necrotic region.

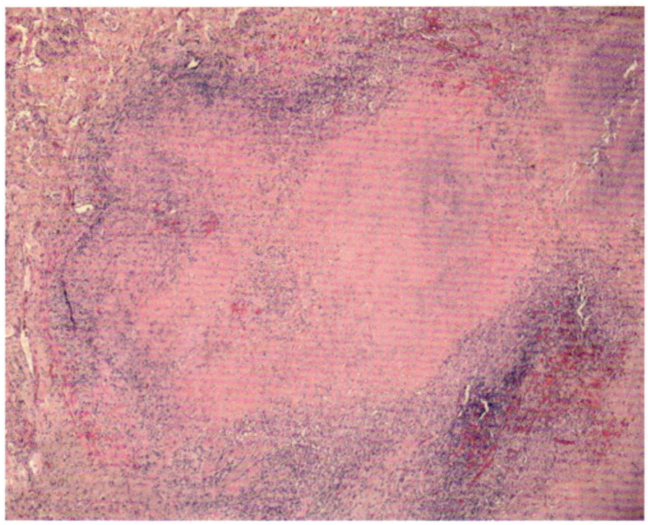

Figure 48.6 Mycobacteria infection: In this example of mycobacterial disease, the necrosis is less nodular and more irregular, mimicking the geographic necrosis of GPA. However, acid-fast stains and cultures confirmed mycobacteria tuberculosis.

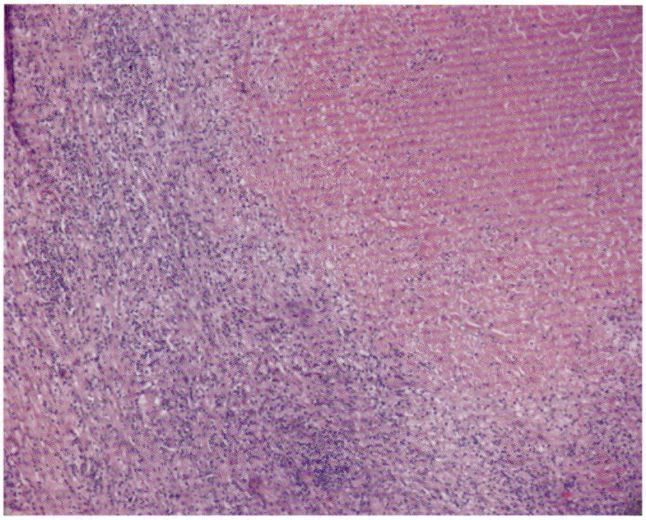

Figure 48.7 Mycobacteria infection: Higher-power of necrosis (also called "caseous," which refers to the chalky or cheese-like appearance of the necrosis on gross examination) with the surrounding wall of chronic inflammation, epithelioid histiocytes, giant cells, and fibrosis.

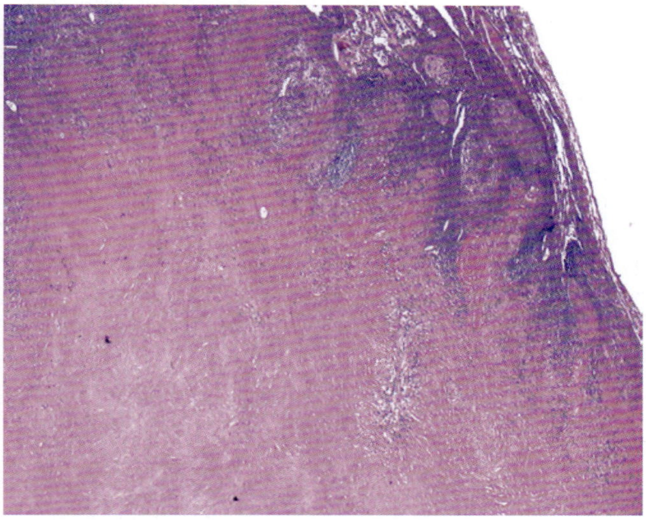

Figure 48.8 Mycobacteria infection: In this example, the necrotic region has fibrosed, but is still surrounded by well-formed, nonnecrotizing granulomas, some of which coalesce—much like the granulomas of sarcoidosis. Acid-fast stains rarely identify organisms in areas of fibrosis or calcification.

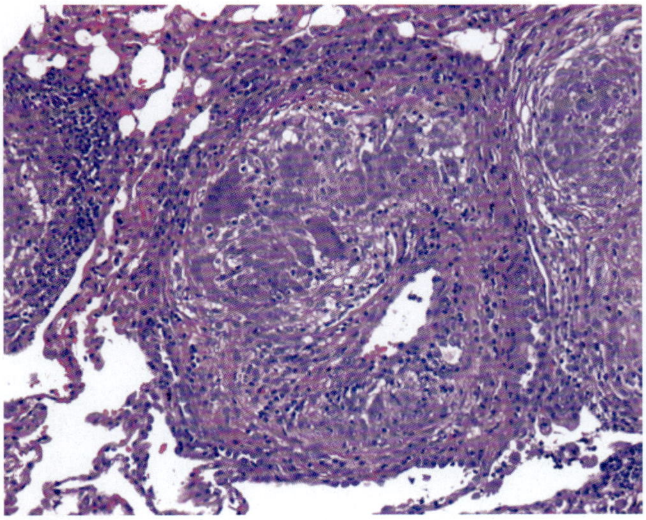

Figure 48.9 Mycobacteria infection: Although vessels are often involved, as in this example, true necrotizing vasculitis usually does not occur. However, there can be significant overlap between mycobacterial vascular involvement and the granulomatous vasculitis of GPA, thus necessitating acid-fast staining and cultures in all cases of granulomatous lung disease.

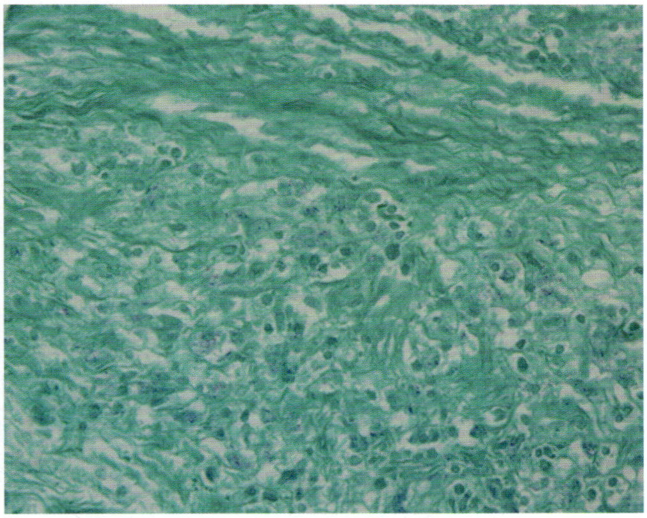

Figure 48.10 Mycobacteria infection: Example of acid-fast stain (Ziehl–Neelsen) in mycobacterial disease. The waxy cell walls of mycobacteria retain the carbol fuchsin (red dye), even after application of acid solvents. Even one red bacillus organism is highly specific for mycobacteria. However, the absence of organisms on acid-fast staining does not rule out mycobacteria. Cultures or molecular assays are necessary to not only confirm the absence (or presence) of organisms but also speciate mycobacteria. Immunofluorescence stains are also available for identifying mycobacterial bacilli, but although more sensitive than acid-fast stains, they are not as specific.

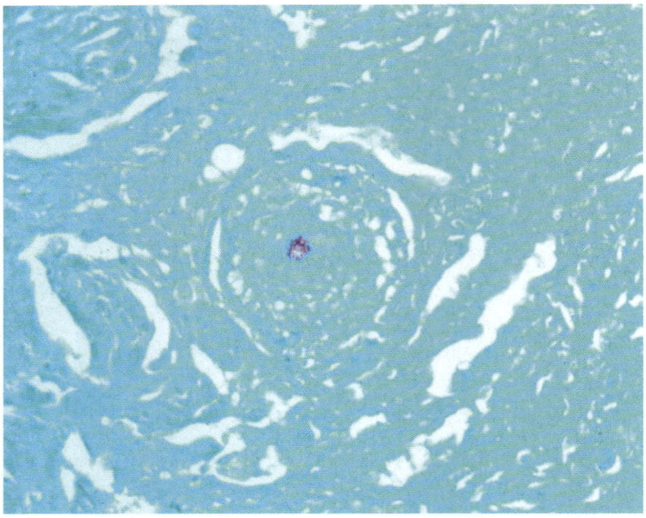

Figure 48.11 Mycobacteria infection: Another example of mycobacteria identified with acid-fast stain.

49 GRANULOMATOSIS WITH POLYANGIITIS VS. RHEUMATOID NODULE

	Granulomatosis with Polyangiitis (GPA; Wegener Granulomatosis)	Rheumatoid Nodule
Age	Adults, mean age 40, but can affect adolescents and, rarely, children.	All ages, but incidence increases with age into the seventh decade of life.
Location	Systemic necrotizing vasculitis with a classic triad of upper airways (sinusitis/otitis, upper airway ulceration), lower respiratory tract, and kidney (glomerulonephritis) involvement. May also affect other organs, including eye, middle ear, nervous system, joints, and skin. May solely involve the lung (limited or localized GPA). Involves small- to medium-sized arteries and veins, as well as capillaries.	Often subpleural or paraseptal.
Symptoms	Constitutional: fever, weight loss, malaise, fatigue. Pulmonary: cough, chest pain, shortness of breath, hemoptysis. Other symptoms depend on organ system involved.	Usually asymptomatic, unless rupture occurs, then hemoptysis.
Signs	Nonspecific lung findings with inspiratory crackles most common. If acute, may have increased diffusing capacity of the lungs for carbon monoxide (DLCO); if chronic, may have restriction and gas exchange abnormalities. Chest x-ray may show multiple bilateral opacities. High-resolution computed tomography (HRCT) often shows bilateral ground-glass opacities or patchy consolidation; occasionally, centrilobular nodules are noted. Cavitation of nodules, diffuse ground-glass opacities (especially with diffuse alveolar hemorrhage [DAH]), atelectasis, and airway complications such as stenosis and ulcerations may also be seen. Bronchoalveolar lavage (BAL) is useful as there are increased red blood cell counts in subsequent aliquots, even in patients without clinical hemoptysis. Laboratory findings usually include anemia and leukocytosis. Positive c-ANCA and anti-proteinase 3 (PR3) autoantibodies are usually present in active disease, but are not present in nearly one-third of patients with limited disease.	Incidental finding in $<1\%$ of rheumatoid arthritis (RA) patients. Radiographically, single or multiple nodules. May rarely precede systemic disease, but usually patients have high titers of rheumatoid factor. Often, have concurrent subcutaneous nodules.
Etiology	The cause is unknown; however, it is clearly mediated by the immune system, resulting in cytoplasmic antineutrophil cytoplasmic antibodies (c-ANCA) directed against specific proteins in white blood cells—proteinase 3 (PR3) in the case of GPA. Another name for ANCA-associated disease is ANCA-associated vasculitis (AAV).	Autoimmune. Nodules may develop secondary to a hypersensitivity reaction to inhaled dust, possibly amplified by immunologic overactivity. Caplan syndrome consists of rheumatoid nodules associated with coal worker's pneumoconiosis or silicosis.
Histology	Characteristically, the major histologic features include (1) lung parenchymal necrosis, (2) vasculitis (generally involving small- to medium-sized arteries, and occasionally veins and capillaries), and (3) granulomatous inflammation.	Well-circumscribed, nonserpiginous, nongeographic nodule composed of palisading epithelioid histiocytes surrounding an acellular necrotic center. The nodule is often surrounded by fibrosis and chronic inflammation *(Figs. 49.5–49.9)*.

	Granulomatosis with Polyangiitis (GPA; Wegener Granulomatosis)	Rheumatoid Nodule
	Often large serpiginous necrotic zones replace lung parenchyma, resulting in the so-called geographic necrosis (deeply basophilic areas with irregular jagged borders) *(Fig. 49.1)*. May have smaller microscopic foci of microabscesses with irregular to round borders *(Fig. 49.2)*. Palisading histiocytes and scattered multinucleated giant cells can be found associated with areas of abscess. The giant cells do not form sarcoid-like granulomas and have a pyknotic quality *(Fig. 49.3)*. Necrotizing vasculitis, which can involve both arteries and veins, characterized by foci of necrosis and granulomatous inflammation. Partial involvement of vessel walls by microabscesses may be seen. Fibrinoid necrosis is usually present *(Fig. 49.4)*. Variant cases may show capillaritis with DAH as the sole histologic abnormalities. Capillaritis is inferred if there are neutrophils with nuclear debris (indicative of apoptosis) within the alveolar septa and there is some evidence of injury—fibrin exudates, pneumocyte reactivity, organization. Although eosinophils are usually inconspicuous, occasionally may have eosinophil-rich variants. Must differentiate from polyangiitis with eosinophils (Churg–Strauss syndrome). Rarely (1%), bronchocentric variant is present. Differentiation from bronchocentric granulomatosis is based on the presence or absence of necrotizing vasculitis.	Vasculitis (usually nonnecrotizing) may be present in the surrounding parenchyma. The differentiation between rheumatoid nodules and GPA may be difficult when there is vasculitis. The presence of numerous multinucleated giant cells, neutrophils, and eosinophils within the infiltrate favors GPA, whereas extension of the lesion through the visceral pleura is characteristic of rheumatoid nodules but less common in GPA. Rarely, diffuse infiltration by small nodules has been reported.
Special studies	Elastic tissue stains or pentachrome (Movat) stain may be used to evaluate vessel walls.	Acid-fast and fungal stains must be performed to rule out infectious etiologies. Elastic tissue stains can help with assessing the presence or absence of necrotizing vasculitis.
Prognosis	5-y survival of 75% with appropriately treated disease.	Good, unless hemorrhage, rupture, or bronchopleural fistulae form.

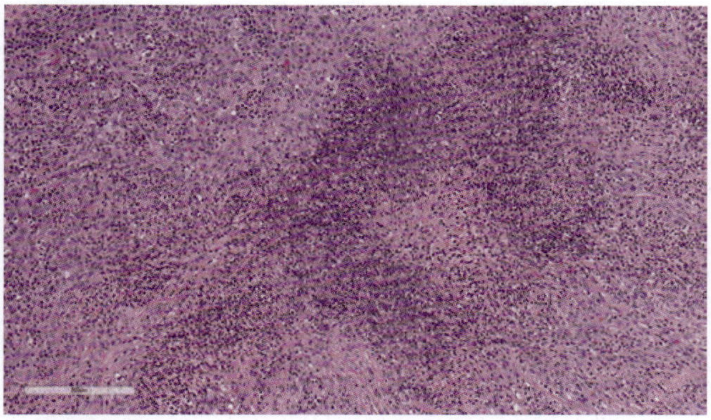

Figure 49.1 GPA: Early geographic basophilic necrosis in an irregular outline.

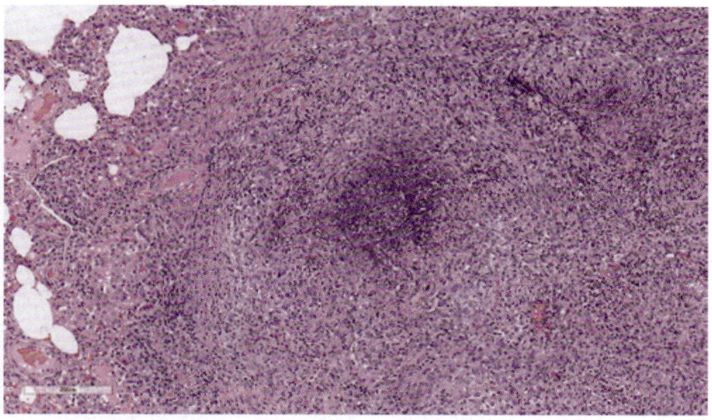

Figure 49.2 GPA: Microabscess with somewhat rounded borders surrounded by palisading histiocytes and other chronic inflammatory cells.

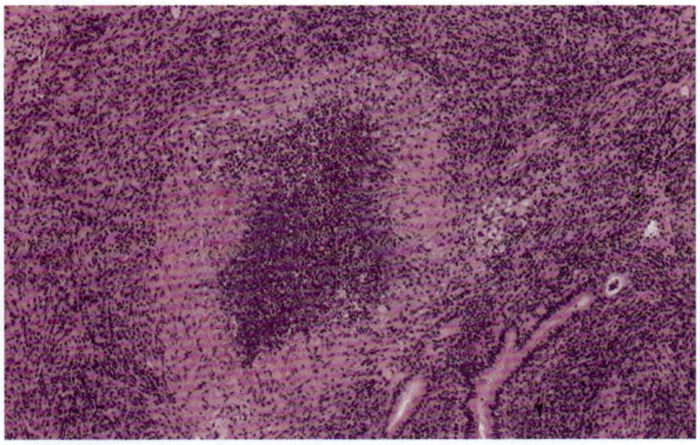

Figure 49.3 GPA: Neutrophils and necrosis, surrounded by palisading histiocytes.

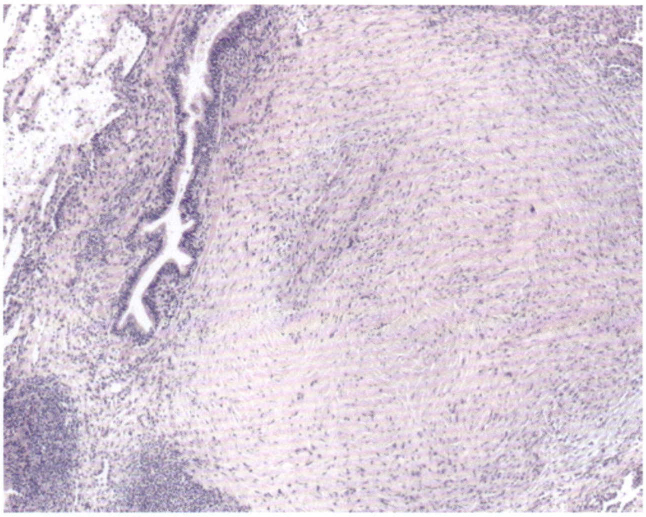

Figure 49.4 GPA: In this example of GPA, although there is no fibrinoid necrosis, there is obvious scarring of the artery (cicatricial changes).

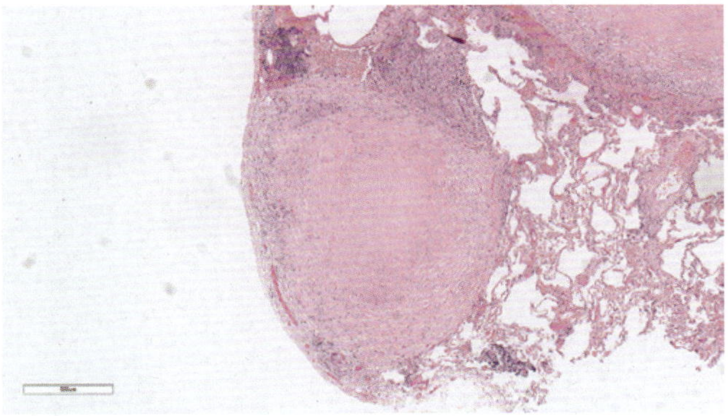

Figure 49.5 Rheumatoid nodule: Low-power image of a subpleural rheumatoid nodule, characterized by a central zone of acellular necrosis surrounded by a rim of histiocytes, occasional multinucleated giant cells, chronic inflammation, and fibrosis. A pleural location favors rheumatoid nodule over GPA, as GPA rarely involves the pleura.

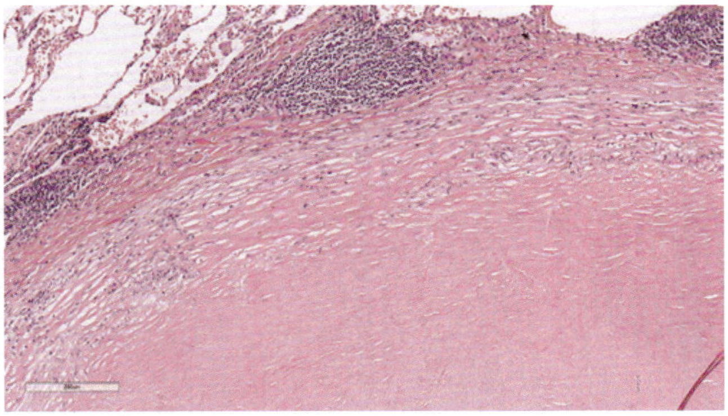

Figure 49.6 Rheumatoid nodule: High-power image showing the eosinophilic necrosis ("necrobiosis") bound by a rim of histiocytes, which in turn are surrounded by lymphocytes and plasma cells. Rheumatoid nodules have fewer giant cells, neutrophils, and eosinophils than do the necrotizing lesions of GPA.

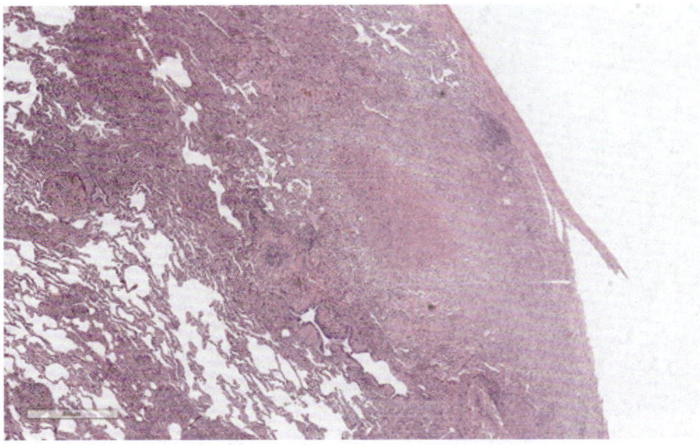

Figure 49.7 Rheumatoid nodule: Subpleural necrobiotic nodule surrounded by a rim of histiocytes.

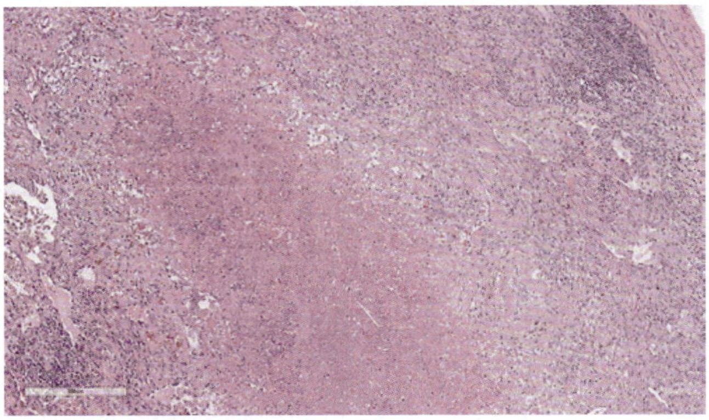

Figure 49.8 Rheumatoid nodule: High-power image demonstrates the necrobiosis surrounded by palisading histiocytes and lymphocytes.

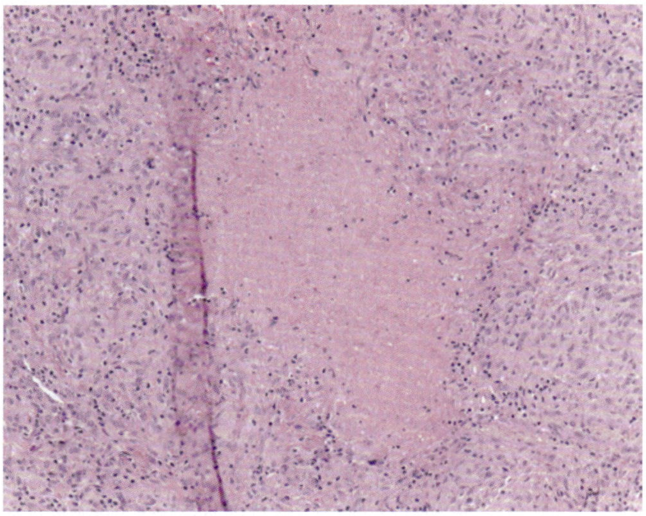

Figure 49.9 Rheumatoid nodule: Another high-power image of necrobiosis.

50 NODULAR SILICOSIS VS. SILICATOSIS

	Nodular Silicosis	Silicatosis
Age	>40 y, usually after several years of exposure.	Incidence increases with age and exposure.
Location	Upper lobe predominance.	Upper and middle lobe predominance.
Symptoms	Slowly progressive chronic cough, exertional dyspnea, fatigue.	Usually asymptomatic. With severe disease, may have symptoms of interstitial lung disease.
Signs	Tachypnea; cor pulmonale with advanced disease. Pulmonary function tests (PFTs) may be normal or may show a combination of mixed restrictive and obstructive defects. Imaging shows well-circumscribed, upper lobe nodules, usually <5 mm in diameter. If coalescent, may form large masses >1 cm, consistent with progressive massive fibrosis (complicated silicosis). Lab findings are nonspecific; Elevated rheumatoid factor (RF), antinuclear antibodies (ANA), and polyclonal increase in Igs may be seen.	Radiographically, small rounded opacities. Rarely progresses to progressive massive fibrosis (PMF). Pleural plaques common in talc and mica pneumoconioses.
Etiology	Usually, exposure to occupational sources of dust with >10% crystalline silica (usually quartz). Crystalline silica is highly fibrogenic.	Usually requires long, heavy exposure to non-asbestos mineral silicates.
Histology	Well-circumscribed nodules with hyalinized whorled collagen centrally and cellular periphery of lymphocytes and dust-laden macrophages *(Figs. 50.1–50.7)*. May have central necrosis with calcifications. Weakly birefringent silica particles in the center and strongly birefringent silicates (silica combined with various cations) toward the periphery. Usually no giant cells or granulomas; if present, should raise concern for associated mycobacterial infection. Background lung parenchyma may show dust macules *(Fig. 50.8)* and mixed-dust fibrotic nodules. Coalescing lesions (PMF) may obliterate lung parenchyma and cavitate. Hilar lymph nodes often involved by silicotic nodules.	The histology varies depending on the mineral present, and there can be considerable overlap in histologic features due to frequent exposure to mixtures of dusts. Often, there are dust macules characterized by dust and dust-laden histiocytes involving distal small airways and alveolar ducts with relatively little fibrosis *(Figs. 50.9 and 50.10)*. Mineral dust airway disease is characterized by dust macules with a greater degree of fibrosis, usually centered on airways, imparting a stellate appearance, and imparting a "Medusa head" appearance similar to the nodules of mixed dust pneumoconiosis *(Fig. 50.11)*. Granulomatous reaction can be seen with exposure to talc, kaolin, feldspars, and others. Granulomas consist of giant cells mixed with fibrosis and dust particles. If talc, then usually innumerable brightly birefringent plate-like material, usually less than 5 µm in diameter are seen *(Fig. 50.12)*. Nodules, <1 cm, gray, brown, blue, or black, with stellate appearance, similar to mixed-dust pneumoconiosis. PMF may result with coalescence of nodules. Diffuse interstitial fibrosis. Pleural fibrosis and thickening.

	Nodular Silicosis	Silicatosis
Special studies	Polarized light used to evaluate silica (weakly birefringent) and silicate particles (strongly birefringent).	Polarized light used to highlight strongly birefringent silicate particles. Analytical transmission and scanning electron microscopic (TEM/SEM) and energy-dispersive x-ray (EDXA) spectra may be performed to identify the dust particles.
Prognosis	Progression is slow; disease can be indolent and disabling. May require transplantation in younger patients.	Slowly progressive without significant mortality or morbidity.

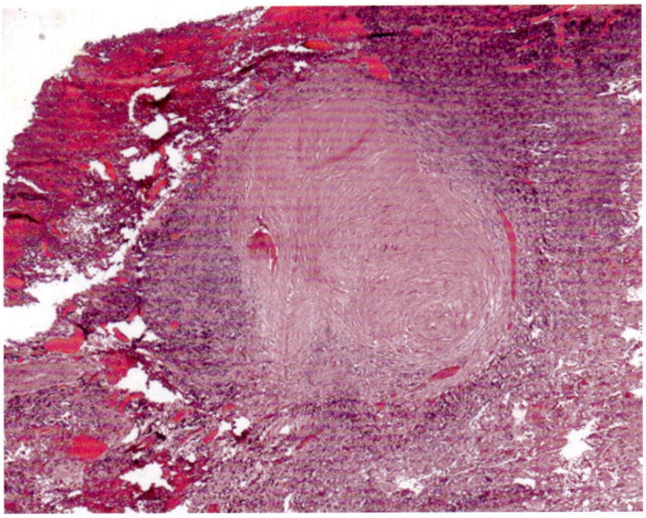

Figure 50.1 Nodular silicosis: Concentrically arrayed, hyalinized bundles of collagen, surrounded by dust-filled histiocytes and lymphocytes. The older the lesion, the more collagenized the nodule. Earlier lesions may show a predominance of fibroblasts and histiocytes. The lesions are usually airway centered. Polarization reveals refractile particles 1–2 μm in diameter, but not all lesions show polarizable material. Necrosis is not a prominent feature.

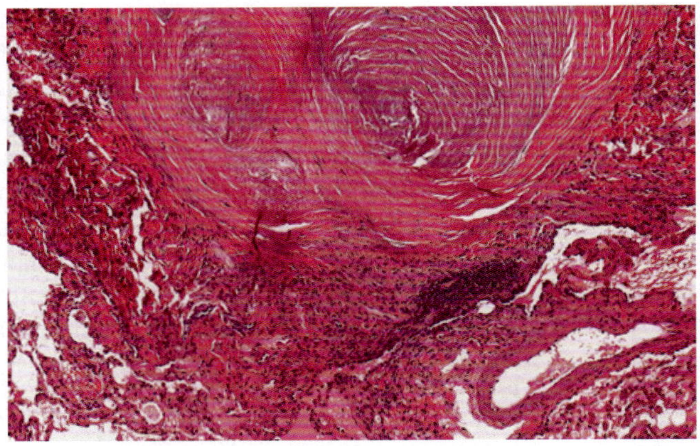

Figure 50.2 Nodular silicosis: Dense collagen surrounded by dust-filled histiocytes.

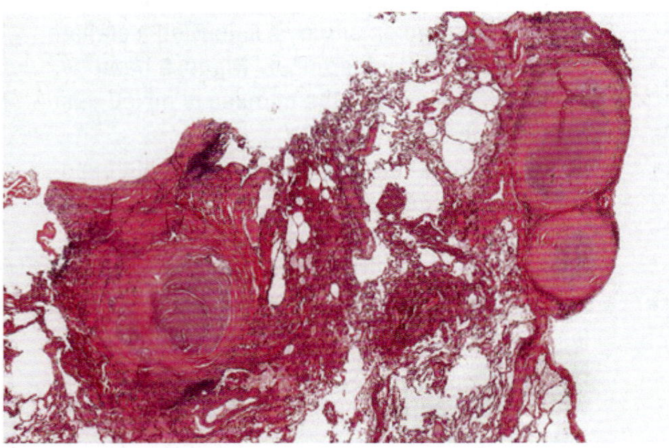

Figure 50.3 Nodular silicosis: Multiple coalescent silicotic nodules.

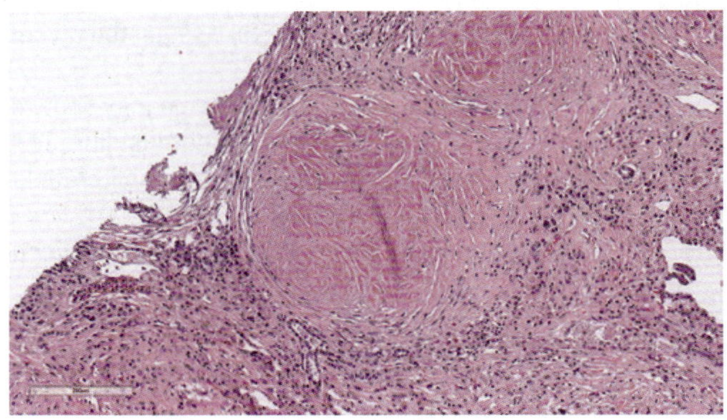

Figure 50.4 Nodular silicosis: High-power image of silicotic nodule.

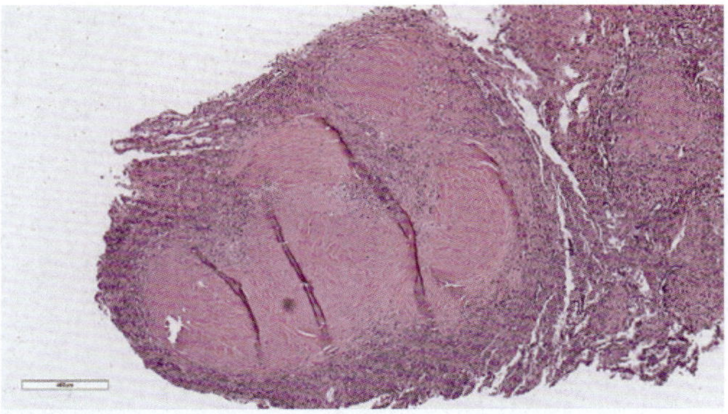

Figure 50.5 Nodular silicosis: Coalescing silicotic nodules.

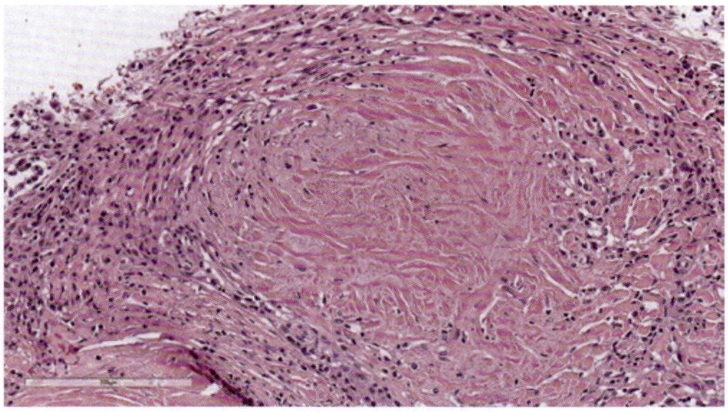

Figure 50.6 Nodular silicosis: Higher-power showing dense collagen surrounded by chronic inflammatory cells.

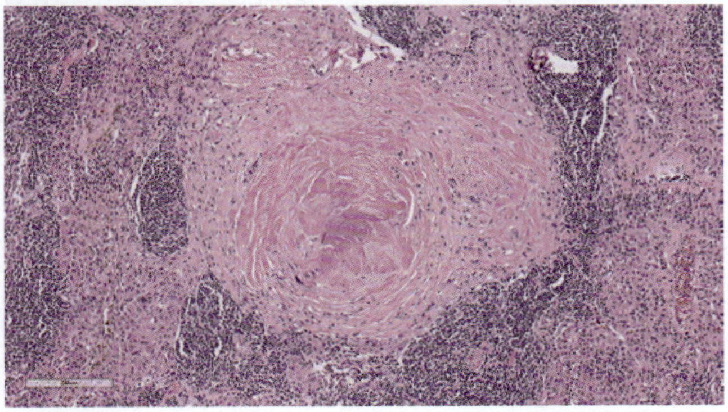

Figure 50.7 Nodular silicosis: Silicotic nodule surrounded by dense chronic inflammation, including histiocytes.

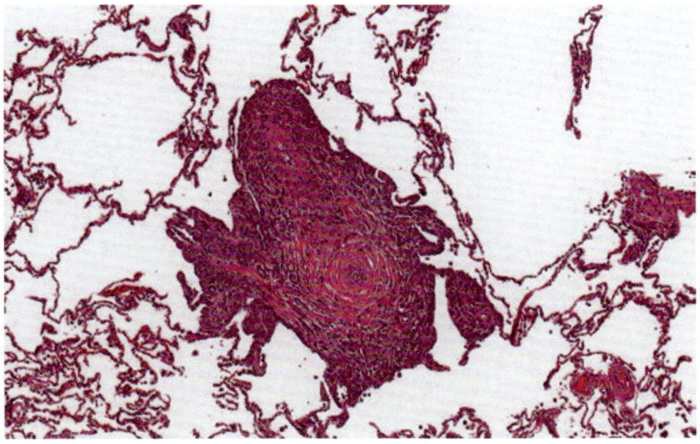

Figure 50.8 Nodular silicosis: Dust macule characterized by interstitial collections of dust-filled histiocytes with mild fibrosis.

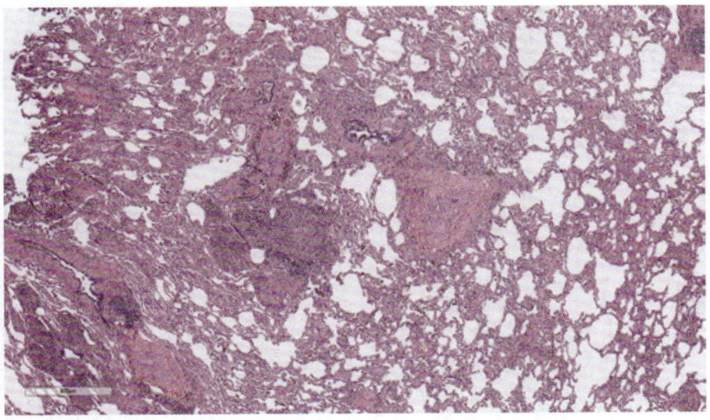

Figure 50.9 Silicatosis: Dust macules centered on airways.

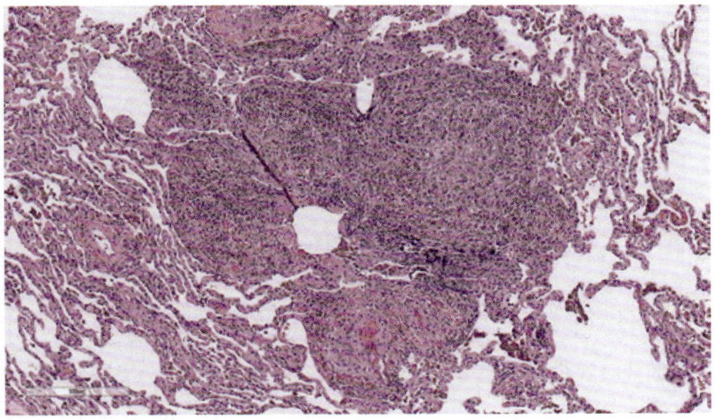

Figure 50.10 Silicatosis: Higher-power of dust macule.

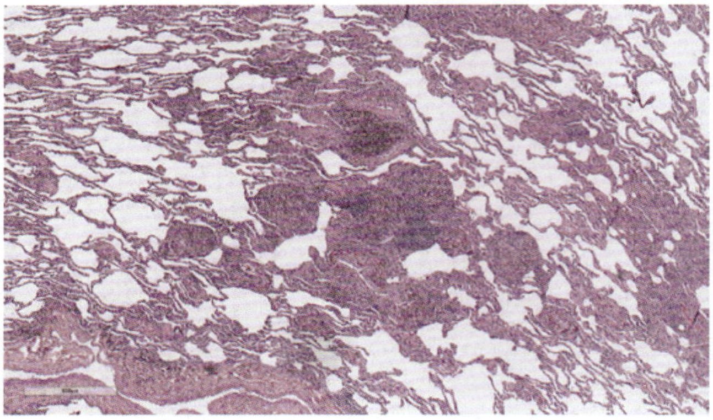

Figure 50.11 Silicatosis: Stellate appearance of early mixed-dust fibrosis with variable numbers of pigmented histiocytes and fibroblasts.

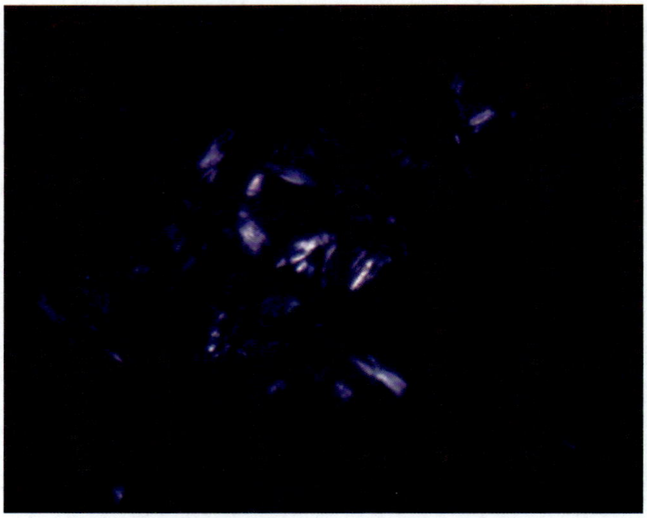

Figure 50.12 Silicatosis: Polarization shows plate-like birefringent particles associated with talc silicatosis.

51 AMYLOID NODULE VS. PULMONARY HYALINIZING GRANULOMA

	Amyloid Nodule	Pulmonary Hyalinizing Granuloma (PHG)
Age	Seventh decade of life.	Young to middle-aged adults (average 45 years of age).
Location	Solitary or multiple nodules that are often peripherally located.	Usually multiple bilateral nodules throughout the lung.
Symptoms	Usually asymptomatic.	Mild cough, fatigue, fever, and/or pleuritic chest pain. One-fourth of the patients are asymptomatic.
Signs	Radiographically, small rounded peripheral nodules, ranging in size from 0.5 to 1.5 cm. May show calcification. Rarely cavitate.	Radiographically, multiple "cotton ball"–type masses from 2 to 4 cm. Usually no calcification or cavitation.
Etiology	Primary (idiopathic) in 80% of cases. Associated with lymphoproliferative diseases (e.g., plasma cell myeloma, primary pulmonary lymphoma) in 20% of cases.	Uncertain, but may be related to sclerosing mediastinitis—possible fibrotic response to latent *Histoplasma* infection.
Histology	Sharply bordered nodules (usually less than 1.5 cm, but can be up to 15 cm) within parenchyma. Characteristic amyloid appearance—eosinophilic, amorphous, globular *(Figs. 51.1 and 51.2)*. Congo red stain highlights the amyloid material *(Figs. 51.3 and 51.4)* and shows an apple-green birefringence with polarized light *(Fig. 51.5)*. Amyloid appears light to medium blue-gray with Mallory trichrome stain *(Fig. 51.6)*. Multinucleated foreign body–type giant cells may surround and ingest amyloid at the periphery *(Figs. 51.7 and 51.8)*. May have foci of calcification and ossification. Plasma cells may be increased.	Nodules composed of thick, acellular collagen bundles arrayed in a whorled, concentric pattern *(Figs. 51.9 and 51.10)*. Collagen "donut" *(Fig. 51.11)*. No refractile, polarizable particles. No apple-green birefringence on Congo red stain. Deep blue color on Mallory trichrome stain. Not truly a granulomatous disease. No foreign body giant cells. No calcification or ossification. No increased plasma cells *(Fig. 51.12)*.
Special studies	Congo red stain *(Figs. 51.3–51.5)*. Electron microscopy shows haphazardly arranged thin fibrils characteristic of amyloid. Amyloid can be classified by biochemical studies. The most common type in nodular amyloidosis is amyloid light chain (AL). Cases that have morphologic features typical of amyloid, but are Congo red negative (amyloid-like nodules) may occur in patients with light chain deposition disease, which by immunohistochemistry studies, are shown to contain immunoglobulin light chain deposits rather than true amyloid. Immunohistochemical stains for plasma cells, and kappa and lambda light chains to rule out monoclonal plasmacytosis. Some amyloid nodules in the lung may be related to forms of low grade lymphoma and additional lymphoma work up may be necessary.	Polarized light to rule out silica and silicate particles. Congo red stain, if necessary, to rule out amyloid. Acid-fast and fungal stains to rule out mycobacterial and fungal diseases, respectively.
Prognosis	Stable for years. Resection rarely necessary.	Excellent prognosis; complete surgical resection is the treatment of choice.

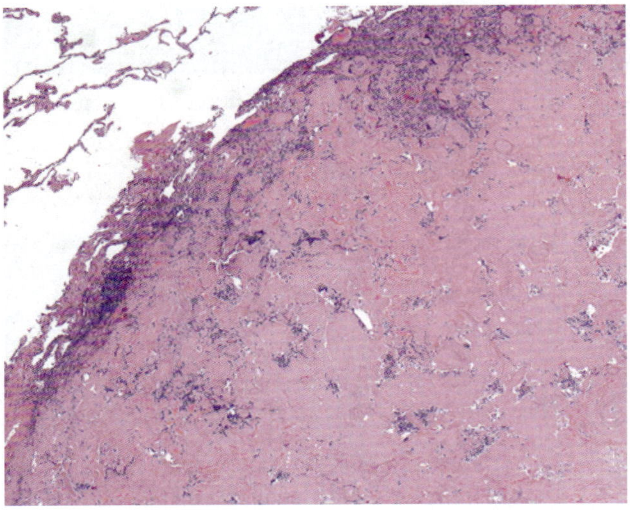

Figure 51.1 Amyloid nodule (low power): Nodule of amyloid consisting of dense, amorphous eosinophilic material. Note the sharp demarcation from the surrounding lung. Note aggregates of inflammatory cells (dark blue) within the nodule, that are in fact composed of plasma cells and lymphocytes.

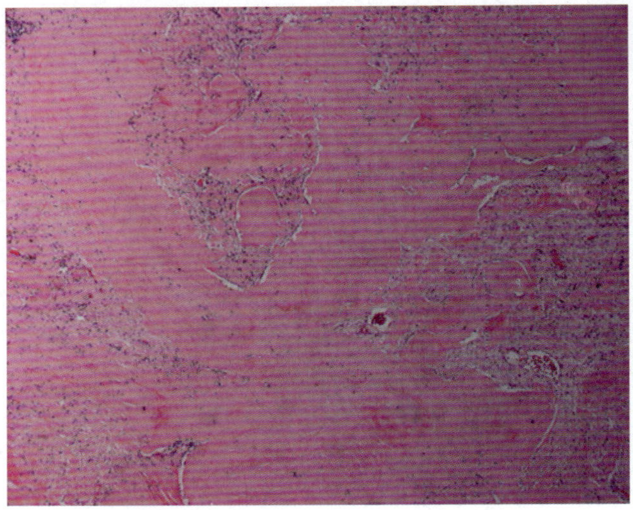

Figure 51.2 Amyloid nodule: Higher-power of the amorphous appearance of amyloid.

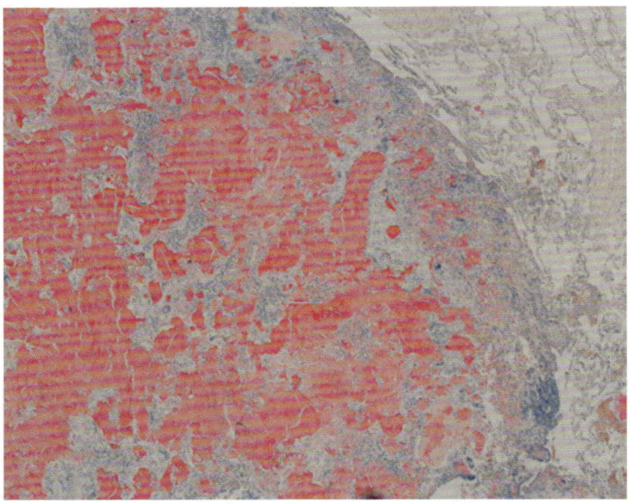

Figure 51.3 Amyloid nodule: Congo red stain highlights the congophilic amyloid material.

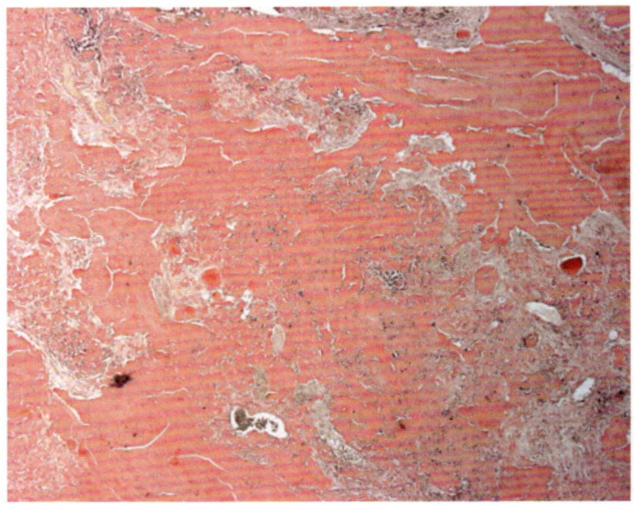

Figure 51.4 Amyloid nodule: Higher-power of Congo red staining of amyloid nodule.

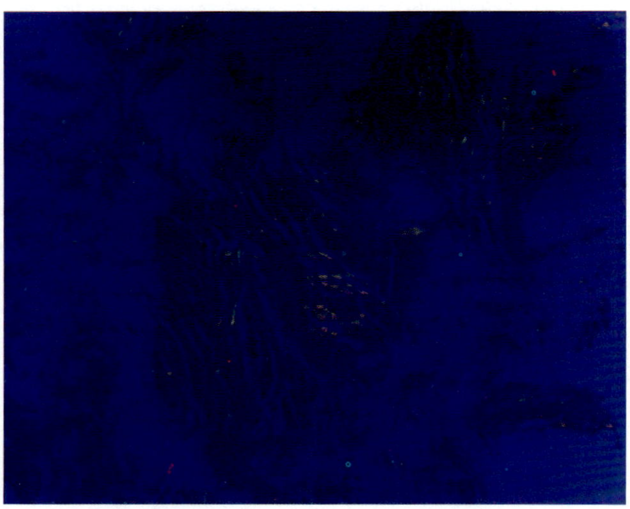

Figure 51.5 Amyloid nodule: With polarized light, the amyloid material shows apple-green birefringence.

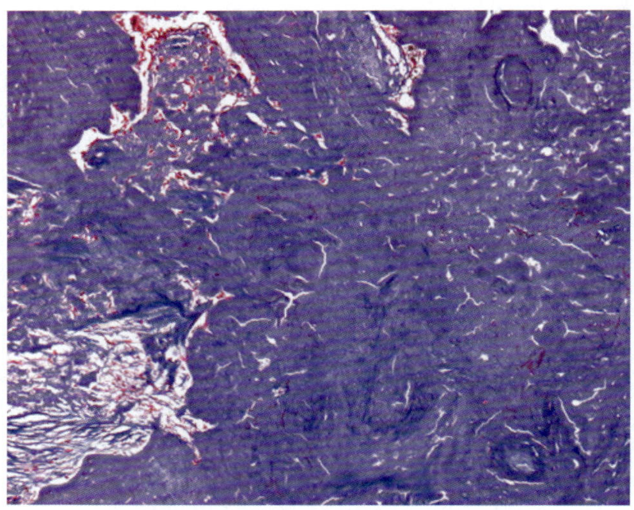

Figure 51.6 Amyloid nodule: Amyloid appears light to medium blue-gray with Mallory trichrome stain in contrast to dark/deep blue pattern of staining seen in dense collagen deposition of PHG.

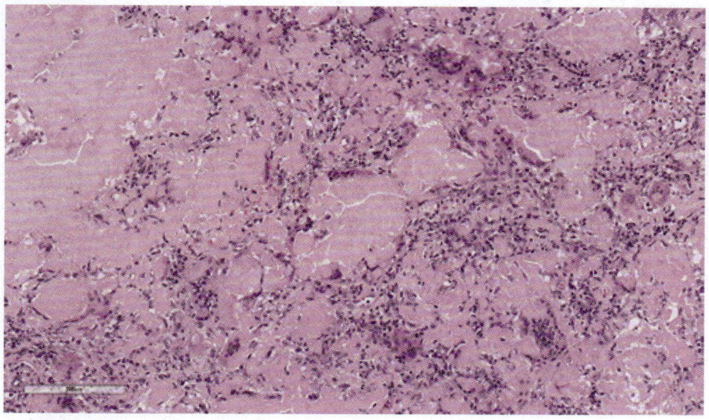

Figure 51.7 Amyloid nodule: There may be a foreign body–type giant cell reaction to amyloid.

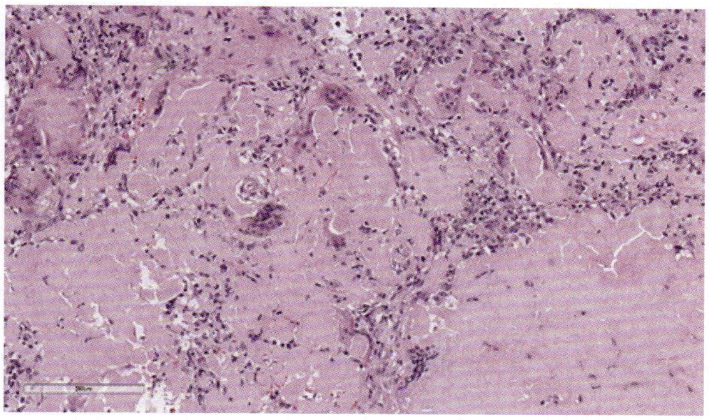

Figure 51.8 Amyloid nodule: The giant cells appear to ingest the amyloid material.

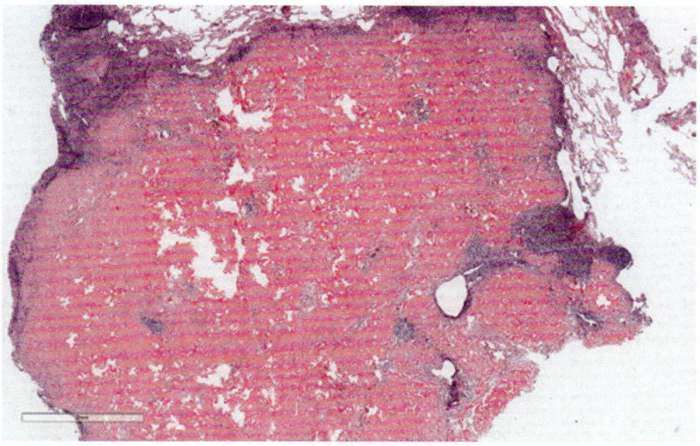

Figure 51.9 PHG (low power): Similarity to nodular amyloidosis, in that there is an acellular eosinophilic appearance.

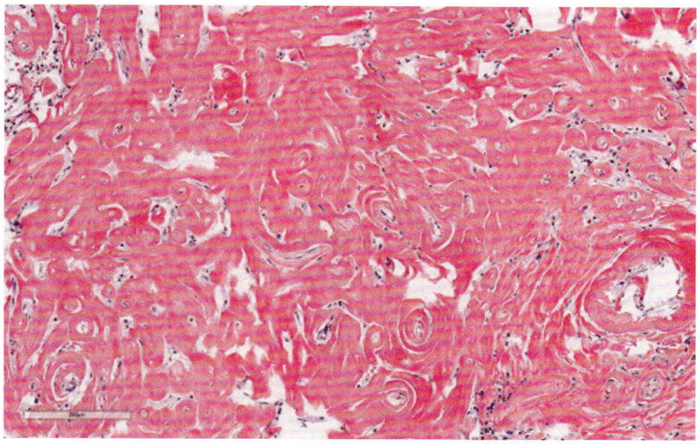

Figure 51.10 PHG (higher power): Composed of thick, acellular collagen bundles arranged in a whorled pattern.

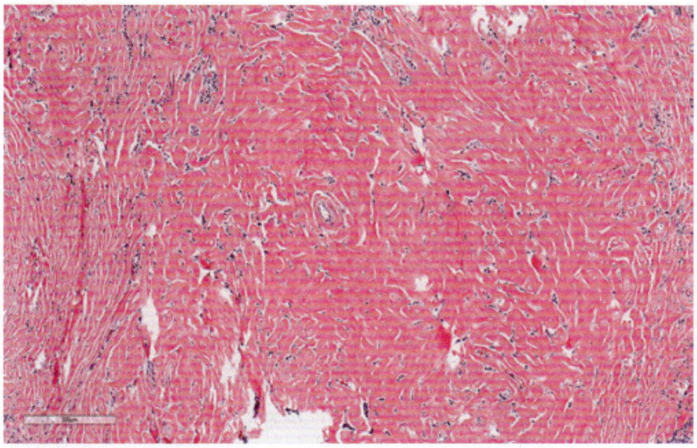

Figure 51.11 PHG: The thick bundles of collagen fibers often form around a vessel, imparting the so-called collagen "donut" appearance.

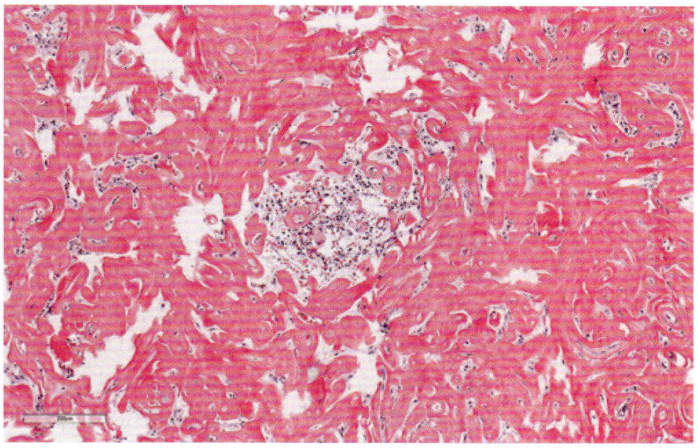

Figure 51.12 PHG: Lymphocytes and plasma cells may be present, but are less prominent than in nodular amyloidosis.

52 ASBESTOSIS VS. USUAL INTERSTITIAL PNEUMONIA/IDIOPATHIC PULMONARY FIBROSIS

	Asbestosis	Usual Interstitial Pneumonia/Idiopathic Pulmonary Fibrosis (UIP/IPF)
Age	Onset usually in middle-aged or elderly people.	>50 y.
Location	Lower lobe predominance, frequent coexisting pleural changes.	Basilar, peripheral lower lobe predominance.
Symptoms	Insidious with dyspnea and cough.	Insidious onset of dyspnea and cough.
Signs	Fine crackles over base of lungs. Clubbing. Restrictive pattern on pulmonary function tests (PFTs). Small, irregular, bilateral lower zone opacities on CT imaging. Pleural plaques and calcifications also seen on CT. With advanced disease—honeycombing evident.	Late inspiratory fine crackles. PFTs show restrictive pattern with gas exchange abnormalities. Radiographically, bilateral reticular pattern, mainly in lower lobes, with honeycombing and ground-glass attenuation.
Etiology	Inhalational exposure to asbestos dust (fibrous silicates). Amphibole groups (e.g., amosite and crocidolite) cause much greater disease than serpentine groups (e.g., chrysotile), as they persist in the lung. Latency period of 15–20 y. Disease may progress even in the absence of exposure (partly related to persistence of asbestos fibers).	Unknown.
Histology	Early manifestation of peribronchiolar fibrosis *(Fig. 52.1)*. Later, extensive interstitial fibrosis with collagen deposition and scant, chronic inflammatory cells *(Figs. 52.2 and 52.3)*. Honeycomb changes in advanced disease. Unlike usual interstitial pneumonia, no significant temporal heterogeneity, no significant fibroblast foci. Asbestos body (iron-coated asbestos fiber—clear central core coated with golden-brown iron protein material) in the presence of diffuse interstitial pulmonary fibrosis is diagnostic of the presence of asbestos *(Figs. 52.4 and 52.5)*. Asbestos bodies often have a beaded appearance. Uncoated asbestos fibers are not visible on hematoxylin and eosin or iron stains. Granulomas uncommon. Often, coexisting pleural plaques *(Figs. 52.6 and 52.7)*.	Interstitial fibrosis and chronic inflammation with fibroblast foci and peripheral accentuation—temporal and spatial heterogeneity *(Figs. 52.8–52.12)*. Honeycombing—characterized by cystic spaces, surrounded by fibrosis and chronic inflammation, lined by flat-to-columnar epithelium, and often filled with mucus and inflammatory debris *(Fig. 52.9)*. No granulomas, although may have airspace multinucleated cells.

	Asbestosis	Usual Interstitial Pneumonia/Idiopathic Pulmonary Fibrosis (UIP/IPF)
Special studies	If asbestos bodies are not visible on H&E, iron stain can be performed. An asbestos body is a type of ferruginous body (iron-coated particle), and thus shows bright blue with iron stain. It must have a clear central core of asbestos, as other particulate matter may be coated with iron. Additional techniques (e.g., mass spectrometry) are necessary to assess uncoated asbestos fibers. Pentachrome (Movat stain) may be used to confirm peribronchiolar accentuation of fibrosis as well as the paucity of fibroblast foci (which appear blue to blue-green on pentachrome stain).	Pentachrome (Movat) stain highlights the temporal heterogeneity with yellow representing dense collagen and blue/blue-green representing the immature collagen of fibroblast foci.
Prognosis	Slowly progressive. Increased risk of lung cancer.	Poor. Median length of survival from diagnosis is 2.5–3.5 y.

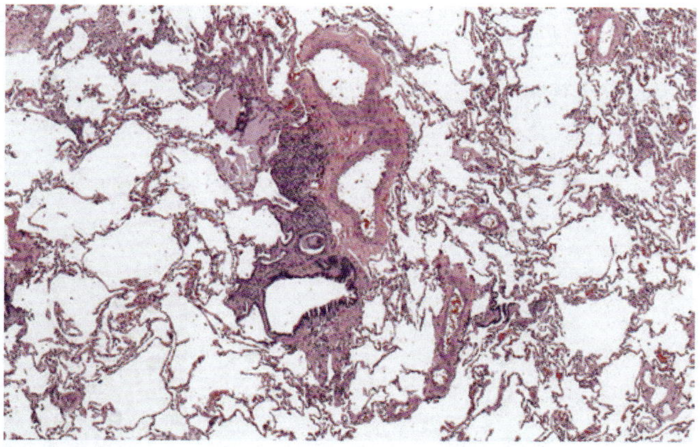

Figure 52.1 Asbestosis: Airway-centered interstitial fibrosis admixed with variable chronic inflammation. The fibrosis is restricted to the airways and does not disrupt the lung architecture. However, this appearance is not specific to asbestosis.

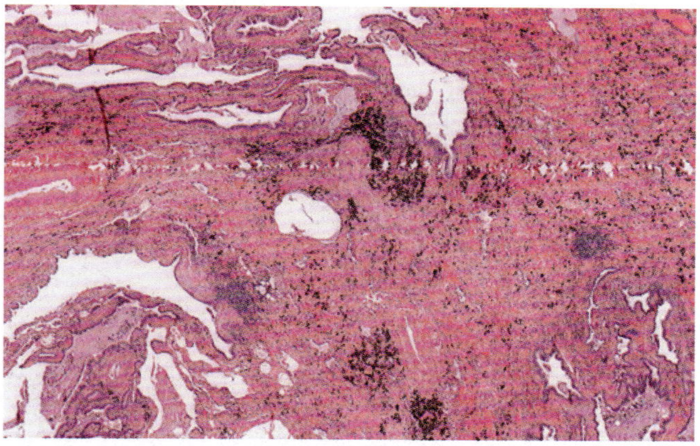

Figure 52.2 Asbestosis: Later in disease, the fibrosis can be extensive and can overlap with UIP. This image demonstrates marked interstitial fibrosis with disruption of the lung architecture. Anthracosis is also evident. There is minimal-to-mild chronic inflammation. Rare fibroblastic foci can be present.

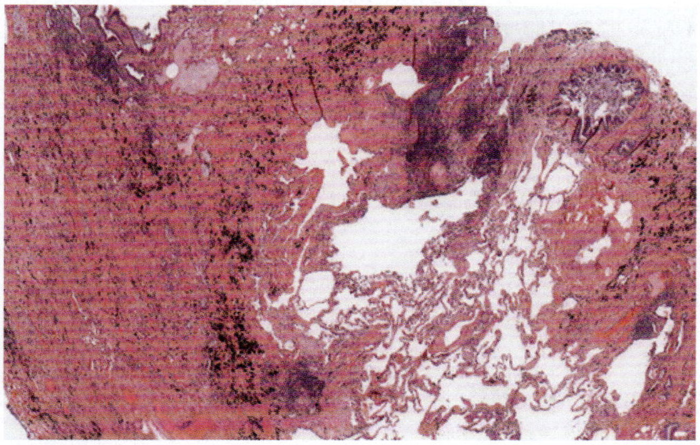

Figure 52.3 Asbestosis: Dense eosinophilic fibrosis, anthracosis, and rare fibroblastic foci. Occasional lymphoid aggregates are present. Although there is overlap with UIP, the fibrosis tends to be more homogeneous and with fewer fibroblast foci.

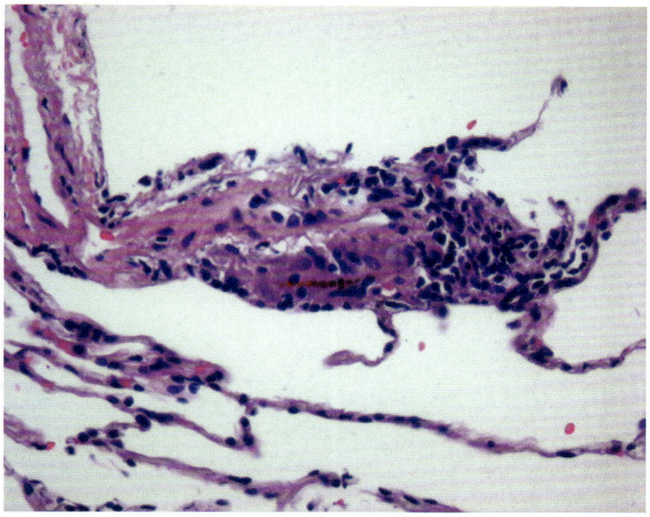

Figure 52.4 Asbestosis: In other areas of the same biopsy as above, the classic asbestos body is visible. The clear central core is coated by iron-containing material, imparting a beaded appearance.

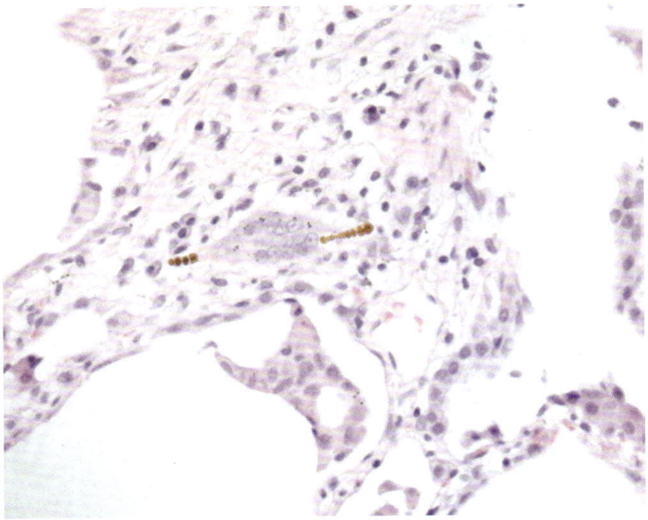

Figure 52.5 Asbestosis: An iron-coated, beaded asbestos body partially engulfed by a multinucleated giant cell. An asbestos body is a subset of a ferruginous body, which is *any* iron-coated particle.

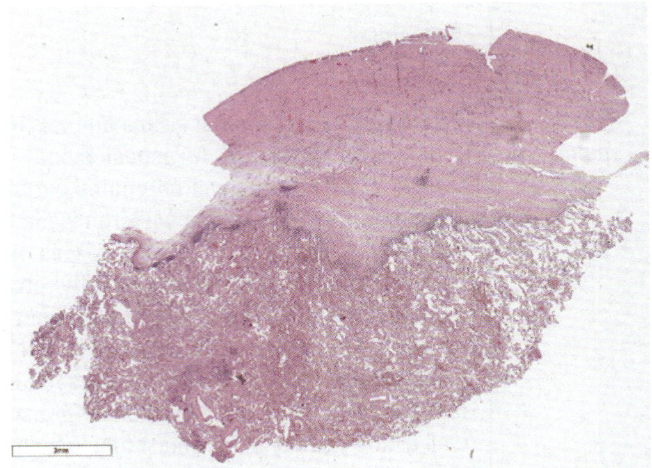

Figure 52.6 Asbestosis: Pleural plaque at low power, demonstrating the thick, collagenized appearance with a parallel to basket-weave arrangement of fibers. Asbestos bodies are rarely found in pleural plaques, but uncoated asbestos fibers can be identified using mineral analysis techniques.

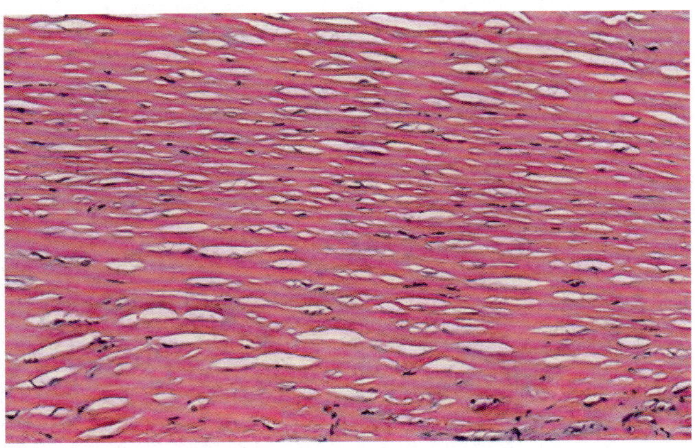

Figure 52.7 Asbestosis: Higher-power of collagen fibers with basket-weave appearance.

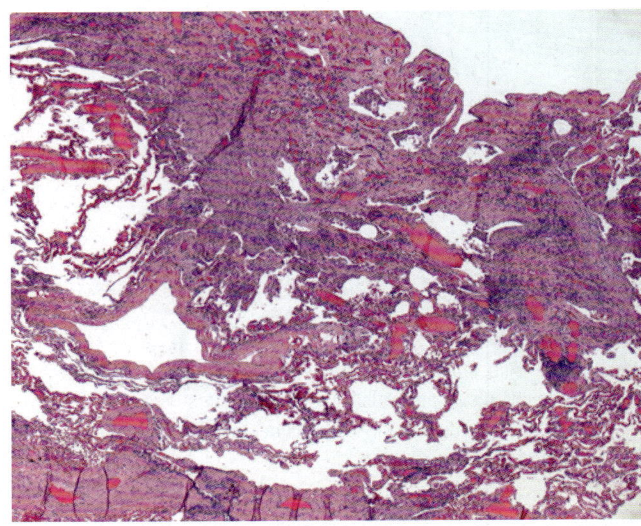

Figure 52.8 UIP/IPF: Upper lobe biopsy from patient with UIP demonstrating a subpleural interstitial process characterized by early fibrosis, extensive fibroblastic activity, and chronic inflammation.

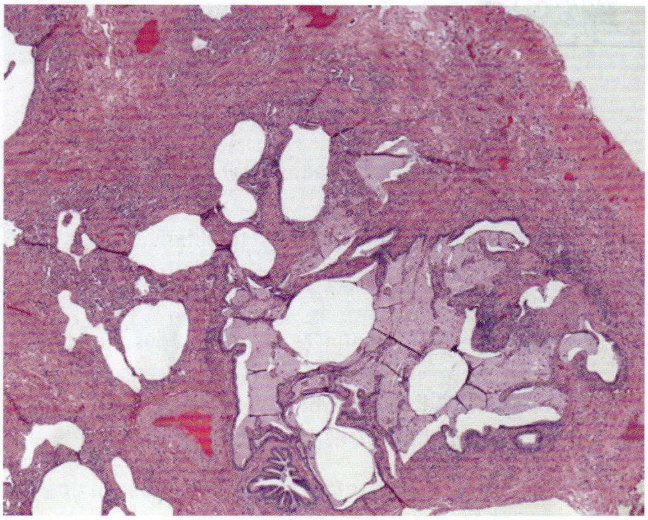

Figure 52.9 UIP/IPF: The lower lobe biopsy from the same patient with UIP demonstrating honeycomb changes characterized by cystic spaces with thick fibrotic walls. The airspaces are lined by cuboidal to ciliated columnar epithelium. The lumens are filled with inspissated mucus and mixed inflammatory cells.

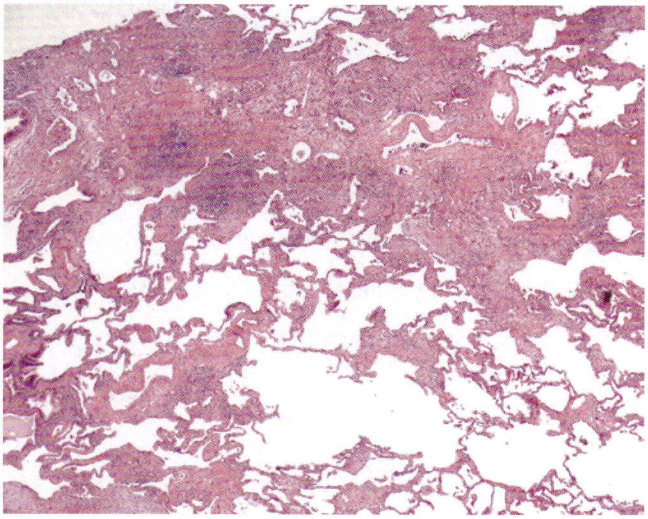

Figure 52.10 UIP/IPF: UIP fibrosis with subpleural accentuation and temporal heterogeneity. Fibroblast foci are subepithelial small aggregates of myofibroblasts/fibroblasts, which stain light pink on H&E.

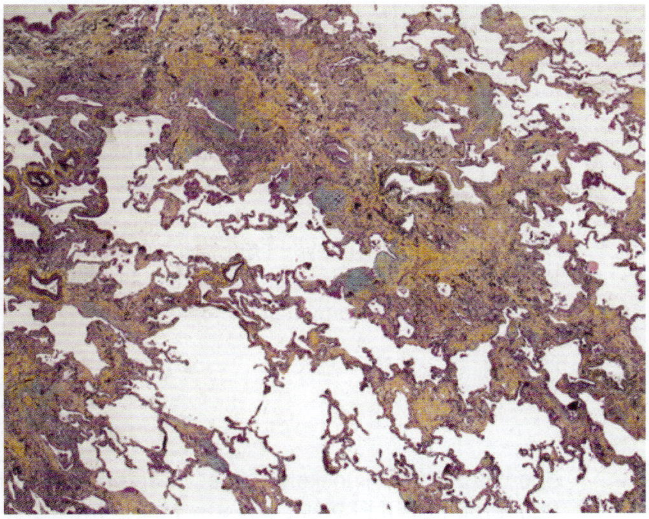

Figure 52.11 UIP/IPF: Movat (pentachrome)–stained serial section from the same patient as above, demonstrating the blue-green hue of the fibroblast foci. The dense collagen stains yellow. The Movat stain is helpful in assessing the heterogeneity of the interstitial process.

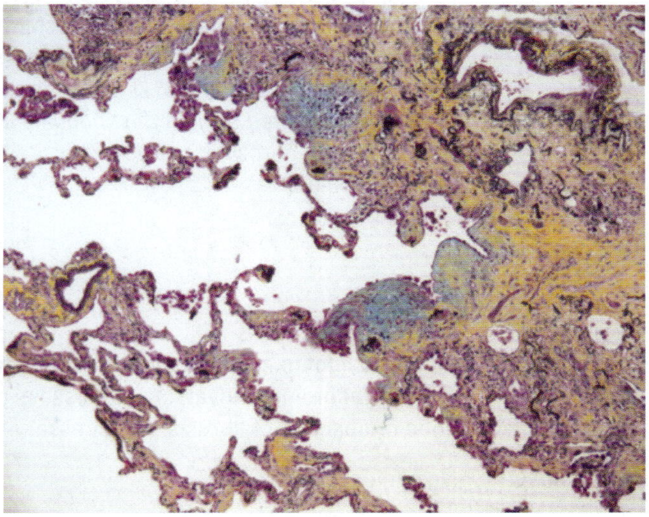

Figure 52.12 UIP/IPF: Higher-power of the fibroblast foci.

53 ANTHRACOTIC DUST MACULES VS. COAL WORKERS' PNEUMOCONIOSIS

	Anthracotic Dust Macules	Coal Workers' Pneumoconiosis
Age	Onset increases with age and exposure.	Onset usually in middle-aged to elderly people.
Location	Upper lobe predominance.	Upper lobe predominance.
Symptoms	Asymptomatic.	May be asymptomatic. May develop dyspnea and cough with black sputum. If progression to progressive massive fibrosis (PMF), which is rare, then symptoms correspondingly increase.
Signs	No clinical signs or functional deficits. May have radiographic abnormalities.	Radiographically, small rounded opacities in upper lobes. Rarely progresses to PMF.
Etiology	Exposure to inert dust. May be seen in urban dwellers as well as in miners.	Exposure to coal dust, which contains not only carbon but also varying concentrations of silica, silicates, and trace elements such as titanium and beryllium.
Histology	Interstitial accumulation of nonpalpable, black, dust-filled macrophages in walls of respiratory bronchioles and alveolar ducts, usually less than 3 mm in size *(Figs. 53.1 and 53.2)*. Collections larger than 3 mm are often termed *dust nodules (Fig. 53.3)*. No associated fibrosis. No granulomas.	Nonpalpable, small airway-centered dust macules *(Figs. 53.4* and *53.5)*. Also have palpable dust nodules, which are stellate to rounded fibrotic nodules, larger than dust macules *(Figs. 53.6–53.8)*. Anthracotic (black) appearance of interlobular septa, pleura, and bronchial, hilar, and mediastinal lymph nodes *(Fig. 53.9)*. Often, coexisting emphysema *(Figs. 53.10 and 53.11)*. PMF lesions (nodules >1 cm) may result from coalescence of dust nodules.
Special studies	Polarized light to evaluate for birefringent material. Pentachrome (Movat) stain to assess presence or absence of fibrosis, as necessary.	None.
Prognosis	No clinical disease.	Good; progression unlikely with early detection. Poor prognosis if PMF develops.

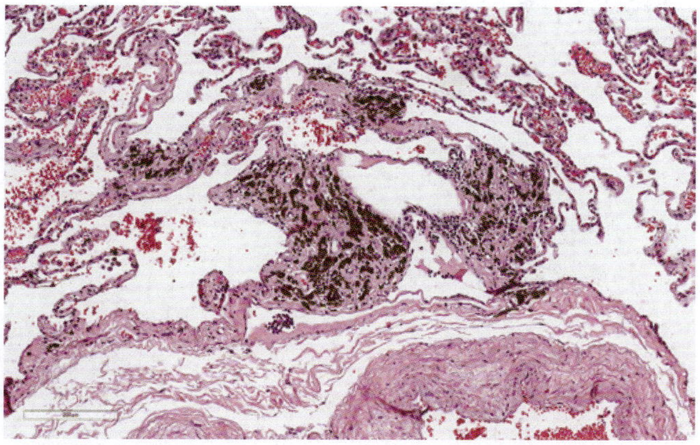

Figure 53.1 Anthracotic dust macule: Dust macule characterized by black to gray particles collecting in interstitial peri-airway-centered locations. Usually not palpable because they are small (<3 mm) and there is no significant associated interstitial fibrosis.

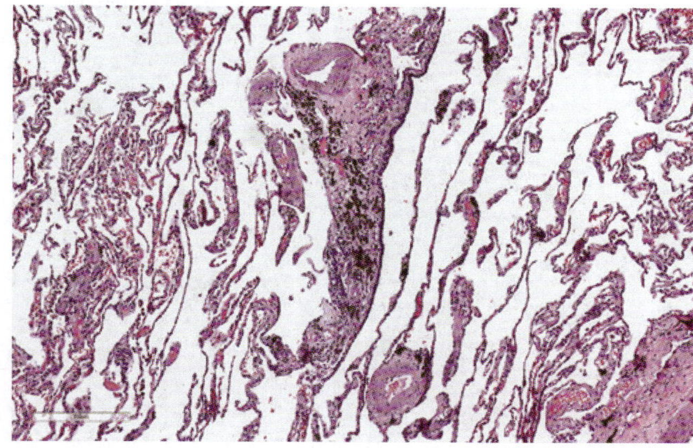

Figure 53.2 Anthracotic dust macule: Another peri-airway accumulation of black particles.

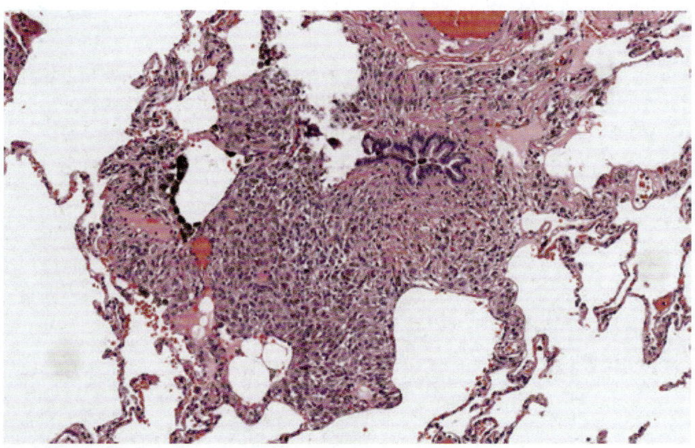

Figure 53.3 Anthracotic dust macule: Early stellate-shaped, "Medusa-head" pattern typical of a larger mixed dust nodule.

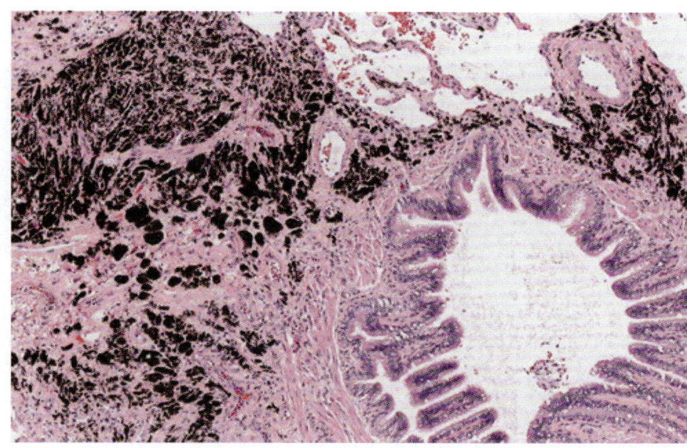

Figure 53.4 Coal workers' pneumoconiosis: Dust macules in coal workers' pneumoconiosis are similar to those in anthracotic dust macules. Carbon particles are present both in macrophages and in tissue.

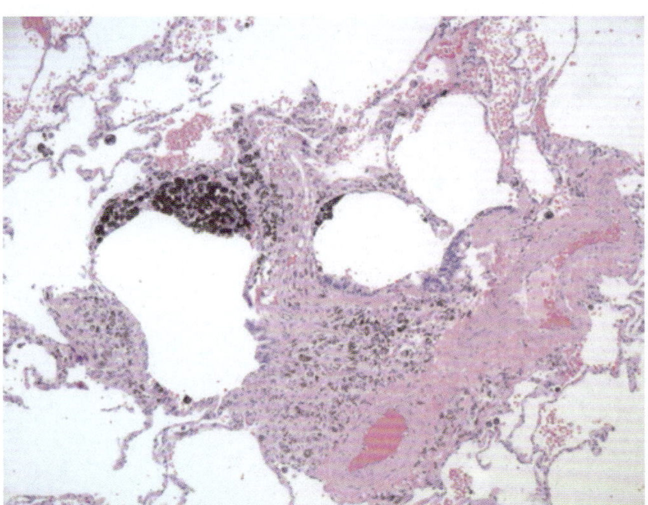

Figure 53.5 Coal workers' pneumoconiosis: Dense anthracosis and dust around an airway. Early fibrotic changes are present.

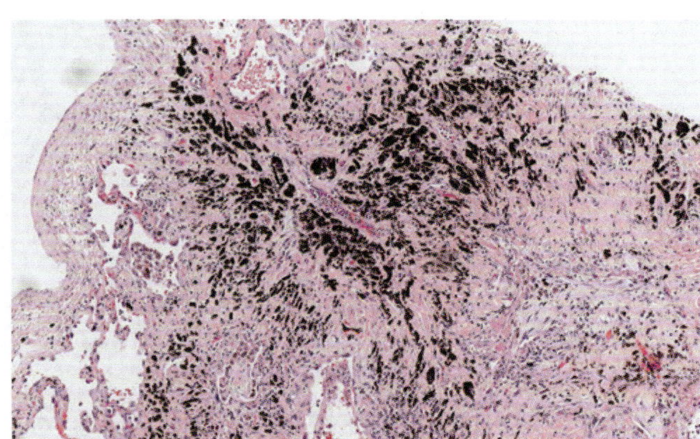

Figure 53.6 Coal workers' pneumoconiosis: Dust nodule with increased collagen.

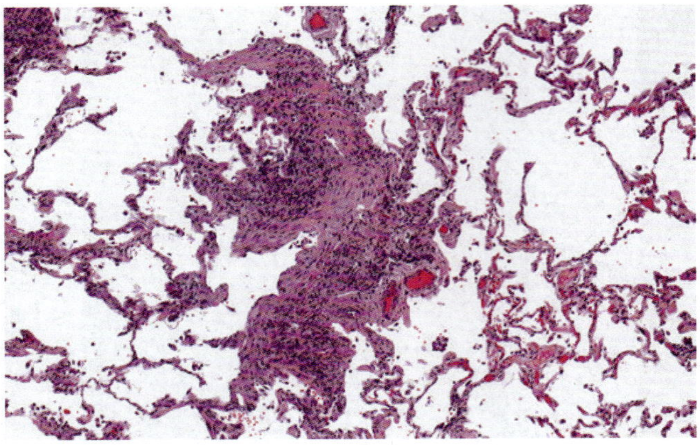

Figure 53.7 Coal workers' pneumoconiosis: Dust macule/nodule with fibroblasts and collagen evident.

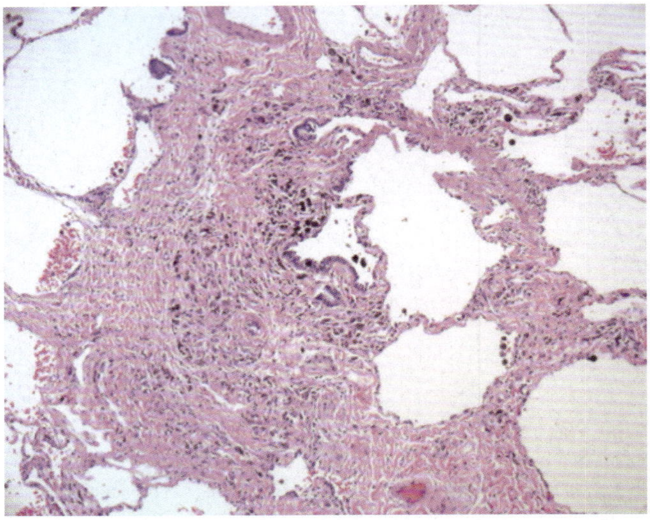

Figure 53.8 Coal workers' pneumoconiosis: Dust nodule associated with collagen around an airway.

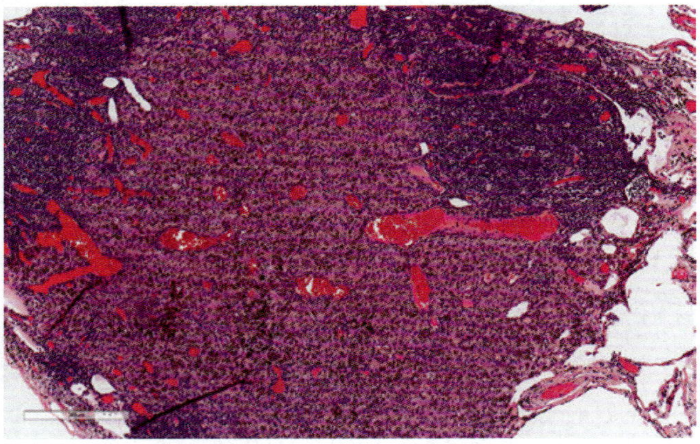

Figure 53.9 Coal workers' pneumoconiosis: Intraparenchymal lymph node demonstrating anthracosis within histiocytes.

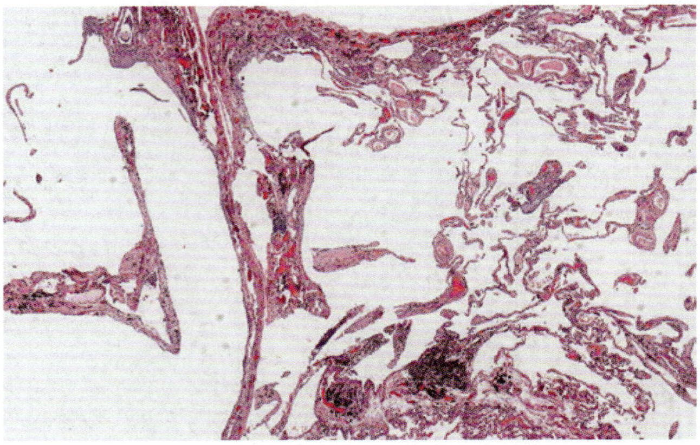

Figure 53.10 Coal workers' pneumoconiosis: Centrilobular emphysema is often present. Here, because of the large emphysematous spaces, the parenchyma is collapsed.

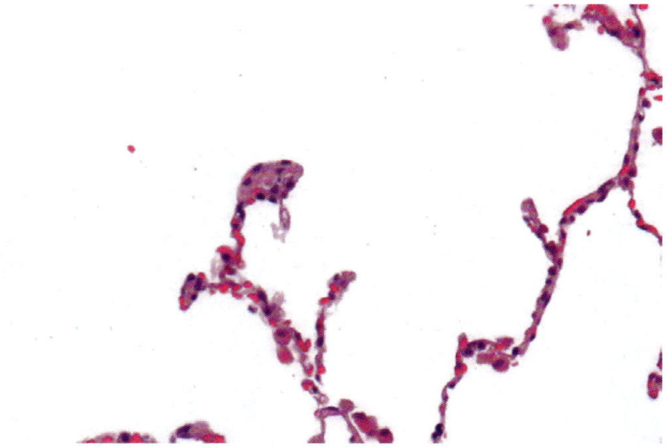

Figure 53.11 Coal workers' pneumoconiosis: High-power view of the typical broken, club-shaped alveolar tip of emphysema.

54 BLEOMYCIN TOXICITY VS. AMIODARONE TOXICITY

	Bleomycin Toxicity	Amiodarone Toxicity
Age	Any, but toxicity increases in older than 70 y.	Toxicity increases with age (especially > 60 y).
Location	Lung bases.	Initially, upper lobe predominant. May become diffuse with continuation of drug.
Symptoms	Nonproductive cough, exertional dyspnea, occasionally fever. With development of interstitial disease, dyspnea at rest.	Insidious dyspnea and dry cough. Occasionally, low-grade fever and malaise.
Signs	Tachypnea, cyanosis, fine bibasilar crackles early, with progression to rhonchi. Pulmonary function tests (PFTs) may be normal or may show a combination of mixed restrictive and obstructive defects. Chest x-ray shows bilateral, bibasilar infiltrates. Occasionally, unilateral and focal. CT imaging shows small linear and subpleural nodular lesions in the lung bases.	Crackles on examination. PFTs show decrease in diffusing capacity of the lungs for carbon monoxide (DLCO). Chest x-ray shows bilateral, bibasilar infiltrates. Occasionally, unilateral and focal. CT imaging shows small linear and subpleural nodular lesions in the lung bases. Amiodarone is an iodinated compound and is radiopaque and hence shows up particularly well on CT. Bronchoalveolar lavage (BAL) shows foamy macrophages. Laboratory studies may show mildly elevated leukocytes and increased erythrocyte sedimentation rate (ESR).
Etiology	Endothelial damage, induction of free radicals. Lung and skin lack the inactivating enzyme (bleomycin hydroxylase), predisposing to toxic side effects.	Mechanism unknown, but toxicity is dose related.
Histology	Early changes of vascular endothelial injury, edema, and pneumocyte damage. Reactive pneumocyte hyperplasia with marked atypia may be present *(Fig. 54.1)*. Fibroblast proliferation (organizing diffuse alveolar damage) and subsequent interstitial, temporally homogeneous, fibrosis may follow *(Fig. 54.2)*. May have concurrent fibrin exudates and/or organizing pneumonia *(Figs. 54.3 and 54.4)*. No giant cells or granulomas.	Foamy, lipid-laden macrophages accumulate in airspaces *(Figs. 54.5* and *54.6)*—however, presence merely reflects drug use, not necessarily toxicity. Cytoplasmic lipid vacuoles may be seen in pneumocytes, endothelial cells, and interstitial cells *(Fig. 54.7)*. Type 2 cells, macrophages, endothelial cells, and interstitial cells show lamellar inclusions (tightly packed whorls of thin lamellae) on electron microscopy (EM). Variable interstitial inflammatory infiltrate. Organizing pneumonia may be present *(Fig. 54.8)*. Diffuse alveolar damage (DAD) is uncommon in amiodarone-induced lung injury.
Special studies	None.	EM for identification of lamellar bodies.
Prognosis	20% of patients develop lung disease; overall mortality of 3%.	Discontinuation of drug and treatment with corticosteroids usually resolves lung injury; however, in hospitalized patients, mortality reaches 33%.

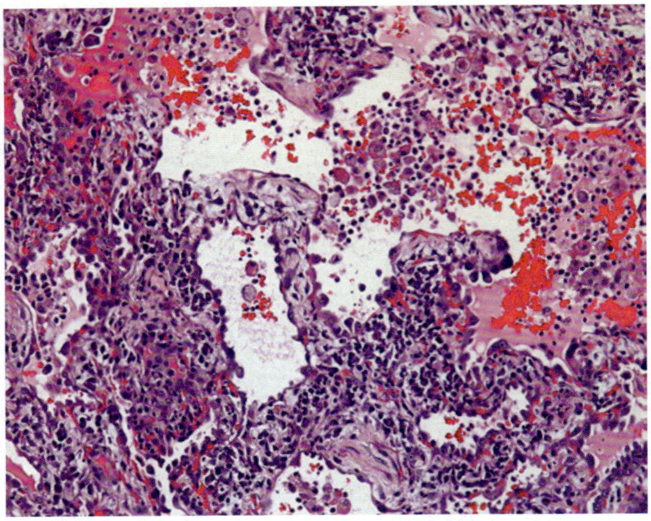

Figure 54.1 Bleomycin toxicity: Alveolar septal thickening by fibroblastic tissue with hyperplasia and reactive atypia of type 2 pneumocytes.

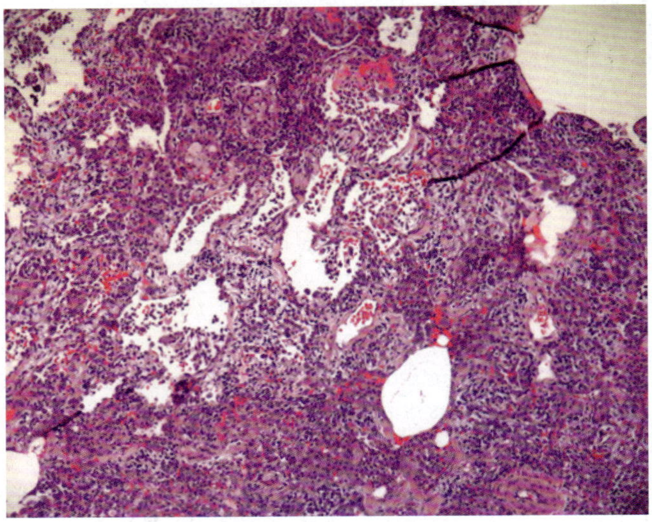

Figure 54.2 Bleomycin toxicity: Low-power view from same patient demonstrating the developing injury pattern with alveolar septa thickened by fibroblastic tissue.

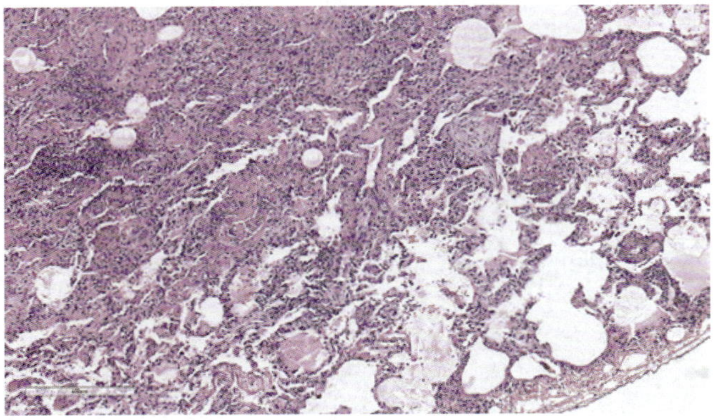

Figure 54.3 Bleomycin toxicity: Acute and organizing lung injury characterized by hyaline membranes, fibrin exudates, and organizing pneumonia.

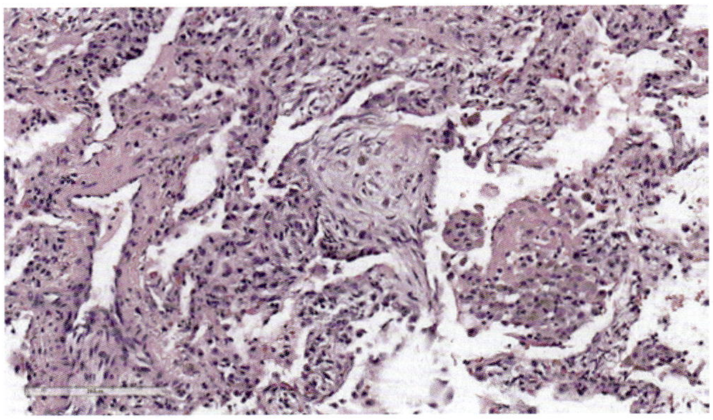

Figure 54.4 Bleomycin toxicity: Fibrin is incorporated into the plug of organizing pneumonia.

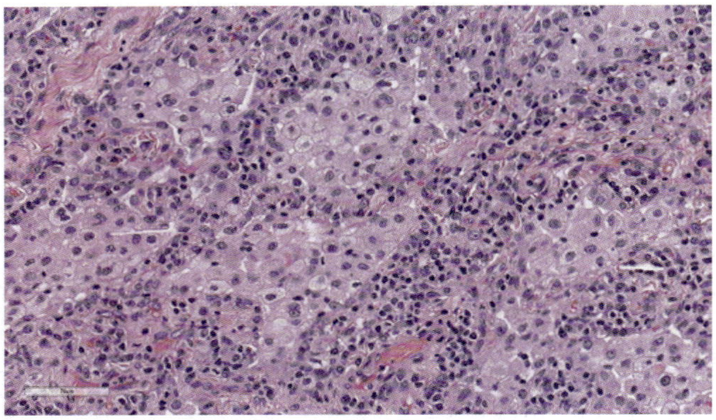

Figure 54.5 Amiodarone toxicity: Prominent foamy alveolar macrophages, characterized by finely vacuolated cytoplasm, in a patient with amiodarone-induced lung injury. There is a mild interstitial chronic inflammatory component. The foamy macrophages indicate usage, not necessarily toxicity, as they can be seen in patients without drug-induced lung disease.

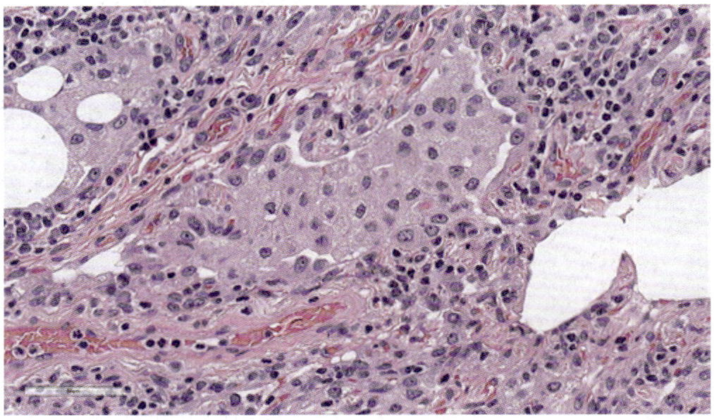

Figure 54.6 Amiodarone toxicity: Higher-power of foamy macrophages.

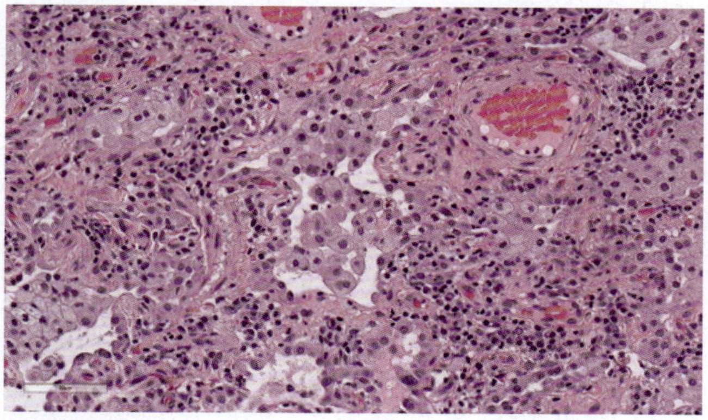

Figure 54.7 Amiodarone toxicity: In this image, there are not only intra-alveolar foamy macrophages, but also some foamy changes of the type 2 reactive pneumocytes. Also, note the mild chronic interstitial inflammatory infiltrate consisting of lymphocytes and plasma cells.

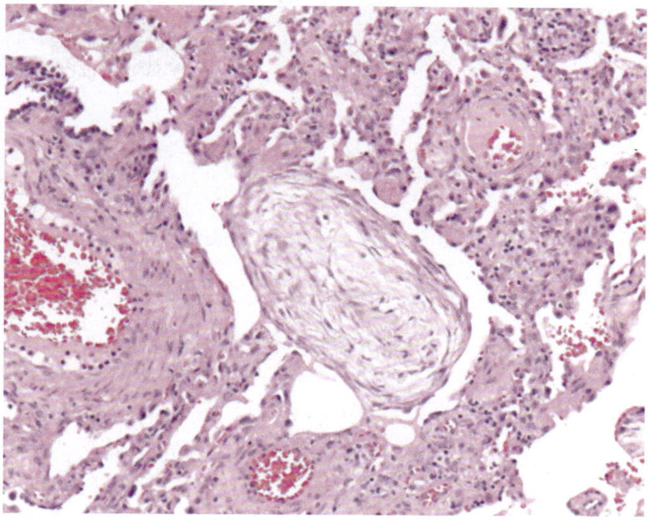

Figure 54.8 Amiodarone toxicity: Organizing pneumonia may be seen, but is a less common manifestation of amiodarone-induced injury.

55 BLEOMYCIN TOXICITY VS. METHOTREXATE TOXICITY

	Bleomycin Toxicity	Methotrexate Toxicity
Age	Any, but toxicity increases in those older than 70 y.	Any.
Location	Lung bases.	Bilateral, throughout the lung.
Symptoms	Nonproductive cough, exertional dyspnea, occasionally fever. With development of interstitial disease, dyspnea at rest.	Dyspnea, nonproductive cough, and fever, usually within days to weeks after therapy initiation.
Signs	Tachypnea, cyanosis, fine bibasilar crackles early, with progression to rhonchi. Pulmonary function tests may be normal or may show a combination of mixed restrictive and obstructive defects. Chest x-ray shows bilateral, bibasilar infiltrates. Occasionally, unilateral and focal. CT imaging shows small linear and subpleural nodular lesions in the lung bases.	Imaging studies show homogeneous opacities, bilateral interstitial infiltrates, and occasionally alveolar infiltrates. Bronchoalveolar lavage shows lymphocytosis. Peripheral eosinophilia in one-third of patients.
Etiology	Endothelial damage, induction of free radicals. Lung and skin lack the inactivating enzyme (bleomycin hydroxylase), predisposing to toxic side effects.	Methotrexate interferes with folic acid metabolism and thus targets replicating cells. Pulmonary toxicity develops in about 10% of patients.
Histology	Early changes of vascular endothelial injury, edema, and pneumocyte damage. Reactive pneumocyte hyperplasia with marked atypia may be present *(Fig. 55.1)*. Fibroblast proliferation (organizing diffuse alveolar damage) *(Fig. 55.2)* and subsequent interstitial, temporally homogeneous, fibrosis may follow. May have concurrent organizing pneumonia. No giant cells or granulomas.	Mononuclear interstitial inflammatory infiltrate and fibrosis *(Figs. 55.3* and *55.4)*. Multinucleated giant cells and poorly formed granulomas may be present (an unusual feature in a drug-related injury) *(Figs. 55.5–55.8)*. Scattered foci of organizing pneumonia *(Fig. 55.9)*. Hyaline membranes may form if diffuse alveolar damage (DAD) pattern develops *(Fig. 55.10)*. Eosinophils in about one-half.
Special studies	None.	If granulomas present, acid-fast and fungal stains to rule out mycobacterial and fungal disease, respectively.
Prognosis	20% of patients develop lung disease; overall mortality of 3%.	Usually reversible with corticosteroids; mortality $<$10%. May reinstitute drug without triggering recurrence.

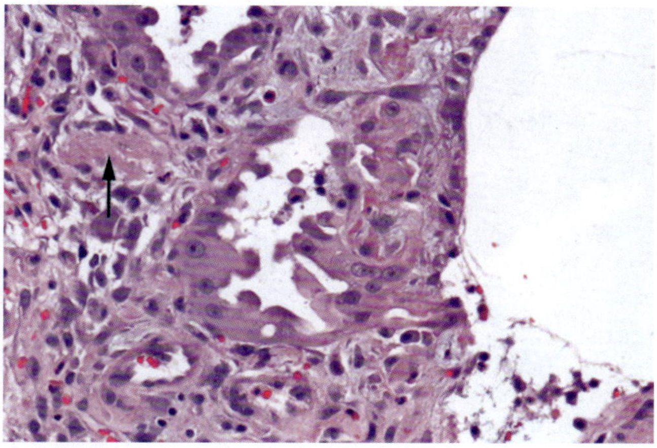

Figure 55.1 Bleomycin toxicity: Markedly reactive type 2 pneumocytes line alveolar spaces. Hyaline membranes can be seen incorporating into the thickened septa (*arrow*).

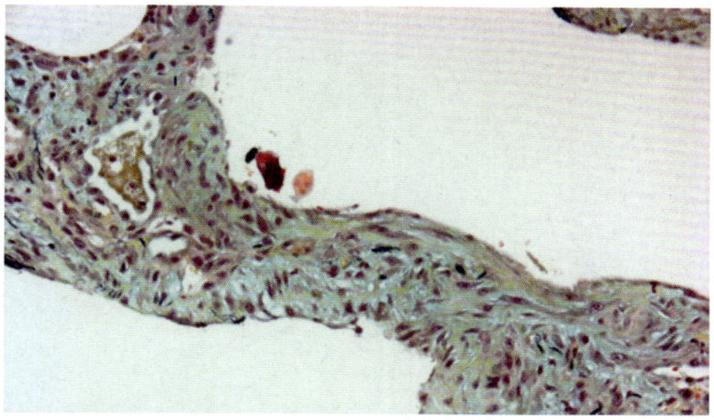

Figure 55.2 Bleomycin toxicity: Movat stain highlights the blue-green appearance of the fibroblastic tissue expanding the septa (organizing DAD).

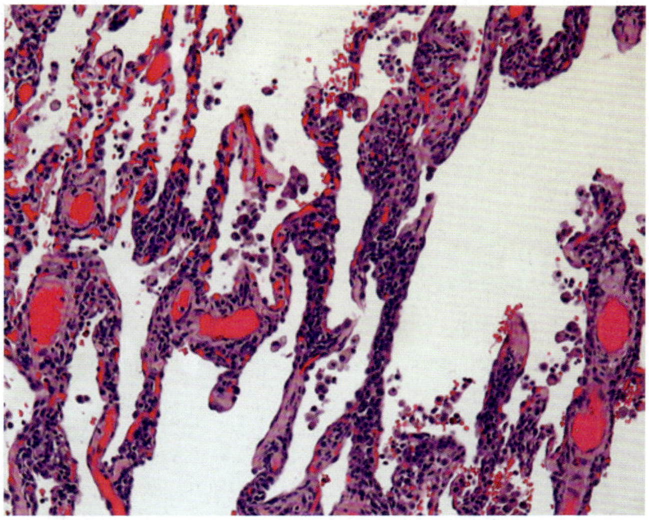

Figure 55.3 Methotrexate toxicity: Chronic interstitial pneumonia in methotrexate drug injury consisting predominantly of lymphocytes, with occasional plasma cells and histiocytes.

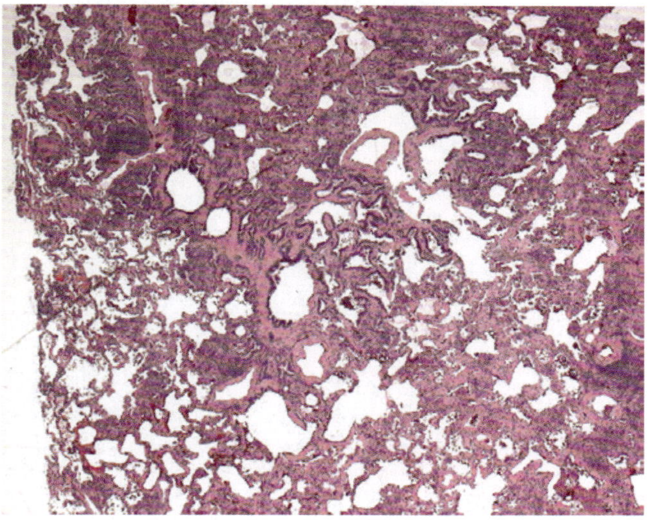

Figure 55.4 Methotrexate toxicity: Chronic interstitial pneumonia with fibrosis.

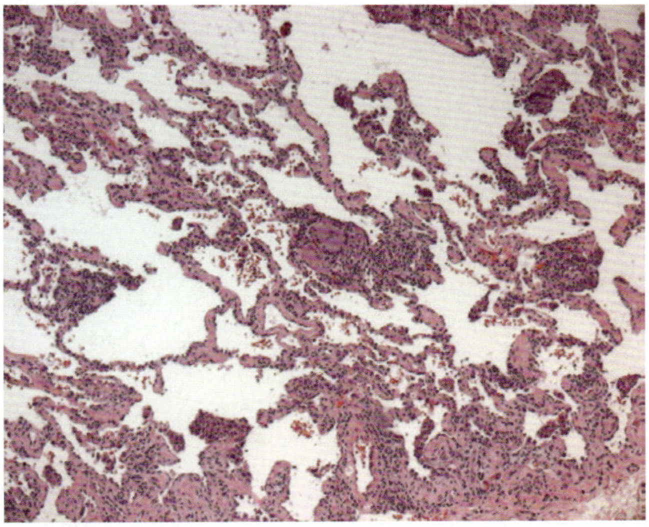

Figure 55.5 Methotrexate toxicity: Interstitial cluster of multinucleated giant cells and epithelioid histiocytes with surrounding septa mildly expanded by chronic inflammation.

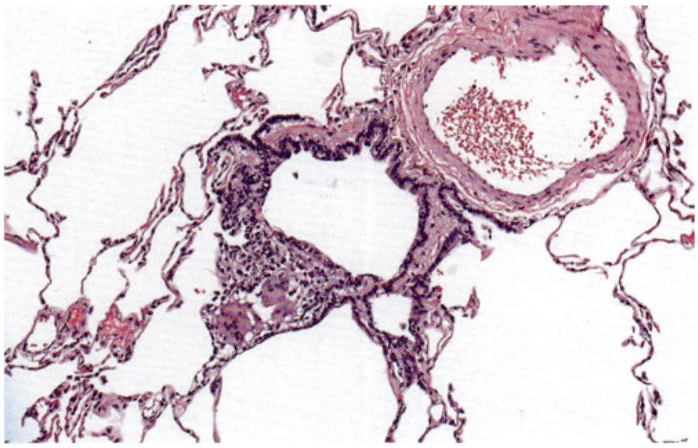

Figure 55.6 Methotrexate toxicity: The granulomas are similar in appearance to those found in hypersensitivity pneumonia (i.e., poorly formed) and often show a bronchiolocentric distribution.

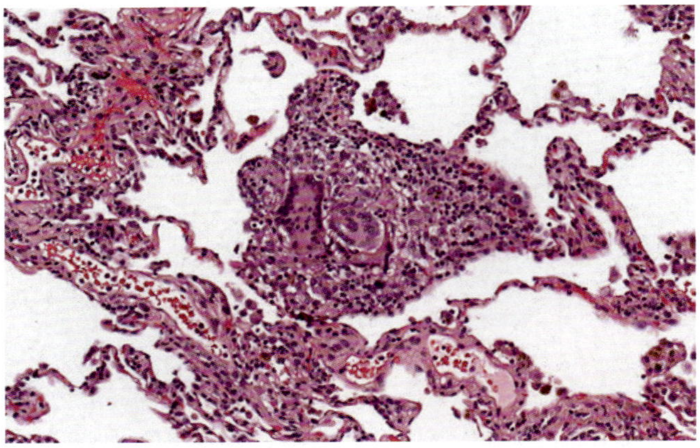

Figure 55.7 Methotrexate toxicity: Small interstitial cluster of multinucleated giant cells and epithelioid histiocytes surrounded by chronic inflammatory cells.

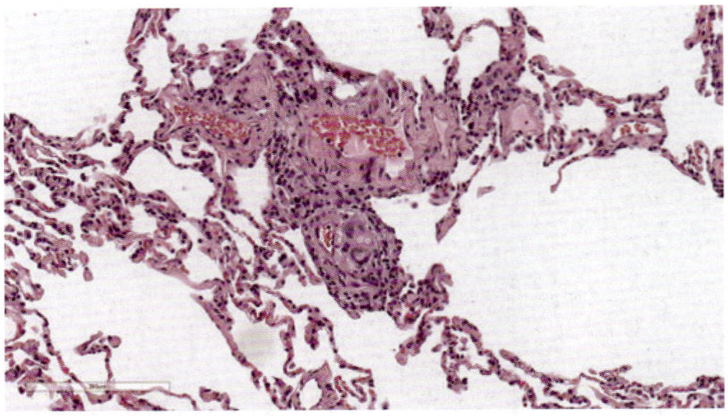

Figure 55.8 Methotrexate toxicity: Occasionally, the granulomas are in a perivascular distribution.

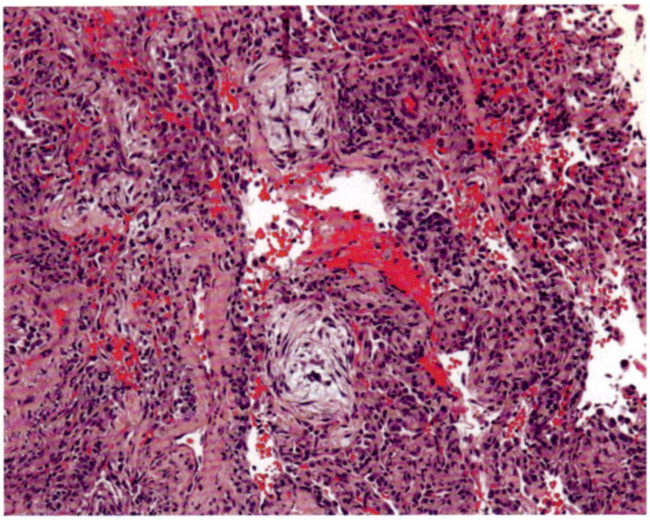

Figure 55.9 Methotrexate toxicity: Organizing pneumonia in a patient with methotrexate toxicity.

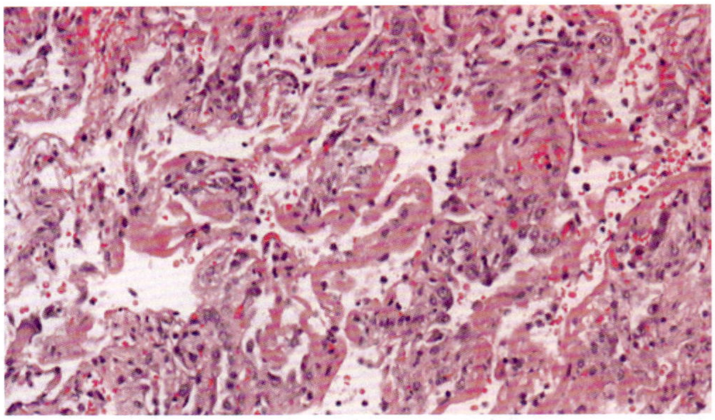

Figure 55.10 Methotrexate toxicity: In some patients, hyaline membranes form, indicating DAD.

56 PULMONARY VENO-OCCLUSIVE DISEASE VS. PULMONARY CAPILLARY HEMANGIOMATOSIS

	Pulmonary Veno-Occlusive Disease (PVOD)	Pulmonary Capillary Hemangiomatosis (PCH)
Age	Any age, but typically children and young adults.	Adults, most commonly, ages 20–40.
Location	Small pulmonary veins and venules located in the interlobular septa.	Bilateral, and patchy throughout the lung.
Symptoms	Exertional dyspnea and fatigue. With progression of disease, there are increasing symptoms of right-sided heart failure including exertional syncope, chest pain, cyanosis, and hepatosplenic congestion.	Hemoptysis.
Signs	Clubbing. Pulmonary function tests (PFTs) show decrease in diffusing capacity of the lungs for carbon monoxide (DLCO). Like severe idiopathic pulmonary arterial hypertension (IPAH), PVOD demonstrates enlarged central pulmonary arteries on chest x-ray or CT. CT imaging additionally demonstrates interstitial pulmonary edema and small bilateral pleural effusions.	Chest x-ray demonstrates enlarged central pulmonary arteries. On CT, enlarged pulmonary arteries and bilateral, multiple, small, poorly defined nodules are seen. V/Q scan often demonstrates matched defects.
Etiology	Likely a pattern of injury from a variety of etiologies, including drugs, bone marrow transplantation, viruses, toxins, radiation, autoimmune diseases, and pregnancy. Overlapping histology in some cases with PCH. In fact, the current WHO classification combines PCH and PVOD in the same group.	Congenital, familial (autosomal recessive), and sporadic forms have all been reported. There is considerable overlap with PVOD; may be a separate phenotypic expression of the same disease.
Histology	Veins within the interlobular septa show luminal narrowing or occlusion by eccentric or concentric intimal fibrosis *(Figs. 56.1–56.4)*. Over time, the veins may become arterialized, mimicking pulmonary arteries *(Fig. 56.5)*; however, the location within the interlobular septa should aid in their differentiation. Small infarcts may be seen adjacent to interlobular septa containing occluded veins (venous infarcts). The interlobular septa are usually edematous and the lymphatics dilated. Arteries and arterioles can show medial hypertrophy, arterial thrombi, or evidence of recanalization. Surrounding lung parenchyma shows hemorrhage and edema. Hemosiderin-laden macrophages may be prominent adjacent to involved interlobular septa. With long-standing hemosiderin deposition, endogenous pneumoconiosis may develop *(Figs. 56.6 and 56.7)*. No plexiform lesions. Foci of interstitial fibrosis may be present. PCH areas may be noted.	At low power, lungs have a peculiar patchy, multifocal "congested" appearance, which on higher power are actually dense proliferations of capillary-like endothelial-lined vessels (at least two capillary layers thick) *(Figs. 56.8 and 56.9)*. Capillary-like proliferations also invade the interlobular septa, peribronchial/bronchiolar interstitium, perivascular connective tissue, and pleura. May also have PVOD change (venous changes, medial hypertrophy, hemosiderin-laden macrophages in airspaces). If septa are expanded sufficiently by the capillary-like proliferation, may mimic an interstitial lung disease at low power *(Fig. 56.10)*. If extensive hemosiderosis is present, may have septal thickening by collagen.

	Pulmonary Veno-Occlusive Disease (PVOD)	Pulmonary Capillary Hemangiomatosis (PCH)
Special studies	Pentachrome (Movat) stain or elastic tissue stain crucial for evaluating venous disease. Both stains identify the vessel as venous rather than arterial (since veins contain one elastic lamina and arteries two), and differentiate fibrosed veins from background septal fibrosis.	Endothelial cell markers (e.g., CD31) can aid in examining the capillary-like proliferations vs. congestion *(Figs. 56.11–56.13)*. Pentachrome (Movat) stain helpful in assessing venous and arterial involvement, as well as distinguishing true interstitial collagen deposition from interstitial thickening secondary to proliferations of capillary-like vessels.
Prognosis	Poor, most patients die within 2 y without lung transplantation.	Similar to PVOD, poor prognosis with median survival of 3 y from the time of diagnosis. Prostacyclin contraindicated because of massive pulmonary edema and possible sudden death.

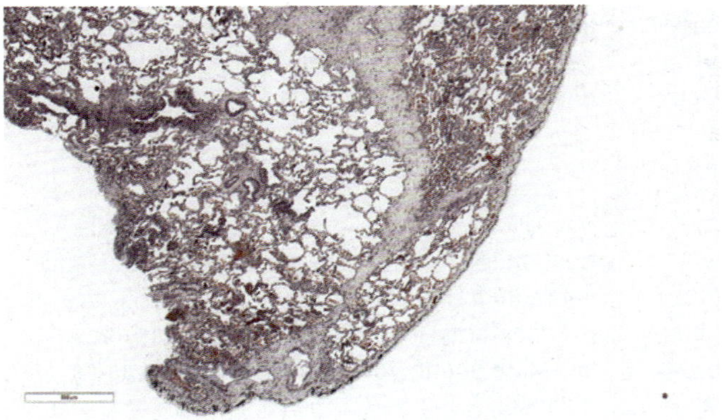

Figure 56.1 PVOD: Low-power image showing the interlobular septal thickening and fibrosis that characterize PVOD (elastic tissue stain).

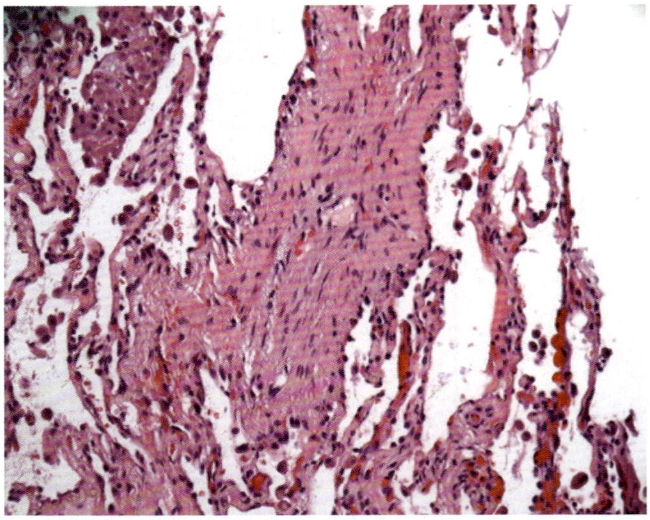

Figure 56.2 PVOD: H&E stain demonstrates the subtle appearance of an occluded vein.

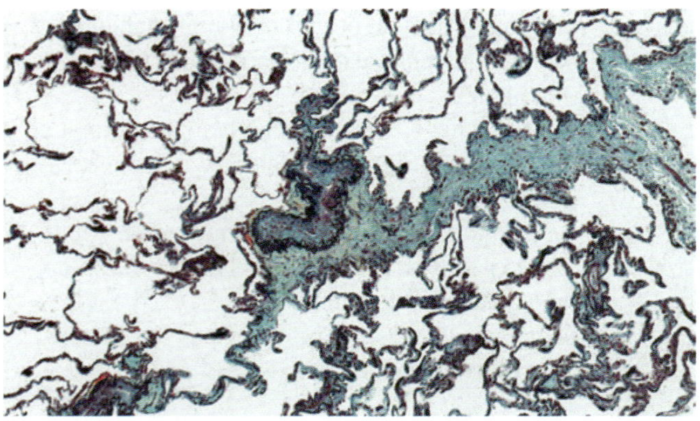

Figure 56.3 PVOD: Movat stain is helpful in assessing the degree of occlusion and/or muscularization of the interlobular veins.

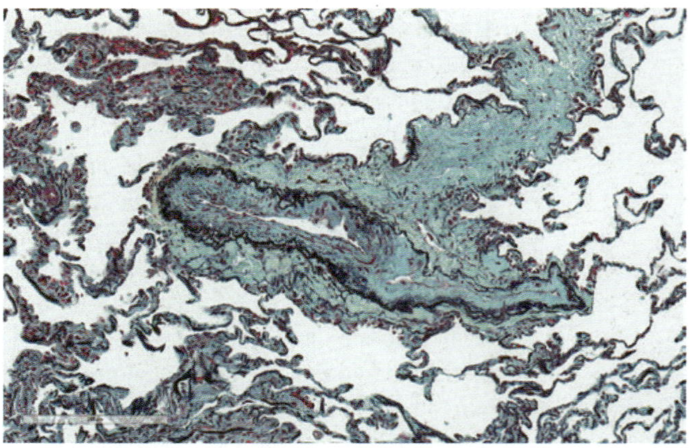

Figure 56.4 PVOD: Movat stain showing another vein with partial occlusion of its lumen. Note the presence of single elastic lamina, confirming the vessel is a vein rather than an artery.

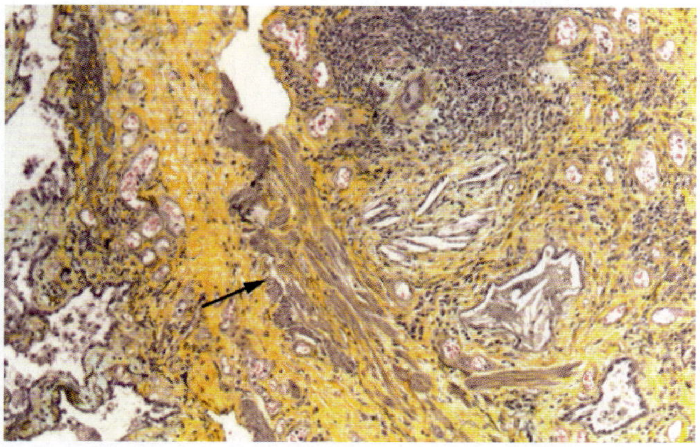

Figure 56.5 PVOD: Muscularization of a pulmonary vein (*arrow*), highlighted by Movat stain.

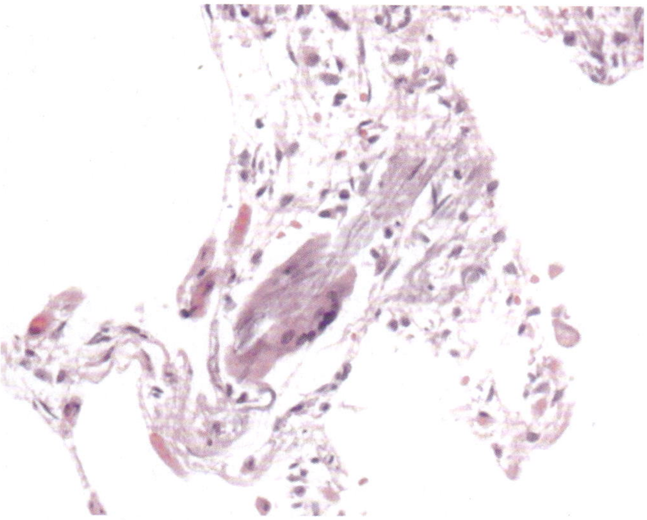

Figure 56.6 PVOD: Foreign body giant cell engulfs iron-encrusted, fragmented elastic fibers, which appear gray-brown on H&E stain.

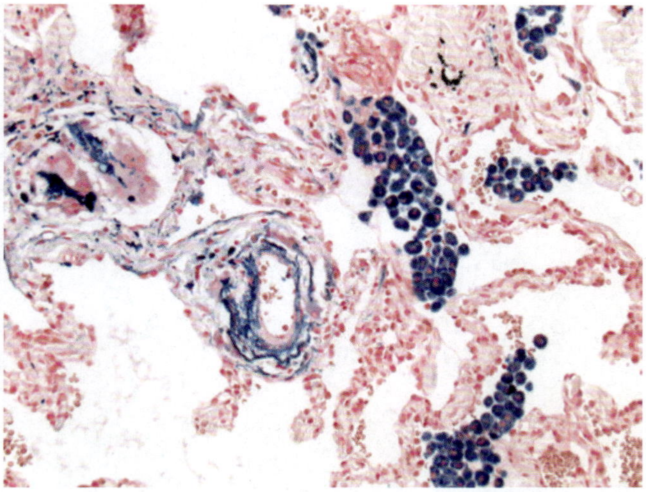

Figure 56.7 PVOD: An iron stain highlights the iron-coated elastic fibers (endogenous pneumoconiosis).

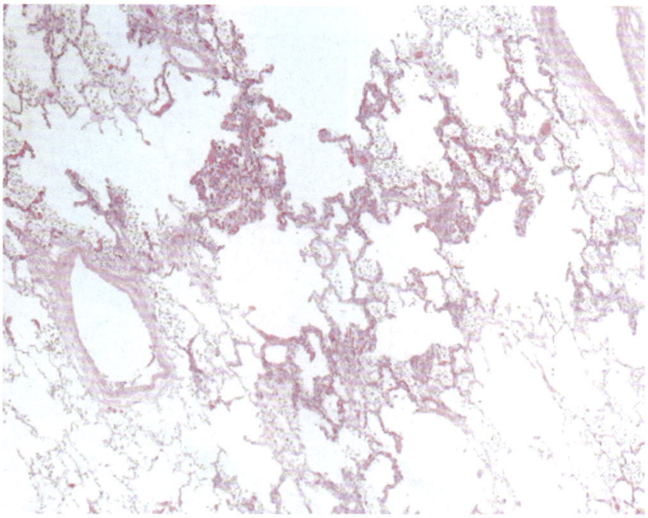

Figure 56.8 PCH: In contrast to normal congestion, which shows diffuse septal vascular congestion, PCH can be appreciated at low power by the patchy appearance of the "congestion." The patchy areas of apparent congestion are actually the areas of septal thickening by proliferation of capillaries.

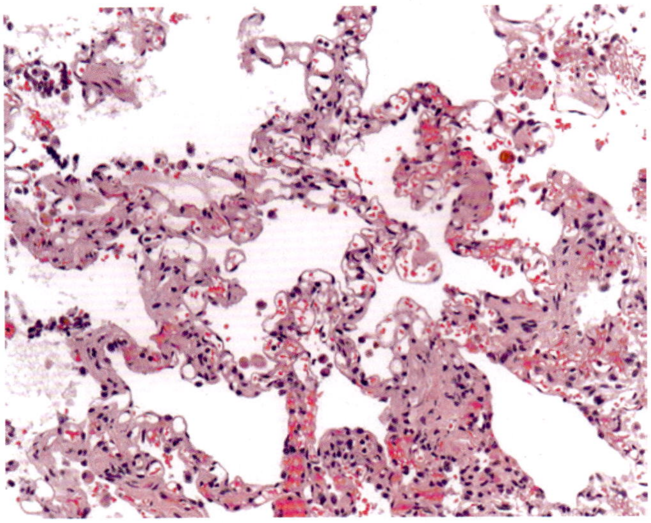

Figure 56.9 PCH: High-power image showing the dilated abnormal capillary-sized vascular proliferations within the alveolar septa.

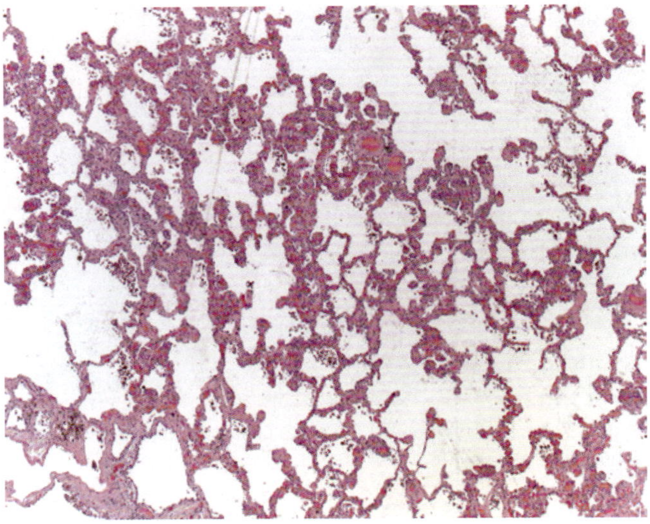

Figure 56.10 PCH: Low-power view demonstrating a relatively diffuse interstitial thickening, which may mimic nonspecific interstitial pneumonia (NSIP).

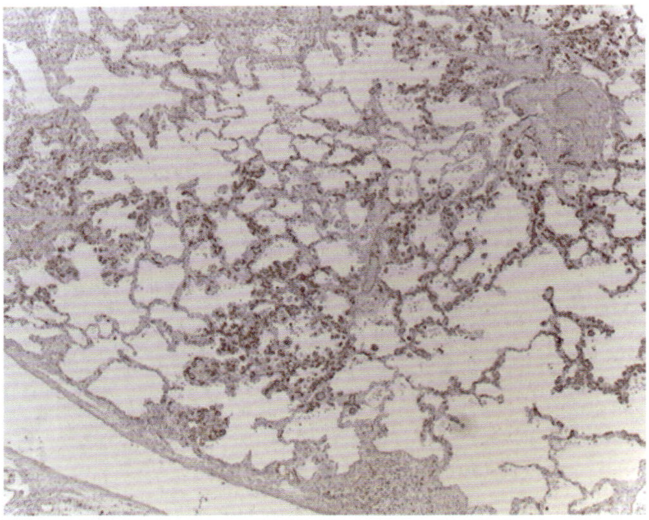

Figure 56.11 PCH: The same case as in Figure 56.10, demonstrating the capillary-like interstitial proliferation, highlighted by an endothelial cell marker (CD31).

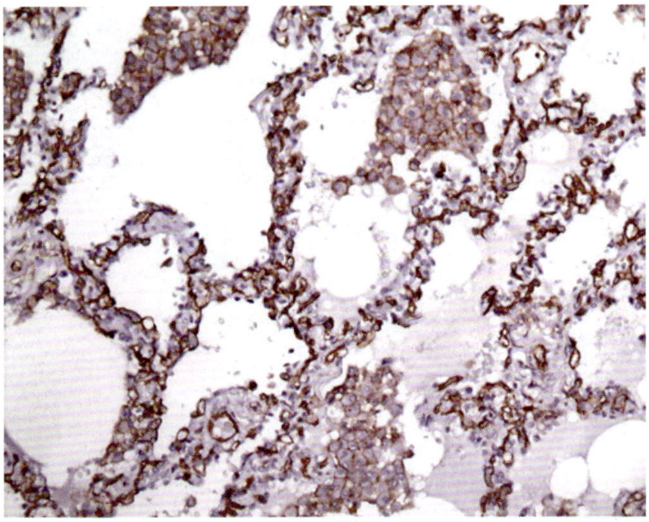

Figure 56.12 PCH: CD31 immunohistochemical stains, as noted above, can be quite helpful in recognizing the vascular nature of the interstitial process. CD31 can also highlight airspace macrophages, as in this case.

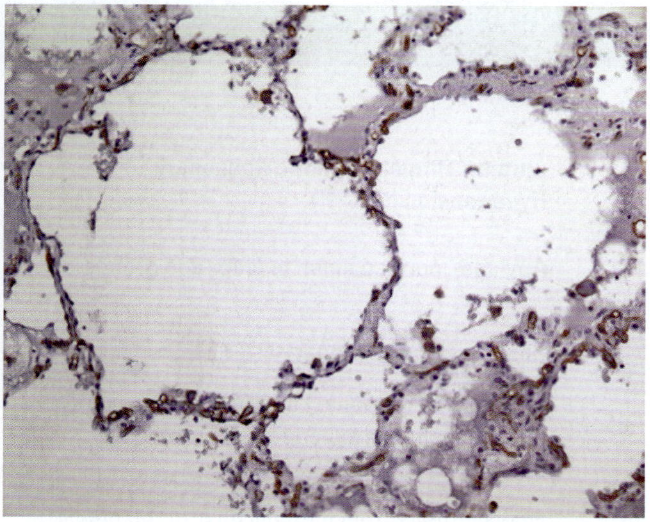

Figure 56.13 PCH: An area of normal alveolar septa from the same patient with PCH, showing single layer of septal capillaries. In PCH, there is interstitial expansion by at least two layers of capillary-type vessels.

57 IDIOPATHIC PULMONARY ARTERIAL HYPERTENSION VS. CHRONIC THROMBOEMBOLIC PULMONARY HYPERTENSION

	Idiopathic Pulmonary Arterial Hypertension (IPAH)	Chronic Thromboembolic Pulmonary Hypertension (CTEPH)
Age	Any age, most commonly in young females. Mean age 36 y.	Any age, more common in older age groups.
Location	Small- to medium-sized pulmonary arteries.	Small to large pulmonary arteries.
Symptoms	Dyspnea, fatigue, and weakness. Substernal chest pain. Syncope with exertion.	Progressive dyspnea. Later in disease, exertional chest pain, syncope, lower extremity edema.
Signs	Cor pulmonale develops late in disease. Cyanosis may develop. Usually no clubbing. Various abnormal heart sounds and regurgitation murmurs on auscultation. Pulmonary function tests (PFTs) show mild restrictive changes with low diffusing capacity of the lungs for carbon monoxide (DLCO). Chest x-ray shows enlargement of pulmonary artery and heart. CT imaging confirms enlarged pulmonary artery and can help rule out other diseases. Echocardiogram and right-heart catheterization confirm increased pulmonary artery pressures (mean pulmonary artery pressure, mPAP, >25 mm Hg). Symptoms may not develop until the mPAP exceeds 60 mm Hg.	Flow murmurs from partially obstructed pulmonary arteries may be heard over lung fields. PFTs often normal. Chest x-ray may be normal or show enlargement of central pulmonary arteries. CT imaging shows enlarged central pulmonary arteries, patchy decreased vascularity, and right-heart enlargement. Echocardiogram shows pulmonary hypertension. Ventilation/perfusion V/Q lung scans show mismatched defects. Right-heart catheterization and pulmonary angiography necessary to define extent of disease and accessibility for surgical intervention.
Etiology	Idiopathic. Familial cases account for <6%—autosomal dominant inheritance pattern with incomplete penetrance is seen. Germline mutations in bone morphogenetic protein receptor type 2 (*BMPR2*) have been identified in patients with familial pulmonary alveolar hypertension (PAH).	Mechanism is unclear, but usually related to prior acute pulmonary emboli (PE) or deep vein thrombosis (DVT). Size of initial PE, recurrent PE, idiopathic PE, and PE at a young age are all risk factors (among others) for developing CTEPH. Emboli of substances other than clots also can cause pulmonary hypertension, including tumor emboli, foreign intravenous injected material by drug addicts or iatrogenically through intravenous infusions, and parasites such as schistosomes. Half of the patients present with CTEPH without any initial PE clinically recognized. Lupus anticoagulant is reportedly present in up to 50% of patients.
Histology	Plexiform lesions, characterized by intraluminal, cellular proliferations of small- to medium-sized pulmonary artery intima, are the hallmark of severe PAH. The lumen of the artery becomes essentially occluded by the glomeruloid-like plexus, which is characterized by multiple, irregular, slit-like vascular lumina *(Figs. 57.1–57.4)*.	Recanalization of pulmonary arteries, characterized by more rigid, "punched-out" lumina than are seen in IPAH plexiform lesions *(Figs. 57.8–57.10)*.

	Idiopathic Pulmonary Arterial Hypertension (IPAH)	Chronic Thromboembolic Pulmonary Hypertension (CTEPH)
	Not all cases of severe PAH demonstrate plexiform lesions. Additional lesions include concentric laminar intimal fibrosis (often in an onionskin appearance), cellular intimal hyperplasia, muscular medial hypertrophy, and muscularization of arterioles *(Figs. 57.5 and 57.6)*. Occasionally, dilatation lesions occur distal to plexiform lesions *(Fig. 57.7)*.	Eccentric intimal fibrosis of pulmonary arteries, varying from mild-to-nearly total obliteration of lumen *(Fig. 57.11)*. Large elastic arteries show intravascular fibrous septa or webs *(Fig. 57.12)*.
Histology	No interstitial lung disease in idiopathic or familial PAH.	Can see evidence of recent or organizing thromboemboli *(Fig. 57.13)*. Mild medial hypertrophy or pulmonary arteries (nonspecific finding). May see evidence of subpleural, wedge-shaped parenchymal infarcts.
Special studies	Can perform immunohistochemistry for endothelial cells (CD34, CD31, etc.) to highlight plexiform lesions, as the lesions may be sparse.	Pentachrome (Movat) stain or elastic tissue stain helpful in distinguishing recanalized and eccentric intimal lesions from plexiform and concentric intimal lesions of IPAH.
Prognosis	Without treatment, median survival is $<$3 y. Newer treatments have improved survival, but lung transplantation may be necessary.	Poor, 5-y survival is 30%. Pulmonary thromboendarterectomy performed in patients with accessible lesions, but mortality rates range from 2% to 20%.

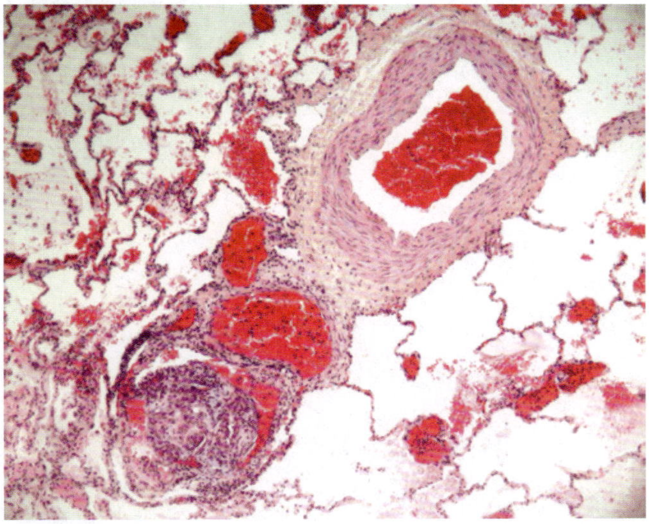

Figure 57.1 IPAH: Low-power view of a plexiform lesion arising from a pulmonary artery.

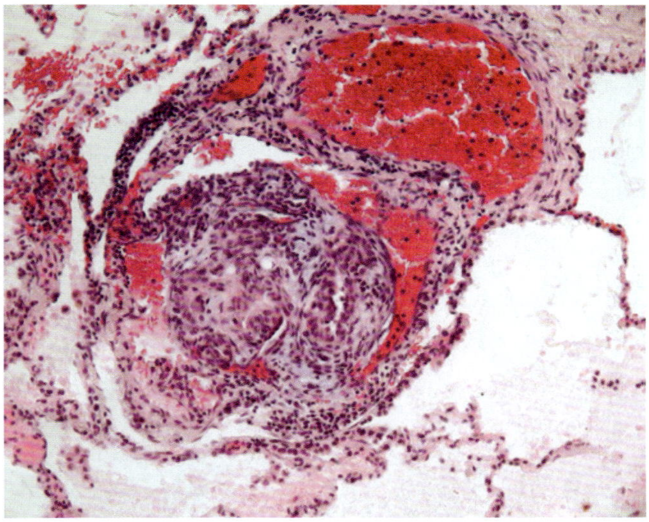

Figure 57.2 IPAH: High-power view of the same plexiform seen in Figure 57.1 showing a proliferation of small vascular channels. Note the appearance, which is similar to a glomerulus.

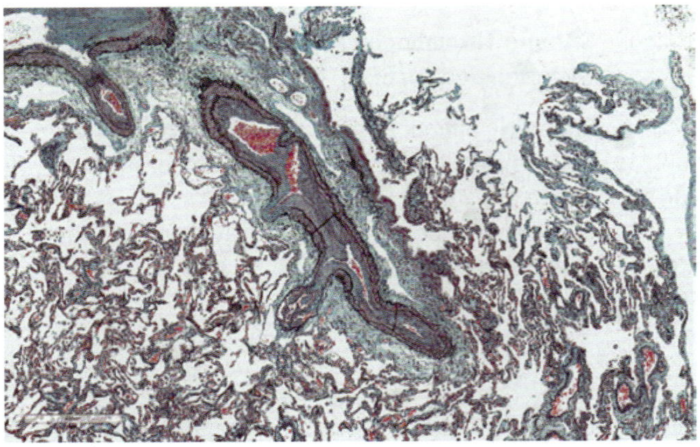

Figure 57.3 IPAH: In this image of a plexiform lesion, the Movat stain highlights the location of the plexiform lesion in relation to the "parent" artery. Plexiform lesions are often found just distal to the bifurcation or branch points of arteries.

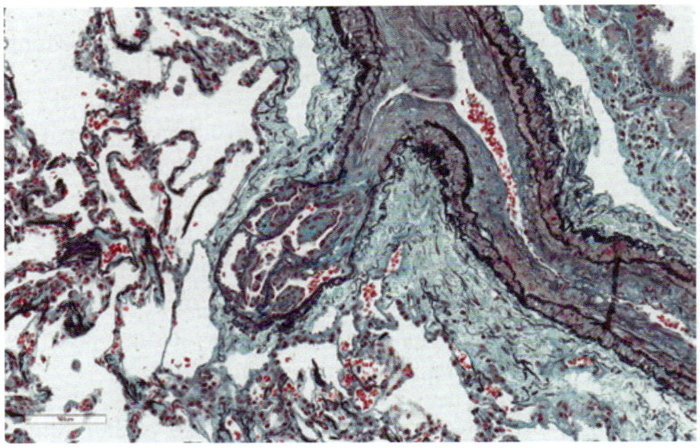

Figure 57.4 IPAH: Higher-power of Figure 57.3 demonstrating a plexiform lesion with readily identifiable slit-like vascular lumina.

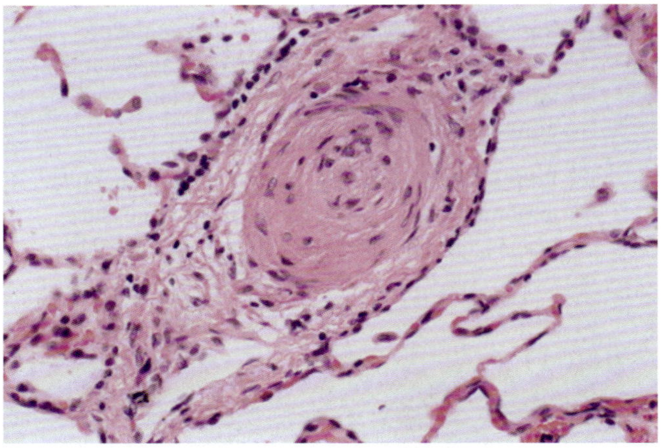

Figure 57.5 IPAH: This image illustrates a concentric laminar lesion characterized by intimal thickening.

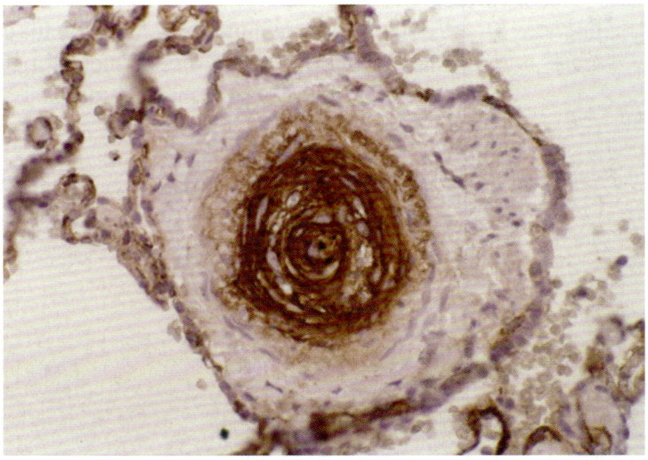

Figure 57.6 IPAH: Factor VIII immunoperoxidase stain (endothelial marker) highlights the concentric onionskin appearance.

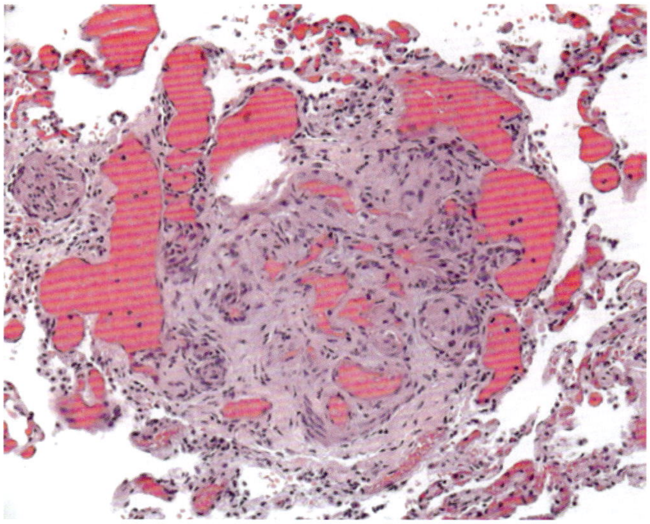

Figure 57.7 IPAH: Dilatation lesions are characterized by small, thin-walled, dilated, blood-filled vascular channels surrounding the plexiform lesion.

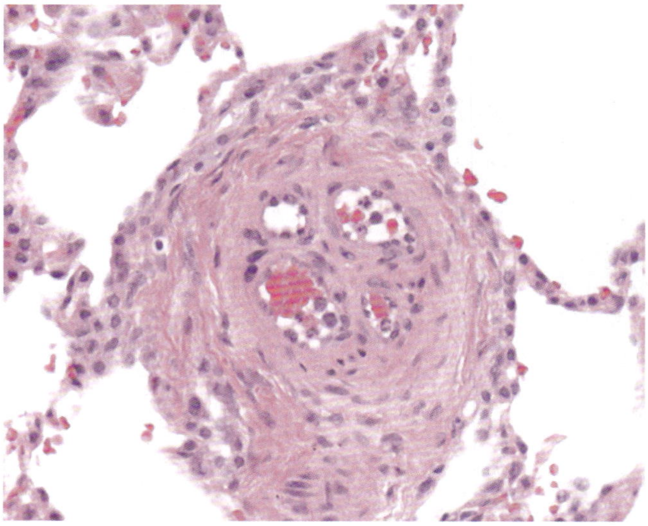

Figure 57.8 CTEPH: Relatively rigid-appearing, "punched-out" vascular lumina typical of recanalized small arteries.

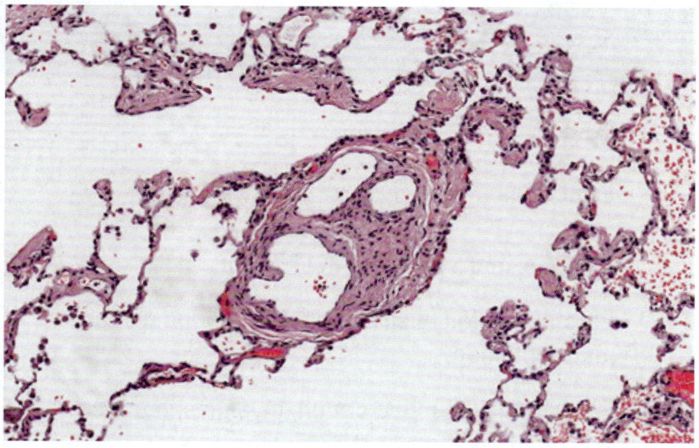

Figure 57.9 CTEPH: Another example of recanalized small vessel.

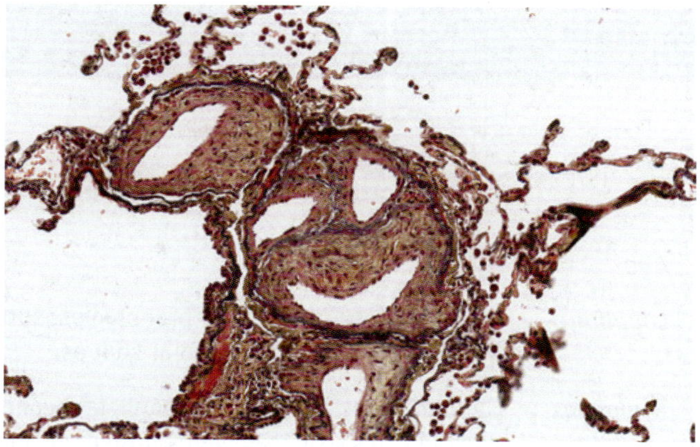

Figure 57.10 CTEPH: The Movat stain highlights the intraluminal nature of the neolumina. Contrast this image with the plexiform lesions in Figures 57.1–57.4. Plexiform lesions are more cellular, irregular, and tortuous than recanalized vessels.

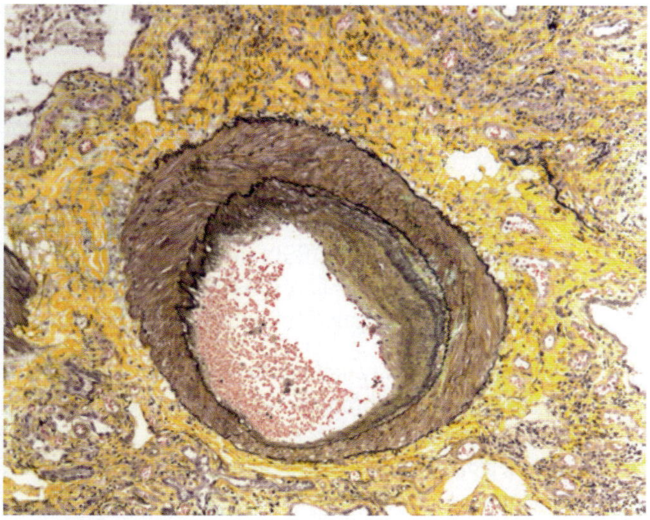

Figure 57.11 CTEPH: Unlike the concentric intimal thickening of PAH, the intimal fibrosis in CTEPH is eccentric, as demonstrated in this Movat-stained section.

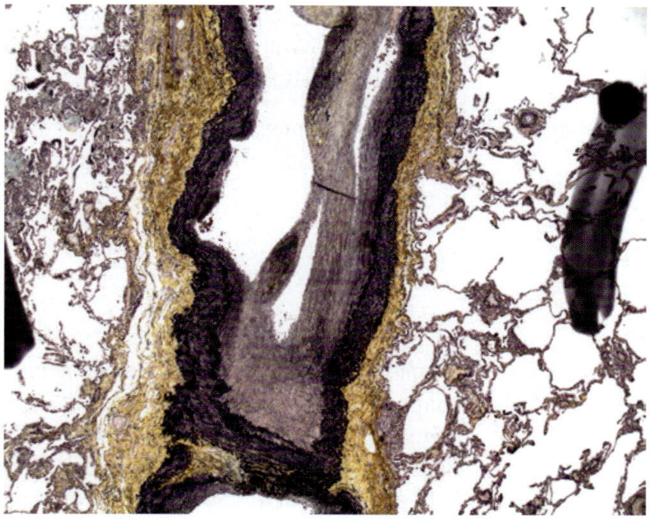

Figure 57.12 CTEPH: Larger arteries demonstrate webs of fibrous tissue that divide the lumen into multiple chambers.

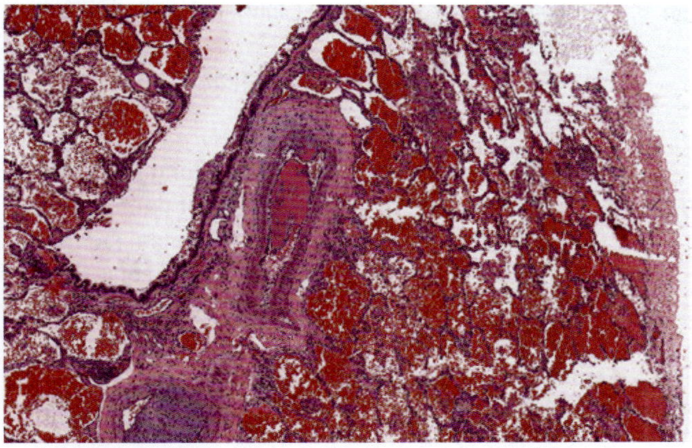

Figure 57.13 CTEPH: Recent thromboembolus is characterized by plugging of vascular lumen by a fibrin clot.

58 ACUTE BACTERIAL BRONCHOPNEUMONIA VS. VIRAL PNEUMONIA

	Acute Bacterial Bronchopneumonia	Viral Pneumonia
Age	All ages.	All ages; more common in children.
Location	Centrilobular—respiratory bronchioles, surrounding alveolar ducts and alveolar spaces.	Patchy, random distribution. Upper lobe disease more common.
Symptoms	Sudden onset. Fever, rigor, cough, tachypnea, dyspnea, malaise; may have purulent or rusty sputum, pleuritic chest pain.	Fever, nonproductive cough, myalgias, fatigue, and headache are common.
Signs	Tachypnea. Rales/crackles, rhonchi, or wheezes. Pleural friction rub. Chest x-ray typically shows patchy infiltrates and poorly defined opacities. Patient may develop cavitary disease if disease progresses. Pleural effusions may be seen. Usually marked leukocytosis.	Similar to bacterial bronchopneumonia with rales/crackles, rhonchi, or wheezes. Radiographically, the lungs are often involved bilaterally. Viral cultures, antigen detection (e.g., nasal swabs), and polymerase chain reaction (PCR) may all be used for detecting specific viruses, depending on the suspected virus.
Etiology	Bacteria—the most common cause of bronchopneumonia is *Staphylococcus* species.	Both DNA and RNA viruses cause viral pneumonias. The most common cause is influenza virus, but others are respiratory syncytial virus, parainfluenza virus, adenoviruses, coronaviruses (e.g., severe acute respiratory syndrome [SARS]), and in the immunosuppressed, herpes simplex virus (HSV), varicella zoster virus, cytomegalovirus, and Epstein–Barr virus.
Histology	Prominent neutrophilic infiltrate within airspaces—an acute exudative infiltrate *(Figs. 58.1 and 58.2)*. Adjacent septa may show neutrophils in septa, but neutrophils in airspaces should outnumber those in airspaces (helpful in differentiating capillaritis from bronchopneumonia). May have acute lung injury with hyaline membranes and fibrin exudates *(Fig. 58.3)*. Depending on the stage of bronchopneumonia, foci of organizing pneumonia may be seen *(Fig. 58.4)*. Empyema may be present.	Initial changes may include expansion of alveolar septa adjacent to bronchioles by a chronic inflammatory process. Often, biopsies will show features of diffuse alveolar damage—hyaline membranes, type 2 pneumocyte hyperplasia, and fibrin exudates *(Figs. 58.5 and 58.6)*. There may be interstitial expansion by chronic inflammation and edema. Some viruses (e.g., cytomegalovirus [CMV], HSV, adenovirus) may show classic intranuclear and intracytoplasmic inclusions *(Figs. 58.7–58.12)*. Airspace neutrophils are not typical of viral infections.
Special studies	Cultures are necessary to identify specific bacterial organisms. Mycobacterial, fungal, and bacterial stains should also be performed.	Always perform mycobacterial and fungal stains if the histology shows diffuse alveolar damage (DAD). Additionally, immunohistochemical stains are available for many of the more common viruses that cause disease (e.g., CMV, HSV, adenovirus). Correlation with cultures, serologies, or other special studies is necessary.
Prognosis	Excellent with treatment; however, high mortality with complications of bacteremia, cavitation, and empyema.	Depending on the virulence of the organisms and the patient's comorbid conditions, may be mild and self-limiting to life-threatening, especially in the elderly and the immunocompromised.

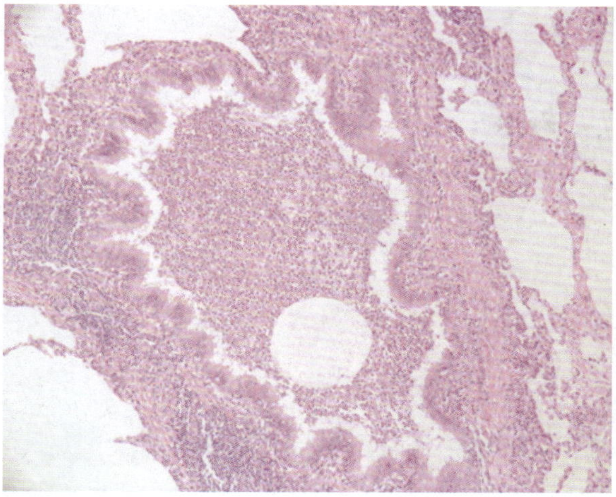

Figure 58.1 Acute bacterial bronchopneumonia: Classically, sheets of neutrophils within the bronchiolar lumen extend out into the adjacent alveolar spaces.

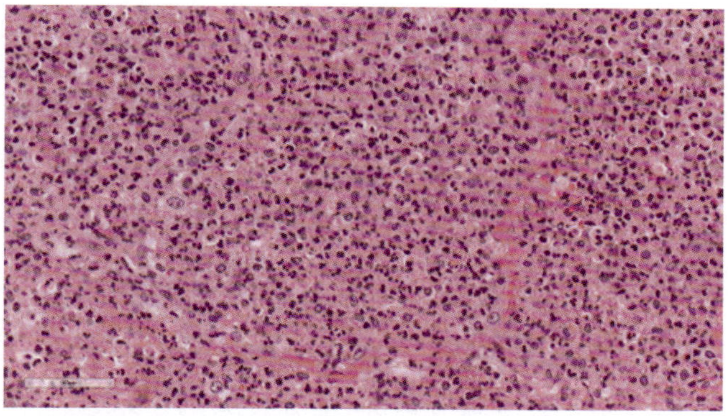

Figure 58.2 Acute bacterial bronchopneumonia: Higher-power showing alveolar spaces filled by marked neutrophilic inflammatory cell infiltrate.

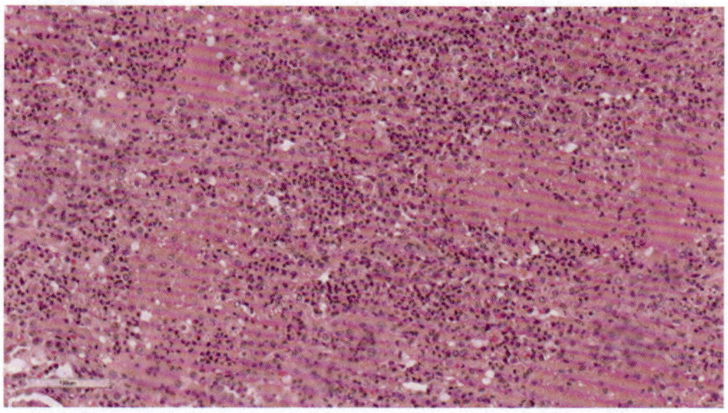

Figure 58.3 Acute bacterial bronchopneumonia: Alveolar fibrinous exudates can be seen. Neutrophils may be present in the alveolar septa (as they traverse the capillaries), but the overwhelming majority of neutrophils are seen within alveolar spaces and lumens of airways.

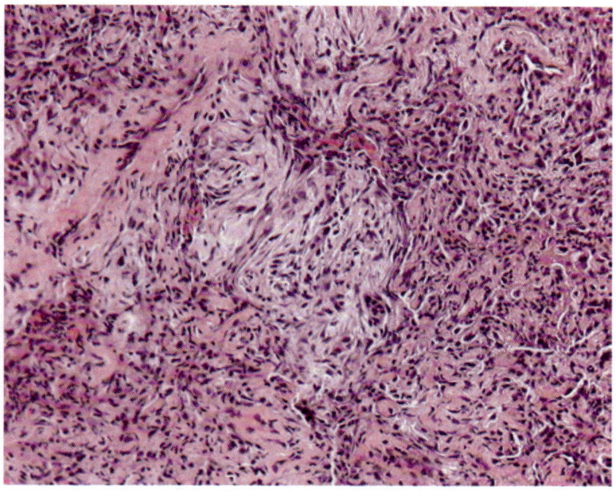

Figure 58.4 Acute bacterial bronchopneumonia: Organizing pneumonia may be seen in the later stage of bronchopneumonia and is characterized by plugs of organizing fibroblastic tissue filling the airspaces.

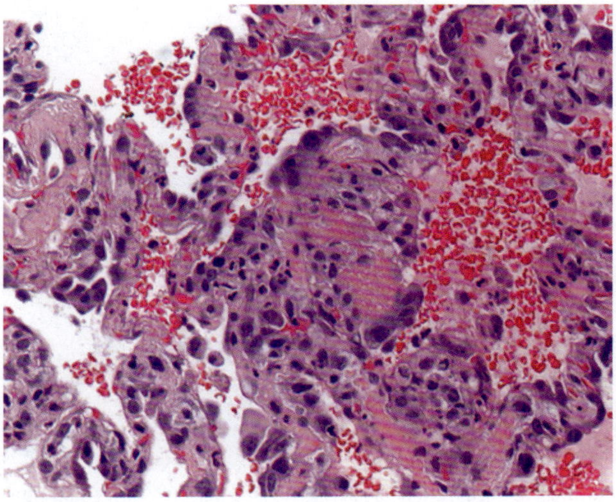

Figure 58.5 Viral pneumonia: Fibrin exudate associated with reactive pneumocytes lining the alveolar spaces.

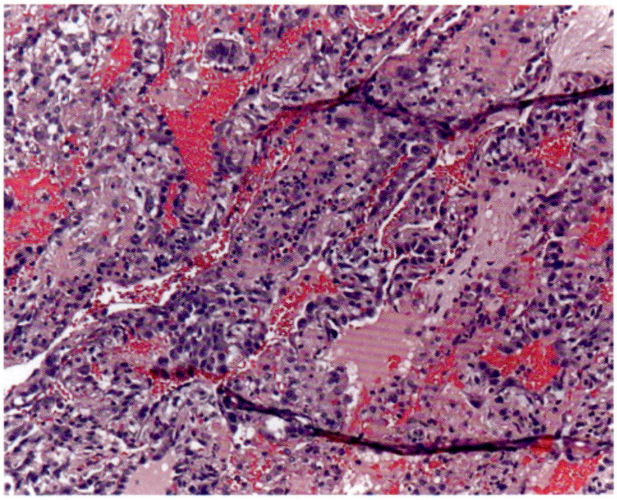

Figure 58.6 Viral pneumonia: Features of organizing diffuse alveolar damage are characterized by the presence of interstitial and intra-alveolar edema, incorporation of fibrin into the alveolar septa, and sparse alveolar septal mononuclear inflammation associated with patchy fibroblastic/myofibroblastic proliferation (early organization).

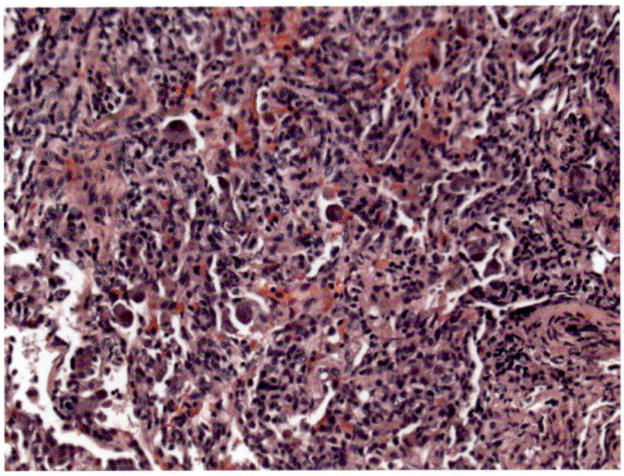

Figure 58.7 Viral pneumonia: CMV inclusions showing intranuclear and intracytoplasmic inclusions. The intranuclear inclusions are dark purple. Cytomegaly is evident.

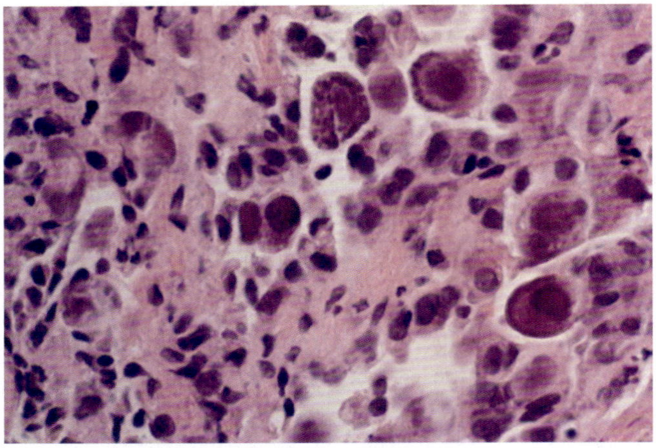

Figure 58.8 Viral pneumonia: Intranuclear inclusions, which are often surrounded by a halo, and coarse, basophilic cytoplasmic granules of CMV.

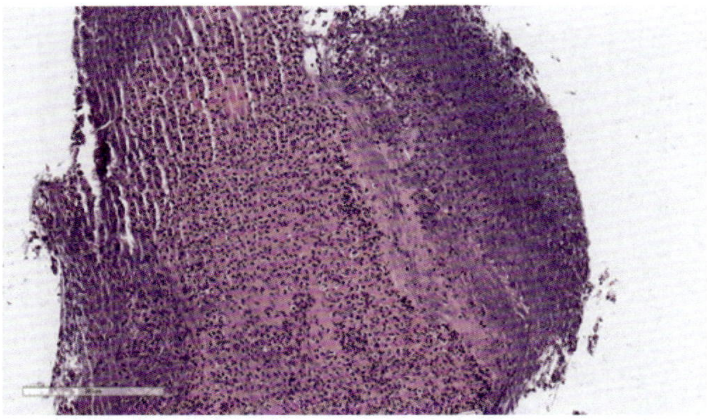

Figure 58.9 Viral pneumonia: Herpes pneumonia often shows a necrotizing bronchopneumonia.

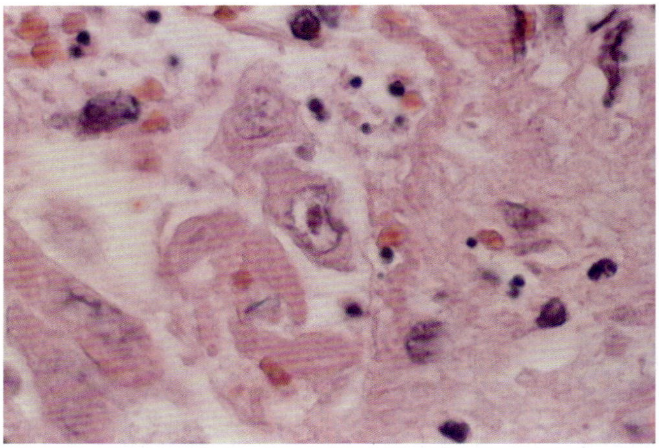

Figure 58.10 Viral pneumonia: HSV shows Cowdry type A inclusion that consists of a somewhat refractile eosinophilic nuclear inclusion surrounded by a clear halo. There is a rim of condensed chromatin at the periphery of the nucleus.

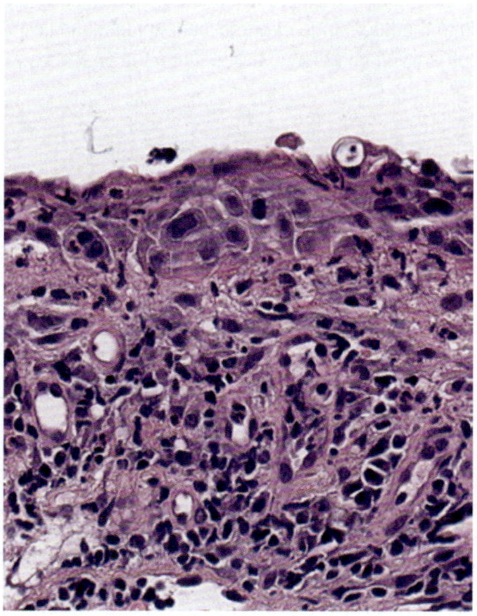

Figure 58.11 Viral pneumonia: The other characteristic inclusion of HSV is the so-called ground-glass appearance of the nuclei. Although this can bear a superficial resemblance to CMV inclusions, there is no significant cytomegaly associated with the HSV inclusion. Additionally, cytoplasmic inclusions are absent in HSV.

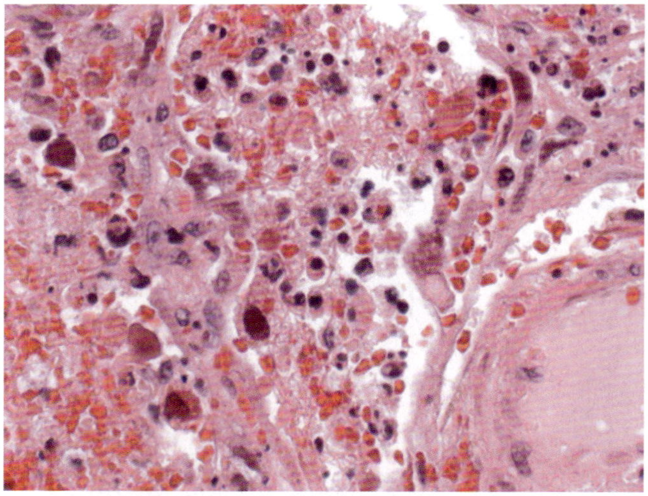

Figure 58.12 Viral pneumonia: Like HSV, adenovirus shows only intranuclear inclusions. The classic appearance is the smudge cell consisting of a basophilic to amphophilic, slightly enlarged nucleus with a smudgy nuclear outline. Adenovirus may also demonstrate small eosinophilic nuclear inclusions surrounded by clear halos, similar to Cowdry type A inclusions of HSV.

59 ACTINOMYCOSIS VS. NOCARDIOSIS

	Actinomycosis	Nocardiosis
Age	All ages, but more common in young to middle-aged adults.	Adults.
Location	Usually unilateral and may extend to pleura and adjacent chest walls. Actinomyces can cross barriers and involve adjacent bones.	Bilateral.
Symptoms	Insidious. Cough, productive sputum, fever, weight loss, occasionally hemoptysis.	Indolent. Fatigue, low-grade fever, weight loss, productive cough. Rarely, pleuritic chest pain, hemoptysis, dyspnea.
Signs	Chest x-ray typically shows localized consolidation with extension to pleura and chest wall. CT imaging often shows infiltrative mass, which may demonstrate cavitation. Peripheral ring-like enhancement can be seen with contrast studies. Patient may have empyema. Peripheral blood shows mild leukocytosis and anemia.	Chest x-ray demonstrates bilateral infiltrates, which can progress to abscesses. Pleural involvement may be present.
Etiology	Anaerobic to microaerophilic gram-positive branching, filamentous bacteria. Often due to aspiration.	Aerobic gram-positive filamentous bacilli. Mycelial form found in soil or organic matter, especially in warmer climates. Infection more common in immunocompromised patients.
Histology	Initially, acute bronchopneumonia and abscess formation, with a prominent surrounding histiocytic response *(Figs. 59.1 and 59.2)*. Sulfur granules (easily identified on hematoxylin and eosin stain) are formed by radially arrayed organisms, which are surrounded by eosinophilic club-like material (Splendore-Hoeppli phenomenon). Sulfur granules are nearly pathognomonic for actinomyces *(Figs. 59.3–59.5)*. Gram-positive beaded, branching (often right-angled), filamentous bacteria <1 µm in diameter. Organisms positive on Gomori methenamine silver (GMS) and Gram stain (similar to *Nocardia*); negative on modified acid-fast (Fite) stain *(Fig. 59.6)*. Although multinucleated giant cells may be seen, usually there is no granuloma formation. Empyema may be present.	Multiple abscesses, may show confluence, with associated necrosis *(Fig. 59.7)*. In chronic cases, may have surrounding epithelioid histiocytes and multinucleated giant cells *(Fig. 59.8)*. Long, thin, beaded filamentous organisms, approximately 1 µm in thickness, with extensive, usually right-angle, random branching (so-called "Chinese character pattern"). Organisms positive on Gram, GMS, and modified acid-fast (Fite) stains *(Figs. 59.9–59.13)*. Does not form sulfur granules. Empyema may be present.
Special studies	Acid-fast stain, modified acid-fast stain, GMS, and tissue Gram stains. Gram stain may be weak and irregular; occasionally may appear gram-negative.	Acid-fast stain, modified acid-fast stain, GMS, and tissue Gram stains. May be difficult to see and can be easily overlooked. Notoriously difficult to culture and may take up to 2 weeks for results.
Prognosis	Excellent with treatment (high-dose penicillin cures >90% of patients).	Excellent prognosis with sulfonamide treatment.

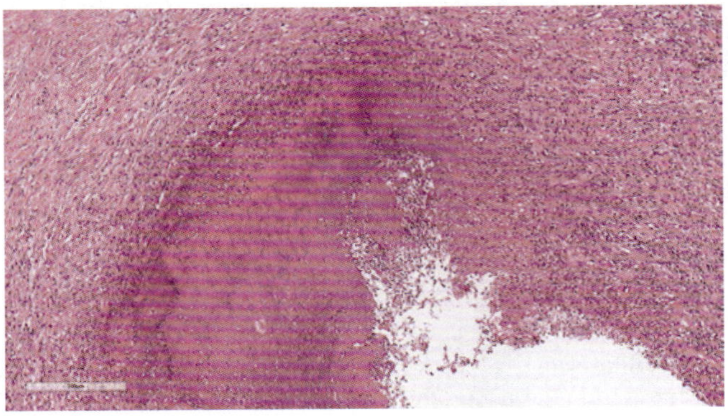

Figure 59.1 Actinomycosis: Necrosis and abscess formation in actinomyces infection can result in extensive tissue destruction. Usually, there is a thick zone of fibroblasts, collagen, and chronic inflammation surrounding the necrotic abscess material.

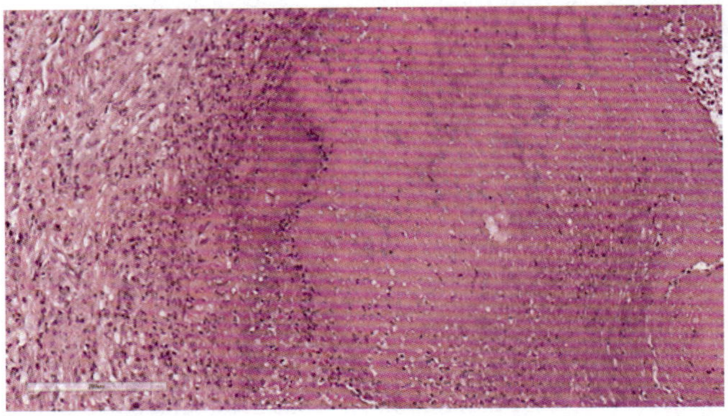

Figure 59.2 Actinomycosis: Higher-power image of necrosis with surrounding fibroblasts, collagen, and chronic inflammation.

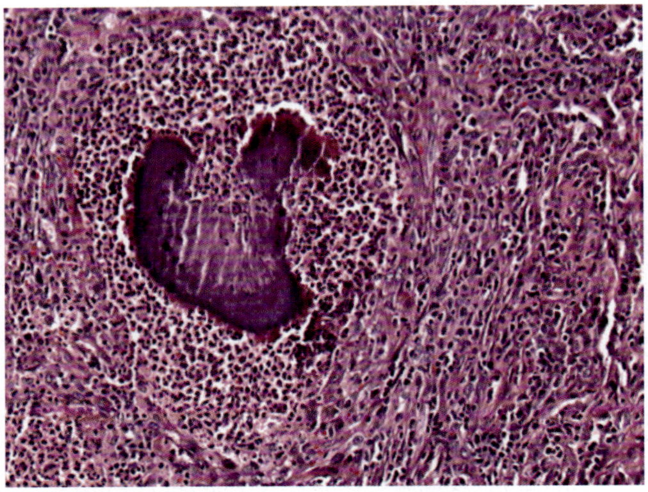

Figure 59.3 Actinomycosis: Sulfur granules surrounded by dense acute inflammation.

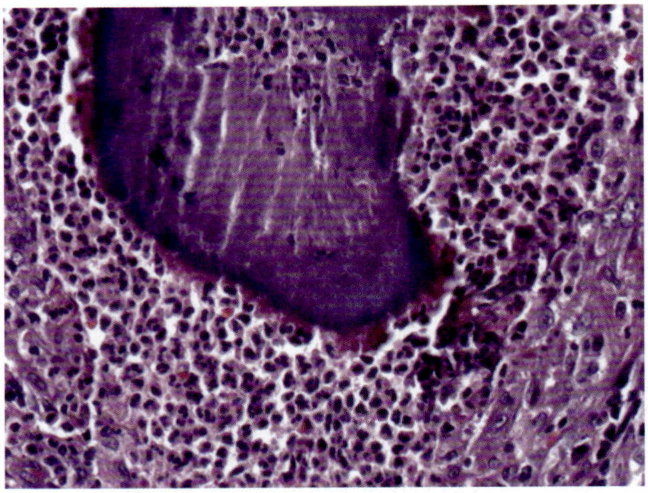

Figure 59.4 Actinomycosis: High magnification of sulfur granules with club-like projections (Splendore-Hoeppli).

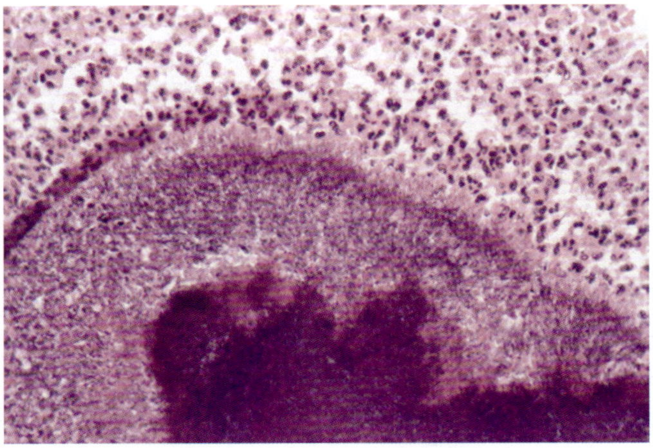

Figure 59.5 Actinomycosis: The Splendore-Hoeppli phenomenon, seen at the periphery, is caused by the accumulation of amorphous, eosinophilic, proteinaceous exudate on the surface of the bacterial colony, as the result of local antigen–antibody complexes precipitation.

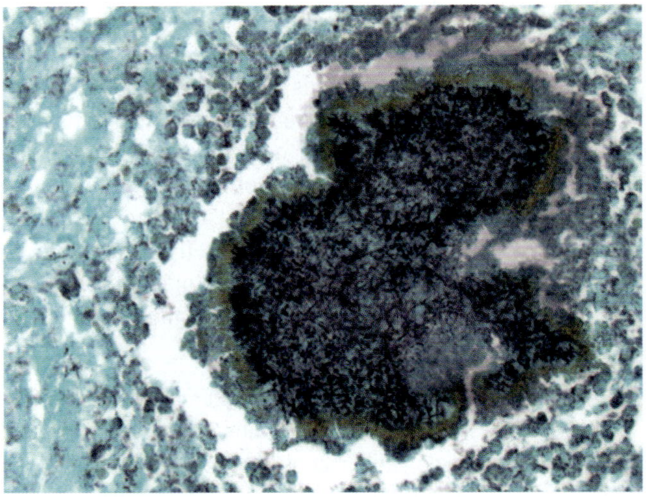

Figure 59.6 Actinomycosis: GMS stain highlights the filamentous branching bacteria. At the periphery of the colony, the Splendore-Hoeppli phenomenon of clubbing is evident.

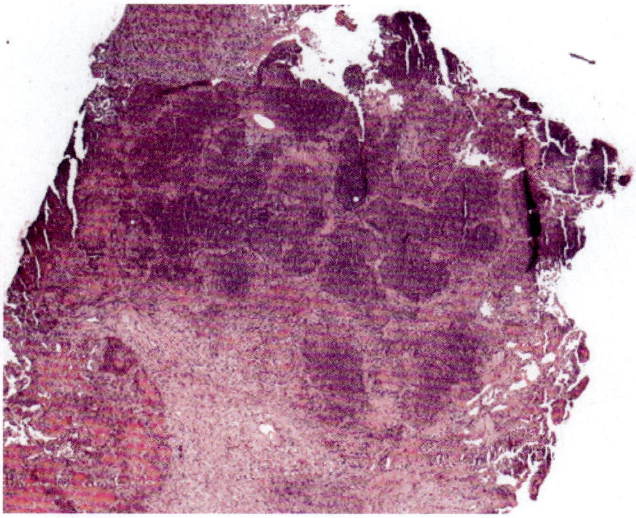

Figure 59.7 Nocardia: Confluent abscesses in nocardia infection.

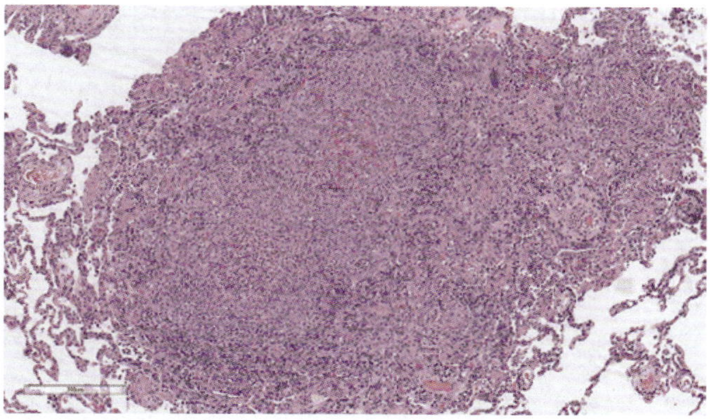

Figure 59.8 Nocardia: This image shows a prominent histiocytic response surrounding the small abscess.

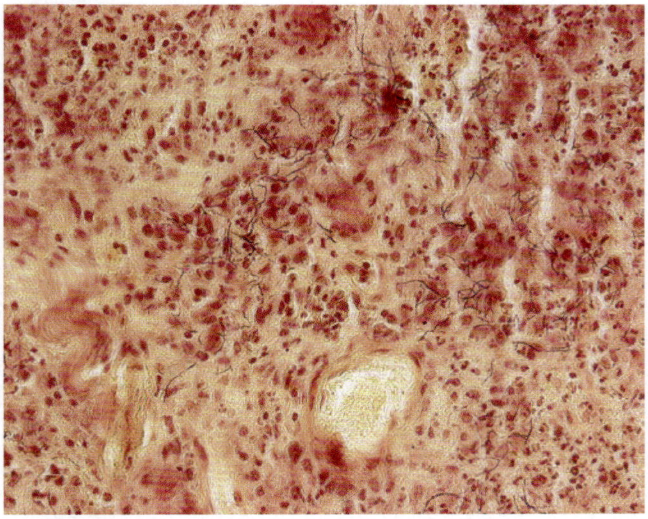

Figure 59.9 Nocardia: *Nocardia and Actinomyces* are indistinguishable on tissue Gram stain. Both show gram-positive, filamentous branching, thin (1 μm) bacteria.

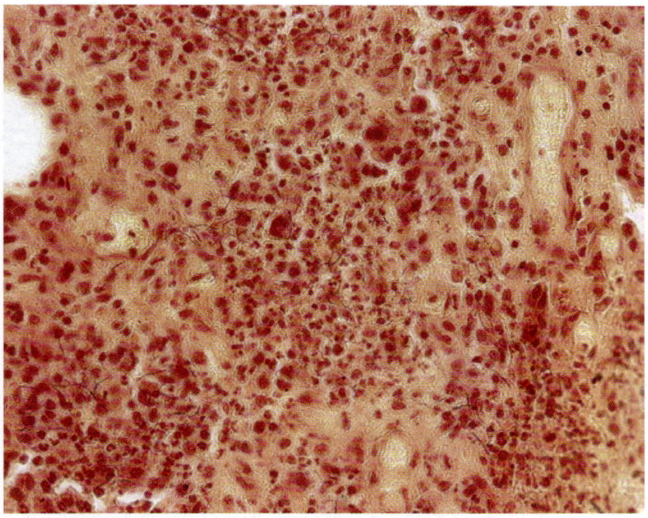

Figure 59.10 Nocardia: The filamentous organisms can be subtle on Gram stain.

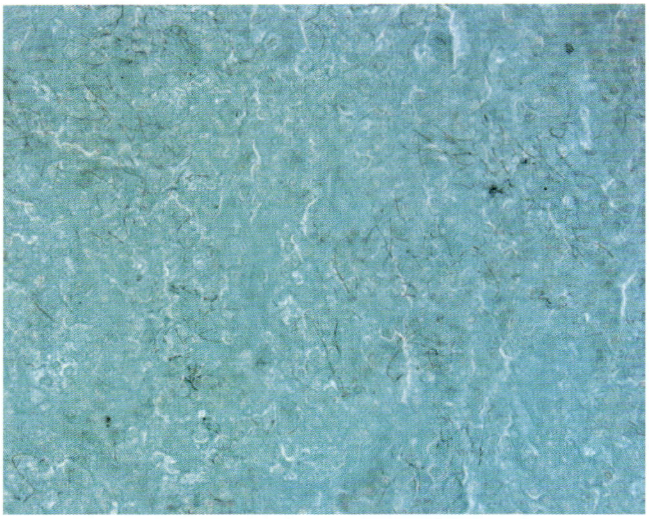

Figure 59.11 Nocardia: *Nocardia and Actinomyces* are both thin (1 μm), filamentous, branching bacteria decorated by GMS stain. However, nocardia does not show the Splendore-Hoeppli phenomenon as seen in actinomyces.

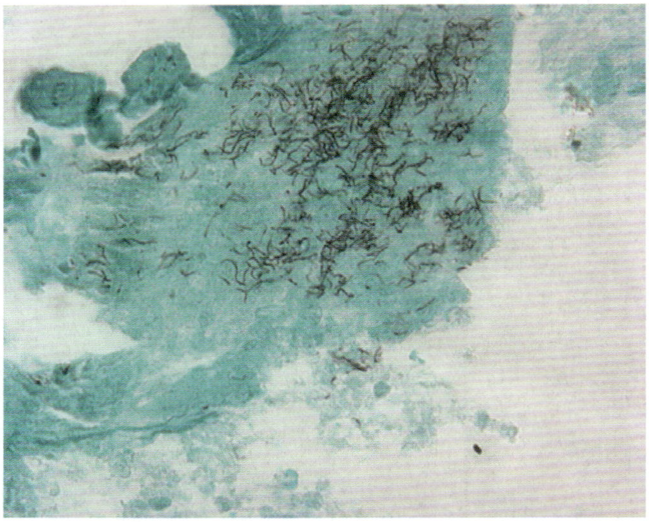

Figure 59.12 Abundant filamentous branching organisms on GMS stain.

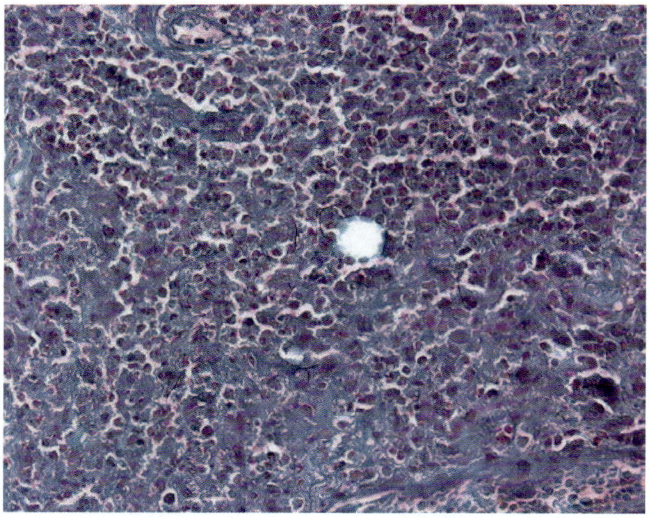

Figure 59.13 Nocardia: Distinguished from actinomyces by its weak acid-fast staining (Fite stain).

60 ASPERGILLOSIS VS. MUCORMYCOSIS

	Aspergillosis	Mucormycosis (Zygomycosis)
Age	All ages.	All ages.
Location	Typically, upper lung fields.	Unilateral or bilateral.
Symptoms	Patient may be asymptomatic or may have cough, fever, hemoptysis (may be life-threatening).	Often acute and severe onset in neutropenic patients. Similar to invasive aspergillosis—fever, cough, dyspnea, and hemoptysis. Onset more subacute in diabetics.
Signs	Variable clinical signs depending on type of infection (i.e., aspergilloma/fungus ball, angioinvasive aspergillosis, chronic necrotizing aspergillosis and allergic bronchopulmonary aspergillosis). Chest x-ray of aspergilloma classically shows apical thin-walled cavities with intracavitary opacities; however, negative radiographs are seen in up to one-third of the patients. Adjacent pleura may be thickened. On CT, invasive aspergillosis may show multifocal pulmonary opacities surrounded by ground-glass opacities, suggestive of intra-alveolar hemorrhage (though not diagnostic of angioinvasion). Neutropenia common with invasive disease.	Chest x-ray shows patchy infiltrates, solitary or multiple opacities. CT imaging may show nodular opacities surrounded by halo of ground-glass opacities, similar to invasive aspergillosis; cavitation may also occur. More than 10 pulmonary nodules and pleural effusions favor invasive pulmonary mucormycosis over invasive aspergillosis.
Etiology	*Aspergillus* (usually *A. fumigatus, A. flavus*, or *A. niger*). Ubiquitous molds found worldwide. Most commonly infects immunocompromised patients, but causes a wide variety of disease in others, including allergic reactions in hypersensitive hosts and colonization.	Zygomycete class of fungi. Most commonly, *Rhizopus, Absidia, Mucor, Rhizomucor*. Widely distributed in nature, found in soil and decaying organic material. Uncommon in immunocompetent host. Infects patients with poorly controlled diabetes mellitus, neutropenia, and immunocompromised patients.
Histology	Organism morphology: typically, 45° branching, septated hyphae, from 3 to 6 µm wide, uniform in shape (parallel contours). Dichotomous branching (branches with same size as parent hyphae) *(Figs. 60.1–60.4)*. Fungus ball (mycetoma; aspergilloma) contains masses of mycelial organisms surrounded by cavitary wall; fruiting bodies and conidial heads may be seen if high oxygen tension is present. Organisms often grow in concentric layers in a radial pattern *(Fig. 60.5)*. With acute invasive aspergillosis, angioinvasion is present—blood vessels occluded by mass of organisms, often with associated parenchymal infarct *(Fig. 60.6)*. With chronic necrotizing aspergillosis, necrotizing granulomatous pneumonia is often seen, with fungal hyphae invading parenchyma. Organizing pneumonia at the periphery can be seen.	Organism morphology: pleomorphic, broad hyphae (5–25 µm wide), with right-angle branching, inconspicuous septations, and "ribbon-like" (folded, wrinkled) appearance. Irregular, not dichotomous, branching pattern *(Figs. 60.8–60.10)*. With angioinvasion, vascular thrombosis, infarcts, and possibly granulomatous vasculitis may be seen.

	Aspergillosis	Mucormycosis (Zygomycosis)
Special studies	GMS or PAS stains *(Fig. 60.7)* to confirm morphology, although organisms also easily visible on H&E. Pentachrome (Movat) or elastic tissue stain to evaluate for angioinvasion.	GMS or PAS stains to confirm morphology; organisms may be visible on H&E *(Figs. 60.11–60.13)*. Pentachrome (Movat) or elastic tissue stain to evaluate for angioinvasion.
Prognosis	Excellent with treatment; aspergillomas and localized infections may require surgical excision.	High mortality rate.

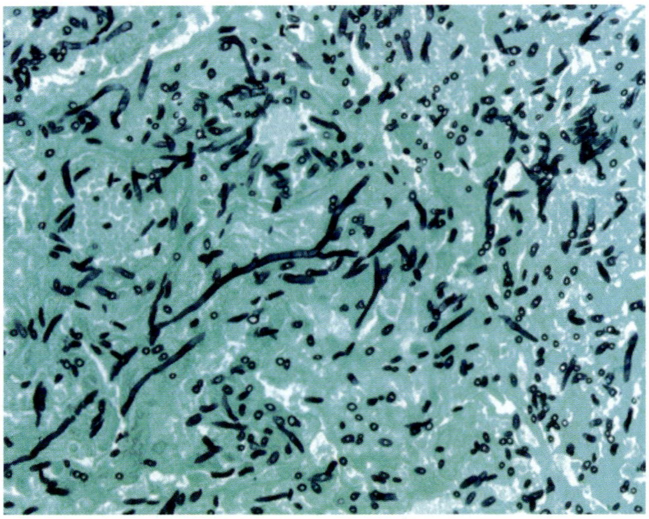

Figure 60.1 Aspergillosis: *Aspergillus* on GMS stain demonstrates branching uniform hyphae (average 4 μm diameter) that are septated at regular intervals. Dichotomous branching at 45° angles. Often they are arrayed in a somewhat parallel manner.

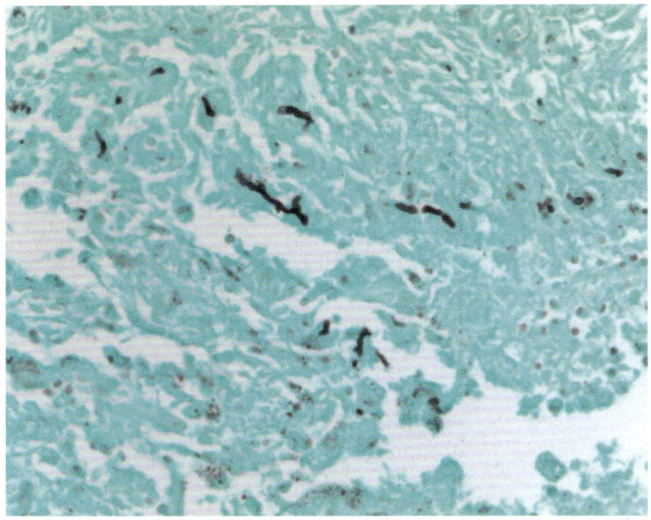

Figure 60.2 Aspergillosis: GMS stain shows rare organisms, but the uniform branching hyphae are still visible.

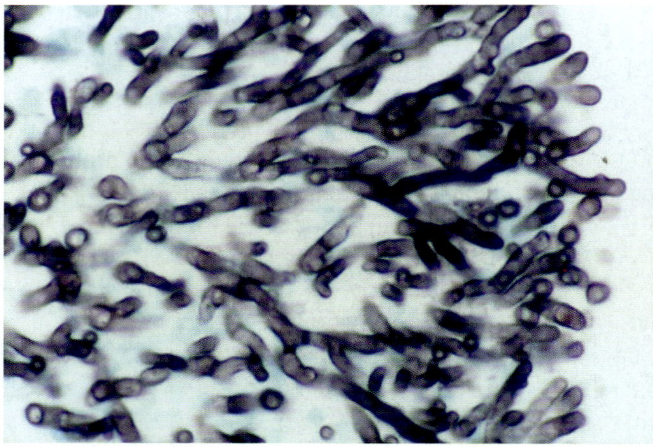

Figure 60.3 Aspergillosis: High-power image of GMS stain showing classic dichotomous branching and septated hyphae.

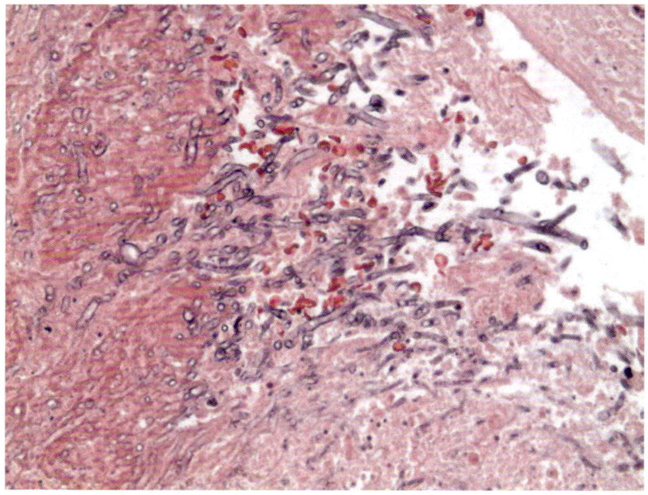

Figure 60.4 Aspergillosis: *Aspergillus* organisms are often visible on H&E stained sections as basophilic elements.

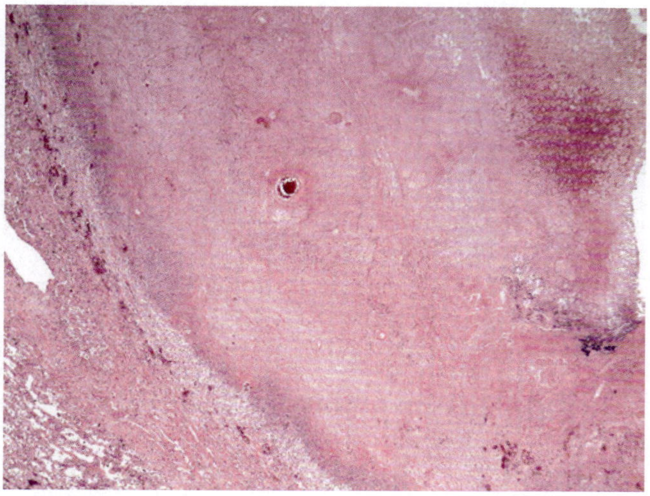

Figure 60.5 Aspergillosis: Fungal ball with mass of *Aspergillus* organisms. The outer edge of the fungal ball is arrayed radially (H&E).

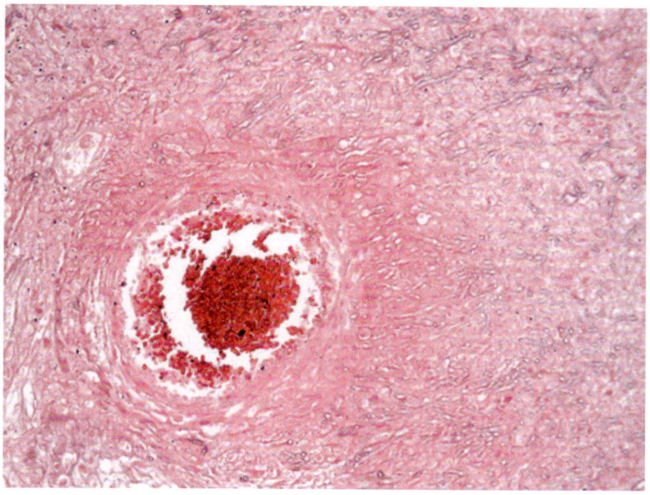

Figure 60.6 Aspergillosis: Small artery infiltrated by *Aspergillus* organisms. The vessel wall appears infarcted (H&E).

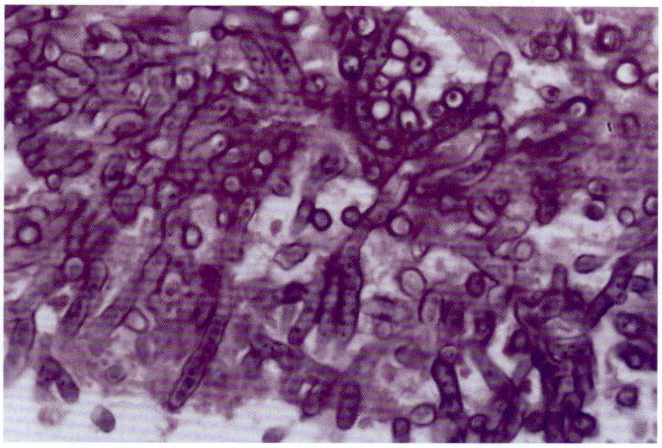

Figure 60.7 Aspergillosis: PAS stain highlights the branching septated forms of *Aspergillus*.

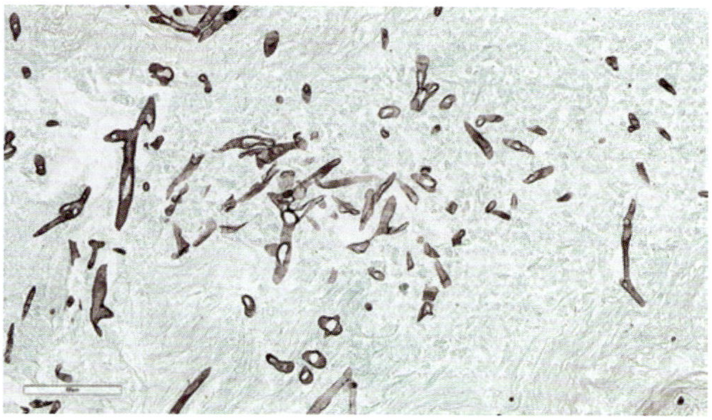

Figure 60.8 Mucormycosis: In contrast to *Aspergillus* organisms, *Mucor* shows broad, irregular (5–15 μm diameter), ribbon-like, nonseptated hyphae (GMS stain). However, twists or folds in the organisms may cause pseudoseptation. Branching is irregular, but often at 90°. Mucor organisms may appear fragmented. They are haphazardly arrayed, unlike the parallel appearance of *Aspergillus*.

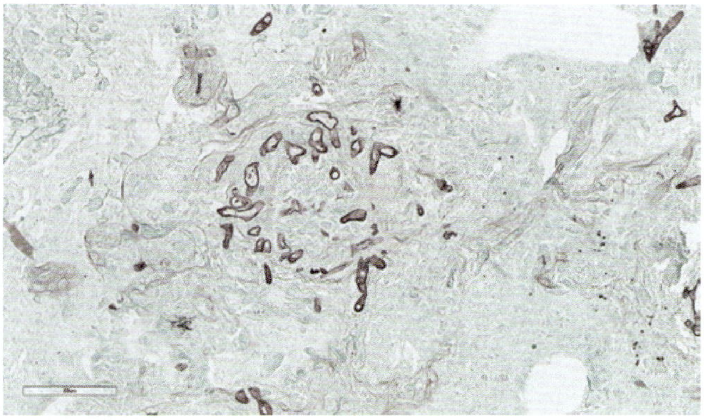

Figure 60.9 Mucormycosis: Haphazardly arrayed fragmented wide hyphae of *Mucor* (GMS stain).

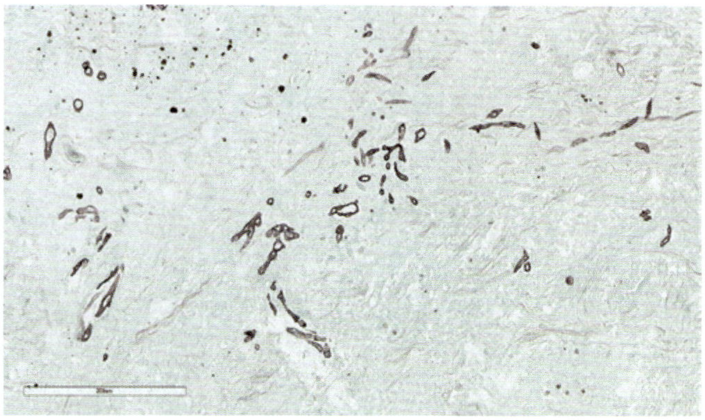

Figure 60.10 Mucormycosis: Another image of the fragmented forms of Mucor (GMS stain).

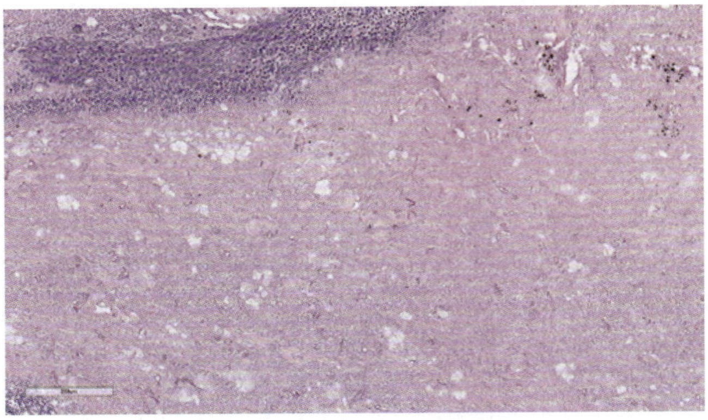

Figure 60.11 Mucormycosis: Like *Aspergillus*, *Mucor* is often readily identified on standard H&E stains.

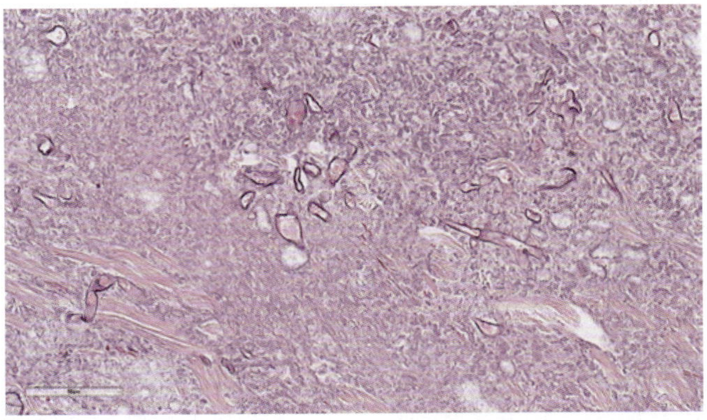

Figure 60.12 Mucormycosis: H&E stain (higher magnification) of *Mucor* organisms.

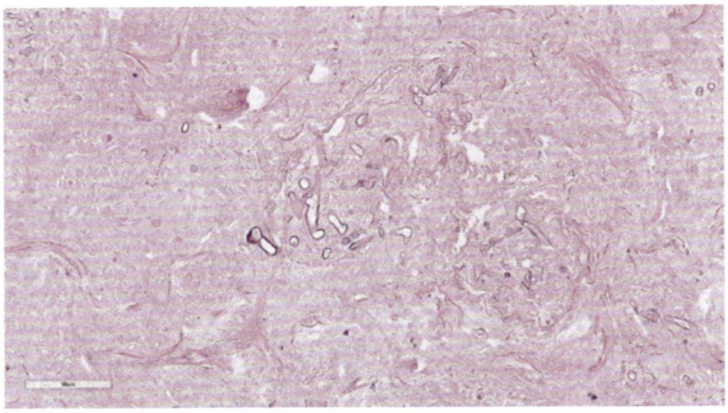

Figure 60.13 Mucormycosis: High-power image of H&E stain showing the fragmented, irregular, aseptated, wide hyphae of *Mucor*.

61 HISTOPLASMOSIS VS. CRYPTOCOCCOSIS

	Histoplasmosis	Cryptococcosis
Age	All ages; chronic disease more common in adults.	All ages.
Location	More common in upper lobes.	More common in upper lobes.
Symptoms	75% of the patients have asymptomatic, self-limiting disease. 25% develop disease, including acute and chronic pulmonary disease. Acute: Flulike fever, cough, myalgia, nonproductive cough, headache, chest pain. Chronic: Indolent with TB-like symptoms—increasing cough, fever, weight loss, dyspnea. Chronic disease more common in patients with COPD/emphysema. Can also develop disseminated disease and fibrosing mediastinitis with variable symptoms (has high mortality in disseminated disease).	Patients may be asymptomatic. Progressive infection (more common in immunosuppressed), can be asymptomatic or can present with mild fever, cough, weight loss, pleuritic chest pain.
Signs	Acute: chest x-ray shows hilar lymphadenopathy and focal pulmonary infiltrate (similar to Ghon complex in TB). With progression of disease, patchy nodular infiltrates and pleural effusion are seen. Chronic: has variable patterns including infiltrative, cavitary, fibrosis with emphysema, and histoplasmoma.	Chest x-ray findings are varied, but may show focal or diffuse pulmonary nodules or patchy air space consolidation. Immunosuppressed patients show more extensive disease (e.g., cavitation, consolidation) than do immunocompetent patients (opposite of TB).
Etiology	*Histoplasma capsulatum*. Dimorphic fungus with yeast and hyphal forms, found in soil; endemic to South Central United States. Disease due to inhalation of infected soil/dust, commonly from bird droppings.	*Cryptococcus neoformans*. Organism found worldwide in soil and bird excreta, especially pigeon. Usually only disseminates in immunocompromised host. Virulence related to its polysaccharide capsule. Different from *Histoplasma*, which is a dimorphic organism, Cryptococcus only shows yeast form.
Histology	Organism morphology: Yeast form in formalin-fixed, paraffin-embedded (FFPE) tissue, 2–4 μm diameter, spherical to oval, with narrow-based budding *(Figs. 61.1 and 61.2)*. Budding may be difficult to identify. Halo may be visible on H&E (due to retraction artifact as, notwithstanding the name, the organism does not have a capsule) *(Fig. 61.3)*. Although *Histoplasma capsulatum* is a dimorphic organism, the hyphal form is usually seen in tissue cultures rather than in FFPE tissue. Classically, shows granulomatous reaction, both necrotizing and nonnecrotizing, with surrounding chronic inflammation *(Figs. 61.4 and 61.5)*. Occasionally, may mimic sarcoidosis. With acute infection, acute fibrinous pneumonia without granulomas may be seen. Organisms cluster within macrophages *(Fig. 61.3)*. Stains strongly with GMS. Occasional darkly stained foci may mimic pneumocystis jiroveci pneumonia (PJP) organisms, but lacks foamy exudate typical of PJP infection *(Fig. 61.6)*.	Organism morphology: Pleomorphic yeast, 2–20 μm diameter, spherical to oval, narrow-based budding. Budding may be single or multiple. Thick mucinous capsule *(Figs. 61.7–61.10)*. If patient is immunocompetent and/or the strain is capsule-deficient, then there is a necrotizing granulomatous inflammatory response *(Fig. 61.11)*. Capsule-deficient organisms may be similar in size to *Histoplasma* organisms (2–4 μm), but should show some mucin positivity. If patient is immunosuppressed, then profusely multiplying yeast forms in alveolar walls, airspaces, and capillaries may be seen. Very little host response.

	Histoplasmosis	Cryptococcosis
Special studies	Strongly positive on GMS and other silver stains. Negative on mucicarmine or other mucin stain.	Positive on GMS and other silver stains. Capsule stains with mucin stains, such as mucicarmine and Alcian blue. Even capsule-deficient organisms will show some positive mucin staining. These are the only pathogenic fungal organisms that stain with mucin stains Additionally, India ink cannot penetrate the capsule, leading to a ghost appearance *(Fig. 61.12)*.
Prognosis	Usually benign and self-limited. Good prognosis with treatment.	Depends on patient's immune status and severity of infection.

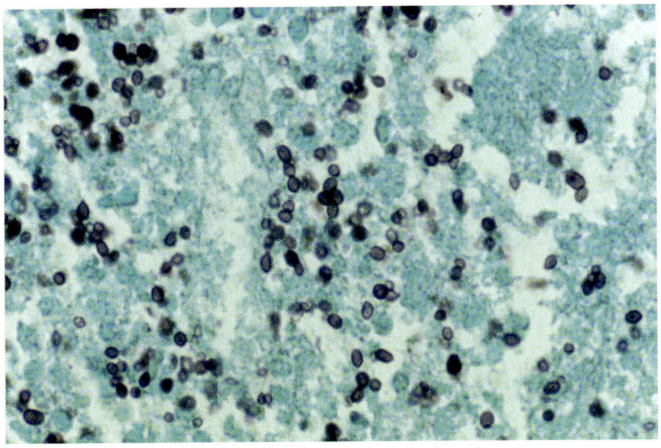

Figure 61.1 Histoplasmosis: Small, oval-to-round yeasts of *Histoplasma*. May show prominent clustering because they are often intracellular within histiocytes. Budding may be inconspicuous, but if seen, is narrow-based (GMS stain).

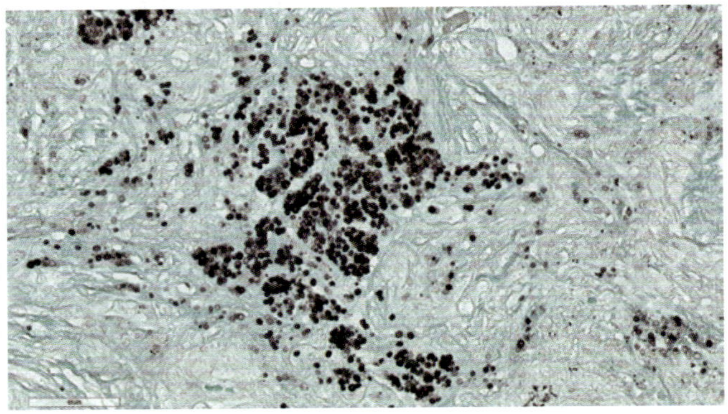

Figure 61.2 Histoplasmosis: Clustering of organisms is evident (GMS stain).

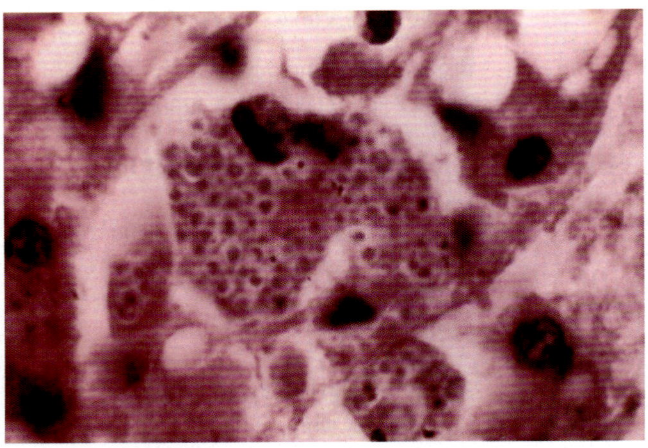

Figure 61.3 Histoplasmosis: Intracellular growth of yeast within histiocytes. Note the artifactual halo around the organisms (H&E).

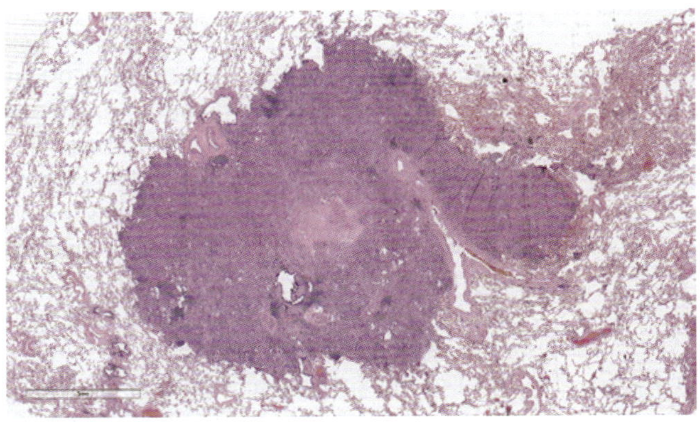

Figure 61.4 Histoplasmosis: Granulomatous inflammation characterized by central necrosis surrounded by chronic inflammation, including histiocytes, is typical of *Histoplasma* infection.

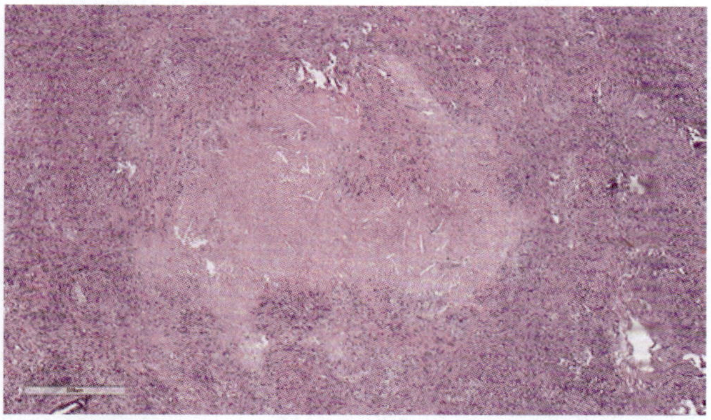

Figure 61.5 Histoplasmosis: High-power image of central necrosis surrounded by histiocytic inflammation.

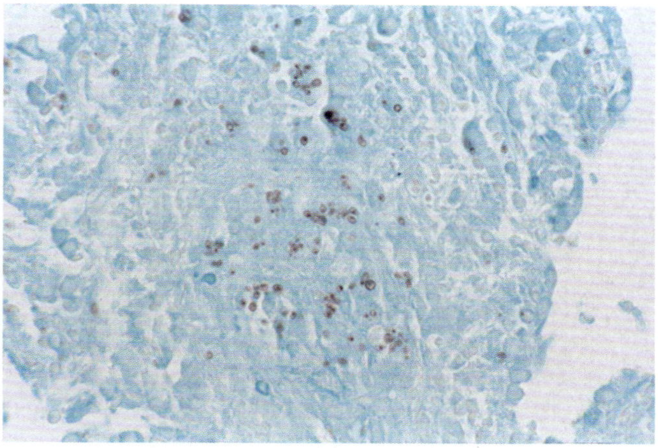

Figure 61.6 Histoplasmosis: Some *Histoplasma* organisms may demonstrate an eccentric, darkly stained dot, similar to PJP infection. The narrow-based budding forms of histoplasmosis can aid in distinguishing the two organisms (GMS stain).

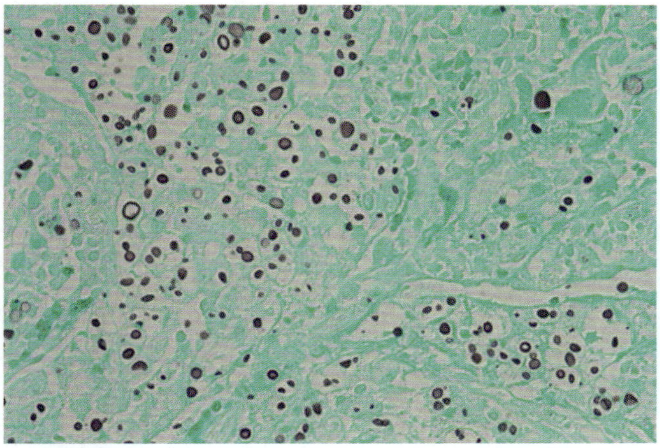

Figure 61.7 Cryptococcosis: Although there is overlap in the morphology of *Cryptococcus* and *Histoplasma* organisms, *Cryptococcus* shows marked variability in size (GMS).

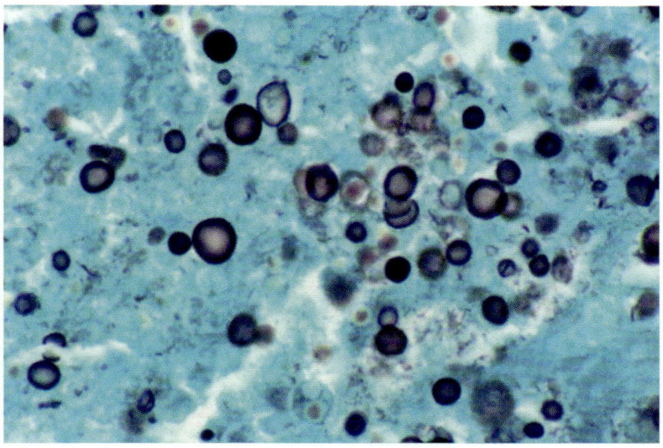

Figure 61.8 Cryptococcosis: Higher-power image highlighting the variability in size.

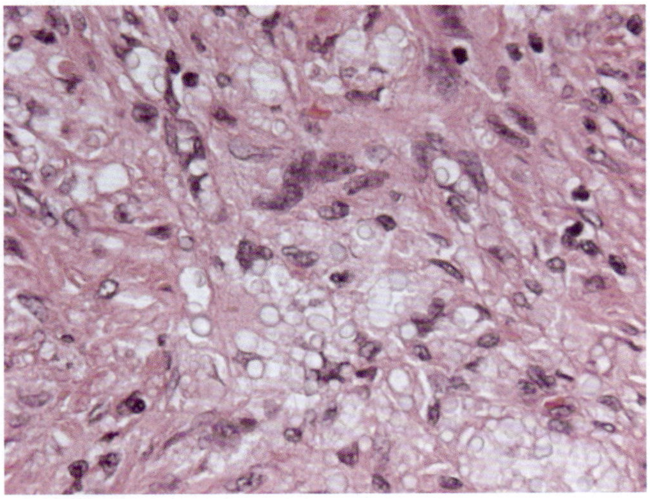

Figure 61.9 Cryptococcosis: On H&E stain, *Cryptococcus* organisms have a characteristic pale blue yeast form with a thick capsule.

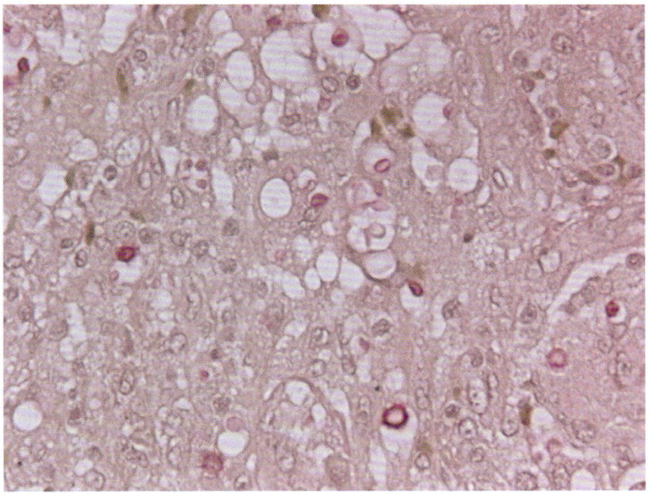

Figure 61.10 Cryptococcosis: Mucin stain decorates the organisms and thick mucinous capsule in bright red. Mucin stains are extremely helpful in separating cryptococcosis from histoplasmosis.

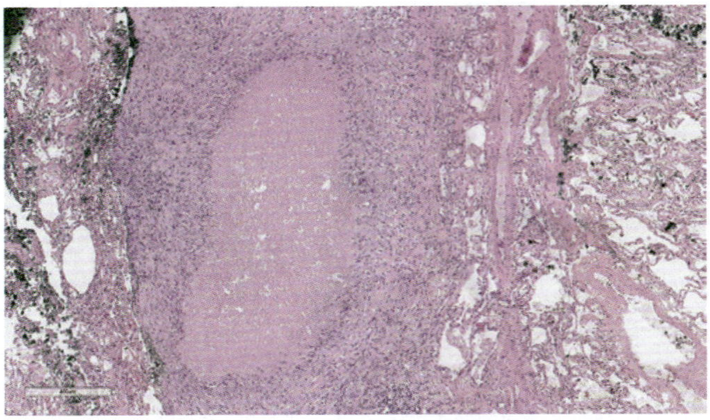

Figure 61.11 Cryptococcosis: Necrotizing granuloma in cryptococcosis. Organisms are often found in the central necrotic region of the necrotizing granuloma.

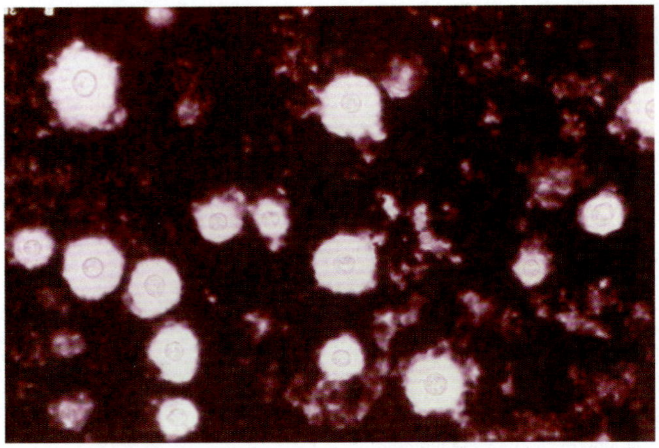

Figure 61.12. Cryptococcosis: India ink stain demonstrates the absence of capsule staining and the ghost-like appearance of the organism.

62 BLASTOMYCOSIS VS. COCCIDIOIDOMYCOSIS

	Blastomycosis	Coccidioidomycosis
Age	All ages, most frequently in young men (probably as a result of increased exposure).	All ages.
Location	Any lobes, but more common in lower lobes.	More common in upper lobes.
Symptoms	May be asymptomatic. Acute infection can present with flulike symptoms that progress to pneumonia with high fever and pleuritic chest pain. Chronic infection (often symptoms >2 mo) causes fever, weight loss, night sweats, cough, hemoptysis, and chest pain.	Often asymptomatic. Otherwise, flulike with fever, nonproductive cough, myalgias, arthralgias, headaches, and pleuritic chest pain. Erythema nodosum in 20% of patients—often portends a better prognosis.
Signs	Acute: Chest x-ray shows focal or diffuse airspace consolidation (even in asymptomatic patients), often bilateral. Chronic: Has variable patterns, including linear infiltrates, fibronodular densities with cavitations, and mediastinal lymphadenopathy. Small pleural effusions are common. CT imaging may show localized mass, often large, and parenchymal consolidation. Cavitation is often evident.	May be normal or may show solitary or multiple nodules, cavitary lesions, hilar lymphadenopathy, and pleural effusions. In chronic disease, biapical pulmonary nodular lesions with cavities may be seen. Can develop a coccidioidoma—usually a solitary coin lesion, which may mimic malignancy on CT imaging.
Etiology	*Blastomyces dermatitidis*. Dimorphic fungus endemic to North America, found in soil mainly along the Mississippi, Ohio, and Missouri river valley and in regions near the Great Lakes. Also reported in other areas of the world. Disease due to inhalation of infected soil.	*Coccidioides immitis*. Dimorphic fungus. Also known as San Joaquin Valley fever. Grows best in arid to semiarid climates; arthroconidial (specialized spore) form can survive for extended periods in desert soil. Exposure increases with soil disturbance (e.g., agriculture, dust storms, construction). Endemic in Southwestern United States, and parts of Central and South America. Causes disease in immunocompetent and immunosuppressed hosts, with more severe disease in the immunosuppressed. Disseminated disease also more common in pregnant women and people of African descent.
Histology	Dimorphic fungi with yeast and hyphal forms. Hyphal forms are usually seen in tissue cultures. In tissue sections, classically appear as 8–15 μm diameter (however, microforms, 2–4 μm, can also be present), spherical to oval, with broad-based budding and a thick cell wall. Organisms are multinucleate and may be identified on H&E by their thick, double-contoured wall *(Figs. 62.1–62.4)*.	Like *B. dermatitidis*, *C. immitis* is also a dimorphic organism with yeast and hyphal forms, but the hyphal forms are usually seen in tissue cultures. In tissue sections, *C. immitis* classically appears as sporulating thick-walled spherule (30–100 μm diameter), with internal septations and endospores (2–5 μm diameter). Immature spherules lack endospores and may be confused with *Blastomyces* organisms. Often ruptured spherules releasing numerous endospores can be seen. Each endospore can potentially develop into a spherule, repeating the cycle *(Figs. 62.6–62.10)*.

	Blastomycosis	Coccidioidomycosis
	Classically, shows neutrophilic microabscesses surrounded by palisading epithelioid histiocytes and multinucleated giant cells (suppurative necrotizing granuloma) *(Fig. 62.5)*. May show acute pneumonia pattern with neutrophils filling alveolar spaces. Positive for GMS and other silver stains. Usually negative for mucicarmine or other mucin stains; if positive, then positive in cell wall, not capsule.	Early histology shows acute suppurative pneumonia. Necrotizing granulomas develop, consisting of fibrocaseous nodules with giant cells and epithelioid histiocytes *(Fig. 62.11)*. Splendore–Hoeppli reaction may be seen around spherules. Vegetative forms, which are usually seen in tissue cultures, consist of 2–4 μm thick septate hyphae and chains of barrel-shaped arthroconidia. Morphology best demonstrated with GMS stain, which stains both the spherules and the endospores. PAS stain highlights endospores, but not the spherules. Negative for mucin stains (mucicarmine, Alcian blue). No budding.
Special studies	Positive on GMS and other silver stain. Negative on mucicarmine or other mucin stain.	GMS to highlight spherules and endospores; PAS to highlight endospores.
Prognosis	Usually benign and self-limited. Long-term follow-up necessary as patients may develop extrapulmonary lesions months to years later.	In general, excellent prognosis, unless disseminated disease (especially in HIV patients).

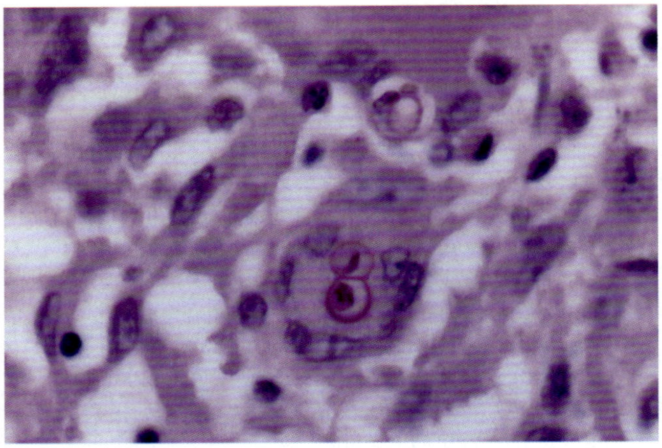

Figure 62.1 Blastomycosis: H&E classic BBBB (broad-based budding blastomycosis) yeast appearance of *B. dermatitidis*.

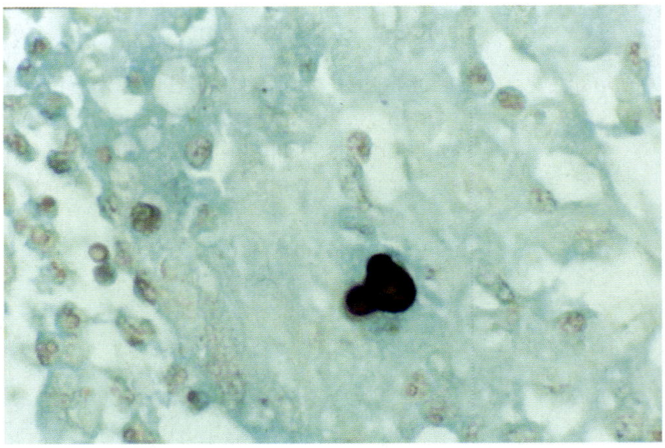

Figure 62.2 Blastomycosis: High-power image of budding yeast organisms on GMS stain.

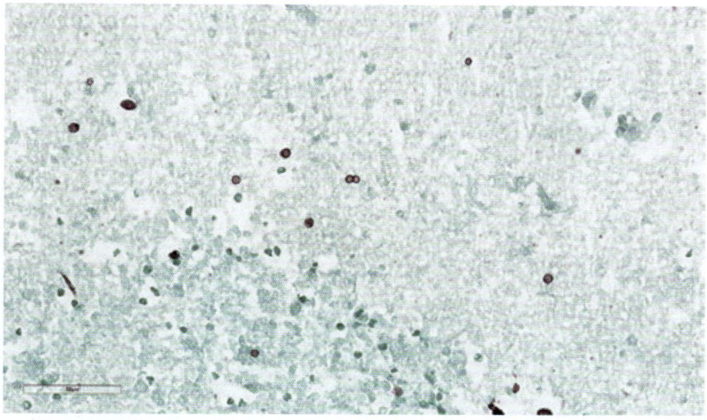

Figure 62.3 Blastomycosis: Microforms of blastomycosis on GMS stain. Broad-based budding is evident.

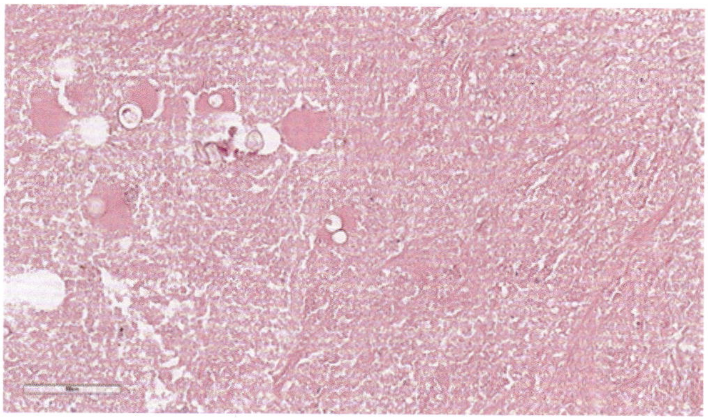

Figure 62.4 Blastomycosis: Broad-based budding visible on H&E stain.

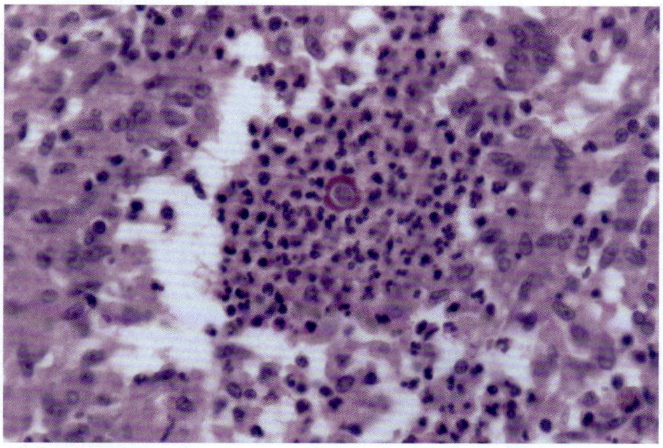

Figure 62.5 Blastomycosis: Microabscess surrounded by epithelioid histiocytes and scattered dispersed lymphocytes. Note characteristic thick cell wall of *B. dermatitidis*. H&E stain.

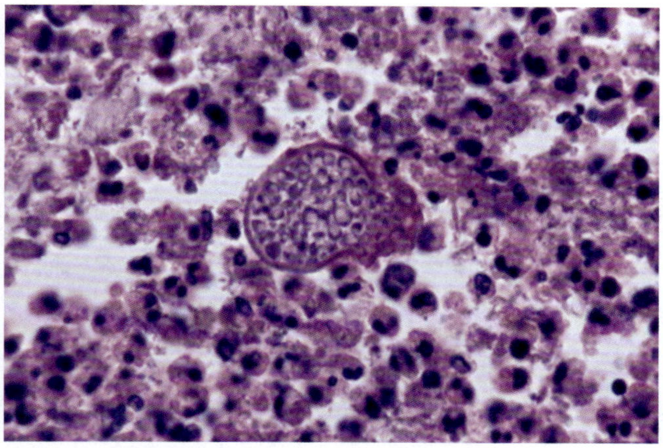

Figure 62.6 Coccidioidomycosis: Spherule containing endospores is visible on H&E stain. Note the surrounding necrosis. Endospores are often better visualized on GMS stain.

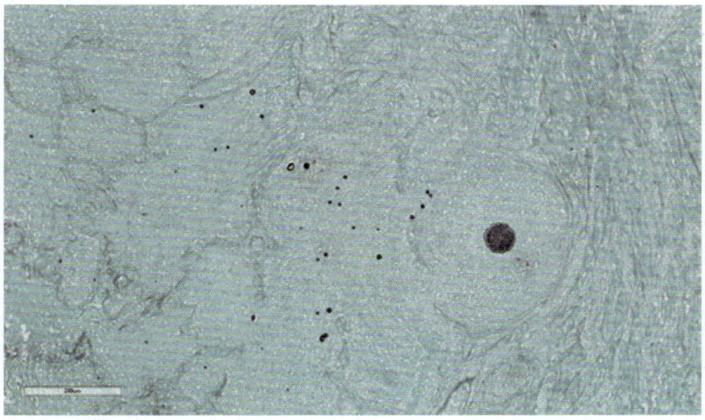

Figure 62.7 Coccidioidomycosis: GMS stain of coccidioidomycosis organisms. At the right side of the field, there is a large spherule filled with endospores. This image also shows immature spherules and released endospores. Although the endospores can resemble *Histoplasma* or *Cryptococci*, the endospores lack budding. Immature spherules can likewise resemble *Blastomyces*, but the absence of broad-based budding favors the immature spherules of coccidioidomycosis.

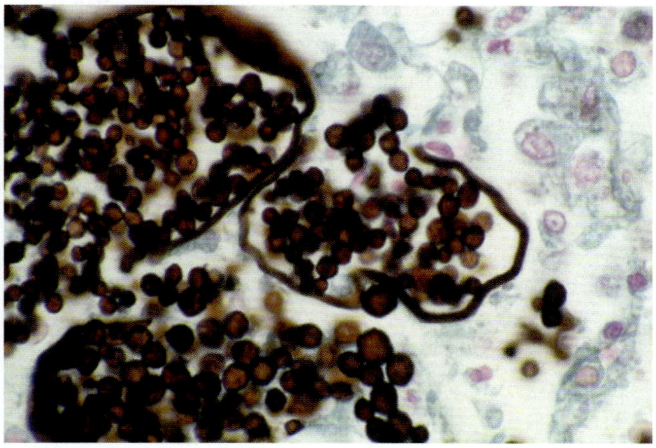

Figure 62.8 Coccidioidomycosis: High-power image of spherule containing multiple endospores.

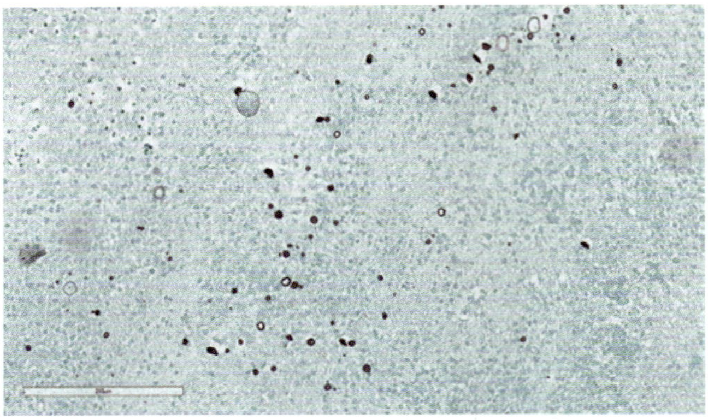

Figure 62.9 Coccidioidomycosis: This GMS-stained image also shows mature spherules, immature spherules, and released endospores.

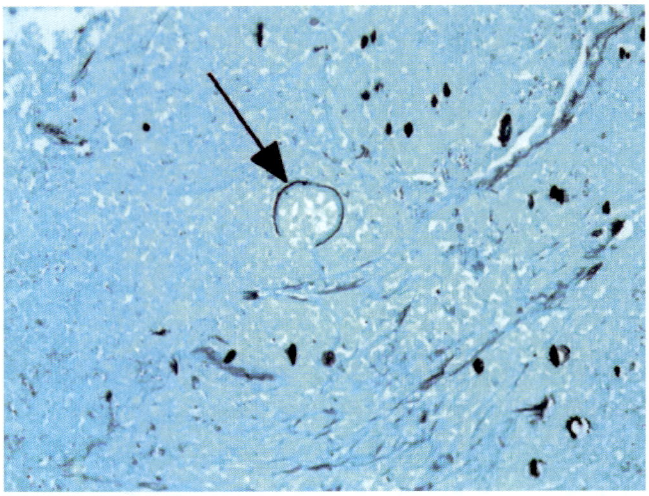

Figure 62.10 Coccidioidomycosis: Here is a ruptured, empty (*arrow*) cyst with scattered free endospores in the surrounding tissue.

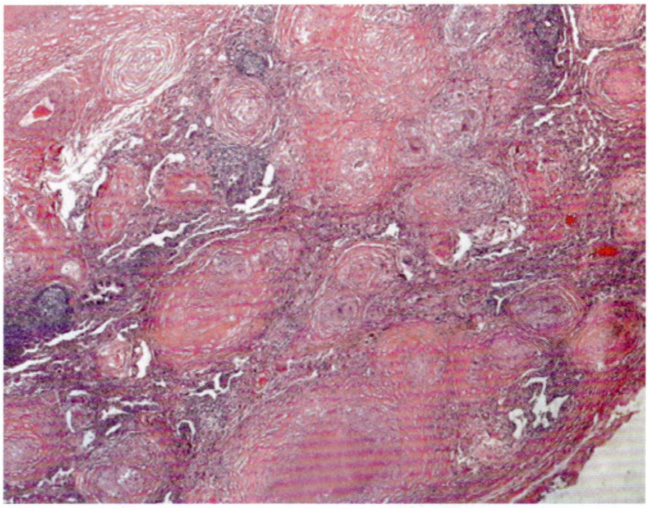

Figure 62.11 Coccidioidomycosis: Typical granulomatous appearance of coccidioidomycosis with necrotizing and nonnecrotizing granulomas evident.

63 PNEUMOCYSTIS JIROVECI PNEUMONIA VS. PULMONARY EDEMA

	Pneumocystis Jiroveci Pneumonia (PJP)	Pulmonary Edema
Age	All ages.	Any age.
Location	Often bilateral.	Bilateral.
Symptoms	Exertional dyspnea, fever, and nonproductive cough most common.	If acute, breathlessness, anxiety, and feelings of drowning. If more gradual, dyspnea on exertion, orthopnea, cough. If severe, frothy sputum may be seen.
Signs	Tachypnea, hypoxemia, decreased DLCO. Chest x-ray may be normal early in disease and may progress to diffuse bilateral infiltrates. CT shows patchy ground-glass opacities with interlobular septal thickening. Elevated LDH (level correlates with degree of lung injury).	Classic chest x-ray shows bilateral infiltrates in a butterfly pattern with pleural effusions.
Etiology	*Pneumocystis jiroveci.* Unicellular fungus. Most common opportunistic infection in HIV-infected patients. Also infects patients with primary immune deficiencies, those undergoing long-term immunosuppression, the severely malnourished, and people with malignancies.	Cardiogenic (most common) and permeability (injury to capillary endothelial cells) causes.
Histology	Organism morphology: round to oval, 5–7 µm cysts, often with prominent grooves or folds *(Fig. 63.1).* Classically, intra-alveolar foamy exudates, finely vacuolated "bubbled" appearance. The bubbles represent the organisms *(Figs. 63.2 and 63.3).* Usually no cholesterol clefts or globular material *(Figs. 63.4 and 63.5).* GMS or other silver stain highlights the PCP cysts. Small darkly stained focus in center may be seen *(Figs. 63.6 and 63.7).* Usually, there is a mild chronic interstitial pneumonia and type 2 cell hyperplasia. Some patients may show an organizing pneumonia pattern on biopsy. Especially in AIDS patients, organizing diffuse alveolar damage (DAD) and/or granulomatous inflammation may be seen (mainly nonnecrotizing).	Acellular, homogeneous eosinophilic material within alveolar spaces—lacks bubbly, foamy appearance of PJP infection *(Figs. 63.8 and 63.9).* No cholesterol clefts or globular material. GMS or other silver stain negative. No chronic interstitial pneumonia or type 2 cell hyperplasia.

	Pneumocystis Jiroveci Pneumonia (PJP)	Pulmonary Edema
Special studies	Induced sputum may show organisms (moderate sensitivity, high specificity). Bronchoalveolar lavage (BAL) has high sensitivity and specificity for identification of organisms. Lung biopsy has essentially 100% sensitivity and specificity. GMS stain is best for identifying cysts. Also, PCR may be used to distinguish active infection from colonization.	As pulmonary edema is a diagnosis of exclusion, GMS stain must be used to rule out PJP. Also PAS stain must be used to rule out alveolar proteinosis.
Prognosis	Mortality rates up to 50% in non-AIDS patients; up to 20% in AIDS patients.	Prognosis is dependent on the cause.

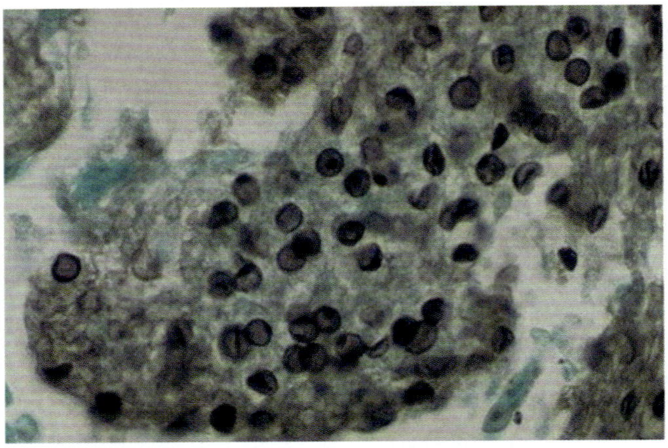

Figure 63.1 PJP: GMS stain highlights the cysts within alveolar spaces.

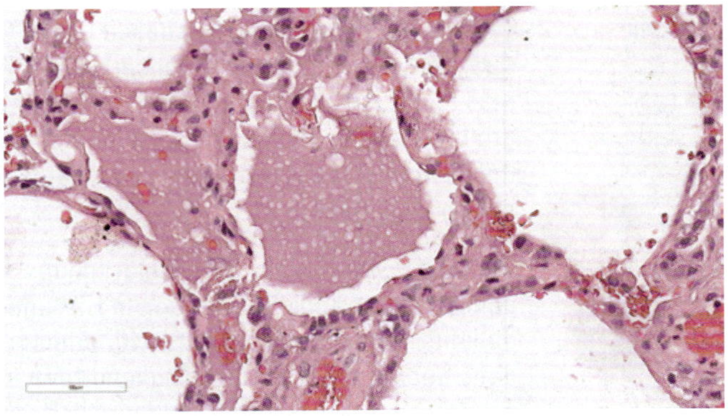

Figure 63.2 PJP: H&E stain of foamy exudate with a frothy appearance.

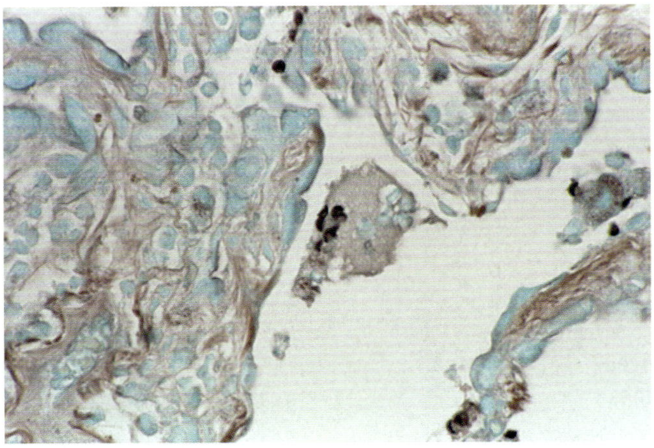

Figure 63.3 PJP: GMS stain shows cysts with a collapsed form, the so-called boat or cup shape.

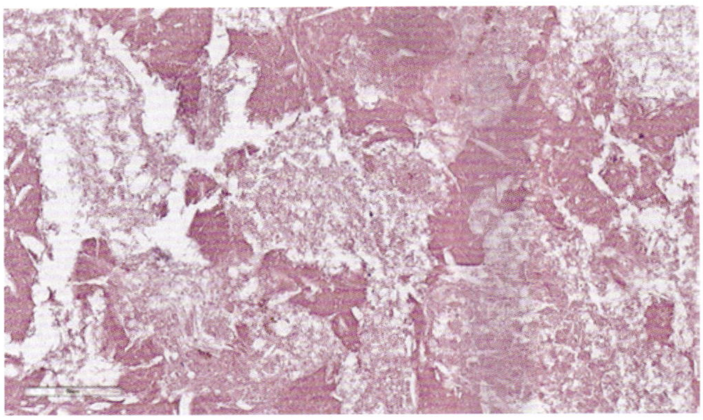

Figure 63.4 PJP: Although typically PJP infection is associated with exudative material lacking cholesterol clefts, in this case, there are clefts evident.

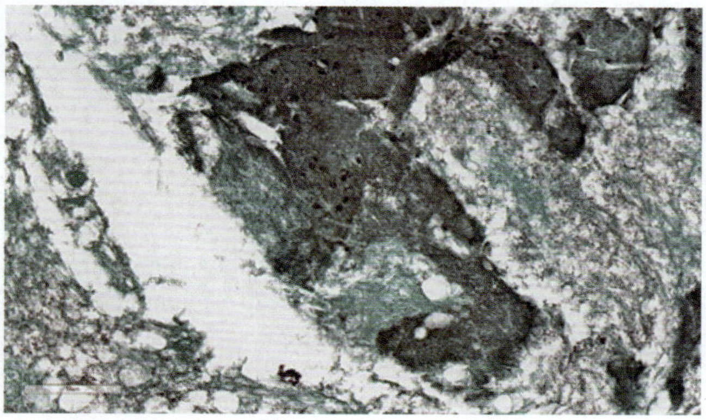

Figure 63.5 PJP: The GMS stain highlights the organisms within the clefted exudative material.

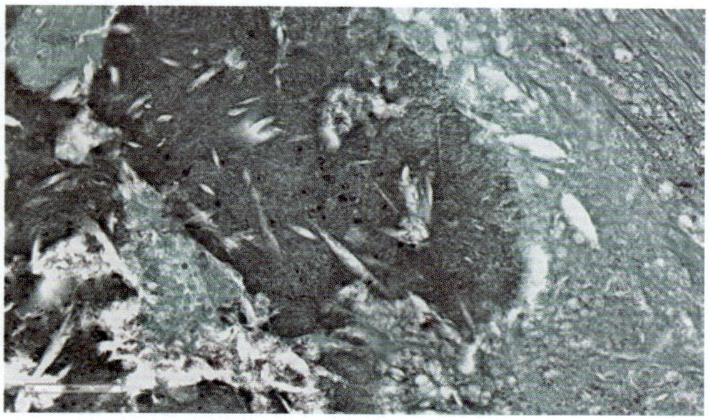

Figure 63.6 PJP: GMS stain from same patient demonstrating the darkly stained foci that can be seen in PJP.

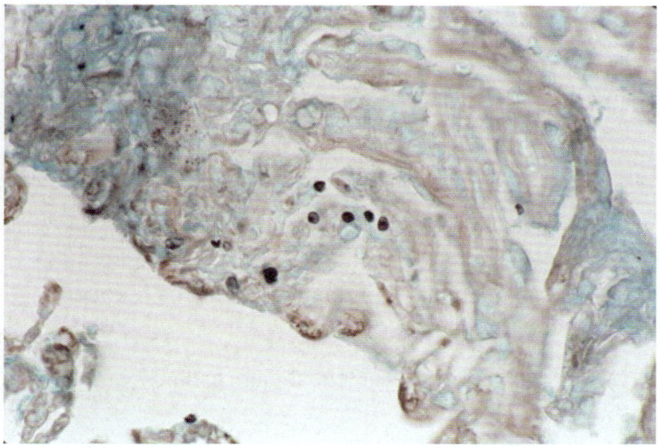

Figure 63.7 PJP: Another patient with the disease. Darkly stained foci are evident.

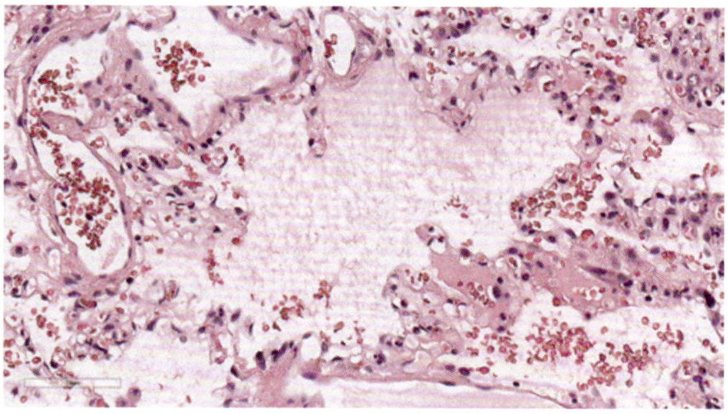

Figure 63.8 Pulmonary edema: Edema fluid has a wispier quality to it than the exudative froth of PJP infection. It also lacks a bubbly appearance and is much more homogeneous in appearance. If in doubt, a GMS stain can be performed to confirm the absence of fungal organisms.

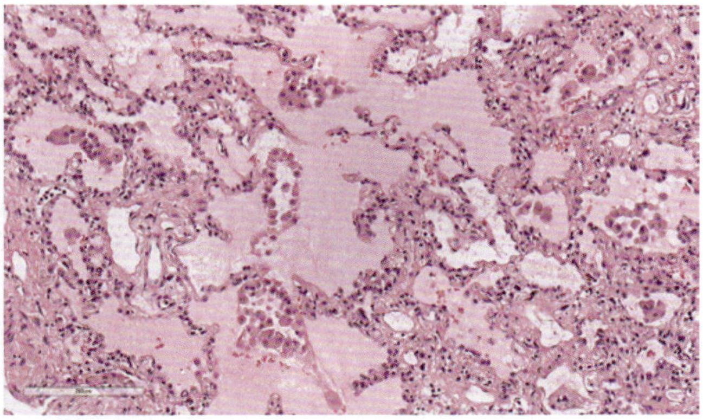

Figure 63.9 Pulmonary edema: Homogeneous, eosinophilic appearance of edema.

64 MYCOBACTERIAL PNEUMONIA VS. SARCOIDOSIS

	Mycobacterial Pneumonia	Sarcoidosis
Age	*Mycobacterium tuberculosis* (MTB) and nontuberculous mycobacteria (NTM) are most commonly seen in men. MTB infection is more commonly diagnosed in the elderly and in people with immunodeficiency. Middle-aged women are most commonly affected with "Lady Windermere syndrome," also known as middle-lobe syndrome, which is caused by *Mycobacterium avium* complex (MAC) infection. Young men and women who use hot tubs, humidifiers, or air conditioners with water contaminated by NTM/MAC may be affected by a hypersensitivity-like pulmonary disease (hot-tub lung).	Sarcoidosis affects patients of all ages, but it occurs most commonly in young adults (20–40 years old), with slight female predominance.
Location	Usually upper lobes. Right middle lobe and lingula in Lady Windermere syndrome.	The disease usually has a lymphatic pattern of distribution in the lung, affecting subpleural zones and coursing along the interlobular septa and bronchovascular bundles.
Symptoms	Cough, shortness of breath, hemoptysis, fatigue, weight loss, fever, and night sweats.	Dyspnea, cough, fever, chest pain, malaise, and weight loss.
Signs	Imaging studies demonstrate nodular lesions, with or without cavitation, which may be unilateral, bilateral, or centrilobular and associated with bronchiectasis and mediastinal or hilar lymphadenopathy.	Imaging studies show interstitial reticular, reticular nodular, or nodular infiltrates following a lymphatic pattern of distribution.
Etiology	MTB and NTM (particularly *Mycobacterium avium* complex [MAC] and *Mycobacterium kansasii*). MTB infection usually occurs in the setting of underlying chronic lung disease (e.g., bronchiectasis, emphysema, malignancy, right middle-lobe syndrome) and in immunocompromised patients.	Uncertain. Current theories consider sarcoidosis to be a disease that in genetically susceptible individuals cause an aberrant immune response driven by an unidentified antigen or antigens. Multiple candidate etiologic agents including mycobacteria, propionibacteria, and environmental agents have been investigated with inconsistent results.

	Mycobacterial Pneumonia	Sarcoidosis
Histology	Randomly distributed nonnecrotizing and necrotizing, well-formed and poorly formed granulomas composed of epithelioid histiocytes and variable amount of multinucleated giant cells associated with a peripheral rim of lymphocytes. The granulomas are present within the airway lumens, alveolar spaces, and interstitial (alveolar septal) spaces *(Figs. 64.1–64.4)*. In AIDS patients, the granulomas are usually poorly formed. Over time, the granulomas will usually become fibrotic and calcified. Vascular involvement may be seen, but true necrotizing vasculitis is uncommon *(Fig. 64.5)*.	Well-formed, coalescent, largely nonnecrotizing granulomas composed of epithelioid histiocytes and variable amount of multinucleated giant cells with a lymphatic pattern of distribution, seen in subpleural zones and coursing along the interlobular septa and bronchovascular bundles. The granulomas are present within the interstitial (alveolar septal) spaces, and there is usually no significant interstitial pneumonia extending into the adjacent lung parenchyma. The granulomas are frequently surrounded by concentric fibrosis, which over time becomes hyalinized with lamellar appearance. In some cases, extensive areas of hyalinized fibrosis replace areas of granulomatous inflammation with distortion of the underlying lung parenchyma architecture *(Figs. 64.7–64.9)*. A variety of nonspecific inclusions may be present, including asteroid bodies *(Fig. 64.10)*, Schaumann/conchoid bodies *(Fig. 64.11)*, Hamazaki–Wesenberg bodies (GMS positive), and birefringent calcium oxalate and calcium carbonate inclusions. Necrosis is unusual except in the so-called nodular necrotizing sarcoidosis, where areas of necrosis are present in a background of confluent, nonnecrotizing, sarcoid-like granulomas. In necrotizing sarcoidosis prominent associated vasculitis may be present, which may be granulomatous *(Fig. 64.12)* or may be characterized by transmural chronic inflammation. Multinucleated giant cells may be prominent *(Fig. 64.13)*, but significant necrosis (necrotizing vasculitis) is usually not a feature.
Special studies	Sputum and tissue cultures, AFB special stain *(Fig. 64.6)*, Auramine-rhodamine fluorescent stain and polymerase chain reaction (PCR)–based molecular testing performed in paraffin-embedded tissues. Culture of water from hot-tub users often yield organisms.	Tissue cultures, AFB special stain, and appropriate molecular testing to exclude infection. Chronic beryllium disease is another condition that can mimic sarcoidosis and the possibility of beryllium exposure should be considered, which may be detected in the blood with the beryllium sensitization test (Blood lymphocyte proliferation test [BeBLPT])
Prognosis	In MTB and NTM, the prognosis is usually good, except for multidrug-resistant organisms and in immunocompromised patients. In patients with hot-tub lung, the prognosis is usually good upon cessation of exposure to contaminated water and/or treatment with corticosteroids.	Spontaneous remission occurs in a large number of cases. A small number of cases develop chronic progressive disease and end-stage fibrosis with honeycombing. Corticosteroids are commonly used for treatment. Nodular and necrotizing sarcoidosis do not appear to have different prognosis.

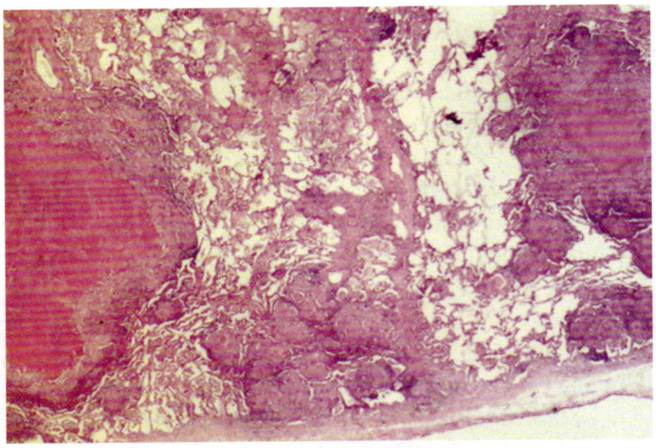

Figure 64.1 Mycobacterial infection: Granulomas with central necrosis (necrotizing granulomas) are seen in the left and right corners of the image. Nonnecrotizing granulomas are seen in the middle lower center of the image.

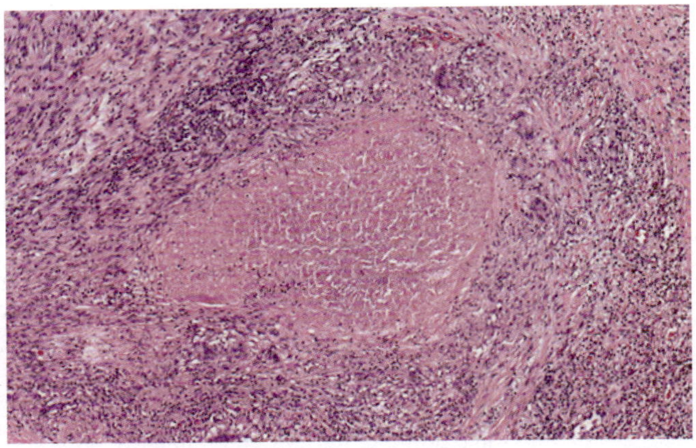

Figure 64.2 Mycobacterial infection: Necrotizing granuloma. The central area of necrosis is surrounded by epithelioid histiocytes admixed with lymphocytes and few multinucleated giant cells. The organisms are usually found within the central necrotic area of the granulomas.

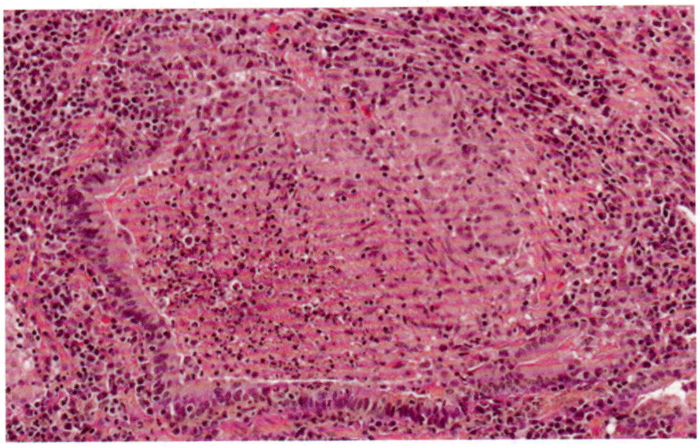

Figure 64.3 Mycobacterial infection: Necrotizing granuloma within an airway lumen.

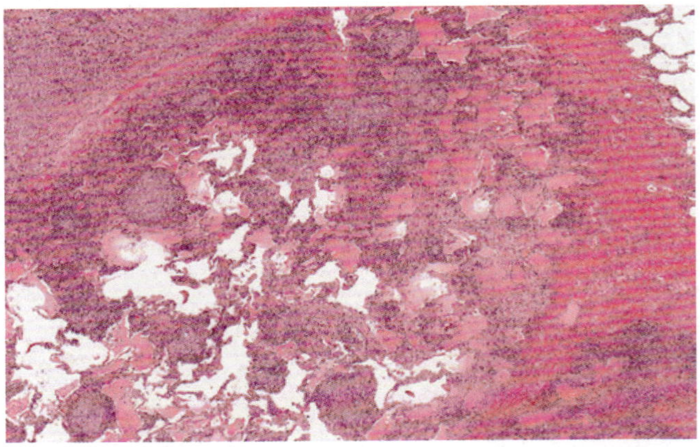

Figure 64.4 Mycobacterial infection: Nonnecrotizing granulomas seen in the interstitium (alveolar septa) and within the alveolar spaces. Note the significant amount of interstitial inflammation extending into the adjacent lung parenchyma. In contrast to sarcoidosis, the granulomas in mycobacterial infection are not surrounded by concentric fibrosis.

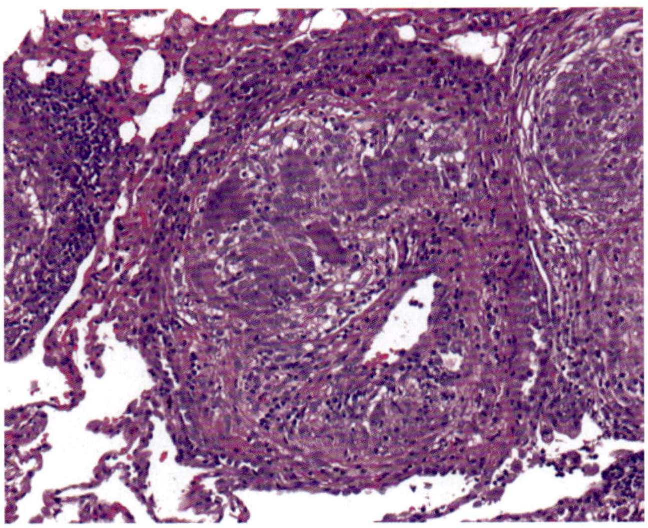

Figure 64.5 Mycobacterial pneumonia: Although vessels may be involved, as in this example, true necrotizing vasculitis usually does not occur.

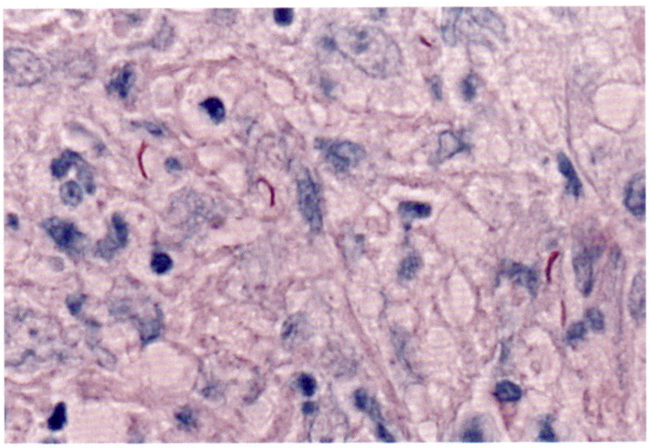

Figure 64.6 Mycobacterial infection: Acid-fast bacilli (AFB) special stain decorates thin red bacilli with a beaded configuration.

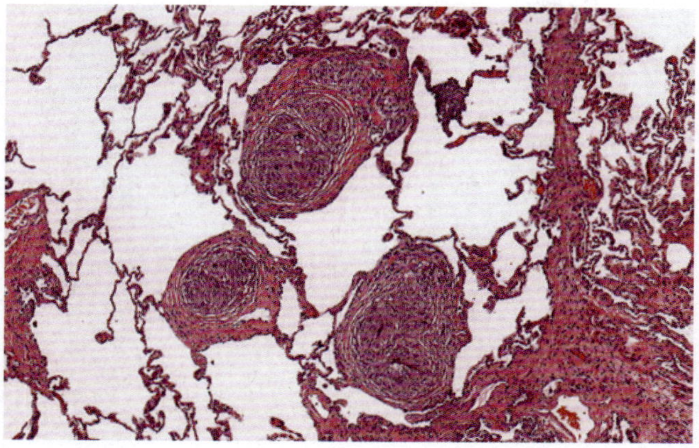

Figure 64.7 Sarcoidosis: Interstitial well-formed nonnecrotizing granulomas composed of epithelioid histiocytes surrounded by characteristic concentric fibrosis. Note that in contrast to mycobacterial infection, in sarcoidosis there is a lack of interstitial pneumonia extending into the adjacent lung parenchyma. The adjacent alveolar septa are usually thin and delicate.

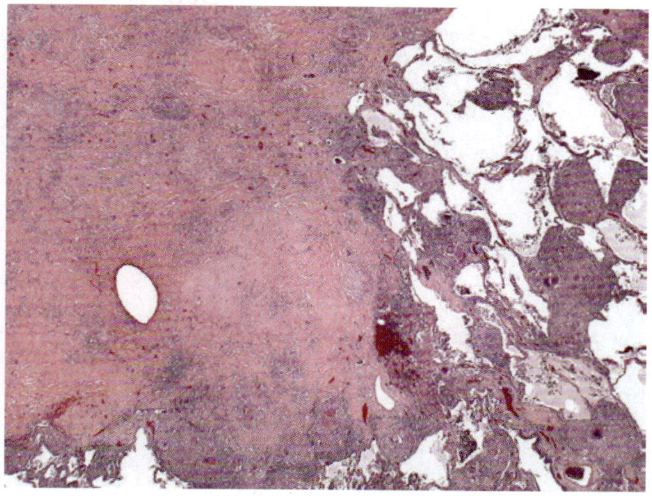

Figure 64.8 Sarcoidosis: In some cases, extensive areas of hyalinized fibrosis replace areas of granulomatous inflammation with distortion of the underlying architecture, which may have a mass-lesion appearance on image studies.

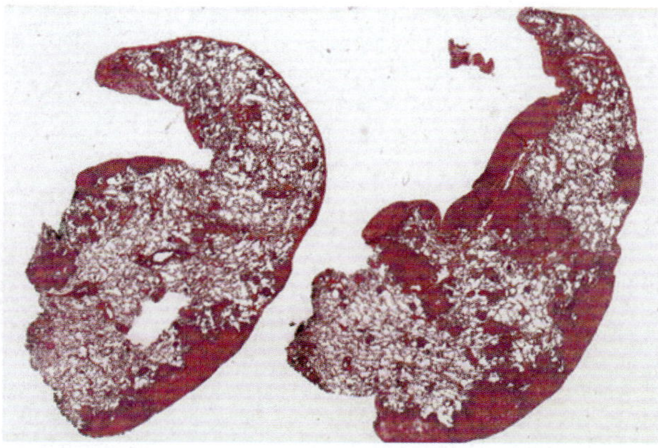

Figure 64.9 Sarcoidosis: Lymphatic pattern of distribution. The granulomas are present in subpleural zones and coursing along the interlobular septa and bronchovascular bundles.

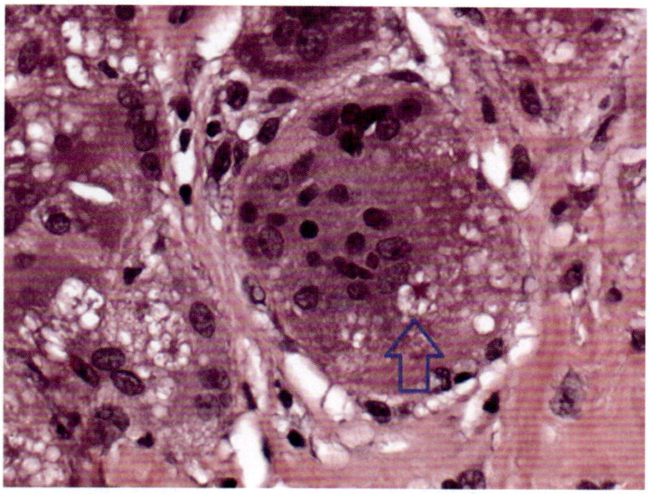

Figure 64.10 Sarcoidosis: A variety of nonspecific inclusions may be present, including asteroid bodies (*arrow*).

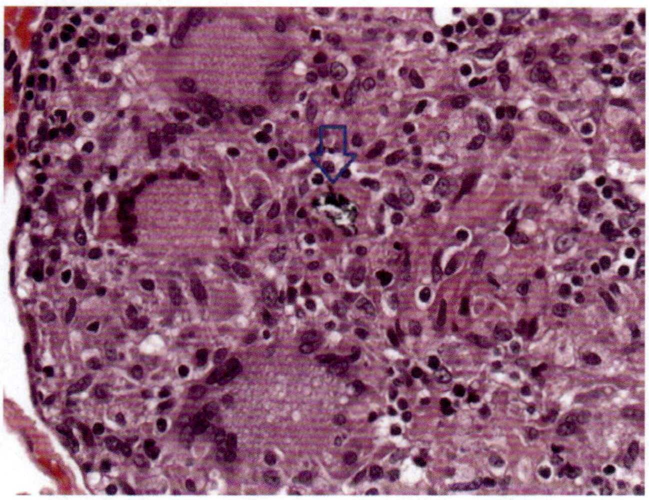

Figure 64.11 Sarcoidosis: Schaumann/conchoid bodies (*arrow*) are another type of nonspecific inclusion seen in sarcoidosis.

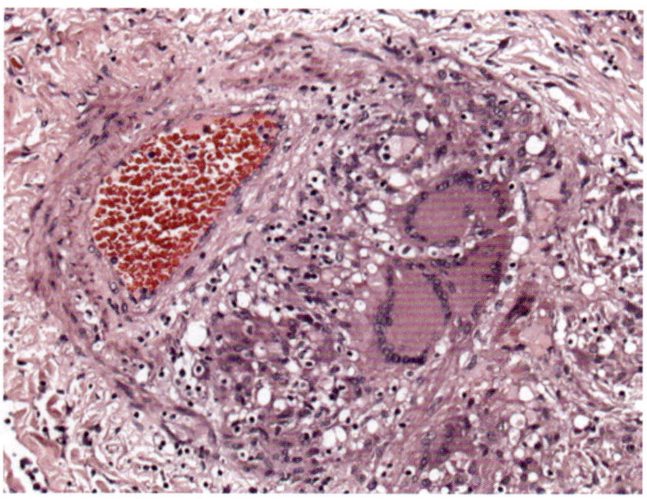

Figure 64.12 Sacoidosis: Granulomatous vasculitis may be present, but necrotizing vasculitis is not a feature of sarcoidosis.

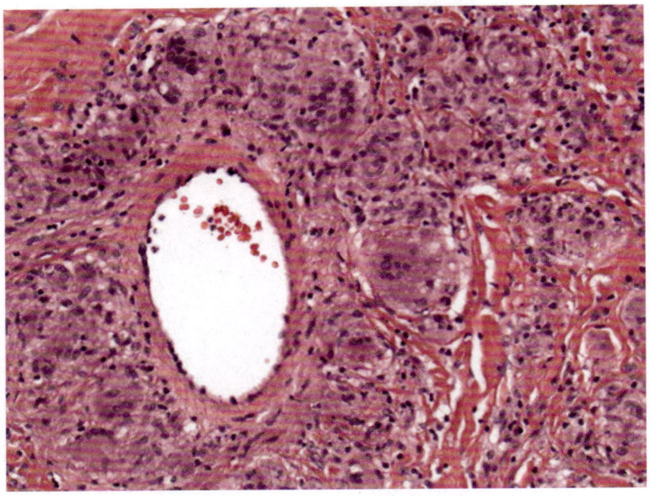

Figure 64.13 Sarcoidosis: Vasculitis with prominent multinucleated giant cells may be present, but necrotizing vasculitis is not a feature of sarcoidosis.

65 PULMONARY INFARCT VS. NECROTIZING GRANULOMA

	Pulmonary Infarct	Necrotizing Granuloma
Age	Any age; usually in adults.	Any age. Age predilection depends on etiologic factor.
Location	Pulmonary arterial infarct is classically described at the periphery of the lung, often giving a subpleural wedge-shaped appearance. However, it may affect any part of the lung. Infarcts related to pulmonary venous obstruction tend to be located near interlobular septa.	Any location, location predilection depends on etiologic factor.
Symptoms	Cough, shortness of breath, chest pain, and hemoptysis or may be asymptomatic.	Symptoms depends on etiologic factor.
Signs	Single or multiple nodular or mass lesions, infiltrates, or consolidation may be seen on chest CT.	Imaging studies show nodular lesions, with or without cavitation, which may be unilateral, bilateral, or centrilobular or have lymphatic pattern of distribution as seen in sarcoidosis.
Etiology	Pulmonary infarct is frequently due to pulmonary thromboembolism, where there is occlusion of pulmonary arteries, usually caused by emboli from deep venous thrombi and less often by in situ thrombosis of small pulmonary arteries. Other causes include angioinvasive infections (e.g., angioinvasive mycoses), angioinfiltrative primary or secondary malignancies, vasculitides, diffuse alveolar damage, amyloidosis, lobar torsion, sickle cell disease, or air, amniotic fluid, or septic emboli or infarcts due to intravascular foreign bodies including iatrogenic ones such as vascular catheters. In rare cases, it is due to pulmonary venous obstruction. Predisposing factors include history of deep venous thrombosis, recent surgery, left-sided heart diseases (e.g., congestive heart failure), and protein C deficiency, among others.	Infections (particularly due to Mycobacterium tuberculosis, nontuberculous mycobacteria, and fungal organisms). Noninfectious necrotizing granulomas as seen in nodular necrotizing sarcoidosis and granulomatosis polyangiitis (Wegener granulomatosis).
Histology	Pulmonary infarct is typically characterized by the presence of wedge, round, geographic or irregular areas showing central coagulative necrosis associated with variable amount of hemorrhage. In these zones, the shadows or ghost of alveolar septal skeleton can be discerned despite the cellular components being largely necrotic. The edge of the areas of necrosis is often surrounded by a palisading layer composed of fibroblasts/myofibroblasts, foamy macrophages, and histiocytes, creating a pseudogranulomatous appearance *(Figs. 65.1–65.3)*. The histiocytes usually lack the epithelioid transformation seen in necrotizing granulomas. Unlike necrotizing granulomas, multinucleated giant cells are usually not present at the edge of the necrosis although they may be seen in adjacent airspaces, usually as cholesterol cleft–laden multinucleated giant cells. Outside the pseudogranulomatous reaction, an inflammatory	Areas of central necrosis surrounded by a palisading layer composed of epithelioid histiocytes and frequent marginal multinucleated giant cells. In granulomatosis with polyangiitis (Wegener granulomatosis), a geographic pattern of basophilic necrosis and vascular inflammation is usually present. The distinct granulomatous reaction of activated epithelioid histiocytes, the presence of frequent marginal giant cells, and absence of areas containing shadows or ghost of alveolar septa and hemorrhage provide clues to distinguish necrotizing granulomas from pulmonary infarcts *(Figs. 65.4–65.6)*.

	Pulmonary Infarct	Necrotizing Granuloma
	margin may be seen in the form of organizing pneumonia associated with lymphoplasmacytic infiltrate, but severe inflammation is usually not a feature. Recent or organizing thrombi or various types of emboli may be found in the adjacent pulmonary arteries. This may be associated with mural inflammation, which should not be mistaken for vasculitis. In the zones of coagulative necrosis, areas of basophilic staining may be seen, composed of granular basophilic karyorrhectic debris originating from neutrophils and necrotic parenchymal cells that often extends to the margin of the pulmonary infarct, which should not be mistaken for granulomatosis with polyangiitis (Wegener granulomatosis). As infarcts organize, they can show various stages of resorption and organization including organizing pneumonia, hemosiderin-laden macrophages, hematoidin pigmentation, dystrophic calcification, squamous cell metaplasia, and alveolar pneumocyte hyperplasia. Of note, squamous cell metaplasia and alveolar pneumocyte hyperplasia are commonly seen around the periphery of the infarct and should not be mistaken for carcinoma. In pleural-based infarcts, the overlying pleura is usually viable, but fibrinous pleuritis or fibrotic pleuritis with adhesions may be seen. As the infarct continues to organize, fibroblastic proliferation, collagen deposition, and scar formation occurs. Evolution and organization depends on the size of the infarct, with large infarcts taking several months to even a year for complete collagenization.	
Special studies	Elastic tissue stains: old or late infarcts may look identical to an old granuloma since they usually round up and form well-circumscribed nodules in which residual collapsed lung parenchyma and alveolar skeleton can be appreciated. GMS and AFB special stains and tissue cultures are helpful to exclude infection.	Elastic tissue stains, which will fail to stain residual collapsed lung parenchyma and alveolar skeleton in the areas of necrosis.
Prognosis	Patients with thromboembolism are treated with anticoagulant therapy. Pulmonary hypertension, cor pulmonale, and sudden death may occur. Thromboendarterectomy can be performed in large vessels.	Prognosis depends on underlying etiology.

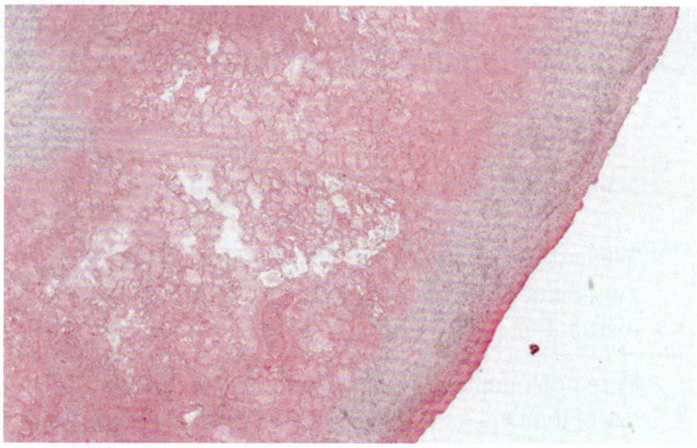

Figure 65.1 Pulmonary infarct (low power): Subpleural-based wedge area showing central coagulative necrosis and shadows or ghost of alveolar septal skeleton. The subpleural edge of the area of necrosis is surrounded by a palisading layer of viable cells.

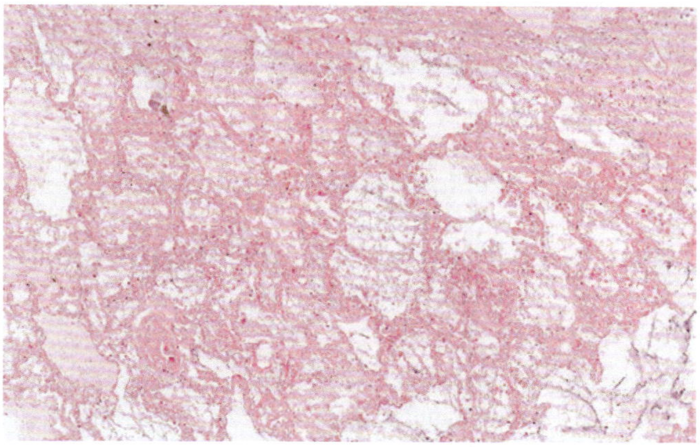

Figure 65.2 Pulmonary infarct (high power): The presence of shadows or ghost of alveolar septal skeleton is typical of pulmonary infarct and not seen in necrotizing granuloma.

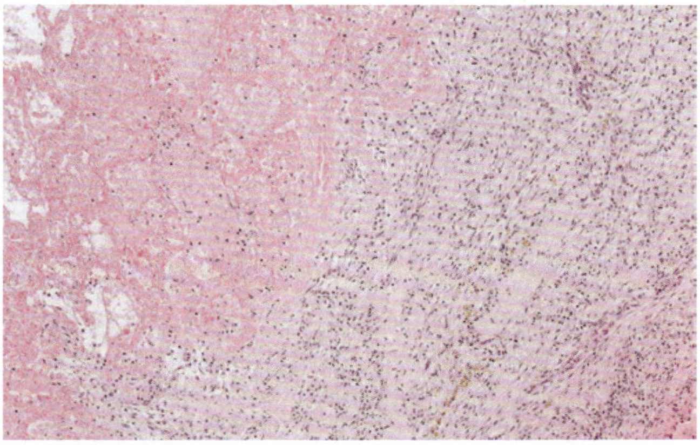

Figure 65.3 Pulmonary infarct (high power): The edge of the area of necrosis is surrounded by a palisading layer composed of fibroblasts/myofibroblasts and histiocytes, creating a pseudogranulomatous appearance. Note the absence of multinucleated giant cells or epithelioid histiocytes.

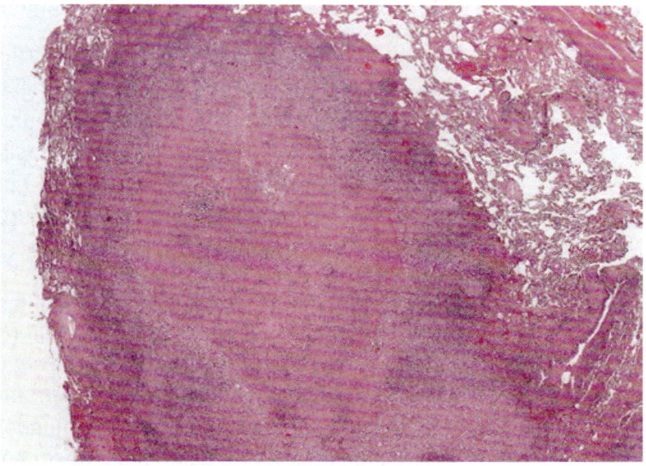

Figure 65.4 Necrotizing granuloma (low power): Central area of necrosis surrounded by a palisading cellular layer. Note the absence of shadows or ghost of alveolar septa skeleton.

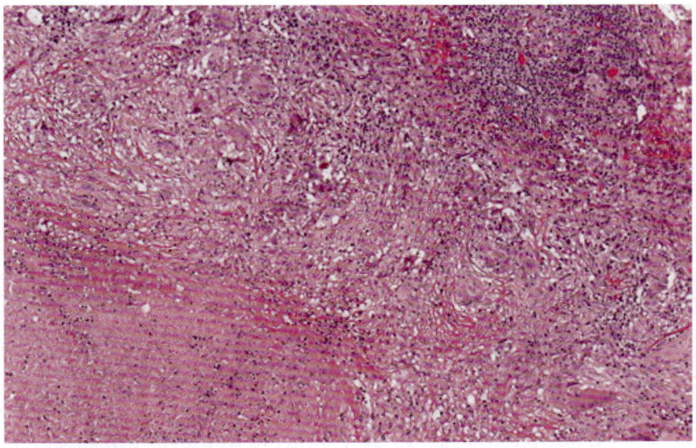

Figure 65.5 Necrotizing granuloma (high power): The central area of necrosis (*lower left corner*), is surrounded by a palisading layer composed of epithelioid histiocytes and frequent marginal multinucleated giant cells.

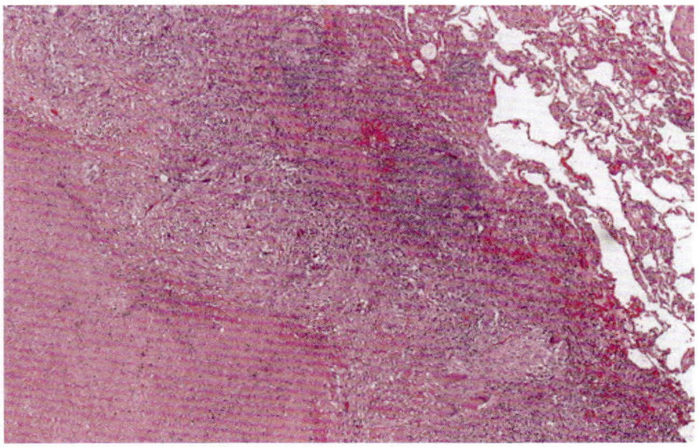

Figure 65.6 Necrotizing granuloma (high power): The presence of frequent marginal multinucleated giant cells in the palisading layer is not a feature of pulmonary infarct.

66 PERIBRONCHIOLAR METAPLASIA VS. NONMUCINOUS ADENOCARCINOMA IN SITU

	Peribronchiolar Metaplasia (PBM)	Nonmucinous Adenocarcinoma In Situ (AIS)
Age	Usually occurs between 40 and 74 y of age, with female predominance.	While there is a wide age distribution, it tends to occur in elderly individuals, with essentially equal sex distribution.
Location	Peribronchiolar/centriacinar lung zones. It may be multifocal.	Pure nonmucinous AIS usually occurs in the periphery of the lung as a solitary lesion, but it may also be multifocal. Nonmucinous AIS may be located in any region of the pulmonary lobule (panlobular), which is different from PBM (usually centrilobular).
Symptoms	Dyspnea, dyspnea on exertion, cough, and shortness of breath; can also be asymptomatic.	May be asymptomatic, and it is usually an incidental finding on CT performed for other medical reasons.
Signs	Pulmonary function tests may show obstructive, restrictive, mixed, or normal patterns. Chest CT may show a wide range of findings including airway wall thickening, bronchiolectasis, air trapping, mosaic attenuation, ground-glass opacities, interstitial thickening, traction bronchiectasis, and honeycomb change.	Chest CT usually shows solitary nonsolid peripheral lesion with ground-glass appearance. Tumors are usually ≤2 cm, but can be up to 3 cm.
Etiology	It is believed to represent a reparative phenomenon resulting from injury to small airways. It can be seen associated with a spectrum of interstitial lung diseases including hypersensitivity pneumonia, usual interstitial pneumonia, nonspecific interstitial pneumonia, desquamative interstitial pneumonia, and respiratory bronchiolitis. It can also be seen in association with connective tissue disease (e.g., rheumatoid arthritis and mixed connective tissue disease), lung cancer, thromboembolism, distal to bronchiectasis, as a component of constrictive bronchiolitis, or idiopathic.	In most cases, a specific cause cannot be identified. It may be seen in never smokers, smokers, and passive smokers. However, it is less commonly associated with smoking than other types of non–small cell lung cancer.
Histology	Proliferation of cuboid to low columnar bronchiolar epithelium (with and without cilia), beyond the respiratory bronchioles along mildly fibrosed peribronchiolar alveolar septa, replacing the normal alveolar cell lining. When the proliferation is prominent, the lesion may assume a nodular shape *(Figs. 66.1–66.3)*.	According to the 2015 WHO classification, "Localized (≤3 cm) tumor with growth restricted to neoplastic cells along preexisting alveolar structures (lepidic growth), lacking stromal, vascular, alveolar space or pleural invasion. Papillary or micropapillary growth patterns or intra-alveolar tumor cells, either within the tumor or spread in the airspaces in the surrounding parenchyma should not be present." The lesion is usually sharply demarcated. The tumor cells are relatively homogeneous; may be cuboidal, flat, or hobnail in shape; and have eosinophilic, slightly foamy cytoplasm. Eosinophilic intranuclear inclusions may or may not be present. Nuclear atypia is minimal, mild, or moderate. There is usually mild alveolar septal widening by fibrosis *(Figs. 66.4* and *66.5)*.

	Peribronchiolar Metaplasia (PBM)	Nonmucinous Adenocarcinoma In Situ (AIS)
Special studies	None.	Immunohistochemical stains for thyroid transcription factor (TTF-1), Napsin-A, and cytokeratin 7 (CK7) show positive immunoexpression. Immunohistochemical stain for cytokeratin 20 (CK20) shows negative immunoexpression.
Prognosis	Many patients are asymptomatic. In symptomatic patients there is variable response to corticosteroids ranging from stabilization and improvement to worsening with persistent progressive disease and death due to disease.	Patients with nonmucinous AIS should be 100% disease free and recurrence free if the lesion is completely excised.

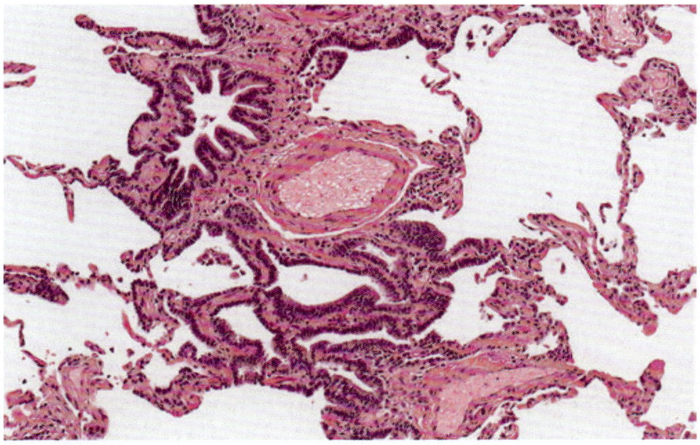

Figure 66.1 PBM: Bronchiolar epithelium proliferating along the alveolar septa.

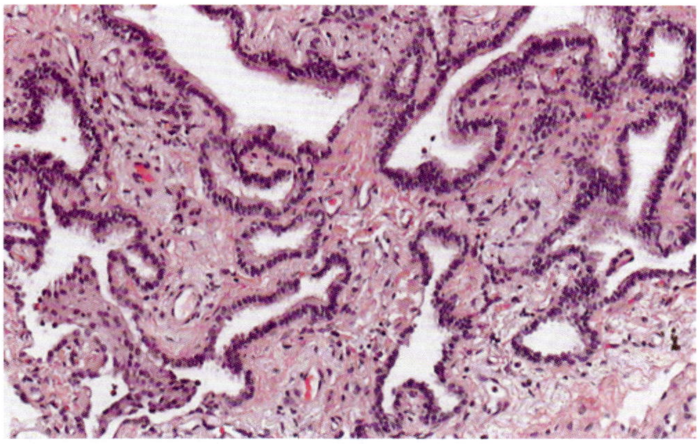

Figure 66.2 PBM: Cuboid to low columnar bronchiolar epithelium proliferating along mildly fibrosed peribronchiolar alveolar septa, replacing the normal alveolar cell lining.

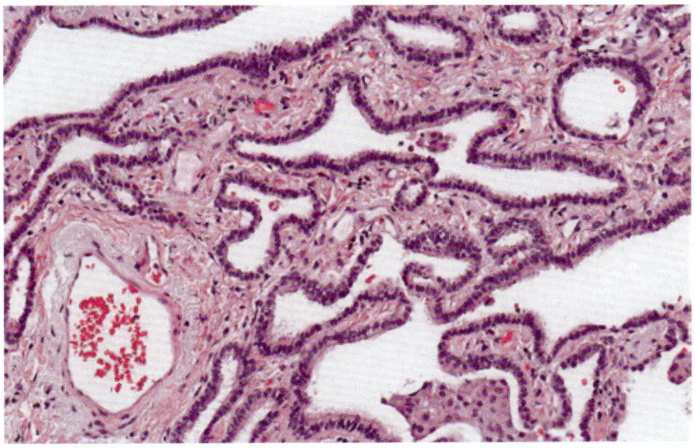

Figure 66.3 PBM: The identification of columnar ciliated epithelium is the diagnostic clue to peribronchiolar metaplasia.

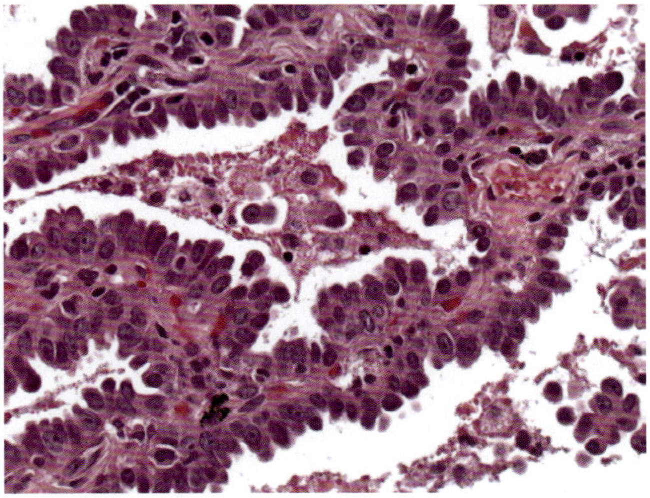

Figure 66.4 Nonmucinous AIS: Monotonous population of atypical cells growing along the alveolar septa (lepidic growth pattern), showing variable amounts of stratification and nuclear overlap, and moderate cytologic atypia. Note the lack of ciliation.

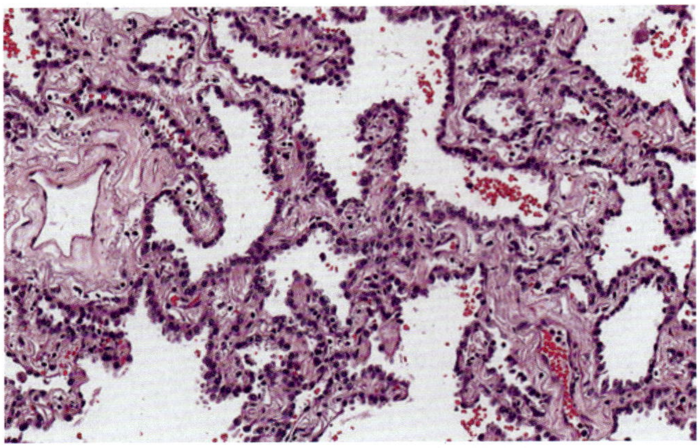

Figure 66.5 Nonmucinous AIS: There is usually mild alveolar septal widening by fibrosis.

67 ATYPICAL ADENOMATOUS HYPERPLASIA VS. NONMUCINOUS ADENOCARCINOMA IN SITU

	Atypical Adenomatous Hyperplasia (AAH)	Nonmucinous Adenocarcinoma In Situ (AIS)
Age	Usually seen in individuals ≥50 y of age. May be more common in women.	While there is a wide age distribution, it tends to occur in elderly individuals, with essentially equal sex distribution.
Location	AAH usually occurs in the periphery of the lung, frequently close to the pleura, as a small localized lesion often arising in the cetrilobular/centriacinar region near respiratory bronchioles.	Pure nonmucinous AIS usually occurs in the periphery of the lung as a solitary lesion, but it may also be multifocal. Nonmucinous AIS may be located in any region of the pulmonary lobule (panlobular), which is different from AAH (usually cetrilobular).
Symptoms	Asymptomatic.	May be asymptomatic, and it is usually an incidental finding on CT performed for other medical reasons.
Signs	AAH is usually not evident on chest CT, but may present as a faint, nonsolid nodule or ground-glass opacification of the lung parenchyma. It is usually ≤0.5 cm.	Chest CT usually shows solitary nonsolid peripheral lesion with ground-glass appearance. Tumors are usually ≤2 cm, but can be up to 3 cm.
Etiology	Unknown. It is a putative precursor of lung adenocarcinoma and is recognized in the 2015 WHO classification of lung tumors as a preinvasive lesion. Ultrastructural and immunohistochemical studies have shown that the cells in AAH can show alveolar pneumocyte or Clara cell differentiation.	In most cases, a specific cause cannot be identified. It may be seen in never smokers, smokers, and passive smokers. However, it is less commonly associated with smoking than other types of non–small cell lung cancer.
Histology	AAH is typically a *poorly demarcated* lesion composed of a single *discontinuous* layer of *heterogeneous* cells proliferating along the alveolar walls. The cells may be flattened, cuboidal, dome shaped, or low columnar. Some cells appear round or globular, and others have apical snouts, sometimes referred to as *hobnail* or "peg cells." Large round cells with double nuclei may be present. *Large gaps between the cells* are usually seen, giving a *discontinuous/interrupted* appearance. Nuclear atypia is variable, ranging from mild to moderate. Occasional tufts of cells may protrude into the alveolar spaces, but true papillae are not seen. The alveolar walls usually show mild thickening by fibrosis *(Figs. 67.1–67.4)*. The lesion is usually ≤0.5 cm but the 0.5-cm size is not an absolute criterion since larger AAHs have been reported, sometimes up to 1.2 cm. It has been proposed that most AAHs will rarely show more than one of the following criteria: (1) marked cell stratification, (2) high cell density with overlapping nuclei and no intercellular gaps, (3) coarse chromatin with prominent nucleoli, (4) "picket fence" pattern of cell	According to the 2015 WHO classification, "Localized (≤3 cm) tumor with growth restricted to neoplastic cells along preexisting alveolar structures (lepidic growth), lacking stromal, vascular, alveolar space or pleural invasion. Papillary or micropapillary growth patterns or intra-alveolar tumor cells, either within the tumor or spread in the airspaces in the surrounding parenchyma should not be present." The lesion is usually *sharply demarcated*. The tumor cells are relatively *homogeneous*; may be cuboidal, flat, or hobnail in shape; and have eosinophilic, slightly foamy cytoplasm. Eosinophilic intranuclear inclusions may or may not be present. Nuclear atypia is minimal, mild, or moderate. There is usually mild alveolar septal widening by fibrosis *(Figs. 67.5–67.8)*. Some lesions demonstrate features intermediate between AAH and nonmucinous AIS and can be problematic. Observation of monotonous population of atypical cells would favor nonmucinous AIS, while a heterogenous cell population

	Atypical Adenomatous Hyperplasia (AAH)	Nonmucinous Adenocarcinoma In Situ (AIS)
	growth, and (5) columnar cells with increased cell height exceeding that of the columnar cells of adjacent terminal bronchioles.	without consistent nuclear atypia would favor AAH. It has been proposed that nonmucinous AIS usually shows three or more of the following criteria: (1) marked cell stratification, (2) high cell density with overlapping nuclei and no intercellular gaps, (3) coarse chromatin with prominent nucleoli, (4) "picket fence" pattern of cell growth, (5) columnar cells with increased cell height exceeding that of the columnar cells of adjacent terminal bronchioles.
Special studies	Not helpful.	Immunoperoxidase stains for thyroid transcription factor 1 (TTF-1), Napsin-A, and cytokeratin 7 (CK7), show positive expression. Immunoperoxidase stain for cytokeratin 20 (CK20), shows negative expression.
Prognosis	Patients with resected AAH are 100% disease free. AAH is frequently found in nonneoplastic lung as an incidental histologic finding in lungs bearing primary cancer, especially adenocarcinoma. The prognosis of lung adenocarcinomas with AAH has not been shown to be different from the prognosis of those without AAH.	Patients with nonmucinous AIS should be 100% disease free and recurrence free if the lesion is completely excised.

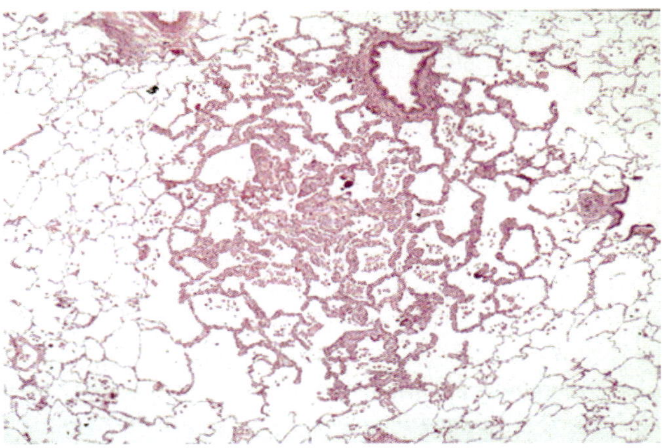

Figure 67.1 AAH (low power): *Poorly* demarcated, *centrilobular* lesion growing along preexisting alveolar structures (lepidic growth pattern).

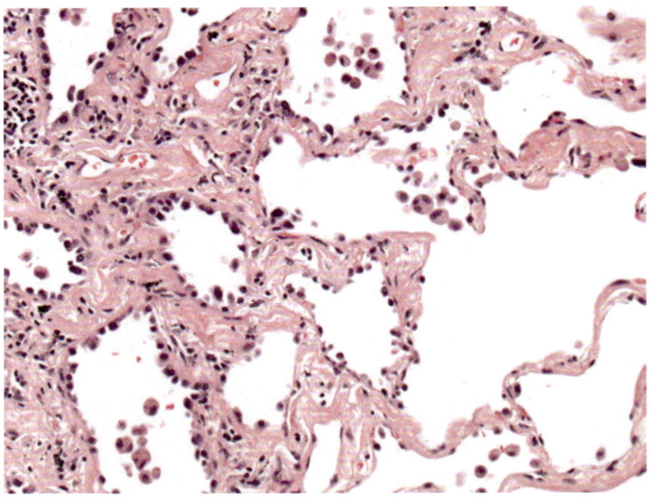

Figure 67.2 AAH: AAH is composed of *heterogeneous* cells growing in a *discontinuous* lepidic growth pattern lacking stromal invasion. The alveolar walls usually show mild thickening by fibrosis.

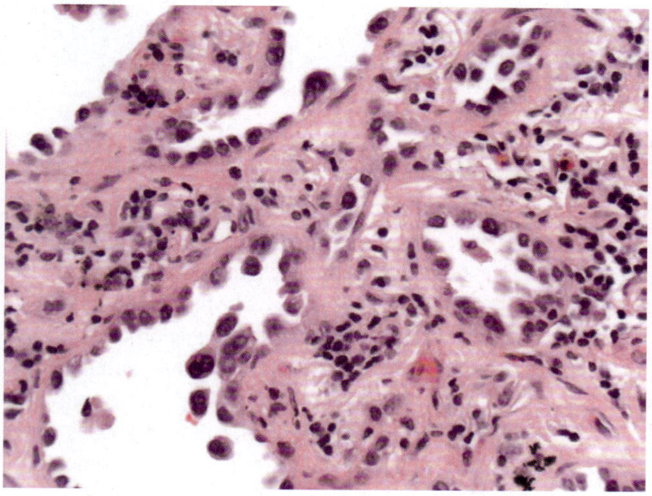

Figure 67.3 AAH: Heterogenous flattened, cuboidal, dome-shaped, low-columnar, and hobnail cells proliferating along the alveolar walls showing no stratification or cell overlap with mild-to-moderate cytologic atypia.

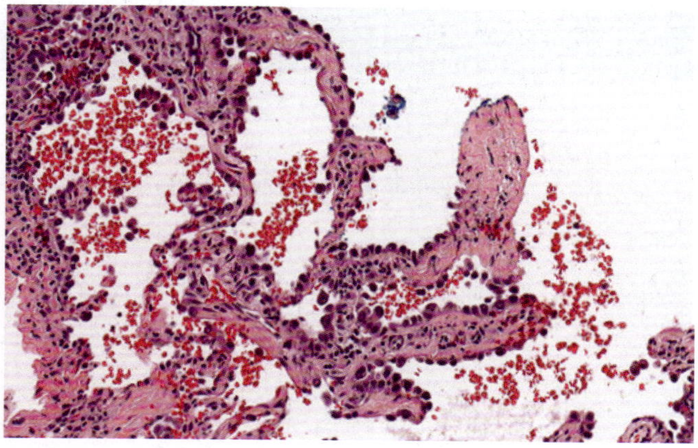

Figure 67.4 AAH: *Heterogeneous* cells growing in a lepidic growth pattern. *Large gaps between the cells* are usually seen, giving a *discontinuous/interrupted* appearance.

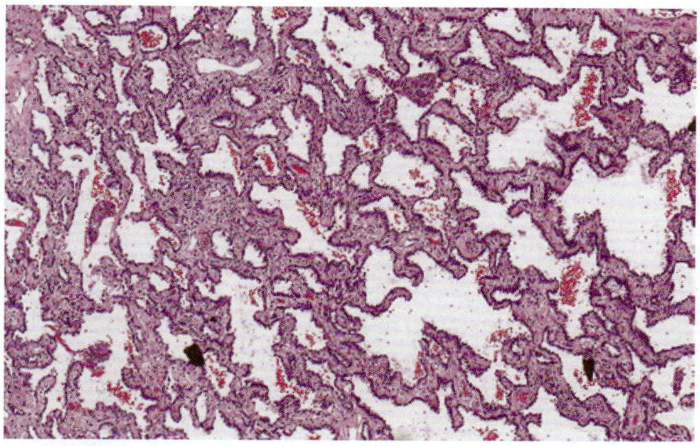

Figure 67.5 Nonmucinous AIS (low power): Usually a *sharply demarcated panlobular* lesion composed of relatively *homogeneous/monotonous* tumor cells growing in a *continuous* lepidic growth pattern lacking stromal invasion is seen.

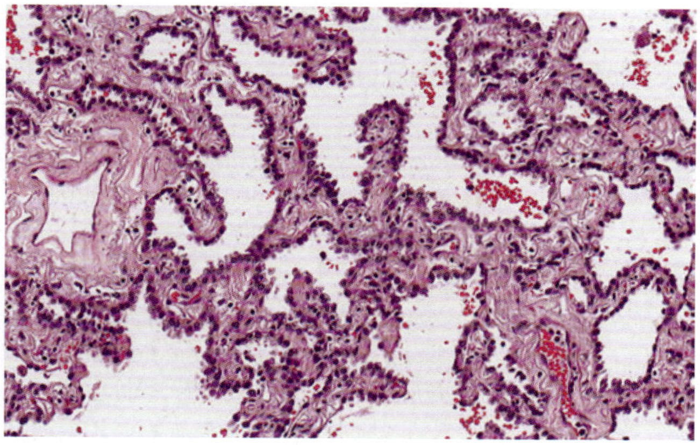

Figure 67.6 Nonmucinous AIS: *Homogeneous/monotonous* crowded cuboidal-shaped tumor cells growing in a continuous lepidic growth pattern. There is usually mild alveolar septal widening by fibrosis.

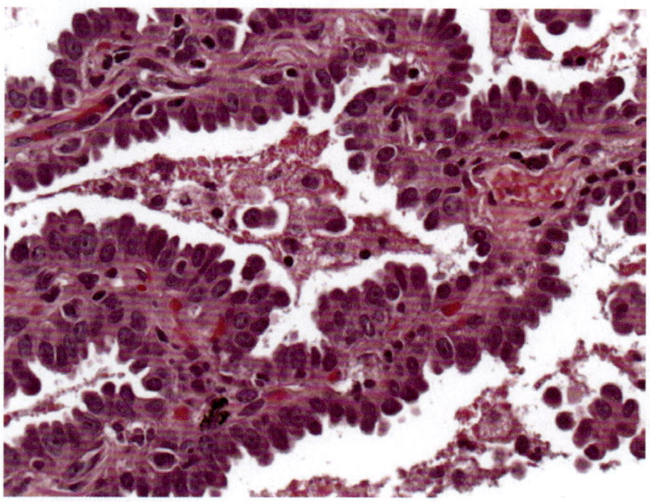

Figure 67.7 Nonmucinous AIS: Monotonous population of atypical cells showing cell stratification and overlapping nuclei. Note lack of intercellular gaps typical of AAH.

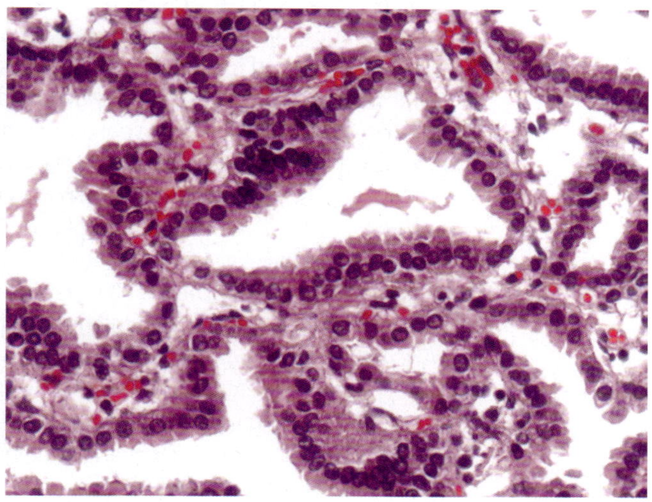

Figure 67.8 Nonmucinous AIS: The presence of continuos monotonous population of atypical cells supports the diagnosis of nonmucinous AIS, in contrast to AAH, which typically shows a discontinuous heterogeneous cell population without consistent nuclear atypia.

68 ATYPICAL ADENOMATOUS HYPERPLASIA VS. MICRONODULAR TYPE II PNEUMOCYTE HYPERPLASIA

	Atypical Adenomatous Hyperplasia (AAH)	Micronodular Type II Pneumocyte Hyperplasia (MNPH)
Age	Usually seen in individuals ≥50 y of age. May be more common in women.	Usually a pulmonary manifestation of tuberous sclerosis (TS), which occurs in association with lymphangioleiomyomatosis (LAM). In this setting, it can occur in men and women. When MNPH occurs in sporadic cases of LAM, it almost always affects childbearing to middle-aged women.
Location	AAH usually occurs in the periphery of the lung, frequently close to the pleura, as a small localized lesion often arising in the cetrilobular/centriacinar region near respiratory bronchioles.	May be seen diffusely and randomly distributed throughout the lungs.
Symptoms	Asymptomatic.	Dyspnea on exertion and pneumothorax if associated with LAM.
Signs	AAH is usually not evident on chest CT, but may present as a faint, nonsolid nodule or ground-glass opacification of the lung parenchyma. It is usually ≤0.5 cm.	High-resolution computed tomography (HRCT) demonstrates multifocal, random, well-defined small nodular parenchymal densities, usually measuring 1–3 mm.
Etiology	Unknown. Ultrastructural and immunohistochemical studies have shown that the cells in AAH can show alveolar pneumocyte or Clara cell differentiation.	Unknown. It is a rare benign hamartomatous proliferation of type II pneumocytes most often found in patients with TS. The lesion can also occur in patients with sporadic lymphangioleyomiomatosis.
Histology	AAH is typically a poorly demarcated lesion composed of a single discontinuous layer of heterogeneous cells proliferating along the alveolar walls. The cells may be flattened, cuboidal, dome shaped, or low columnar. Some cells appear round or globular, and others have apical snouts, sometimes referred to as *hobnail* or "peg cells." Large round cells with double nuclei may be present. Large gaps between the cells are usually seen, giving a discontinuous/interrupted appearance. Nuclear atypia is variable, ranging from mild to moderate. Occasional tufts of cells may protrude into the alveolar spaces, but true papillae are not seen. The alveolar walls usually show mild thickening by fibrosis *(Figs. 68.1–68.4)*. The lesion is usually ≤0.5 cm, but the 0.5-cm size is not an absolute criterion since larger AAHs have been reported, sometimes up to 1.2 cm. It has been proposed that most AAHs will rarely show more than one of the following criteria: (1) marked cell stratification, (2) high cell density with overlapping nuclei and no intercellular gaps, (3) coarse chromatin with prominent nucleoli, (4) "picket fence" pattern of cell growth, and (5) columnar cells with increased cell height exceeding that of the columnar cells of adjacent terminal bronchioles.	Nodular areas composed of a proliferation of homogeneous and plump enlarged cuboidal or hobnail-shaped benign alveolar type II pneumocytes lining a mildly thickened alveolar septa. The adjacent alveolar spaces are small, distorted, and frequently filled by macrophages, giving the lesion a solid appearance *(Figs. 68.5–68.7)*.

	Atypical Adenomatous Hyperplasia (AAH)	Micronodular Type II Pneumocyte Hyperplasia (MNPH)
Special studies	Usually not necessary.	The proliferating type II pneumocytes stain for cytokeratin, EMA, BER-EP4, and often surfactant apoprotein B and tuberin, and are negative for CD1a and HMB-45.
Prognosis	Patients with resected AAH are 100% disease free. AAH is frequently found in nonneoplastic lung as an incidental histologic finding in lungs bearing primary cancer, especially adenocarcinoma. The prognosis of lung adenocarcinomas with AAH has not been shown to be different from the prognosis of those without AAH.	MNPH itself is not progressive and therefore treatment is not required. Prognosis depends on severity of symptoms from underlying TS and/or LAM.

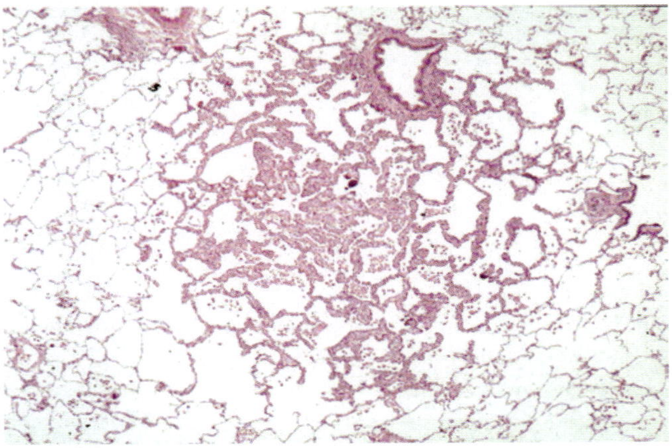

Figure 68.1 AAH (low power): *Poorly* demarcated, *centrilobular* lesion growing along preexisting alveolar structures (lepidic growth pattern).

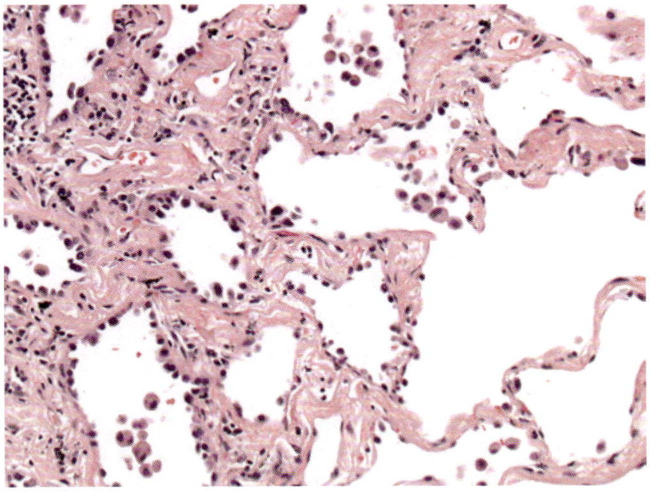

Figure 68.2 AAH: AAH is composed of heterogeneous cells growing in a *discontinuous* lepidic growth pattern lacking stromal invasion. The alveolar walls usually show mild thickening by fibrosis.

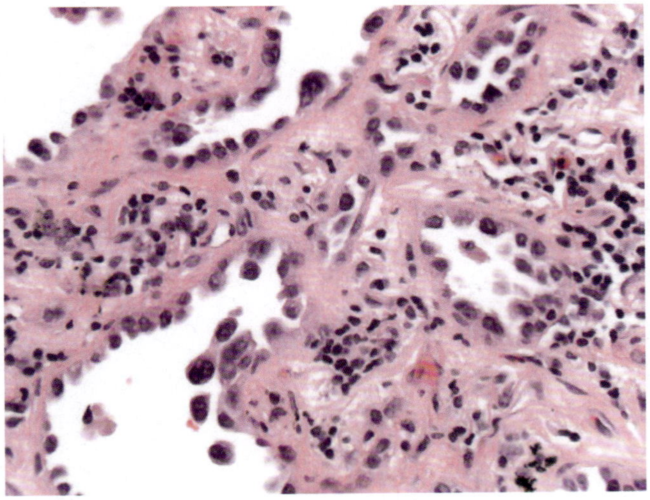

Figure 68.3 AAH: Heterogenous, flattened, cuboidal, dome-shaped, low-columnar, and hobnail cells proliferating along the alveolar walls showing no stratification or cell overlap with mild-to-moderate cytologic atypia.

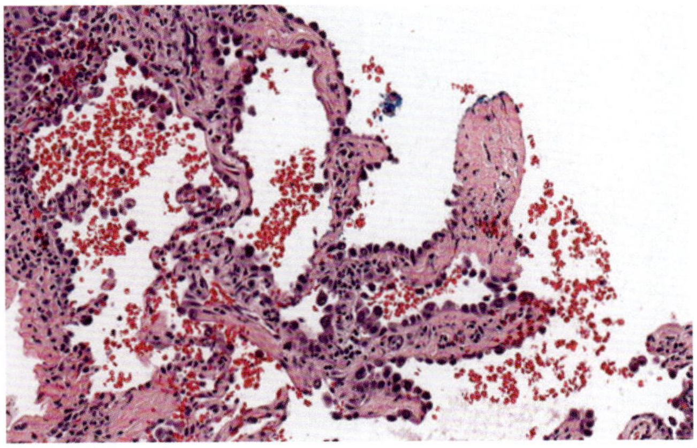

Figure 68.4 AAH: Heterogeneous cells growing in a lepidic growth pattern. *Large gaps between the cells* are usually seen, giving a *discontinuous/interrupted* appearance.

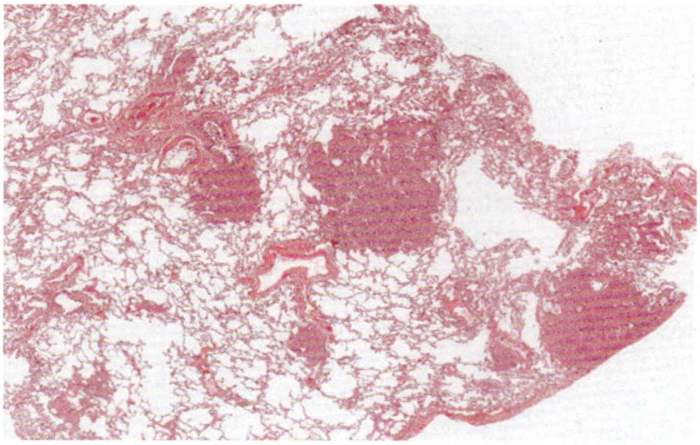

Figure 68.5 MNPH (low power): Cellular nodular lesions.

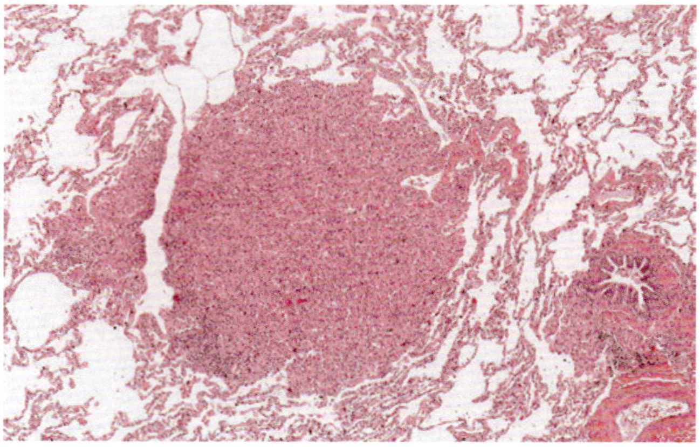

Figure 68.6 MNPH (medium power): The cellular nodular lesion is composed of a proliferation of alveolar type II pneumocytes.

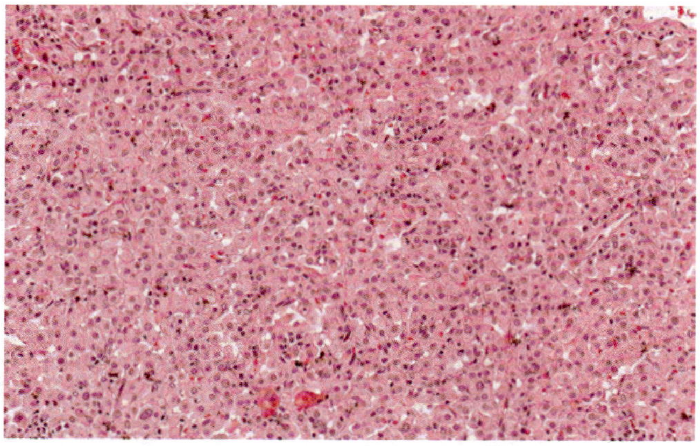

Figure 68.7 MNPH (high power): Cellular nodular proliferation of homogeneous and plump enlarged benign alveolar type II pneumocytes. The alveolar septa may be thickened by scarring and the adjacent small and distorted alveolar spaces are frequently filled by macrophages, giving the lesion a solid appearance.

69 MENINGOTHELIAL-LIKE MICRONODULES VS. CARCINOID TUMORLETS

	Meningothelial-Like Micronodules (MNLMs)	Carcinoid Tumorlets
Age	MNLMs usually occur in adults older than 40 y of age with a mean age in the 60s and female predilection.	Carcinoid tumorlets generally occur in patients around 50–70 y of age, with female predilection.
Location	They occur randomly anywhere in the pulmonary interstitium (alveolar septa), often, but not always, around blood vessels.	Typically located in the wall of bronchioles or in areas of scarring. They are often multifocal and bilateral.
Symptoms	Usually asymptomatic. In the vast majority of cases, pulmonary MNLMs are incidental findings of no clinical significance, encountered in lung biopsies or resection specimens performed for other reasons. In rare cases, however, they are numerous and reported to cause clinical symptoms including dyspnea and cough.	Most patients tend to be asymptomatic at diagnosis. Cases associated with diffuse idiopathic pulmonary neuroendocrine cell hyperplasia (DIPNECH) may be asymptomatic or present with long history of cough and breathlessness.
Signs	Chest CT demonstrates incidental or bilateral micronodules and in rare cases reticulonodular interstitial infiltrates. Pulmonary function tests may show mild restrictive changes.	Carcinoid tumorlets may be seen as small pulmonary nodules on chest CT. Pulmonary function tests in cases associated with DIPNECH may show obstructive or mixed obstructive/restrictive pattern.
Etiology	The origin of these lesions remains uncertain. MNLMs can be encountered in association with virtually any form of lung disease, including various types of chronic interstitial lung disease, organizing pneumonia, diffuse alveolar damage, granulomatous inflammation, malignant tumors, and vascular disease. The similarity of the immunohistochemical staining pattern and the ultrastructural findings in MNLMs to meningiomas along with the lack of neuroendocrine differentiation led to the name meningothelial-like nodule. However, data utilizing loss of heterozygosity (LOH) genotyping analysis have failed to confirm genetic similarity to meningiomas. Whether diffuse pulmonary meningotheliomatosis arises from incidental MNLMs or whether it is a separate disease is not clear.	Unknown. They are usually incidental histologic or radiologic discoveries. They are commonly seen associated with chronic inflammatory pulmonary disease, particularly chronic small and large airway inflammation and within scars. They can also be found in normal lung parenchyma and as part of DIPNECH.

	Meningothelial-Like Micronodules (MNLMs)	Carcinoid Tumorlets
Histology	Meningothelial-like nodules are interstitial cellular proliferations composed of cells with morphologic features that resemble meningothelial cells (e.g., those seen in meningothelial meningiomas) including syncytial sheets, whorl-like pattern, and bland nuclear features. The cells are typically uniform, epithelioid, with round to oval nuclei, abundant cytoplasm, and indistinct cell membranes *(Figs. 69.1 and 69.2)*. There is usually no admixed inflammatory component, but fibrosis may be present in the background. The extremely unusual condition in which patients with innumerable meningothelial-like nodules present with clinical and radiologic evidence of interstitial lung disease has been termed *diffuse pulmonary meningotheliomatosis*. The morphology of diffuse pulmonary meningotheliomatosis lesions is identical to incidental MNLMs.	Small, often multiple nodular proliferations ($<$0.5 cm) of pulmonary neuroendocrine cells within the epithelium with breaching of the basement membrane and extension into adjacent connective tissue. The cells are oval to spindle shaped with coarsely granular (salt-and-pepper) chromatin. They lack mitotic activity and necrosis *(Figs. 69.3–69.6)*.
Special studies	Positive expression for epithelial membrane antigen (EMA), vimentin, and CD56 (weak and patchy). Negative expression for cytokeratin, muscle markers (SMA, desmin), vascular markers (CD34, CD31, F-VIII, D2-40), melanoma markers (HMB45, S100), estrogen receptor (ER), TTF-1, and the neuroendocrine markers synaptophysin and chromogranin.	In contrast to MNLMs, carcinoid tumorlets stain with cytokeratin, synaptophysin, and chromogranin. The use of CD56 as a neuroendocrine marker in this setting may be a pitfall since CD56 stains carcinoid tumorlets and also stains meningothelial-like micronodules. However, CD56 staining in meningothelial-like micronodules is typically weak and patchy, whereas it is usually strong and diffuse in carcinoid tumorlets. Synpatophysin or chromogranin staining will help making the distinction.
Prognosis	Incidental MNLMs have no prognostic significance, and very little follow-up is available for patients with diffuse pulmonary meningotheliomatosis. In those few followed-up cases, the lung lesions appear stable or only slowly progressive.	In many cases, they are incidental histologic findings of no importance or clinical consequences. In cases where carcinoid tumorlets are part of DIPNECH, they can be associated with a chronic slowly progressive disease of either obstructive or mixed obstructive/restrictive pattern or develop progressive constrictive bronchiolitis.

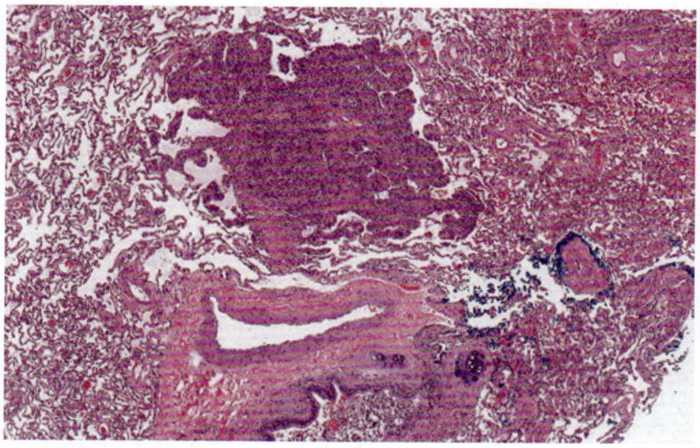

Figure 69.1 MNLM (low power): Stellate-shaped interstitial nodule. They occur randomly anywhere in the pulmonary interstitium (alveolar septa), often but not always around blood vessels.

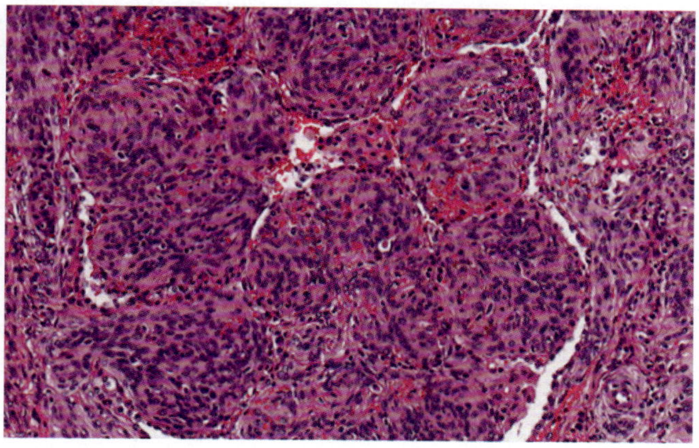

Figure 69.2 MNLM (high power): The nodular lesion is composed of nests of uniform, epithelioid cells with round to oval nuclei, abundant cytoplasm, and indistinct cell membranes.

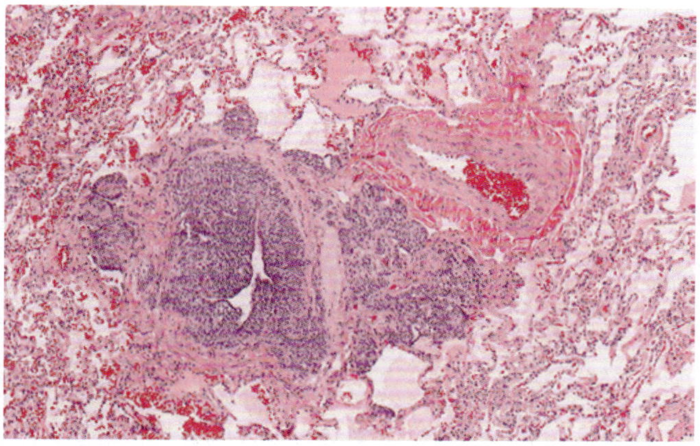

Figure 69.3 Carcinoid tumorlets: It is typically located in the wall of bronchioles or in areas of scarring. There are proliferations of pulmonary neuroendocrine cells within the bronchial epithelium with breaching of the basement membrane and extension into the bronchial wall and adjacent connective tissue.

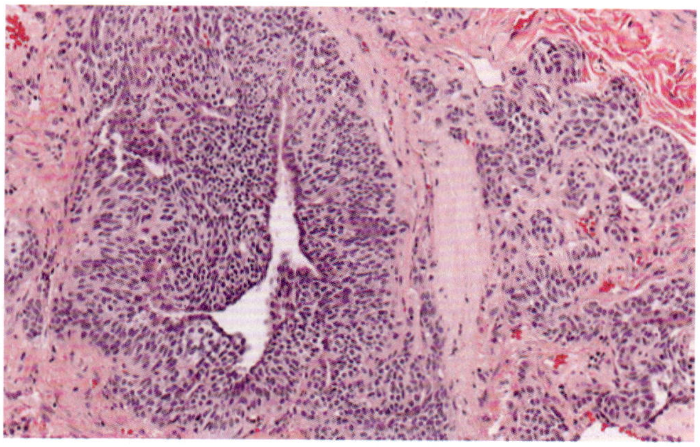

Figure 69.4 Carcinoid tumorlets: The cells are oval to spindle shaped, with coarsely granular (salt-and-pepper) chromatin.

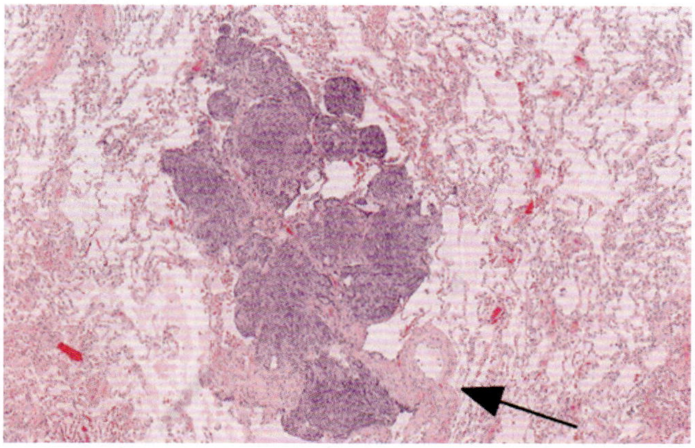

Figure 69.5 Carcinoid tumorlets: Proliferation of spindle-shaped neuroendocrine cells, which obliterate the bronchiole. The corresponding small pulmonary artery is seen in the lower middle field (*arrow*).

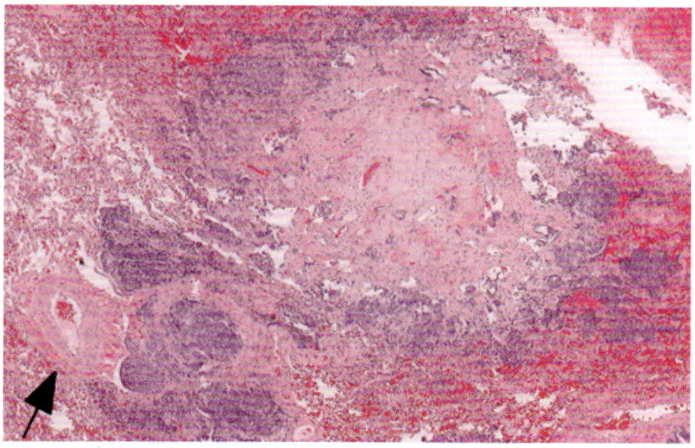

Figure 69.6 Carcinoid tumorlets: Proliferation of neuroendocrine cells associated with scarring that has completely replaced the bronchiole. The corresponding small pulmonary artery is seen in the lower left field (*arrow*).

70 TYPICAL CARCINOID VS. ATYPICAL CARCINOID

	Typical Carcinoid (TC)	Atypical Carcinoid (AC)
Age	TC usually occurs in individuals <60 y of age with an average presentation at 45 y of age. While many studies indicate approximately equal male and female distribution, some studies indicate slight female predominance.	AC occurs in slightly older age group (around 60 y of age) compared with TC, with female predominance.
Location	TC usually presents as a central endobronchial mass, although approximately one-third of TC are peripherally located and may not have an obvious associated airway.	Same as TC. More ACs arise peripherally than TC.
Symptoms	Central tumors may be associated with cough, wheezing, hemoptysis, stridor, or obstructive symptoms, while peripheral tumors may be asymptomatic. Clinical syndromes due to peptide production are uncommon and usually associated with metastasis, but include carcinoid syndrome, Cushing syndrome, and acromegaly. Occasional carcinoids are associated with multiple endocrine neoplasia type 1 (MEN1) syndrome or diffuse idiopathic pulmonary neuroendocrine cell hyperplasia (DIPNECH).	Same as TC.
Signs	Chest CT shows well-circumscribed nodules, usually central and less often peripheral. Calcification can occur. The lesion is usually PET negative.	Same as TC. More ACs arise peripherally than TC.
Etiology	Unknown. Fewer than half of patients with TC are current or former cigarette smokers.	Unknown. While the majority of carcinoid patients are never-smokers or light smokers, AC is more associated with current or former smokers than TC patients. Approximately 60% of patients have clinical history of cigarette smoking.
Histology	TC typically has an organoid pattern of growth with variable arrangement of tumor in single-cell nests, ribbons, or trabeculae growth pattern, which is usually associated with arborizing vascular network. Other patterns include pseudorosettes formation, pseudoglandular growth, follicular growth, or papillary growth. Spindle cell morphology may be seen, particularly in peripheral tumors. The tumor cells are typically uniform, polygonal in shape, with central nuclei, finely granular to coarsely stippled (salt and pepper) nuclear chromatin, inconspicuous nucleoli, and moderate to abundant amount of eosinophilic cytoplasm. Cells with pronounced pleomorphism or prominent nucleoli may be present, which should not be taken as criteria for AC. The stroma may show unusual features such as calcification, ossification, or deposition of amyloid-like material *(Figs. 70.1–70.9)*. According the 2015 WHO classification, the defining features are "≥0.5 cm, lack of necrosis and mitotic rate of 0–1 mitosis/2 mm^2 area of tumor." Carcinoid tumors range in size from 0.5 to 9.5 cm. Nodular neuroendocrine proliferations measuring <0.5 cm are classified as carcinoid tumorlets.	AC generally shows the same range of histological features as TC. The defining features according the 2015 WHO classification are "the presence of 2–10 mitoses/2 mm^2 area of tumor and/or the presence of necrosis or both." As these discriminating features may be present only focally, the absence of these features on a core or bronchoscopic biopsy does not exclude AC. Therefore, small biopsies should be designated as "carcinoid tumor" with final classification left to a resected specimen *(Figs. 70.10 and 70.11)*.

	Typical Carcinoid (TC)	Atypical Carcinoid (AC)
Special studies	Neuroendocrine markers strong expression including CD56, synaptophysin, and chromogranin. 80% of tumor stains for pancytokeratin. TTF-1 is typically negative but may be expressed in one-third of cases, particularly in peripheral tumors. In contrast with small cell lung carcinoma, TTF-1 is considered supportive of primary pulmonary origin in pulmonary carcinoids. The Ki-67 (MIB-1) proliferation marker may show nuclear staining in up to 5% of TC tumor cells.	Same as TC. The Ki-67 (MIB-1) proliferation marker may show nuclear staining in up to 20% of AC tumor cells.
Prognosis	Treatment of TC is generally surgical. TC is in general associated with a favorable prognosis with a 5-y survival rate of 85%–90%. In a small percentage of cases (approximately 15%), metastasis to lymph nodes have been reported.	Like TC, AC is treated surgically. AC has worse prognosis compared with TC, with a 5-y survival rate of 60%–70% and a 10-y survival of 35%–50%. AC is more likely to metastasize than TC. Lymph node metastasis is present at the time of diagnosis in approximately 30%–40% of patients.

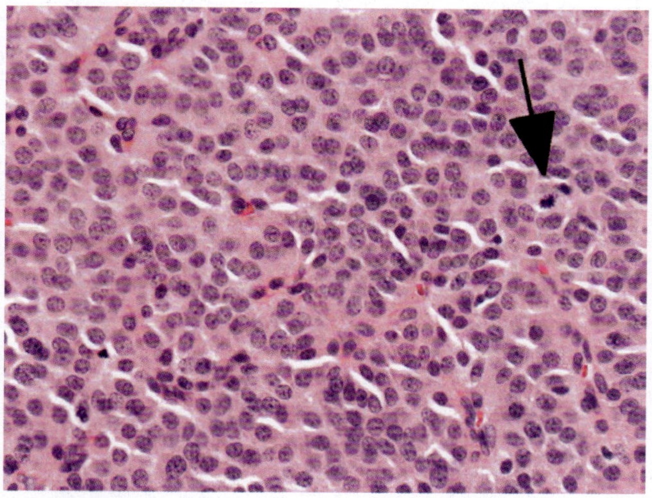

Figure 70.1 TC (high power): The tumor cells in TC and AC have similar morphology showing typically uniform cells, polygonal in shape, with central nuclei, finely granular nuclear chromatin, inconspicuous nucleoli, and moderate to abundant amount of eosinophilic cytoplasm. In this case, note the presence of one mitotic figure (*upper right/arrow*).

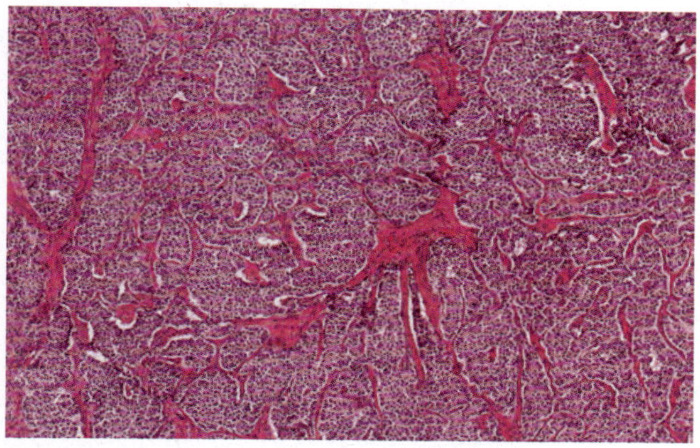

Figure 70.2 TC: TC with cells arranged in a typical organoid growth pattern lying within an arborizing vascular network.

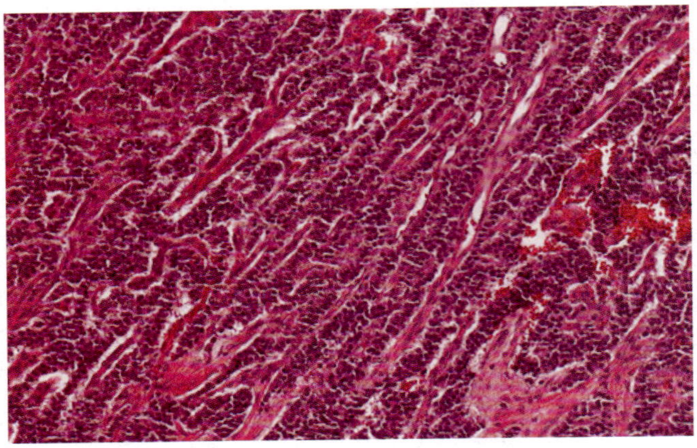

Figure 70.3 TC: TC with trabecular growth pattern.

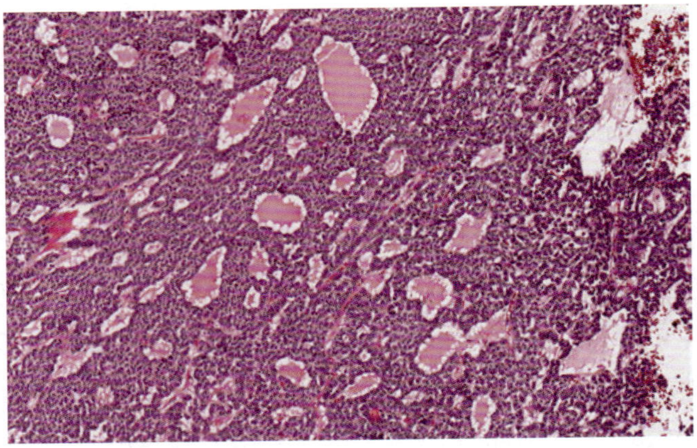

Figure 70.4 TC: TC with follicular growth pattern mimicking the appearance of thyroid follicles.

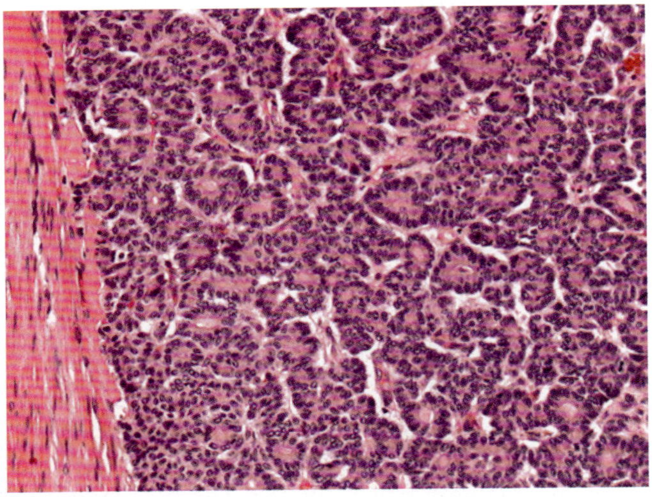

Figure 70.5 TC: TC with pseudorosette formation.

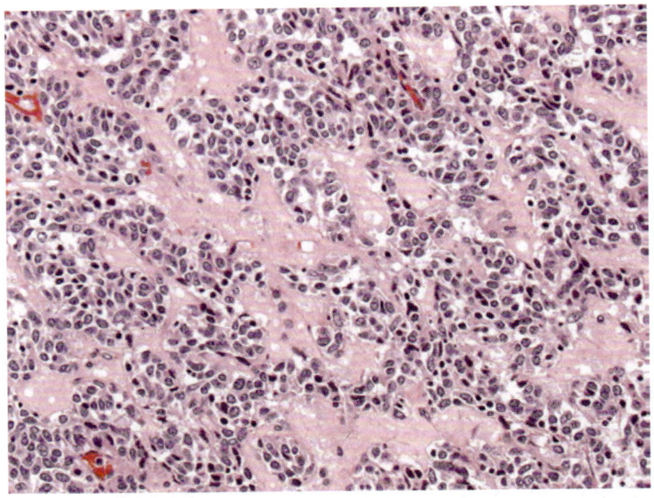

Figure 70.6 TC: TC associated with hyalinized collagenous stroma resembling amyloid.

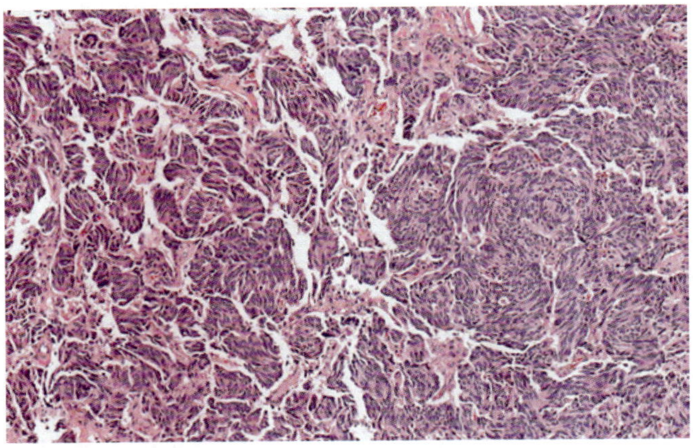

Figure 70.7 TC: TC with spindle cell morphology, which is usually seen in peripheral tumors.

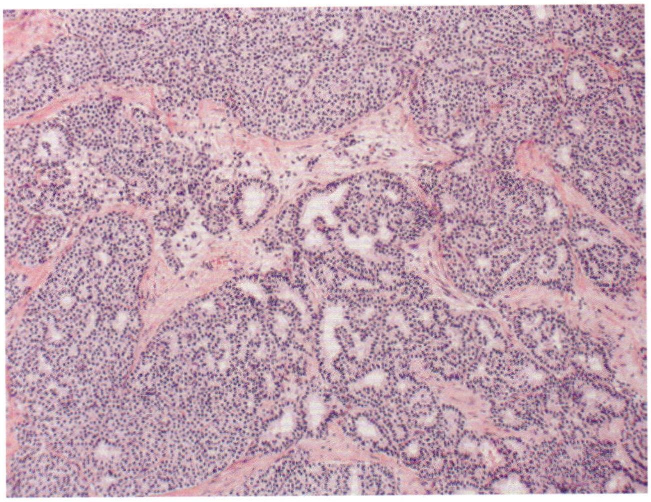

Figure 70.8 TC: TC with pseudoglandular growth pattern. (Courtesy of Dr. Yale Rosen.)

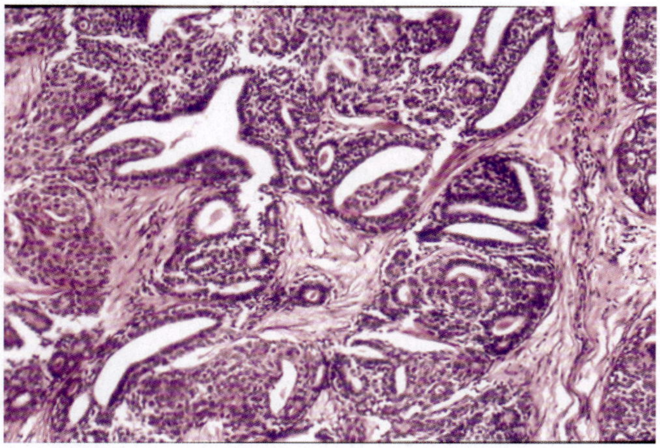

Figure 70.9 TC: Another example of TC with pseudoglandular growth pattern. (Courtesy of Dr. Yale Rosen.)

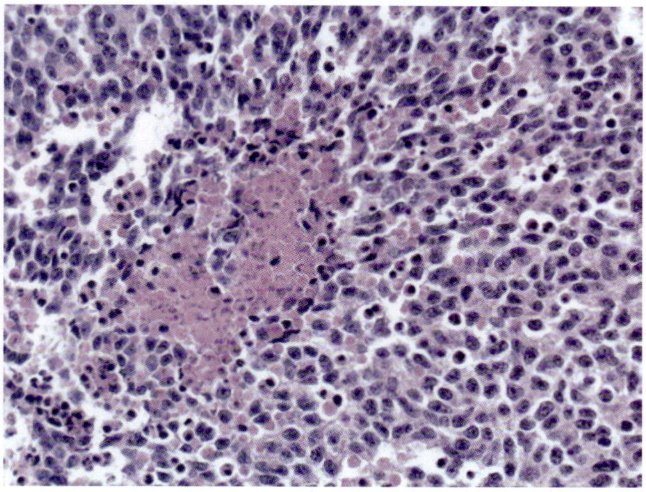

Figure 70.10 AC: Note area of necrosis (*middle field*). Necrosis is not a feature of TC.

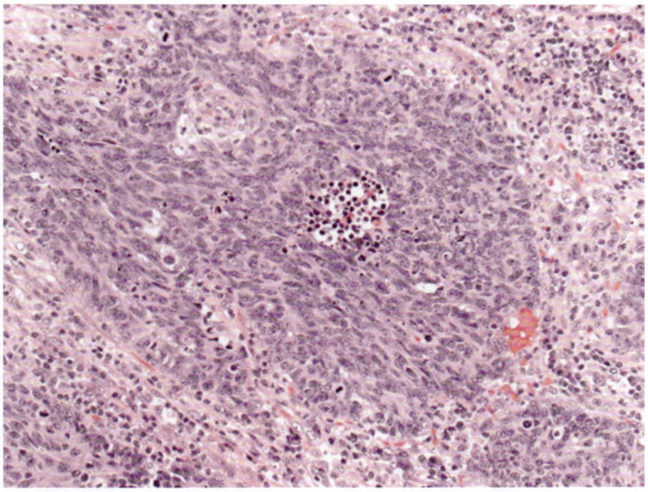

Figure 70.11 AC: Six mitotic figure areas noted. Except for mitotic count (2–10 mitotic figures/2 mm^2) and/or the presence of necrosis, AC tumor cells are histologically similar to those of TC with similar growth patterns.

71 ATYPICAL CARCINOID VS. SMALL CELL LUNG CARCINOMA

	Atypical Carcinoid (AC)	**Small Cell Lung Carcinoma (SCLC)**
Age	AC affects people between 47 and 60 y of age, with predominance in women.	SCLC affects people between 40 and 70 y of age. SCLC is seen almost exclusively in heavy cigarette smokers and is more common in men.
Location	AC may present as a central endobronchial mass or as a peripherally located lesion.	SCLC is usually located centrally in the major airways, but may occur peripherally in the lungs in about 5% of cases.
Symptoms	Central tumors may be associated with cough, wheezing, hemoptysis, stridor, or obstructive symptoms, while peripheral tumors may be asymptomatic. Clinical syndromes due to peptide production are uncommon and usually associated with metastasis, but include carcinoid syndrome, Cushing syndrome, and acromegaly. Occasional ACs are associated with multiple endocrine neoplasia type 1 (MEN1) syndrome or diffuse idiopathic pulmonary neuroendocrine cell hyperplasia (DIPNECH).	Patients often present with rapid onset signs or symptoms due to local intrathoracic tumor growth, extrapulmonary distant spread, paraneoplastic syndromes, or a combination of these features. Symptoms may include cough, dyspnea, hemoptysis, weight loss, or other constitutional symptoms. Superior vena cava syndrome is a presenting finding in 10% of patients. Associated paraneoplastic syndromes such as hyponatremia (due to inappropriate secretion of antidiuretic hormone), Cushing syndrome, Lambert–Eaton myasthenic syndrome, peripheral neuropathy, or limbic encephalopathy may be observed.
Signs	Chest CT shows central or peripherally located well-circumscribed nodules. Calcification can occur. The lesion is usually PET negative.	SCLC classically presents as a large hilar mass with extensive mediastinal lymphadenopathy and lobar collapse on chest CT. A minority of cases may present with peripheral masses.

	Atypical Carcinoid (AC)	Small Cell Lung Carcinoma (SCLC)
Etiology	Unknown. While the majority of carcinoid patients are never-smokers or light smokers, approximately 60% of patients with AC have a clinical history of cigarette smoking.	It is highly linked to tobacco smoking.
Histology	ACs generally show the same range of histologic features of typical carcinoid (refer to chapter 70, Figures 70.1 to 70.9), and usually have an organoid pattern of growth with variable arrangement of tumor in single-cell nests, ribbons, or trabeculae growth pattern, which is usually associated with arborizing vascular network. Other patterns include pseudorosette formation, pseudoglandular growth, follicular growth, or papillary growth. Spindle cell morphology may be seen, particularly in peripheral tumors. The tumor cells are typically uniform, polygonal in shape, with central nuclei, finely granular to coarsely stippled (salt and pepper) nuclear chromatin, inconspicuous nucleoli, and ***moderate-to-abundant amount of eosinophilic cytoplasm***. Cells with pronounced pleomorphism or prominent nucleoli may be present. The stroma may show unusual features such as calcification, ossification, or deposition of amyloid-like material. According to the 2015 WHO classification, the defining features of AC are "the presence of 2–10 mitoses/2 mm^2 area of tumor and/or the presence of necrosis or both" *(Figs. 71.1 and 71.2)*. As these discriminating features may be present only focally, the absence of these features on a core or bronchoscopic biopsy does not exclude AC. Therefore, small biopsies should be designated as "carcinoid tumor," with final classification based on a resected specimen.	Sheet-like growth without a neuroendocrine architecture is the most frequent growth pattern, although trabeculae, peripheral palisading, and rosette formation may be seen. The tumor cells are small sized (generally less than the diameter of 3–4 small lymphocytes), have oval- to spindle-shaped nuclei, ***scant or almost indiscernible cytoplasm***, finely granular nuclear chromatin with a "salt-and-pepper appearance" and absent or faint nucleoli. The nuclear-to-cytoplasmic (N/C) ratio is very high. Nuclear molding, crushing artifact, and encrustation of blood vessels with basophilic material, the so-called Azzopardi phenomenon, may be observed *(Figs. 71.3–71.5)*. While the mitotic rate is by definition (2015 WHO classification) $>$10 mitoses/2 mm^2 area of tumor, it usually ranges from 50 to 60 with a median of 80 mitoses/2 mm^2. On small transbronchial (TBBX) biopsies, SCLC may exhibit significant crushing artifact. Such cases should be interpreted with caution as other tumors including carcinoid, lymphoma, and basaloid squamous cell carcinoma may also show considerable crushing artifact. In needle-core biopsies and larger or resected specimens, the cells of SCLC may appear larger in comparison with their appearance on a TBBX and have slightly more discernable cytoplasm; however, in comparison with lymphocytes, the cells remain proportionally small and the N/C ratios remain very high.

	Atypical Carcinoid (AC)	Small Cell Lung Carcinoma (SCLC)
Special studies	Neuroendocrine markers strong expression including CD56, synaptophysin, and chromogranin. About 80% of tumors stain for pancytokeratin. TTF-1 is typically negative but may be expressed in one-third of cases, particularly in peripheral tumors. In contrast with SCLC, TTF-1 is considered supportive of primary pulmonary origin in carcinoids. The Ki-67 (MIB-1) proliferation marker may show nuclear staining in up to 20% of AC tumor cells.	A panel of neuroendocrine markers including CD56, synaptophysin, and chromogranin A is useful. CD56 is the most sensitive marker, but it is also less specific. Synaptophysin and CD56 can diffusely and strongly stain SCLC, while chromogranin A can be more focal and weak. It should be noted that $<$10% of SCLC can be negative or only focally positive for neuroendocrine marker expression. SCLC usually stains positive for cytokeratin markers (e.g., AE1/AE3, CAM5.3) and characteristically exhibits a dot-like, perinuclear, or diffuse cytoplasmic staining pattern. CK 7 is frequently negative, but may be positive in a minority of cases. CK 20 is consistently negative. TTF-1 is positive in the majority (90%–95%) of SCLC cases but, unlike TTF-1 expression in carcinoid tumors, TTF-1 expression in SCLC does not definitively support a pulmonary origin and may be found in SCLC arising in other locations. Napsin-A is consistently negative. Testing for the Ki-67 (MIB-1) proliferation marker should be performed whenever possible, particularly in small biopsies to avoid misdiagnosing carcinoid tumors in the presence of crushing artifact. The Ki-67 index is much higher than in AC and usually shows nuclear staining in 50%–100% of SCLC tumor cells.
Prognosis	AC is treated surgically. AC has better prognosis compared with SCLC with a 5-y survival rate of 60%–70% and a 10-y survival rate of 35%–50%. Lymph node metastasis is present at the time of diagnosis in approximately 30%–40% of patients.	SCLC frequently presents at an advanced stage and has a poor prognosis with a 2-y survival rate of only 10% with metastatic disease, and a 5-y survival rate of approximately 25% when there is no metastatic involvement. The median overall survival time is 12.7 mo. Chemotherapy is the usual treatment. Surgical resection and chemotherapy are performed in some centers for limited disease.

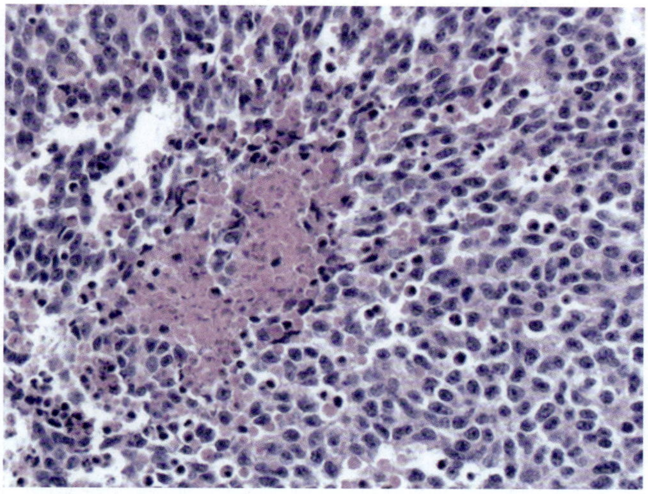

Figure 71.1 AC (low power): AC generally shows the same range of growth patterns and cytologic features seen in TC (seen in chapter 70, Figures 70.1 to 70.9). The defining features of AC are the presence of 2–10 mitoses/2 mm^2 area of tumor and/or the presence of necrosis or both. Note the area of necrosis (*middle left*).

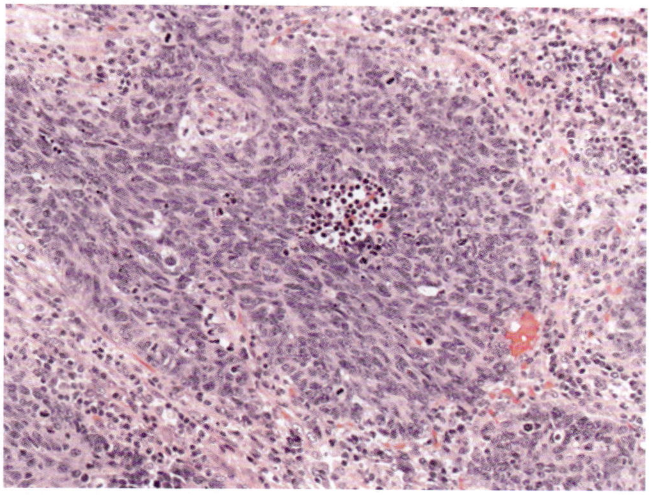

Figure 71.2 AC: The defining features of AC are "the presence of 2–10 mitoses/2 mm^2 area of tumor and/or the presence of necrosis or both." Six mitotic figures are noted in this figure. The amount of eosinophilc (pink)cytoplasm seen in AC tumos cells is greater than the amount of cytoplas seen in SCLC tumor cells, which have characteristic scant or almost indiscernible cytoplasm.

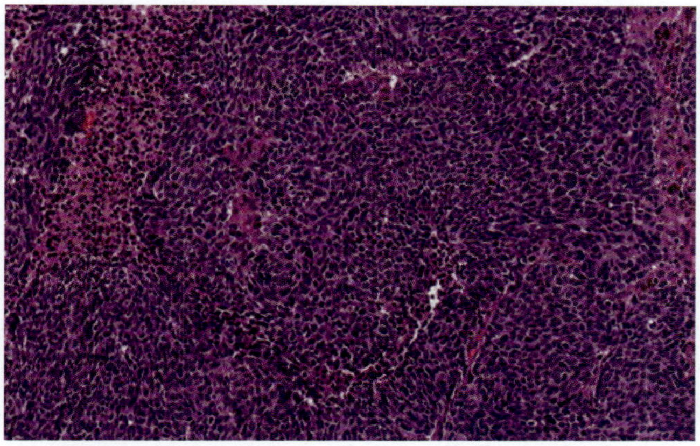

Figure 71.3 SCLC: The tumor cells usually show a sheet-like growth pattern.

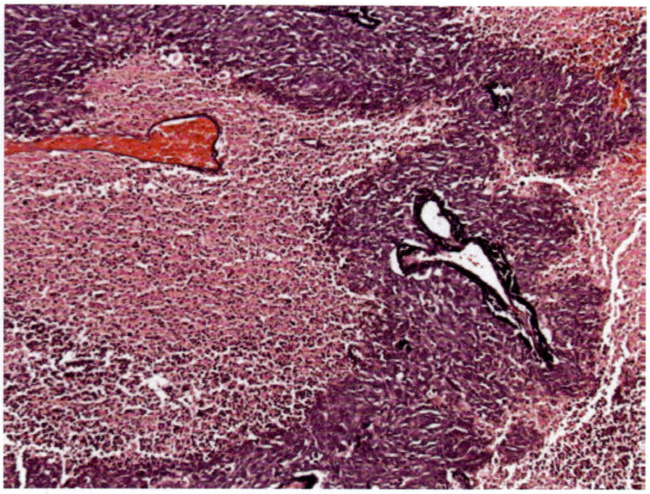

Figure 71.4 SCLC: Extensive area of necrosis is observed. Note Azzopardi effect (*middle right*) characterized by the presence of crushed DNA around a blood vessel in this largely necrotic tumor.

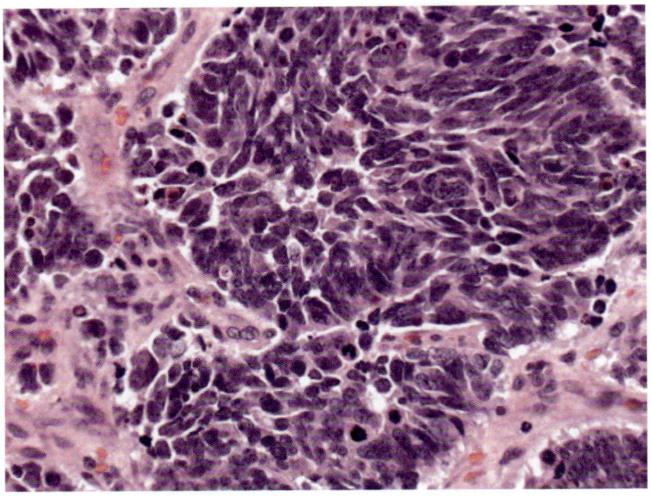

Figure 71.5 SCLC: The tumor cells are small sized (generally less than the diameter of 3–4 small lymphocytes), have oval- to spindle-shaped nuclei, *scant or almost indiscernible cytoplasm*, finely granular nuclear chromatin, and absent nucleoli. The nuclear-to-cytoplasmic (N/C) ratio is very high.

72 ADENOCARCINOMA VS. SQUAMOUS CELL CARCINOMA

	Adenocarcinoma	Squamous Cell Carcinoma (SQCC)
Age	Wide age distribution, ranging from 20 y to more than 70 y. It is the most common cell type of lung cancer in both genders, replacing SQCC over the past several decades.	Wide age distribution, occurs more in men than in women, and is closely correlated with history of tobacco smoking. The incidence has been decreasing compared to adenocarcinomas.
Location	While most (about 75%) pulmonary adenocarcinomas are peripheral parenchymal masses, centrally located adenocarcinomas may also occur.	It is usually centrally located (75% of cases), arising from the proximal bronchi. However, SQCC may originate in the peripheral pulmonary parenchyma.
Symptoms	Wide variety of symptoms. The most common symptoms include progressive shortness of breath, cough, chest pain/pressure, or constitutional symptoms. Due to predominant peripheral location, adenocarcinomas may be discovered as an incidental mass or nodule on image studies performed for other reasons and thus may not present clinical symptoms.	SQCC tends to produce symptoms at an earlier stage than adenocarcinomas. Symptoms may include cough, shortness of breath, chest pain, hemoptysis, and constitutional symptoms. Endobronchial growth may occlude the airway lumen causing bronchiectasis, infection, or bronchopneumonia.
Signs	Image studies usually demonstrate a single peripheral mass or multiple nodular tumors. They may also present as pneumonia-like consolidation on chest image studies. Subpleural tumors may be associated with pleural thickening, pleural space involvement, and pleural effusion. Some rare subpleural tumors may present with predominant growth on the pleural surface and encase the lung in a diffuse malignant mesothelioma-like pattern referred to as *pseudomesotheliomatous carcinoma*.	Image studies usually demonstrate proximal masses in the hilar and perihilar areas or proximal airways.
Etiology	Atypical adenomatous hyperplasia (AAH) is believed to be the precursor lesion of peripheral pulmonary adenocarcinomas, and progression from AAH to adenocarcinoma in situ (AIS) to invasive adenocarcinoma has been proposed. Although most adenocarcinomas are caused by tobacco smoking, it is also the most frequent cell type in patients who have never smoked.	SQCC arises from progressive squamous epithelial dysplasia and has a strong association with tobacco smoking.

	Adenocarcinoma	Squamous Cell Carcinoma (SQCC)
Histology	Adenocarcinomas are defined as carcinomas with gland formation and/or mucin production. The 2015 WHO classification of pulmonary adenocarcinomas includes subtypes of several growth patterns: lepidic, acinar, papillary, micropapillary, and solid *(Figs. 72.1–72.5)*. Some solid poorly differentiated adenocarcinomas have dense eosinophilic cytoplasm that resembles SQCC, but lack diagnostic squamous features such as keratinization, keratin pearls, or intercellular bridges (see *Fig. 72.9*). Other variants include invasive mucinous adenocarcinoma, colloid adenocarcinoma, fetal adenocarcinoma, and enteric adenocarcinoma. If sampled adequately, virtually all pulmonary adenocarcinomas are of mixed subtypes, although one subtype usually predominates. According to the 2011 IASLC/ATS/ERS and 2015 WHO classifications, the classification of invasive adenocarcinoma should include the predominant subtype after comprehensive histological subtyping by semiquantitatively estimating the percentage of the various subtypes present in 5% increments.	SQCC may be keratinizing or nonkeratinizing. Keratinizing SQCC is characterized by the presence of keratinization, keratin pearl formation, and/or intercellular bridges *(Figs. 72.6–72.8)*. In nonkeratinizing SQCC, immunohistochemistry is required to distinguish it from poorly differentiated adenocarcinoma. Some SQCCs may show papillary, clear cell, small cell, and basaloid morphology. According to the 2015 WHO classification, this subtyping classification is no longer recommended, except for the basaloid morphology because at this point there is no evidence to suggest that papillary, small cell, and clear cell morphology have either prognostic or molecular significance.

	Adenocarcinoma	Squamous Cell Carcinoma (SQCC)
Special studies	The most important reason for performing immunostains is to confirm the primary site of origin in the lung and to confirm adenocarcinoma cell type as opposed to SQCC cell type, before starting bevacizumab or pemetrexed therapy. Most pulmonary adenocarcinomas are immunopositive for a variety of cytokeratins including AE1/AE3, CK7, and CAM 5.2, but are usually negative for CK5/6 and p40 (which are usually immunopositive in SQCC), and CK20 (except for mucinous adenocarcinoma and enteric adenocarcinoma). Thyroid transcription factor-1 (TTF-1) shows immunopositivity in 75%–85% of pulmonary adenocarcinomas. Napsin-A has comparable sensitivity with that of TTF-1, although some reports have suggested that TTF-1 is superior for differentiation from SQCC. In poorly differentiated adenocarcinomas with solid growth pattern, the presence of ≥5 tumor cells in at least two high-power fields showing intracytoplasmic mucin droplets or mucin within glandular lumen is also a supportive diagnostic feature, which can be demonstrated with mucicarmine, PAS, or Alcian blue stains. Molecular testing for epidermal growth factor receptor (EGFR) gene mutational analysis and anaplastic lymphoma kinase (ALK) gene rearrangement is important for treatment management. Activating mutations in EGFR gene are clustered in exons 18–21. The two most common EGFR gene mutations are in-frame deletions in exon 19 (45%), followed by point mutation (CTG to CGC) in exon 21 at nucleotide 2573, which result in substitution of leucine by arginine at codon 858 (L858R) (41%). EML4-ALK fusion accounts for >90% of ALK gene rearrangements in lung adenocarcinoma. EGFR gene mutation and ALK gene rearrangement are more commonly found in never-smoker patients with adenocarcinoma. EGFR mutations are more common in Asian patients and women. V-Ki-ras2 Kirsten rat sarcoma (KRAS) gene mutations in codons 12, 13, or 61 are present in 30% of adenocarcinomas and are particularly common in smokers.	Poorly differentiated, solid-type SQCC of the lung may be difficult to distinguish from poorly differentiated, solid-type adenocarcinoma *(Fig. 72.9)*. Differentiation of solid-type SQCC from solid-type adenocarcinoma is very important in selecting appropriate therapeutic agents. For instance, bevacizumab may cause fatal hemorrhage in patients with SQCC. Diffuse positive staining with squamous markers CK5/6 and p40 and negativity for TTF-1 confirm squamous cell type. The squamous marker p63 may be positive in 16-65% of lung adenocarcinomas. Therefore, given p63 low specificity it is not recommended using this marker to distinguish adenocarcinoma from squamous cell carcinoma. According to the 2015 WHO classification, the presence of intracellular mucin in a few cells does not exclude tumors from this category.

	Adenocarcinoma	Squamous Cell Carcinoma (SQCC)
Prognosis	Never-smoking status and female sex are favorable prognostic factors independent from the tumor stage. Tumor size ≥2.5 cm, solid and micropapillary subtypes, and a maximum standardized uptake value (SUV) of ≥7 are predictors of poor disease-free survival. The prognosis for stage I lepidic predominant adenocarcinoma is usually good, unless associated with close margin in limited resection, visceral pleural invasion, and/or angiolymphatic invasion or the presence of micropapillary growth pattern component. Tumors with EGFR mutation may respond favorably to EGFR tyrosine kinase inhibitors (EGFR TKIs) such as gefitinib and erlotinib. Tumors with ALK gene rearrangement may respond favorably to ALK blockade with crizotinib. Of note, in-frame insertion mutations in EGFR exon 20 are associated with primary resistance to EGFR TKI. Acquisition of an additional T790M mutation is the most common cause of secondary resistance to EGFR TKI. However, using more sensitive mutation-detection techniques, it was shown that T790M EGFR mutation may coexist with L858R mutations, which might confer pretreatment (primary) resistance to EGFR TKIs. Amplification of MET gene is another mechanism of EGFR TKIs resistance. The presence of KRAS mutation is usually associated with resistance to EGFR TKIs.	The prognosis of SQCC is mainly dependent on the patient's clinical tumor stage, with the highest stages having the worst prognosis. The 5-y survival rate for SQCC is generally better than that of adenocarcinoma. SQCC tends to metastasize later than other types of non–small cell lung carcinoma.

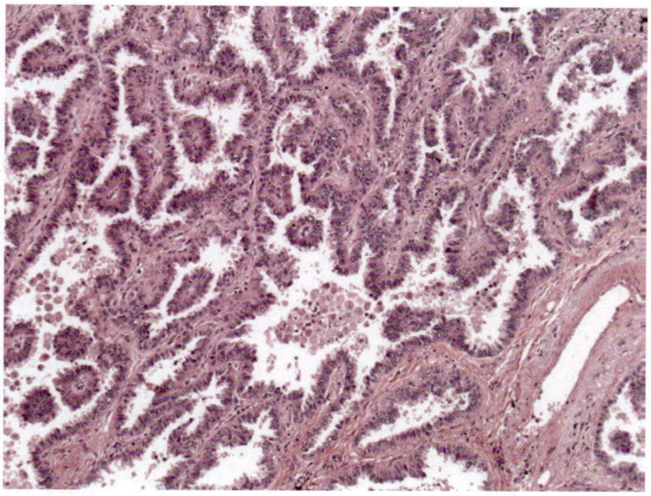

Figure 72.1 Lepidic adenocarcinoma: The tumor cells grow along the surface of the alveolar walls.

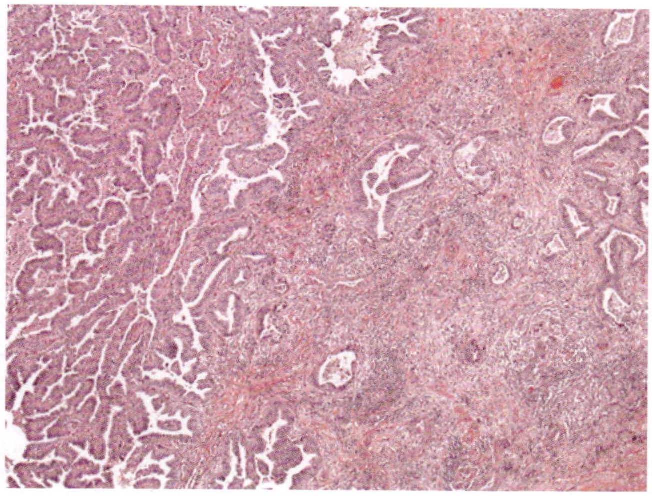

Figure 72.2 Adenocarcinoma: Lepidic adenocarcinoma (*left*) and acinar adenocarcinoma characterized by the presence of malignant glands within a fibro-inflammatory stroma (*right*).

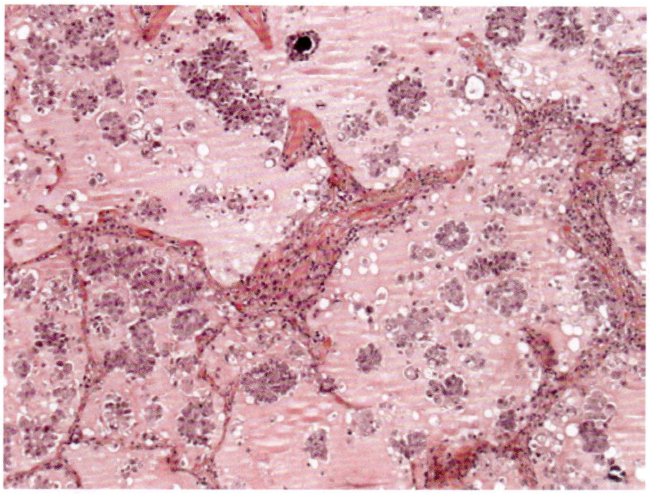

Figures 72.3 Micropapillary adenocarcinoma: Dyscohesive papillary clusters of cytologically malignant cells "float" within the air spaces. The tumor cells form papillae that lack fibrovascular core.

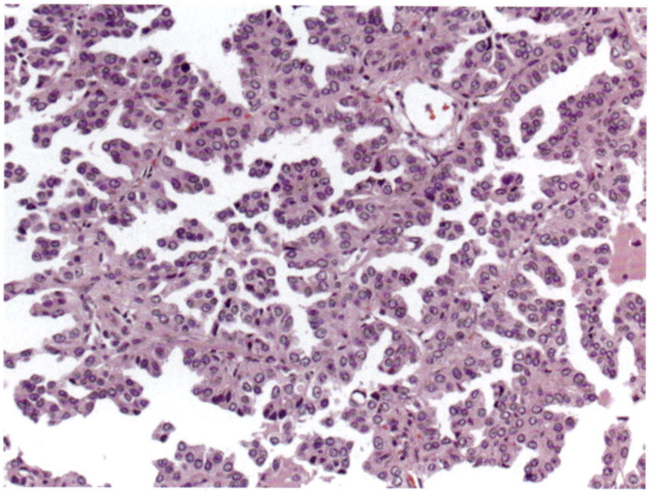

Figure 72.4 Papillary adenocarcinoma: The tumor cells form true papillary structures with papillae lined by glandular epithelium surrounding a fibrovascular core.

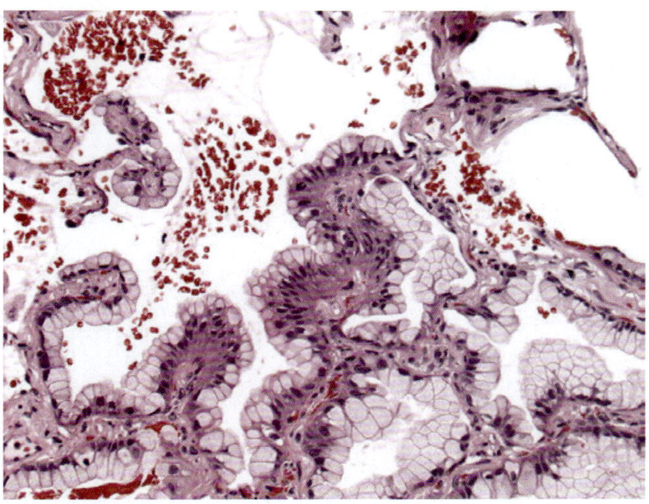

Figure 72.5 Mucinous adenocarcinoma: The columnar mucinous tumor cells grow in a lepidic growth pattern.

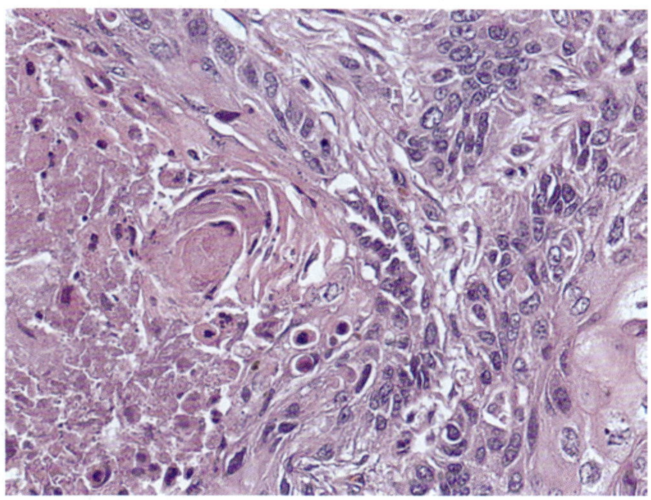

Figure 72.6 SQCC: Squamous differentiation manifesting as keratinization of single cells and keratin pearl formation.

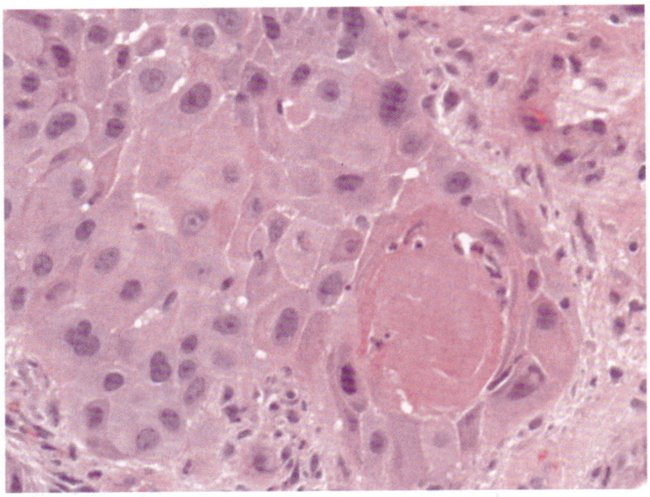

Figure 72.7 SQCC: Squamous differentiation manifesting as keratin pearl formation and intercellular bridges.

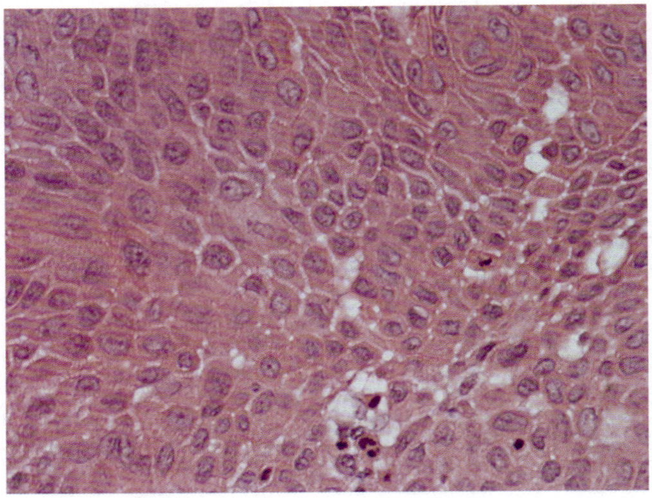

Figure 72.8 SQCC: Squamous differentiation manifesting as intercellular bridges.

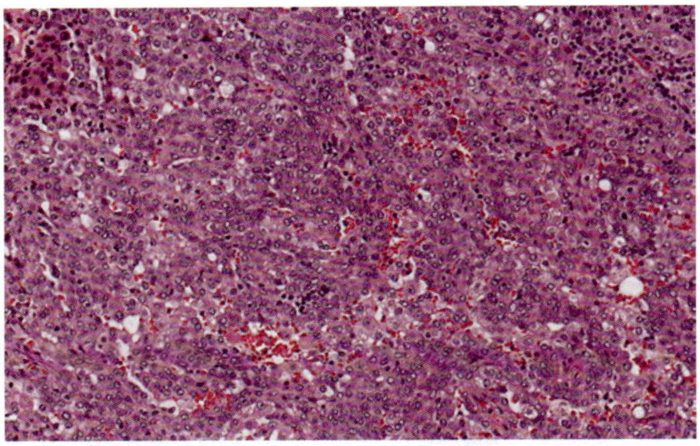

Figure 72.9 Solid adenocarcinoma: Poorly differentiated tumor with no glandular or squamous differentiation. In this poorly differentiated carcinoma with solid growth pattern, immunoperoxidase stains are of paramount importance to differentiate adenocarcinoma solid type from nonkeratinizing poorly differentiated SQCC. In this case, the tumor cells expressed TTF-1, Napsin-A, and cytokeratin 7 but not CK5/6 and p40, supporting the diagnosis of poorly differentiated adenocarcinoma with solid growth pattern/solid adenocarcinoma.

73 ADENOCARCINOMA VS. SCLEROSING PNEUMOCYTOMA

	Adenocarcinoma	Sclerosing Pneumocytoma (SP)
Age	Wide age distribution, ranging from 20 y of age to more than 70 y of age. It is the most common cell type of lung cancer in both genders.	Wide age distribution, ranging from 11–80 y, but is most commonly seen in middle-aged adults. It has a strong female predominance, with F:M ratio of 4–5:1, with 80% of cases occurring in women.
Location	While most (about 75%) pulmonary adenocarcinomas are peripheral parenchymal masses, centrally located adenocarcinomas may also occur.	SPs are typically solitary and peripheral lesions. In rare cases may present as multiple lesions, have visceral pleural or mediastinal involvement or occur as an endobronchial lesion.
Symptoms	Wide variety of symptoms. The most common symptoms include progressive shortness of breath, cough, chest pain/pressure, or constitutional symptoms. Due to its predominant peripheral location, adenocarcinomas may be discovered as an incidental mass or nodule on image studies performed for other reasons and thus may not present clinical symptoms.	Patients are usually asymptomatic. The lesion is typically discovered incidentally and presents as a slowly enlarging, asymptomatic pulmonary nodule.
Signs	Image studies usually demonstrate a single peripheral mass or multiple nodular tumors. They may also present as pneumonia-like consolidation on chest image studies. Subpleural tumors may be associated with pleural thickening, pleural space involvement, and pleural effusion. Some rare subpleural tumors may present with predominant growth on the pleural surface and encase the lung in a diffuse malignant mesothelioma-like pattern referred to as *pseudomesotheliomatous carcinoma.*	Chest x-ray and CT show a solitary, well-circumscribed mass. Cystic change may be present.
Etiology	Atypical adenomatous hyperplasia (AAH) is believed to be the precursor lesion of peripheral pulmonary adenocarcinomas, and progression from AAH to adenocarcinoma in situ (AIS) to invasive adenocarcinoma has been proposed. Although most adenocarcinomas are caused by tobacco smoking, they are also the most frequent cell type in patients who have never smoked.	The tumor was previously considered to be a vascular neoplasm and hence was formerly called sclerosing hemangioma. Currently, on the basis of immunohistochemical data, the tumor is thought to be derived from nonmucinous bronchiolar respiratory epithelium and is therefore called *sclerosing pneumocytoma.*

	Adenocarcinoma	Sclerosing Pneumocytoma (SP)
Histology	Adenocarcinomas are defined as carcinomas with gland formation and/or mucin production. The 2015 WHO classification of pulmonary adenocarcinomas includes subtypes of several growth patterns: lepidic, acinar, papillary, micropapillary, and solid *(Figs. 73.1–73.6)*. Other variants include invasive mucinous adenocarcinoma, colloid adenocarcinoma, fetal adenocarcinoma, and enteric adenocarcinoma. If sampled adequately, virtually all pulmonary adenocarcinomas are of mixed subtypes, although one subtype usually predominates. According to the 2011 IASLC/ATS/ERS and 2015 WHO classifications, the classification of invasive adenocarcinoma should include the predominant subtype after comprehensive histological subtyping by semiquantitatively estimating the percentage of the various subtypes present in 5% increments.	Most tumors have a heterogeneous variegated appearance resulting from a mixture of growth patterns including papillary, sclerotic, solid, and hemorrhagic. The tumor is typically composed of two cell types: cuboidal surface cells and round stromal cells. The cuboidal surface cells have phenotypic features of bronchiolar epithelium and type II pneumocytes. The round stromal cells are round to polygonal in shape and have round-to-oval, centrally located bland nuclei with fine chromatin. The papillary growth pattern is composed of papillary structures lined by cuboidal surface cells. The stalk of the papillae contains round stromal cells instead of true fibrovascular cores. The sclerotic pattern is composed of areas of dense hyaline collagen. The solid pattern is composed of sheets of round stromal cells. Cuboidal surface cells may be present forming small tubules. The hemorrhagic pattern is composed of large blood-filled spaces, which may be lined by epithelial tumor cells. Hemosiderin deposits, foamy macrophages, cholesterol clefts, mast cells, calcifications, and adipose tissue are common secondary findings *(Figs. 73.7–73.13)*. Mitotic figures are rare, and necrosis should not be present. The presence of bland cytologic features, characteristic two-cell population, and distinctive immunostaining profile differentiates this tumor from adenocarcinoma.
Special studies	Most pulmonary adenocarcinomas are immunopositive for a variety of cytokeratins including AE1/AE3, CK7, and CAM 5.2 but are usually negative for CK20 (except for mucinous adenocarcinoma and enteric adenocarcinoma). Thyroid transcription factor-1 (TTF-1) shows immunopositivity in 75%–85% of pulmonary adenocarcinomas. Napsin-A has comparable sensitivity with that of TTF-1. Molecular testing for epidermal growth factor receptor (EGFR) gene mutational analysis and ALK gene rearrangement is important for treatment management. Activating mutations in EGFR gene are clustered in exons 18–21. The two most common EGFR gene mutations are in-frame deletions in exon 19 (45%), followed by point mutation (CTG to CGC) in exon 21 at nucleotide 2573, resulting in substitution of leucine by arginine at codon 858 (L858R) (41%). EML4-ALK fusion accounts for >90% of ALK gene rearrangements in lung adenocarcinoma. EGFR gene mutation and ALK gene rearrangement are more commonly found in never-smokers with adenocarcinoma. EGFR mutations are more common in Asian patients and women. KRAS mutations in codons 12, 13, or 61 are present in 30% of adenocarcinomas and are particularly common in smokers.	The two cell types have slightly different immunophenotype. The cuboidal surface cells show positive expression for pancytokeratin, EMA, CK7, TTF-1, and Napsin-A. The round stromal cells are usually negative for pancytokeratin and only focally positive for CK7. They are positive for EMA and TTF-1. They may rarely be positive for Napsin-A.

	Adenocarcinoma	Sclerosing Pneumocytoma (SP)
Prognosis	Never-smoking status and female sex are favorable prognostic factors independent from the tumor stage. Tumor size ≥2.5 cm, solid and micropapillary subtypes, and a maximum standardized uptake value (SUV) of ≥7 are predictors of poor disease-free survival. The prognosis for stage I lepidic-predominant adenocarcinoma is usually good, unless associated with close margin in limited resection, visceral pleural invasion, and/or angiolymphatic invasion or the presence of micropapillary growth pattern component. Tumors with EGFR mutation may respond favorably to EGFR tyrosine kinase inhibitors (EGFR TKIs) such as gefitinib and erlotinib. Tumors with ALK gene rearrangement may respond favorably to ALK blockade with crizotinib. Of note, in-frame insertions mutations in EGFR, exon 20 are associated with primary resistance to EGFR TKI. Acquisition of an additional T790M mutation is the most common cause of secondary resistance to EGFR TKI. However, using more sensitive mutation-detection techniques, it was shown that T790M EGFR mutation may coexist with L858R mutations, which might confer pretreatment (primary) resistance to EGFR TKIs. Amplification of MET gene is another mechanism of EGFR TKIs resistance. The presence of KRAS mutation is usually associated with resistance to EGFR TKIs.	SP behaves in a clinically benign fashion. No disease-related deaths have been reported at this point. While there have been reports of lymph nodes metastases in a very small percentage of cases, these do not appear to adversely affect prognosis.

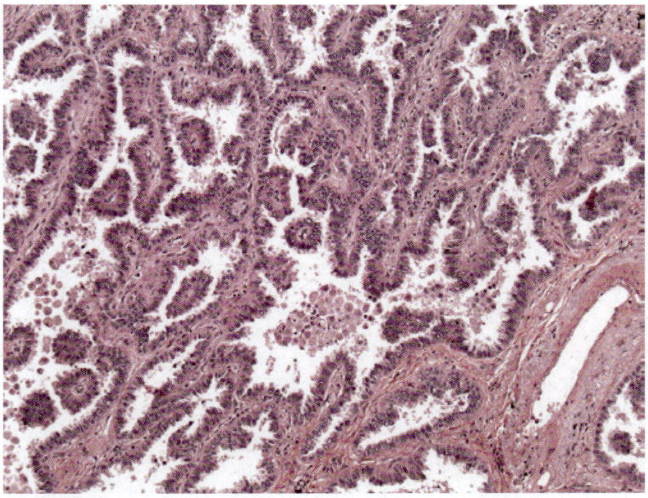

Figure 73.1 Lepidic adenocarcinoma: The tumor cells grow along the alveolar walls surface.

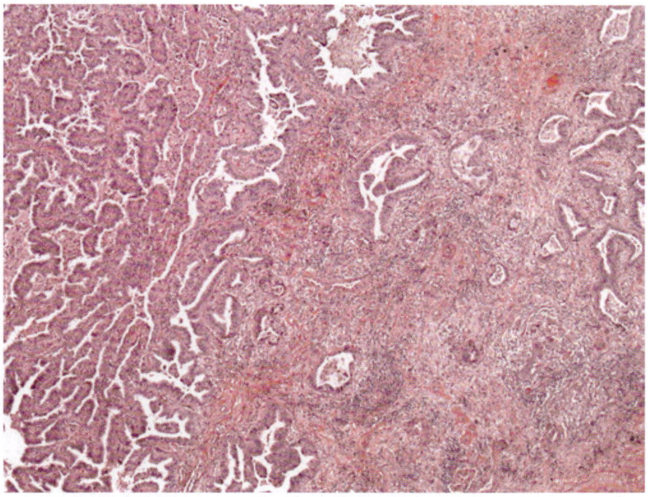

Figure 73.2 Adenocarcinoma: Lepidic adenocarcinoma *(left)* and acinar adenocarcinoma, characterized by the presence of malignant glands within a fibro-inflammatory stroma *(right)*.

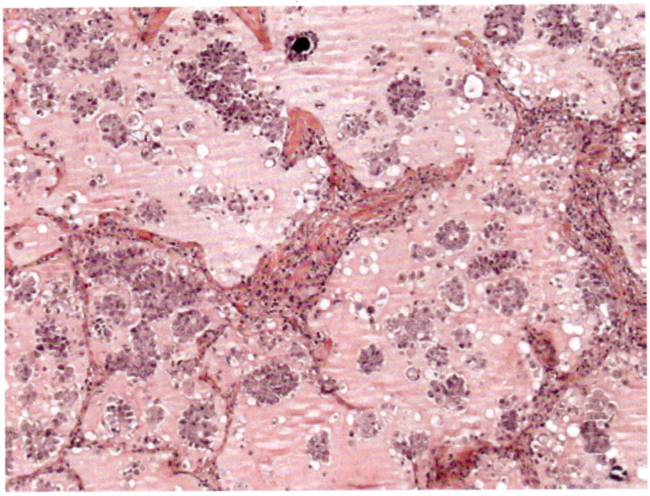

Figure 73.3 Micropapillary adenocarcinoma: Dyscohesive papillary clusters of cytologically malignant cells "float" within the air spaces. The tumor cells form papillae that lack fibrovascular core.

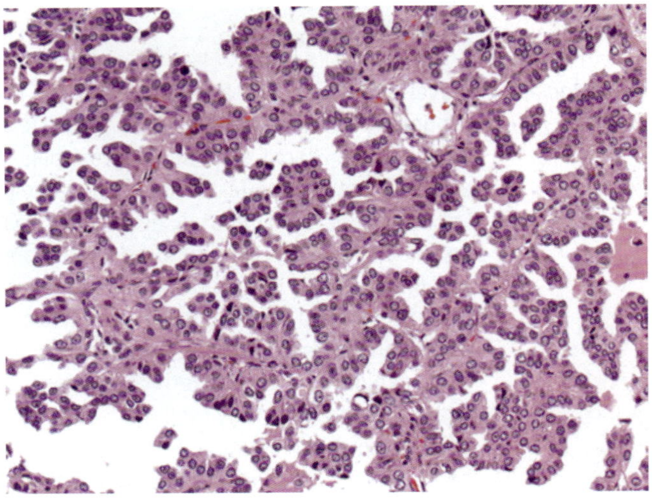

Figure 73.4 Papillary adenocarcinoma: The tumor cells form true papillary structures, with papillae lined by glandular epithelium surrounding a fibrovascular core.

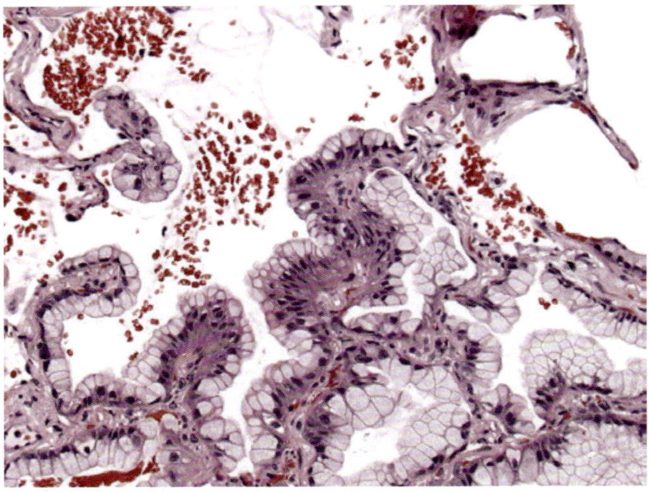

Figure 73.5 Mucinous adenocarcinoma: The columnar mucinous tumor cells grow in a lepidic growth pattern.

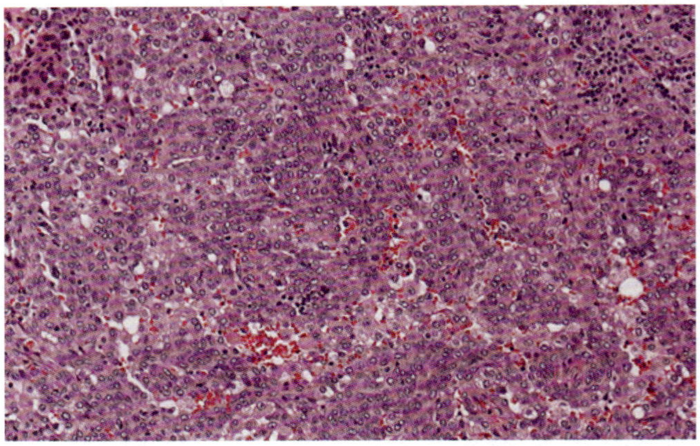

Figure 73.6 Solid adenocarcinoma: In this poorly differentiated adenocarcinoma with solid growth pattern, immunoperoxidase stains are of paramount importance to confirm the diagnosis. In this case, the tumor cells expressed TTF-1, Napsin-A, and cytokeratin 7.

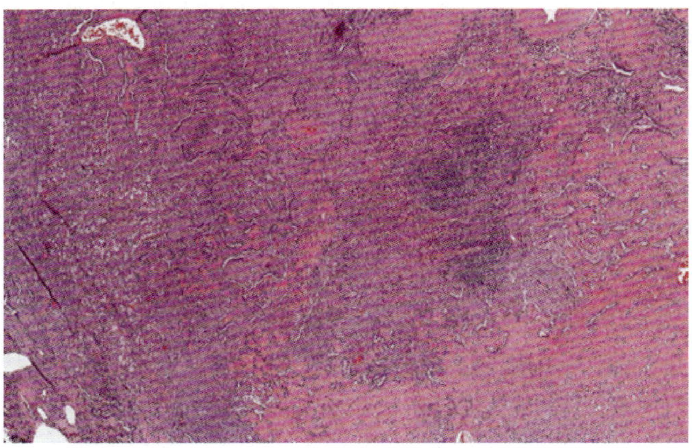

Figure 73.7 SP: Lesion with a typical heterogeneous variegated appearance resulting from a mixture of papillary, sclerotic, and solid growth patterns.

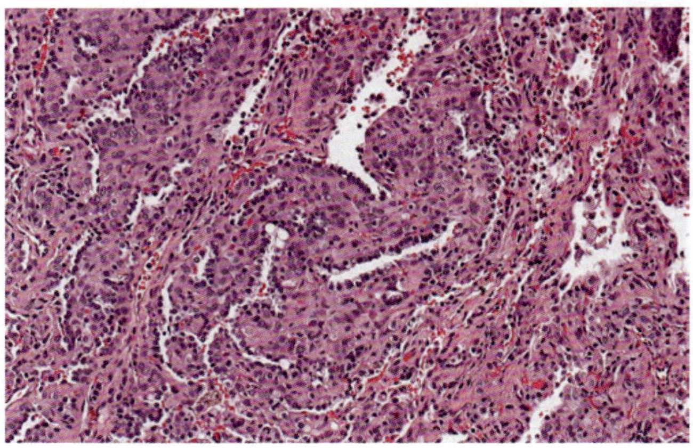

Figure 73.8 SP: The tumor is characteristically composed of two cell types: cuboidal surface cells and round stromal cells. The presence of bland cytological features, characteristic two-cell population, and distinctive immunostaining profile differentiates this tumor from adenocarcinoma.

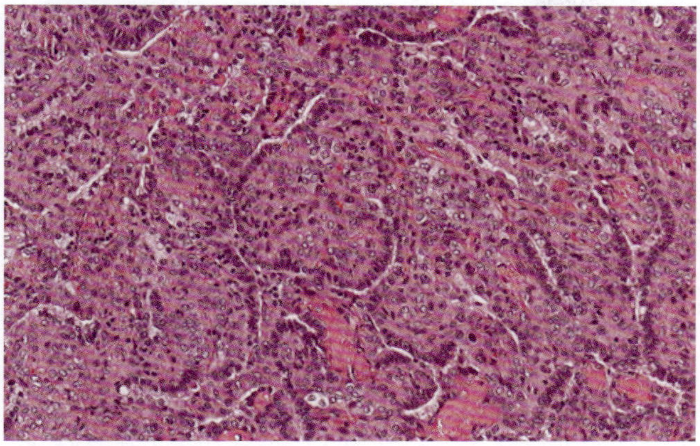

Figure 73.9 SP (papillary growth pattern): The papillae in SP are lined by cuboidal surface cells. In contrast to papillary adenocarcinoma, the stalk of the papillae in SP contains round stromal cells instead of true fibrovascular cores.

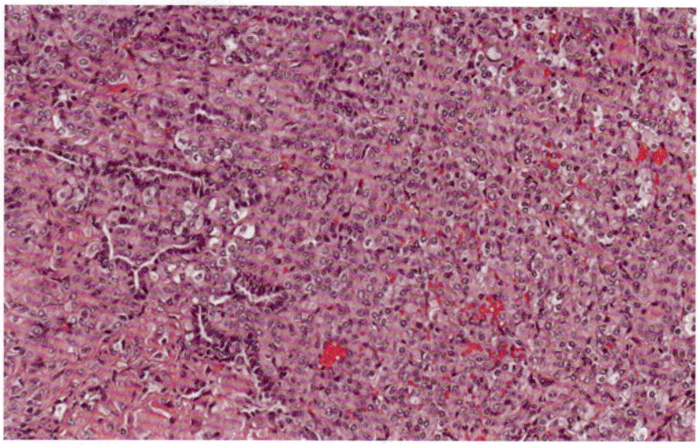

Figure 73.10 SP: Solid growth pattern composed of sheets of round stromal cells. Note cuboidal surface cells forming small tubules on the left side of this image.

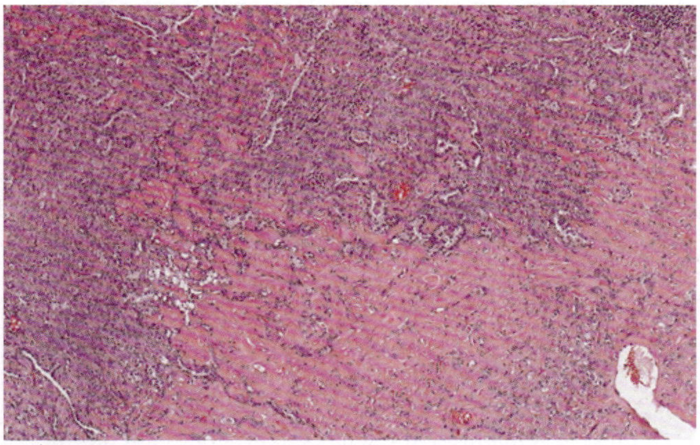

Figure 73.11 SP: Sclerotic pattern composed of dense hyaline collagen.

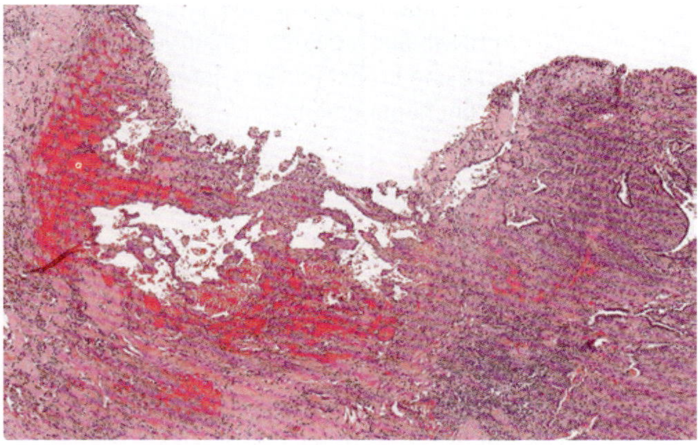

Figure 73.12 SP: Hemorrhagic pattern showing large blood-filled spaces.

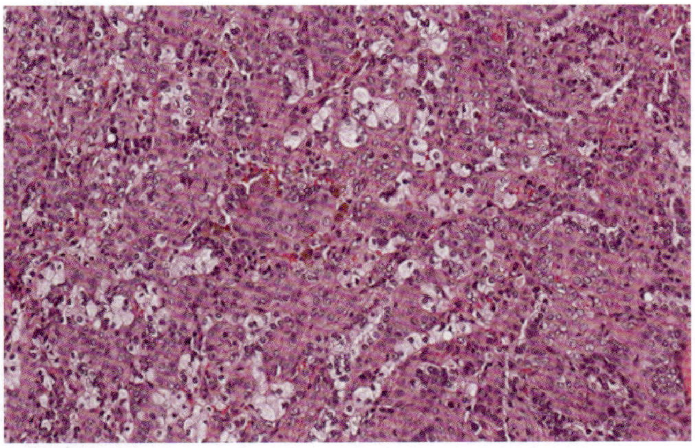

Figure 73.13 SP: Solid growth pattern associated with foamy macrophages, which is a common secondary finding seen in sclerosing hemangioma.

74 BASALOID SQUAMOUS CELL CARCINOMA VS. SMALL CELL CARCINOMA

	Basaloid Squamous Cell Carcinoma (Basaloid SQCC)	Small Cell Lung Carcinoma (SCLC)
Age	Wide age distribution, occurs more in men than in women, and is closely correlated with history of tobacco smoking.	SCLC occurs between 40 and 70 y of age. SCLC is seen almost exclusively in heavy cigarette smokers and is more common in men.
Location	Basaloid SQCC is predominantly centrally located (75% of cases), arising from the proximal bronchi. However, it may originate in the peripheral pulmonary parenchyma.	SCLC is usually located centrally in the major airways, but may occur peripherally in the lungs in about 5% of cases.
Symptoms	Symptoms may include cough, shortness of breath, chest pain, hemoptysis, and constitutional symptoms. Endobronchial growth may occlude the airway lumen causing bronchiectasis, infection, or bronchopneumonia.	Patients often present with rapid onset signs or symptoms due to local intrathoracic tumor growth, extrapulmonary distant spread, paraneoplastic syndromes, or a combination of these features. Symptoms may include cough, dyspnea, hemoptysis, weight loss, or other constitutional symptoms. Superior vena cava syndrome is a presenting finding in 10% of patients. Associated paraneoplastic syndromes such as hyponatremia (due to inappropriate secretion of antidiuretic hormone), Cushing syndrome, Lambert–Eaton myasthenic syndrome, peripheral neuropathy, or limbic encephalopathy may be observed.
Signs	Image studies usually demonstrate proximal masses in the hilar and perihilar areas or proximal airways.	SCLC classically presents as a large hilar mass with extensive mediastinal lymphadenopathy and lobar collapse on chest CT. A minority of cases may present with peripheral masses.
Etiology	Basaloid SQCC arises from progressive squamous epithelial dysplasia and has strong association with tobacco smoking.	Unknown. It is highly linked to tobacco smoking.

	Basaloid Squamous Cell Carcinoma (Basaloid SQCC)	**Small Cell Lung Carcinoma (SCLC)**
Histology	Basaloid SQCC usually shows solid nodular, organoid, or anastomotic trabecular invasive growth pattern associated with marked peripheral palisading of tumor cells nuclei. The tumor cells are relatively small, monomorphic, cuboidal, or fusiform in shape and have finely granular to vesicular chromatin and have inconspicuous to absent nucleoli. The amount of cytoplasm may be scant but nuclear molding is absent. The number of mitotic figures is high ranging from 15 to 50 mitoses/2 mm^2 of tumor. Most basaloid SQCCs have a hyaline or mucoid stroma. Comedo-type necrosis is common, and rosette formation may be present *(Figs. 74.1 and 74.2)*. Extensive carcinoma in situ is usually seen in adjacent bronchial epithelium. According to the 2015 WHO classification, tumors that show keratinizing or nonkeratinizing SQCC features, but have a major basaloid component (>50% of tumor), should be classified as basaloid SQCC.	Sheet-like growth without a neuroendocrine architecture is the most frequent growth pattern, although trabeculae, peripheral palisading, and rosette formation may be seen. The tumor cells are small sized (generally less than the diameter of 3–4 small lymphocytes) and have oval- to spindle-shaped nuclei, scant or almost indiscernible cytoplasm, finely granular nuclear chromatin with a "salt-and-pepper appearance," and absent or inconspicuous nucleoli. The nuclear-to-cytoplasmic (N/C) ratio is extremely high. Nuclear molding, crushing artifact, and encrustation of blood vessels with basophilic material, the so-called Azzopardi phenomenon, may be observed *(Figs. 74.3–74.5)*. While the mitotic rate is by definition (2015 WHO classification) >10 mitoses/2 mm^2 area of tumor, it usually ranges from 50 to 60 with a median of 80 mitoses/2 mm^2. On small transbronchial (TBBX) biopsies, SCLC may exhibit significant crushing artifact. Such cases should be interpreted with caution as other tumors including basaloid SQCC, carcinoid, and lymphoma may also show considerable crushing artifact. In needle-core biopsies and larger or resected specimens, the cells of SCLC may appear larger in comparison with their appearance on a TBBX and have slightly more discernable cytoplasm; however, in comparison with lymphocytes the cells remain proportionally small and the N/C ratios remain very high.
Special studies	Basaloid SQCC express p63, p40, and CK5/6. TTF-1 is never expressed. Neuroendocrine markers (CD56, chromogranin, and synaptophysin) are usually negative but occasionally may be focally positive. The Ki-67 index is high and usually shows nuclear staining in 50%–80% of tumor cells.	p63, p40, and CK5/6 (squamous markers) are negative. A panel of neuroendocrine markers including CD56, synaptophysin, and chromogranin A is useful. CD56 is the most sensitive marker, but it is also less specific. Synaptophysin and CD56 can diffusely and strongly stain SCLC, while chromogranin A can be more focal and weak. It should be noted that <10% of SCLC can be negative or only focally positive for neuroendocrine markers expression. SCLC usually stains positive for cytokeratin markers (e.g., AE1/AE3, CAM5.3) and characteristically exhibits a dot-like, perinuclear, or diffuse cytoplasmic staining pattern. CK 7 is frequently negative, but may be positive in a minority of cases. CK 20 is consistently negative. TTF-1 is positive in the majority (90%–95%) of SCLC cases, but, unlike TTF-1 expression in non small cell lung carcinoma, TTF-1 expression in SCLC does not definitively support a pulmonary origin and may be found in SCLC arising in other locations. Napsin-A is consistently negative. The Ki-67 (MIB-1) proliferation marker index is high and usually shows nuclear staining in 50%–100% of SCLC tumor cells.
Prognosis	Although basaloid SQCC is rare and data are limited, the prognosis is in general considered to be worse than that of other types of non–small cell lung cancer.	SCLC frequently presents at an advanced stage and has a poor prognosis with a 2-y survival rate of only 10% with metastatic disease and a 5-y survival rate of approximately 25% when there is no metastatic involvement. The median overall survival time is 12.7 mo. Chemotherapy is the usual treatment. Surgical resection and chemotherapy are performed in some centers for limited disease.

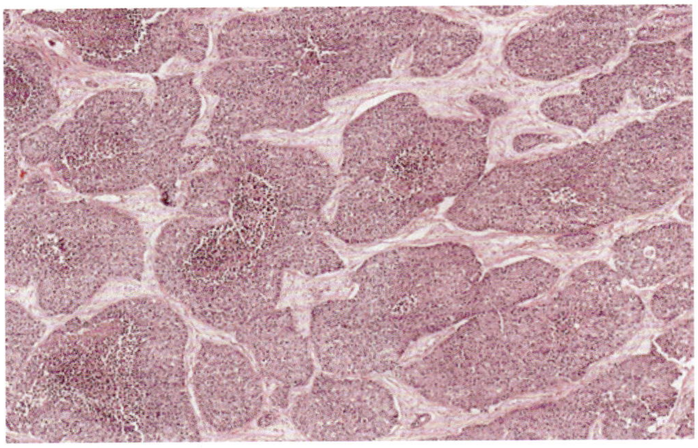

Figure 74.1 Basaloid SQCC: There is solid nodular growth pattern associated with comedo-type necrosis and marked peripheral palisading of tumor cells nuclei, within a mucoid stroma.

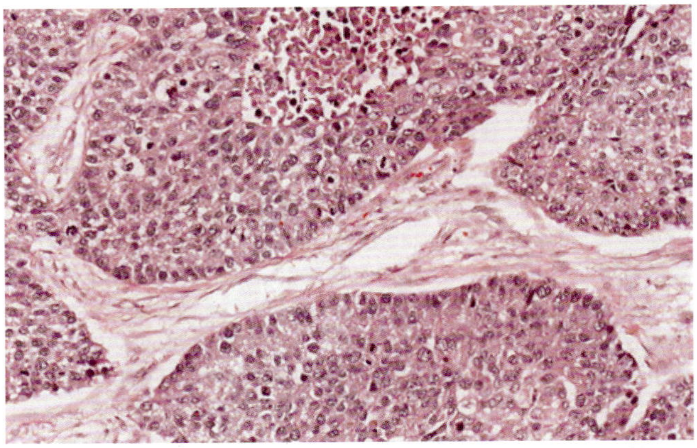

Figure 74.2 Basaloid SQCC (high power): There is characteristic peripheral palisading at the edge of the tumor cells nests. These tumor cells express CK5/6, p63, and p40, and do not express TTF-1 or neuroendocrine markers.

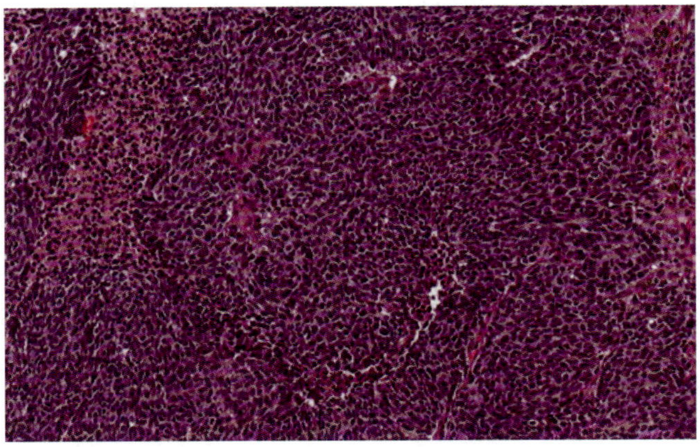

Figure 74.3 SCLC: The tumor cells usually show a sheet-like growth pattern. These tumor cells express TTF-1 and neuroendocrine markers, but fail to express CK5/6, p63, and p40.

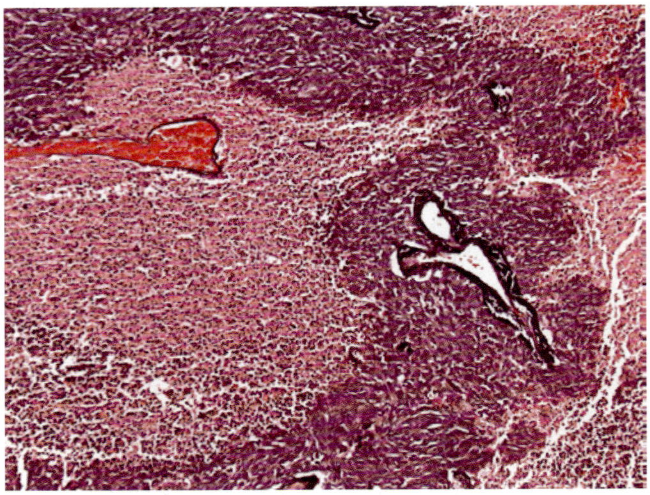

Figure 74.4 SCLC: There is extensive area of necrosis. Note Azzopardi effect *(middle right)* characterized by the presence of crushed DNA around a blood vessel in this largely necrotic tumor.

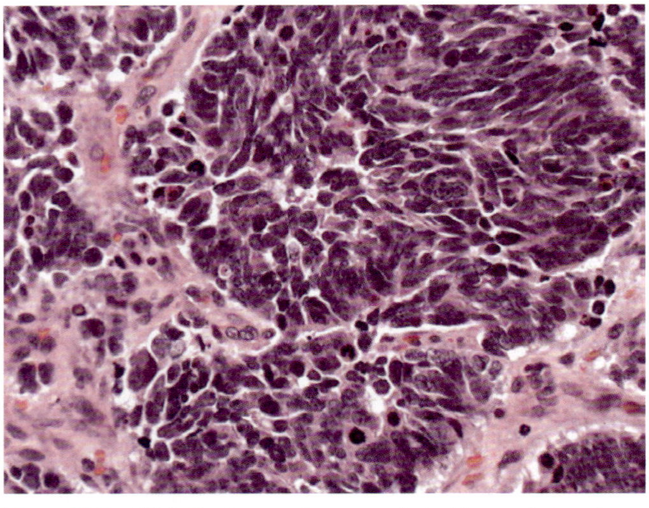

Figure 74.5 SCLC: The tumor cells are small sized (generally less than the diameter of 3–4 small lymphocytes), have oval- to spindle-shaped nuclei, scant or almost indiscernible cytoplasm, finely granular nuclear chromatin, and absent nucleoli. The nuclear-to-cytoplasmic (N/C) ratio is very high.

75 LARGE CELL NEUROENDOCRINE CARCINOMA VS. SMALL CELL LUNG CARCINOMA

	Large Cell Neuroendocrine Carcinoma (LCNEC)	Small Cell Lung Carcinoma (SCLC)
Age	The average age of diagnosis is about 65 y, and most patients are male and smokers.	SCLC occurs between 40 and 70 y of age. SCLC is seen almost exclusively in heavy cigarette smokers and is more common in men.
Location	LCNEC typically arises in the peripheral lung.	SCLC is usually located centrally in the major airways, but may occur peripherally in the lungs in about 5% of cases.
Symptoms	While cough, hemoptysis, dyspnea, pneumonia, and chest pain are common symptoms at presentation, due to the common peripheral location, it may also be asymptomatic. Weight loss, fatigue, or signs and symptoms due to metastatic disease may be the initial presentation. Different from SCLC, paraneoplastic syndromes are not common.	Patients often present with rapid onset signs or symptoms due to local intrathoracic tumor growth, extrapulmonary distant spread, paraneoplastic syndromes, or a combination of these features. Symptoms may include cough, dyspnea, hemoptysis, weight loss, or other constitutional symptoms. Superior vena cava syndrome is a presenting finding in 10% of patients. Associated paraneoplastic syndromes such as hyponatremia (due to inappropriate secretion of antidiuretic hormone), Cushing syndrome, Lambert–Eaton myasthenic syndrome, peripheral neuropathy, or limbic encephalopathy may be encountered.
Signs	Image studies usually demonstrate peripheral lung masses. Despite the frequent peripheral location, associated pleural effusion is rare.	SCLC classically presents as a large hilar mass with extensive mediastinal lymphadenopathy and lobar collapse on chest CT. A minority of cases may present with peripheral masses.
Etiology	Like small cell carcinoma, LCNE is highly related to smoking.	It is highly linked to tobacco smoking.

	Large Cell Neuroendocrine Carcinoma (LCNEC)	Small Cell Lung Carcinoma (SCLC)
Histology	LCNEC was classified as a variant of large cell carcinoma in the 2004 WHO classification, but is classified under neuroendocrine tumors according to the 2015 WHO classification. LCNEC shows morphologic features of neuroendocrine differentiation including organoid nesting, trabecular growth, peripheral palisading of tumor cells, and rosette formation. Central necrosis of tumor cell nests and large areas of necrosis may occur. The tumor cells are larger than SCLC cells and have, in general, polygonal shape, *moderate-to-abundant cytoplasm, coarse-to-vesicular chromatin, and prominent nucleoli* *(Figs. 75.1–75.6)*. Mitotic rate is by definition (2015 WHO classification) >10 mitoses/2 mm^2 area of tumor, with an average of 70–75 mitoses. Nuclei with vesicular chromatin vs. finely granular chromatin, conspicuous nucleoli vs. inconspicuous-to-absent nucleoli, polygonal cell shape vs. more fusiform tumor shape, and moderate-to-abundant vs. markedly scant cytoplasm are morphologic features that help in differentiating LCNEC from SCLC, respectively.	Sheet-like growth without a neuroendocrine architecture is the most frequent growth pattern, although trabeculae, peripheral palisading, and rosette formation may be seen. The tumor cells are small sized (generally less than the diameter of 3–4 small lymphocytes) and have oval- to spindle-shaped nuclei, *scant or almost indiscernible cytoplasm, finely granular nuclear chromatin* with a "salt-and-pepper appearance," *and absent or faint nucleoli. The nuclear-to-cytoplasmic (N/C) ratio is very high*. Nuclear molding, crushing artifact, and encrustation of blood vessels with basophilic material, the so-called Azzopardi phenomenon, may be observed *(Figs. 75.7–75.9)*. While the mitotic rate is by definition (2015 WHO classification) >10 mitoses/2 mm^2 area of tumor, it usually ranges from 50 to 60 with a median of 80 mitoses/2 mm^2. In needle-core biopsies and larger or resected specimens, the cells of SCLC may appear larger in comparison with their appearance on a TBBX and have slightly more discernable cytoplasm; however, in comparison with lymphocytes, the cells remain proportionally small and the N/C ratios remain very high. Small cell carcinoma typically exhibits small-sized tumor cells, less conspicuous nucleoli, more finely granular chromatin, and much less cytoplasm than LCNEC.
Special studies	In addition to neuroendocrine morphology on H&E-stained sections, confirmation of neuroendocrine differentiation is required using immunoperoxidase stains such as chromogranin, synaptophysin, and CD56. LCNECs are typically immunopositive for CK7 and pancytokeratin, with either a dot-like or diffuse cytoplasmic pattern. TTF-1 is immunopositive in approximately 50% of cases, a figure that is generally lower than that of SCLC. The Ki-67 (MIB-1) proliferation index usually shows nuclear staining in 40%–80% of LCNEC tumor cells. Both SCLC and LCNEC show similar immunostaining patterns, and hence immunostaining is of no benefit in differentiating the two tumors.	A panel of neuroendocrine markers including CD56, synaptophysin, and chromogranin A is useful. CD56 is the most sensitive marker, but it is also less specific. Synaptophysin and CD56 can diffusely and strongly stain SCLC, while chromogranin A can be more focal and weak. It should be noted that <10% of SCLC can be negative or only focally positive for neuroendocrine marker expression. SCLC usually stains positive for cytokeratin markers (e.g., AE1/AE3, CAM5.3), and characteristically exhibits a dot-like, perinuclear, or diffuse cytoplasmic staining pattern. CK 7 is frequently negative, but may be positive in a minority of cases. CK 20 is consistently negative. TTF-1 is positive in the majority (90%–95%) of SCLC cases but, unlike TTF-1 expression in LCNEC, TTF-1 expression in SCLC does not definitively support a pulmonary origin and may be found in SCLC arising in other locations. Napsin-A is consistently negative. The Ki-67 index usually shows nuclear staining in 50%–100% of SCLC tumor cells.

	Large Cell Neuroendocrine Carcinoma (LCNEC)	Small Cell Lung Carcinoma (SCLC)
Prognosis	LCNEC are considered aggressive tumors. Patients with this tumor are more likely to develop recurrence and have a shorter survival compared to patients with other types of NSCLC, even in those with stage I disease. In two studies, 5-y survival rates as low as 32.1% and 33%, respectively, have been reported for patients with stage I disease. The clinical efficacy of chemotherapy for unresectable LCNEC has been shown to be comparable with that for extensive small cell lung cancer, and patients may benefit from SCLC-based chemotherapy.	SCLC frequently presents at an advanced stage and has a poor prognosis with a 2-y survival rate of only 10% with metastatic disease, and a 5-y survival rate of approximately 25% when there is no metastatic involvement. The median overall survival time is 12.7 mo. Chemotherapy is the usual treatment. Surgical resection and chemotherapy is performed in some centers for limited disease.

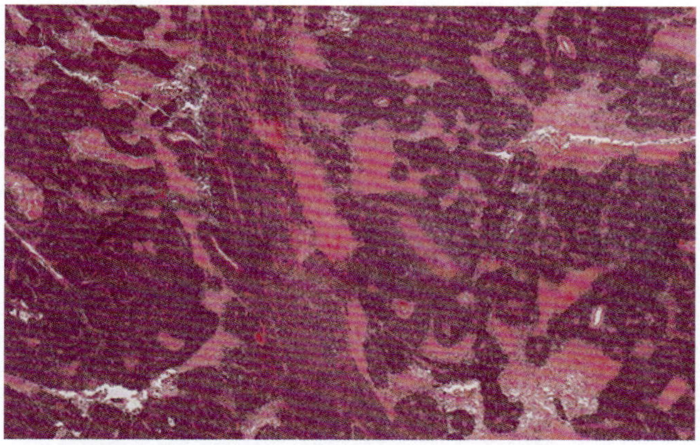

Figure 75.1 LCNEC showing extensive areas of necrosis.

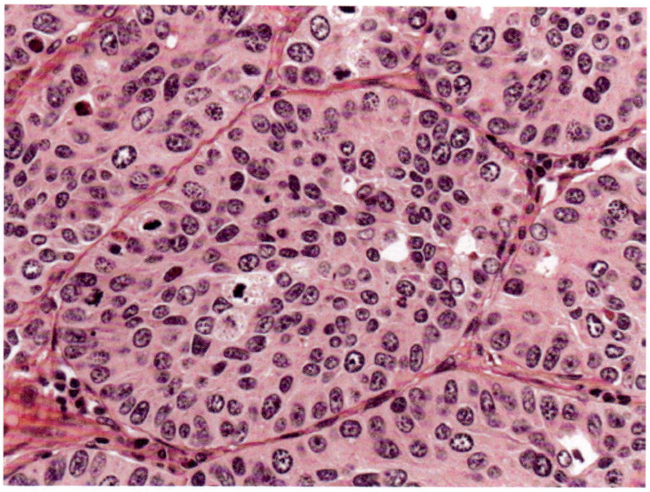

Figure 75.2 LCNEC showing organoid nesting growth pattern.

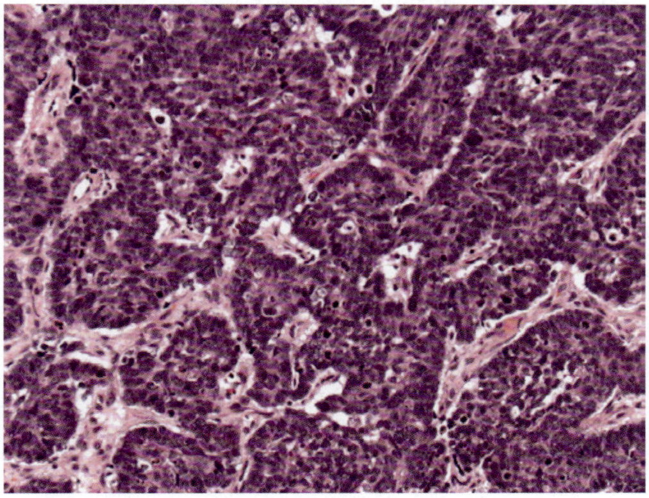

Figure 75.3 LCNEC showing trabecular growth pattern with peripheral nuclear palisading.

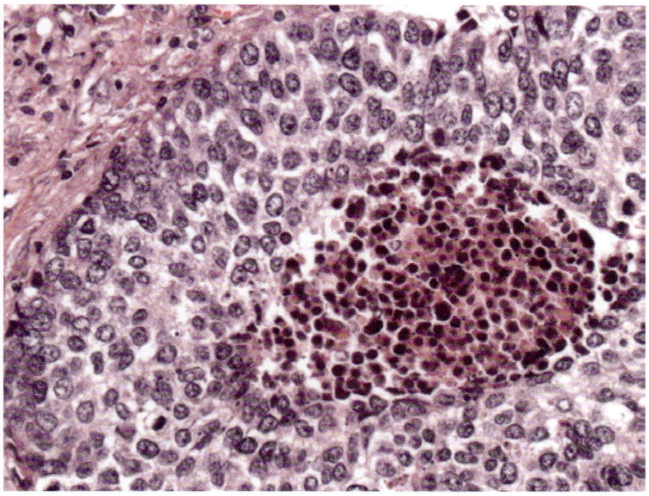

Figure 75.4 LCNEC (with central necrosis): The tumor cells have vesicular chromatin and a fair amount of cytoplasm.

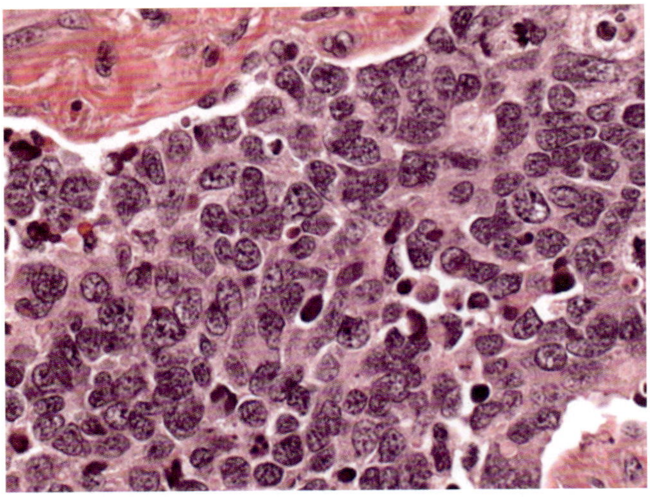

Figure 75.5 LCNEC High power view showing tumor cells with fair amount of cytoplasm. In contrast, SCLC have characteristic scant cytoplasm, nuclear molding and higher N/C.

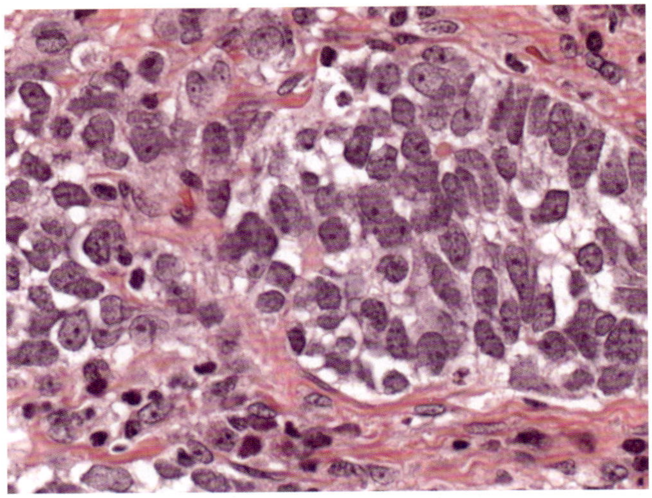

Figure 75.6 LCNEC: Note prominent nucleoli. Nuclei with vesicular chromatin vs finely granular chromatin, conspicuous nucleoli vs inconspicuous to absent nucleoli, polygonal cell shape vs more fusiform tumor shape and moderate to abundant vs markedly scant cytoplasm are morphologic features that help in differentiating LCNEC from SCLC respectively.

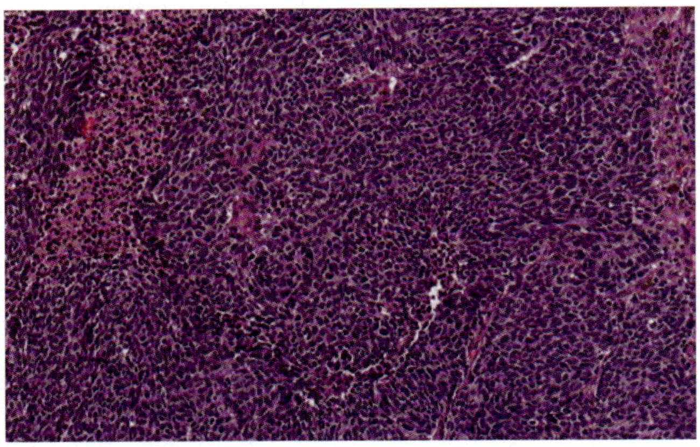

Figure 75.7 SCLC: The tumor cells usually show a sheet-like growth pattern.

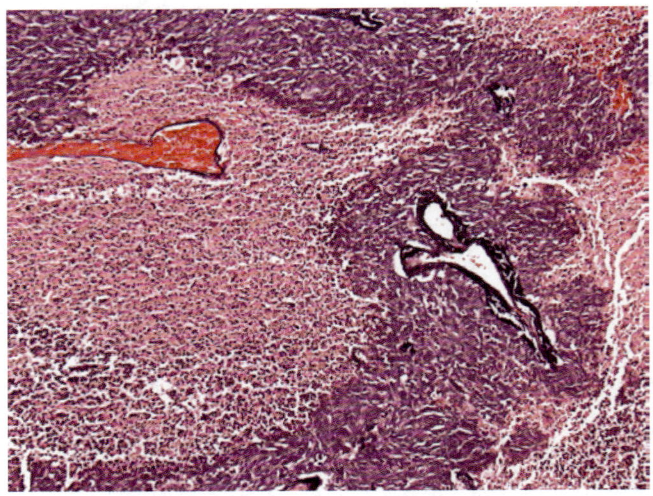

Figure 75.8 SCLC with extensive area of necrosis. Note Azzopardi effect (*middle right*) characterized by the presence of crushed DNA around a blood vessel in this largely necrotic tumor.

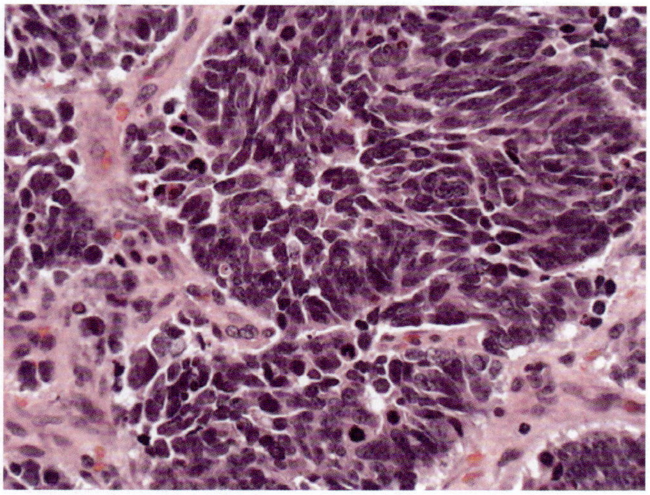

Figure 75.9 SCLC: The tumor cells are small sized (generally less than the diameter of 3–4 small lymphocytes) and have oval- to spindle-shaped nuclei, scant or almost indiscernible cytoplasm, finely granular nuclear chromatin, and absent nucleoli. The nuclear-to-cytoplasmic (N/C) ratio is much higher than that of LCNEC.

76 LARGE CELL CARCINOMA VS. ADENOCARCINOMA WITH SOLID GROWTH PATTERN/SOLID ADENOCARCINOMA

	Large Cell Carcinoma (LCC)	**Adenocarcinoma with Solid Growth Pattern/Solid Adenocarcinoma (SA)**
Age	The average age of diagnosis is about 60 y, and most patients are smokers.	Wide age distribution, ranging from 20 y of age to more than 70 y of age.
Location	LCC usually arises in the peripheral lung.	Although most (about 75%) pulmonary adenocarcinomas are peripheral parenchymal masses, centrally located adenocarcinomas may also occur.
Symptoms	Nonproductive cough, dyspnea and weight loss similar to other non small cell lung carcinomas.	Wide variety of symptoms. The most common symptoms include progressive shortness of breath, cough, chest pain/pressure, or constitutional symptoms. Because of predominant peripheral location, adenocarcinomas may be discovered as an incidental mass or nodule on image studies performed for other reasons and may not present clinical symptoms.
Signs	Image studies usually demonstrate large masses in the periphery of the lung. In some cases, it can be associated with pleural or chest wall invasion.	Image studies usually demonstrate a single peripheral mass or multiple nodular tumors. They may also present as pneumonia-like consolidation on chest image studies. Subpleural tumors may be associated with pleural thickening, pleural space involvement, and pleural effusion. Some rare subpleural tumors may present with predominant growth on the pleural surface and encase the lung in a diffuse, malignant, mesothelioma-like pattern referred to as "pseudomesotheliomatous carcinoma."
Etiology	It is highly related to smoking.	Atypical adenomatous hyperplasia (AAH) is believed to be the precursor lesion of peripheral pulmonary adenocarcinomas, and progression from AAH to adenocarcinoma in situ (AIS) to invasive adenocarcinoma has been proposed. Although most adenocarcinomas are caused by tobacco smoking, adenocarcinoma is the most frequent cell type in patients who have never smoked.
Histology	LCC is an undifferentiated tumor that lacks cytologic, architectural, and immunohistochemical features of adenocarcinoma, squamous cell carcinoma, or small cell carcinoma. LCC is composed of sheets or nests of large polygonal cells with vesicular nuclei, prominent nucleoli, and moderate amounts of cytoplasm *(Fig. 76.1)*. Mucin production should not be present. According to the 2015 WHO classification, the diagnosis of LLC must only be made in thoroughly sampled resection specimens and cannot be made on nonresection specimens or cytology specimens.	SAs are composed of polygonal tumor cells forming nests and sheets that lack recognizable patterns of adenocarcinoma, such as acinar, papillary, micropapillary, or lepidic growth patterns *(Fig. 76.2)*.

	Large Cell Carcinoma (LCC)	Adenocarcinoma with Solid Growth Pattern/Solid Adenocarcinoma (SA)
Special studies	LCCs are immunonegative for TTF-1 and Napsin-A (adenocarcinoma markers), and CK5/6, p63, and p40 (squamous cell carcinoma markers).	SAs are immunopositive for the pneumocyte markers TTF-1 and Napsin-A. Intracytoplasmic mucin droplets should be present in ≥5 tumor cells in at least two high-power fields, confirmed by mucin histochemical stains *(Figs. 76.3–76.5)*.
Prognosis	LCC may be associated with lower disease-free and overall survival when compared with solid-predominant growth pattern adenocarcinomas. Many cases that were previously diagnosed as LCCs have been reclassified as other histologic types (e.g., solid adenocarcinoma, poorly differentiated squamous cell carcinoma, or neuroendocrine tumor/large cell neuroendocrine carcinoma [LCNEC]) according to 2015 WHO classification, and data specific to LCC by the new classification are limited. However, few LCCs by the new classification may harbor adenocarcinoma-associated mutations including KRAS and occasional epidermal growth factor receptor (EGFR) mutations. Therefore, molecular testing is recommended in this subgroup when there is advanced disease and targeted therapy is to be considered.	Never-smoking status and female sex are favorable prognostic factors independent from the tumor stage. Tumor size ≥2.5 cm, solid and micropapillary subtypes, and a maximum standardized uptake value (SUV) of ≥7 are predictors of poor disease-free survival. Tumors with EGFR gene mutation may respond favorably to EGFR tyrosine kinase inhibitors (EGFR TKIs) such as gefitinib and erlotinib. Tumors with ALK gene rearrangement may respond favorably to ALK blockade with crizotinib. Of note, in-frame insertion mutations in EGFR gene exon 20 are associated with primary resistance to EGFR TKI. Acquisition of an additional T790M mutation is the most common cause of secondary resistance to EGFR TKI. However, using more sensitive mutation-detection techniques, it was shown that T790M EGFR gene mutation may coexist with L858R mutations, which might confer pretreatment (primary) resistance to EGFR TKIs. Amplification of MET gene is another mechanism of EGFR TKIs resistance. The presence of KRAS gene mutation is usually associated with resistance to EGFR TKIs.

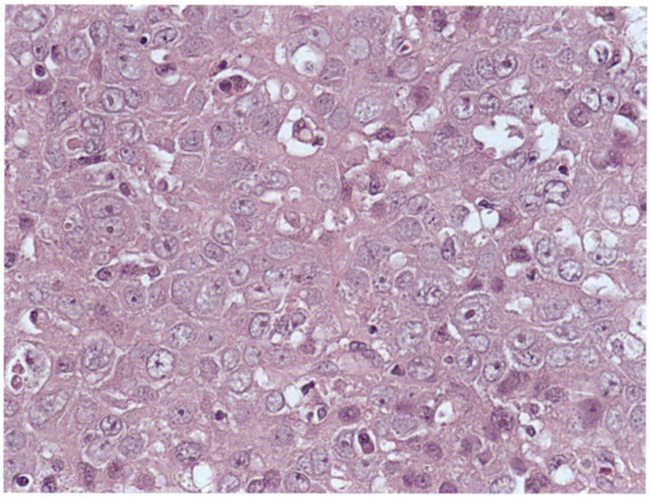

Figure 76.1 LCC showing large polygonal cells with vesicular nuclei, prominent nucleoli, and moderate amounts of cytoplasm. Cytologic, architectural, and immunohistochemical features of adenocarcinoma, squamous cell carcinoma, or small cell carcinoma should not be present.

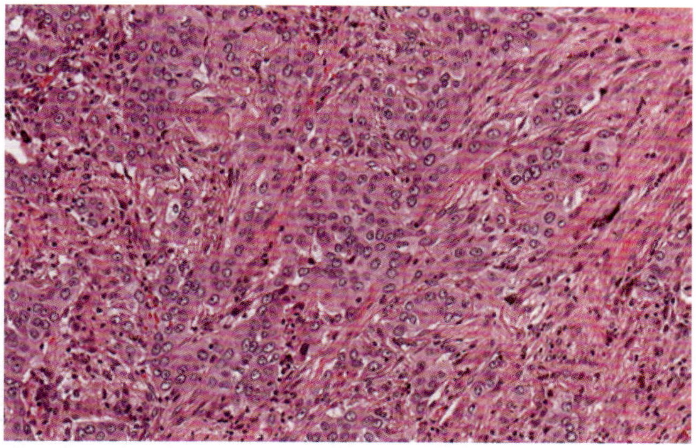

Figure 76.2 SA showing solid nests of large epithelial cells with abundant cytoplasm and prominent nucleoli.

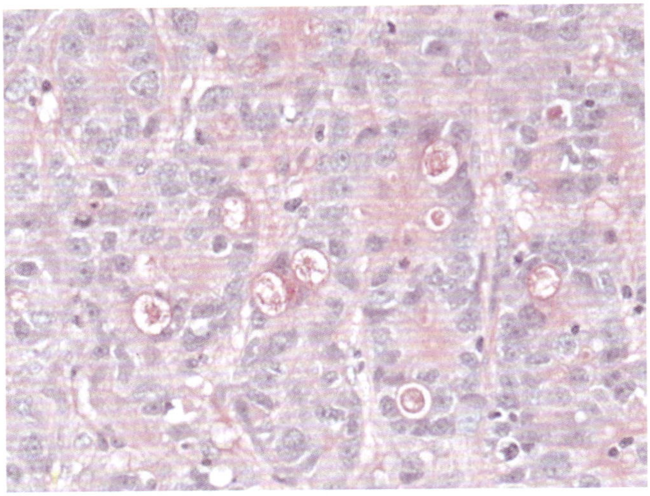

Figure 76.3 SA: Mucin stain decorates intracytoplasmic mucin droplets.

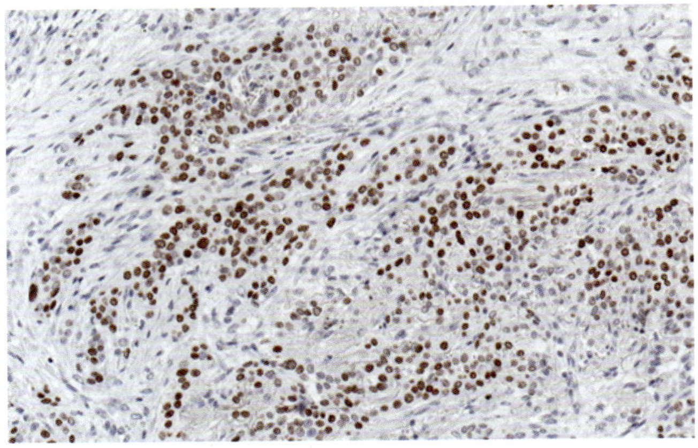

Figure 76.4 SA: Immunopositive for TTF-1.

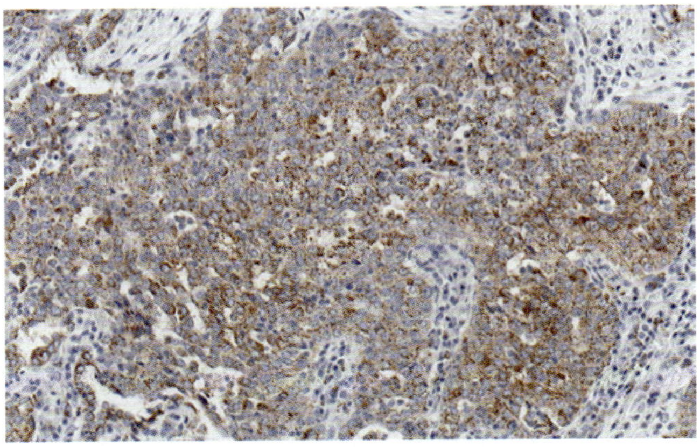

Figure 76.5 SA: Immunopositive for Napsin-A.

77 EPITHELIOID HEMANGIOENDOTHELIOMA VS. PULMONARY HAMARTOMA

	Epithelioid Hemangioendothelioma (EH)	Pulmonary Hamartoma (PH)
Age	EH occurs over a wide age distribution, ranging from 7–81 y, with a median age of 38 y, and has a strong female predilection (60%–80%).	PHs are more common in men, and incidence peaks during the sixth decade of life.
Location	Intraparenchymal pulmonary lesion(s) with no characteristic location. It may arise in more than one site (e.g., lung, liver, bone, and soft tissue), simultaneously or sequentially.	PHs are usually peripheral. Approximately 10% arise endobronchially.
Symptoms	Patients are frequently asymptomatic (50%–70% cases). Pleuritic chest pain is the most common symptom in the majority of the symptomatic patients. Less frequent symptoms include cough, dyspnea, hemoptysis, pleural effusion, and systemic symptoms.	PH is typically asymptomatic, although endobronchial lesions may cause symptoms due to bronchial obstruction.
Signs	In more than 60% of cases, chest CT demonstrates multiple bilateral perivascular nodules (<2 cm in size) that mimic metastatic cancer or granulomas. Between 10% and 19% of cases present as a solitary lung nodule (up to 5 cm). Cavitary or calcified nodules have been described.	Peripheral PH typically presents as a solitary, well-circumscribed nodule on routine chest x-ray. Multiple lesions are rare. Most PH are noncalcified. Occasionally, calcification is present and appears as "popcorn calcification," which is virtually diagnostic. On chest CT, the presence of fatty densities within the lesion are also highly suggestive of the diagnosis.
Etiology	EH is a rare neoplasm of endothelial cells associated with a specific fusion gene (see special studies).	Unknown.
Histology	Low-power examination typically reveals round-to-oval nodules with central hypocellular sclerotic or chondroid zone and cellular peripheral zone *(Fig. 77.1)*. The cellular zone is typically composed of cytologically bland, round-to-slightly spindle-shaped endothelial cells, with intracytoplasmic lumina containing red blood cells, which are usually arranged in strands and solid nests *(Fig. 77.2)*. The intracytoplasmic vacuoles may mimic a signet ring appearance. The stroma may be chondroid, hyaline, mucinous, or myxomatous. EH is typically seen associated with arterioles, venules, or lymphatic vessels. Areas of necrosis, calcification, and ossification may occur. The tumors frequently show an intra-alveolar growth pattern *(Fig. 77.3)*. They may be of low or intermediate grade. The intermediate grade is characterized by the presence of necrosis, increased mitotic activity (mean 2 mitoses per 2 mm^2 area of tumor), and greater nuclear atypia.	PH is usually a lobulated lesion and is composed predominantly of chondroid or chondromyxoid tissue intermixed with variable proportions of other mesenchymal components, including fat, connective tissue, smooth muscle, and bone. Entrapped clefts of respiratory-type epithelium may be present between the lobules of mesenchymal components *(Figs. 77.4 and 77.5)*.

	Epithelioid Hemangioendothelioma (EH)	Pulmonary Hamartoma (PH)
Special studies	The tumor cells are immunopositive for vascular markers such as CD31, CD34, and FLI1. The t(1;3)(p36.3;q25) chromosomal translocation is characteristic of EH, resulting in the WWTR1-CAMTA1 gene fusion, which can be demonstrated by RT-PCR or FISH to confirm the diagnosis. A smaller subset of cases shows a distinct YAP1-TFE3 gene fusion, resulting in overexpression of TFE protein.	The mesenchymal cells are positive for S100 protein, which may be useful in the diagnosis. PHs have a high-frequency translocation t(3;12)(q27-28;q14-15), resulting in the HMGA2-LPP gene fusion.
Prognosis	The 5-y survival rate is 60%. The prognosis is worse for intermediate grade compared with low grade and can be as low as 20%. Negative prognostic factors include extensive intrapulmonary and pleural spread, weight loss, anemia, and hemorrhagic pleural effusions. Most patients with intermediate grade eventually die of respiratory failure secondary to pulmonary parenchyma replacement by tumor cells.	PHs are slowly growing neoplasms with excellent prognosis. Surgical resection is the treatment of choice for endobronchial lesions or symptomatic peripheral lesions. Recurrence or malignant transformations are exceedingly rare.

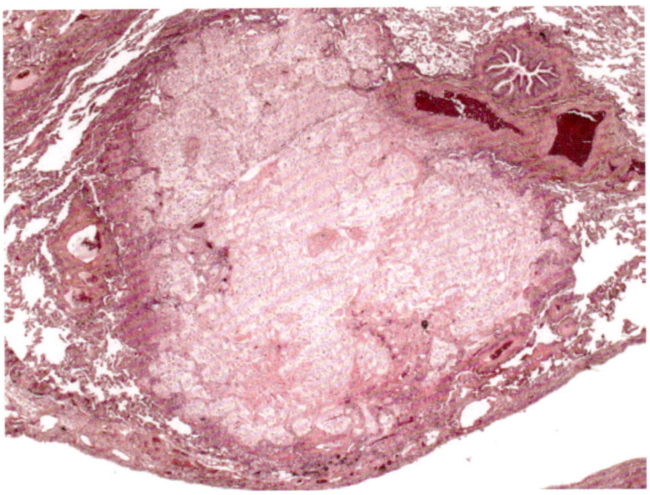

Figure 77.1 EH: Low-power round lesion with hypocellular sclerotic central zone and cellular peripheral zone.

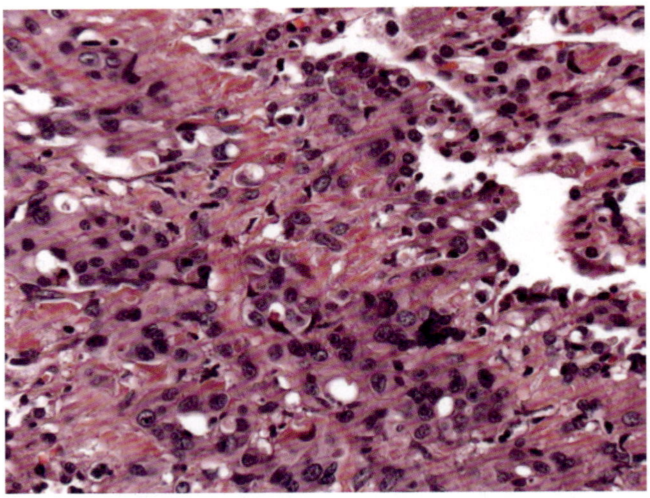

Figure 77.2 EH: The cellular zone is composed of cytologically bland, round-to-slightly spindle-shaped endothelial cells, with intracytoplasmic lumina containing red blood cells. The intracytoplasmic vacuoles may mimic a signet ring appearance.

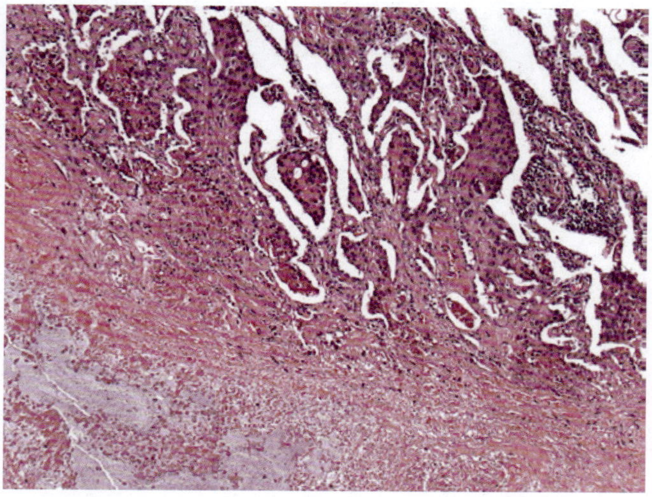

Figure 77.3 EH: The tumor frequently shows an intra-alveolar growth pattern and for that reason was formerly known as intravascular bronchoalveolar tumor (IVBAT).

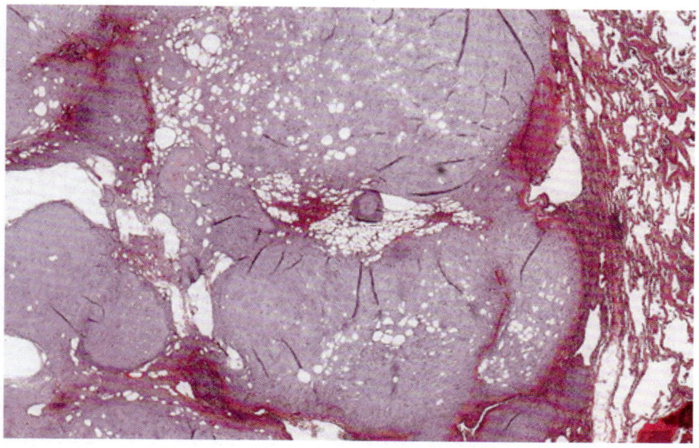

Figure 77.4 PH: Lobulated lesion composed predominantly of chondroid or chondromyxoid tissue intermixed with variable proportions of mature adipose tissue.

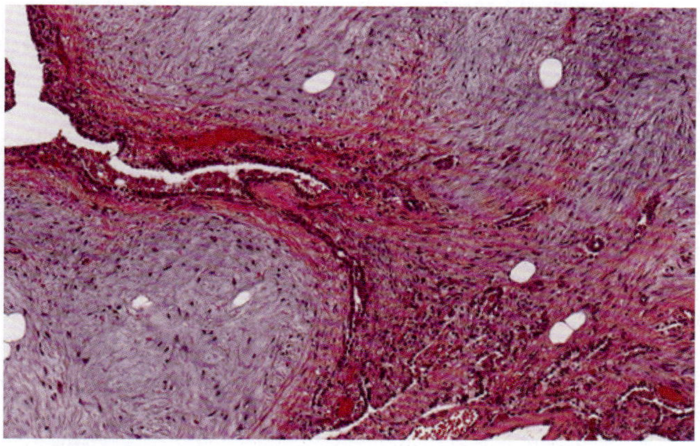

Figure 77.5 PH: High-power lobules of chondromyxoid tissue. Note adjacent entrapped clefts of benign respiratory-type epithelium between the lobules of mesenchymal components (*lower right*).

78 MUCOEPIDERMOID CARCINOMA VS. ADENOSQUAMOUS CARCINOMA

	Mucoepidermoid Carcinoma (MEC)	Adenosquamous Carcinoma (ASC)
Age	MEC occurs between the first and eighth decades of life, with a mean age between 39 and 40 y.	The mean age is around 60 y, with male predominance.
Location	MECs are usually endobronchial lesions that typically arise in central airways.	ASC usually arises in the peripheral pulmonary parenchyma.
Symptoms	Cough, wheezing, hemoptysis, and obstructive pneumonia. More peripheral lesions may be asymptomatic.	Cough, dyspnea, chest pain, hemoptysis, or can be asymptomatic.
Signs	Chest CT usually shows centrally located endobronchial mass. MEC is usually PET-positive.	Chest CT usually shows a peripheral solid mass. Central scarring, peripheral ground-glass opacification, and puckering of the overlying pleura may be seen.
Etiology	MECs originate from the submucosal glands of the tracheobronchial tree. There is no association with smoking.	ASC is associated with smoking.
Histology	MEC is composed of three cell types: mucous secreting, intermediate, and epidermoid (or squamous) cells. Mucous-secreting cells typically show abundant mucin-rich cytoplasm. Epidermoid cells show features of nonkeratinizing squamous cells with eosinophilic cytoplasm and distinct intercellular bridges. Keratinization or keratin pearls formation should not be present. The intermediate cells are smaller than squamous cells, oval or polygonal in shape, with round-to-oval nuclei, and eosinophilic or clear cytoplasm. Cells with clear cell appearance and an oncocytic component may also be seen. MECs are divided into low- and high-grade neoplasms. Low-grade tumors show predominance of mucous-filled cystic areas admixed with a minor component of solid areas. The cystic areas are lined by cytologically bland columnar, goblet, cuboidal, clear, or oncocytic-appearing mucin-producing cells. Mitotic figures are rare. The solid areas are composed of epidermoid and intermediate cells with minimal cytological atypia and rarely necrosis. The stroma is usually edematous with hyalinization, calcification, ossification, and granulomatous reaction adjacent to areas of mucous extravasation. High-grade tumors show predominance of solid areas composed of intermediate and epidermoid cells, with a minor component of mucin-secreting cells. There is nuclear atypia, pleomorphism, hyperchromasia, and frequent mitotic activity and necrosis *(Figs. 78.1–78.5)*.	ASC is characterized by areas of both adenocarcinoma and squamous cell carcinoma, each involving approximately 10% or more of the tumor. The two components may be arranged separately or mixed with each other. The components of squamous cell carcinoma (e.g., single-cell keratinization, keratin pearls, or intercellular bridges) and adenocarcinoma (e.g., acinar, tubular, or papillary structures) should be clearly and unequivocally evident on light microscopy *(Figs. 78.6 and 78.7)*. The degree of differentiation of each component can vary. The diagnosis is more difficult in poorly differentiated solid adenocarcinoma and nonkeratinizing squamous cell carcinoma components. Squamous cell carcinoma in situ can be found in the mucosa adjacent to some ASC, but it is not observed in MEC. Squamous cell carcinoma that entraps benign bronchial glands or adenocarcinoma that entraps metaplastic squamous epithelium should not be confused with ASC.

	Mucoepidermoid Carcinoma (MEC)	**Adenosquamous Carcinoma (ASC)**
Special studies	MEC is TTF-1 and Napsin-A negative. The epidermoid cells express CK5/6. The most characteristic chromosomal abnormality is the t(11;19)(q21;p13) chromosomal translocation, which involves the mucoepidermoid carcinoma translocated 1 (MECT1) and mammalian mastermind-like 2 (MAML2) genes. Fusion gene MECT1-MAML2 (also known as CRTC1-MAML2) occurs in both low- and high-grade tumors, more frequently in low grade.	Immunoperoxidase stains should support the presence of dual population of tumor cells with adenocarcinoma and squamous cell differentiation. TTF-1 is immunopositive in the adenocarcinoma component. P40 and CK5/6 are immunopositive in the squamous carcinoma component. In solid adenocarcinoma component, the presence on mucin stain of more than five cytoplasmic mucin droplets in at least two high-power fields supports the diagnosis of adenocarcinoma. ASCs may harbor epidermal growth factor receptor (EGFR) or KRAS genes mutations. EGFR gene mutations tend to be detected in women and nonsmokers, whereas KRAS gene mutations have been noted in smokers. ASC may also harbor ALK and ROS1 gene rearrangement.
Prognosis	The recommended treatment is surgical resection. Low-grade MEC has good prognosis, while high-grade tumors behave similarly to other non–small cell lung carcinomas. Poor prognosis factors include positive resection margins and lymph node metastasis.	ASC behaves aggressively. The 5-y survival rate after resection is about 40%. The predominant cell-type component within individual tumors has not been shown to have an impact on prognosis.

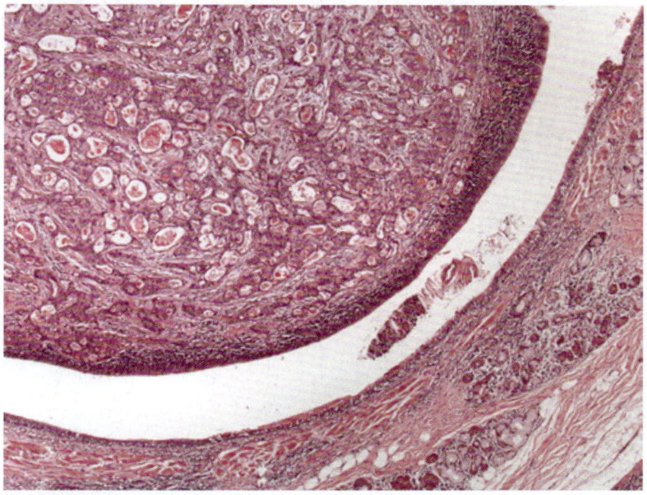

Figure 78.1 MEC (low grade, low power): Low-grade disease characteristically shows multiple cysts with mucous-secreting cells admixed with epidermoid cells and intermediate cells.

Reprinted from Achcar Rde O, Nikiforova MN, Dacic S, et al. Mammalian mastermind like 2 11q21 gene rearrangement in bronchopulmonary mucoepidermoid carcinoma. *Hum Pathol.* 2009 Jun;40(6):854-60, with permission.

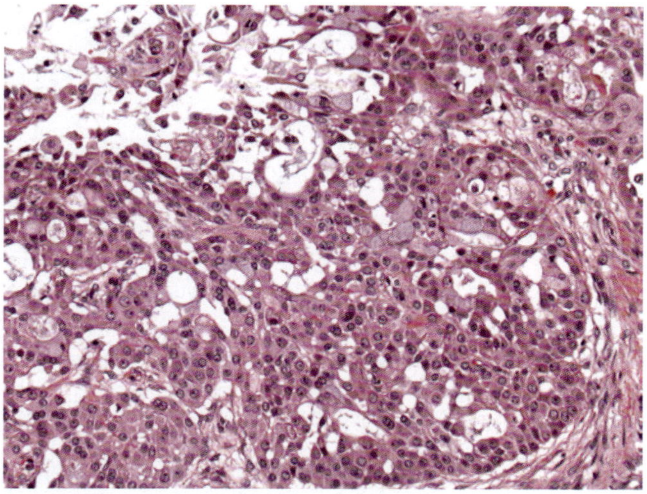

Figure 78.2 MEC (low grade, high power): Mucin-rich cells, cells with squamoid appearance, and cells transitional between the two are observed. Note minimal cytologic atypia.

Reprinted from Achcar Rde O, Nikiforova MN, Dacic S, et al. Mammalian mastermind like 2 11q21 gene rearrangement in bronchopulmonary mucoepidermoid carcinoma. *Hum Pathol.* 2009 Jun;40(6):854-60, with permission.

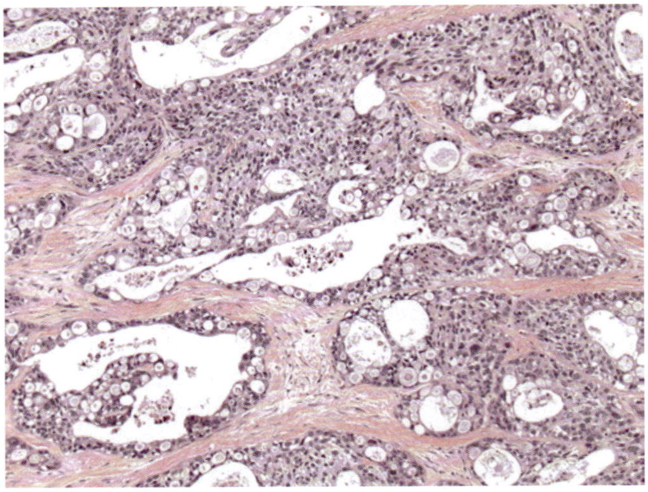

Figure 78.3 MEC (high grade): Disease showing a mixture of cystic and solid areas, although the latter predominate.

Reprinted from Achcar Rde O, Nikiforova MN, Dacic S, et al. Mammalian mastermind like 2 11q21 gene rearrangement in bronchopulmonary mucoepidermoid carcinoma. *Hum Pathol.* 2009 Jun;40(6):854-60, with permission.

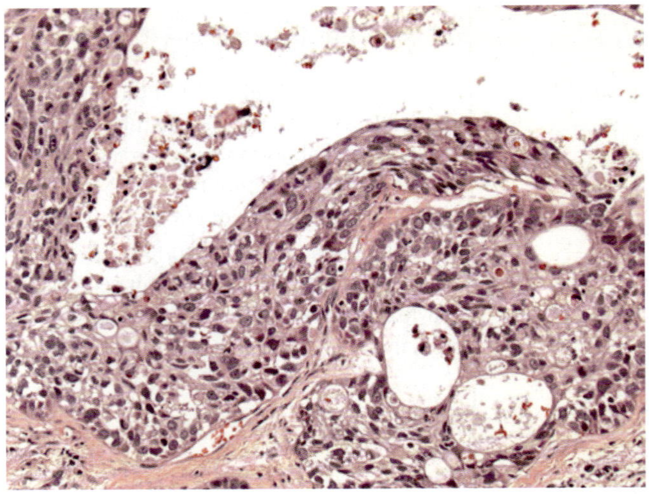

Figure 78.4 MEC (high grade): The cellular elements of mucous-rich, transitional and epidermoid cells show cytologic atypia.

Reprinted from Achcar Rde O, Nikiforova MN, Dacic S, et al. Mammalian mastermind like 2 11q21 gene rearrangement in bronchopulmonary mucoepidermoid carcinoma. *Hum Pathol.* 2009 Jun;40(6):854-60, with permission.

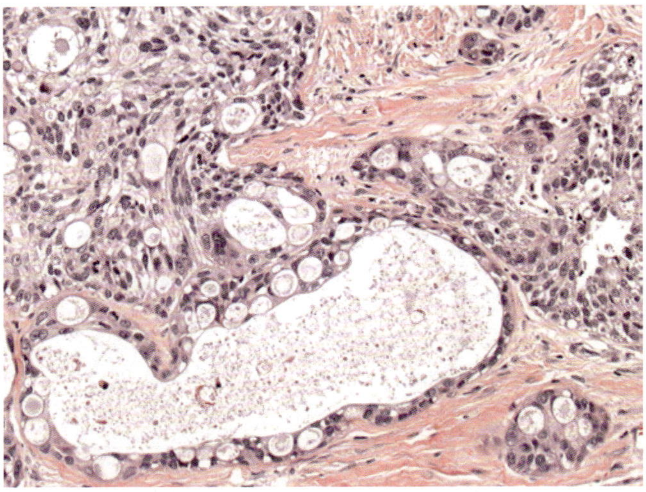

Figure 78.5 MEC (high grade): Disease showing cytologic atypia and necrosis.

Reprinted from Achcar Rde O, Nikiforova MN, Dacic S, et al. Mammalian mastermind like 2 11q21 gene rearrangement in bronchopulmonary mucoepidermoid carcinoma. *Hum Pathol.* 2009 Jun;40(6):854-60, with permission.

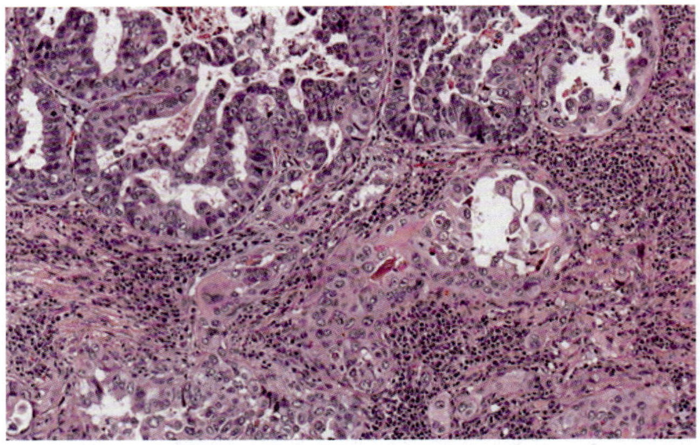

Figure 78.6 ASC: Adenocarcinoma with acinar growth pattern (upper field) and islands of squamous cell carcinoma (lower field) components are seen.

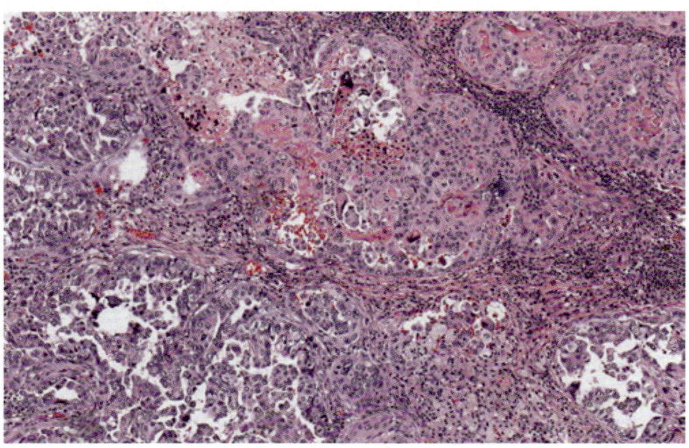

Figure 78.7 ASC: Image shows islands of squamous cell carcinoma (upper field) and adenocarcinoma with acinar and micropapillary growth patterns (lower field).

79 ADENOID CYSTIC CARCINOMA VS. ADENOCARCINOMA

	Adenoid Cystic Carcinoma (ACYSC)	Adenocarcinoma
Age	The average age of presentation is 50 y. There is no gender predominance.	Wide age distribution ranging from 20 y to more than 70 y. It is the most common type of lung cancer in both genders.
Location	ACYSC typically arises as an endobronchial tumor.	Although most (about 75%) pulmonary adenocarcinomas are peripheral parenchymal masses, centrally located adenocarcinomas may also occur.
Symptoms	Cough, wheezing, shortness of breath, and hemoptysis due to airway obstruction.	Wide variety of symptoms. The most common symptoms include progressive shortness of breath, cough, chest pain/pressure, or constitutional symptoms. Because of predominant peripheral location, adenocarcinomas may be discovered as an incidental mass or nodule on image studies performed for other reasons and may not present clinical symptoms.
Signs	Chest CT typically shows centrally located mass.	Image studies usually demonstrate a single peripheral mass or multiple nodular tumors. They may also present as pneumonia-like consolidation on chest image studies. Subpleural tumors may be associated with pleural thickening, pleural space involvement, and pleural effusion. Some rare subpleural tumors may present with predominant growth on the pleural surface and encase the lung in a diffuse, malignant, mesothelioma-like pattern referred to as "pseudomesotheliomatous carcinoma."
Etiology	ACYSC is derived from a primitive cell, presumably of tracheobronchial gland origin, which shows luminal epithelial and myoepithelial cell differentiation. There is no evidence of an association with smoking.	Atypical adenomatous hyperplasia (AAH), is believed to be the precursor lesion of peripheral pulmonary adenocarcinomas, and progression from AAH to adenocarcinoma in situ (AIS) to invasive adenocarcinoma has been proposed. Although most adenocarcinomas are caused by tobacco smoking, adenocarcinoma is the most frequent cell type in patients who have never smoked.
Histology	ACYSC tumor cells grow in three main architectural patterns including cribriform, tubular, and solid growth patterns *(Figs. 79.1–79.3)*. The cribriform growth pattern is the most typical architecture, characterized by the presence of nests of cells arranged around spaces filled with periodic acid-Schiff stain (PAS) positive eosinophilic (basement membrane-like) or basophilic to mucoid material. In the two-to-three-layered tubular growth pattern, the luminal epithelial cells show a cuboidal appearance and the peripheral cells form a myoepithelial layer. In the solid growth pattern, the tumor cells form irregular islands in which cystic-like spaces are absent or scant. The tumor cells are of small size, with scant cytoplasm and	Adenocarcinomas are defined as carcinomas with gland formation and/or mucin production. The 2015 WHO classification of pulmonary adenocarcinomas includes subtypes of several growth patterns: lepidic, acinar, papillary, micropapillary, and solid *(Figs. 79.4–79.9)*. Other variants include invasive mucinous adenocarcinoma, colloid adenocarcinoma, fetal adenocarcinoma, and enteric adenocarcinoma. If sampled adequately, virtually all pulmonary adenocarcinomas are of mixed subtypes, although one subtype usually predominates. According to the 2011 IASLC/ATS/ERS and 2015 WHO classifications, the classification of invasive adenocarcinoma should include the predominant subtype after comprehensive histologic subtyping by semiquantitatively estimating the percentage of the various subtypes present in 5% increments.

	Adenoid Cystic Carcinoma (ACYSC)	Adenocarcinoma
	usually homogeneous, oval-to-angulated hyperchromatic nuclei. Perineural invasion is frequent. Mitotic figures are usually rare or absent. The stroma is eosinophilic, hyalinized, or collagenous.	
Special studies	Immunoperoxidase stains demonstrate that the tumor cells have a variable expression of luminal epithelial and myoepithelial markers including cytokeratin, vimentin, smooth muscle actin, calponin, S-100 protein, p63, and CD117 (C-Kit). The luminal epithelial cells usually express more intense staining for cytokeratins than do myoepithelial cells. TTF-1 and Napsin-A are immunonegative. EGFR and KRAS genes mutation are not identified.	Most pulmonary adenocarcinomas are immunopositive for a variety of cytokeratins, including AE1/AE3, CK7, and CAM 5.2, but are negative for vimentin, smooth muscle actin, calponin, S-100 protein, p63, and C-KIT (myoepithelial markers). TTF-1 shows immunopositivity in 75%–85% of pulmonary adenocarcinomas. Napsin A has comparable sensitivity with that of TTF-1. Molecular testing for epidermal growth factor receptor (EGFR) gene mutational analysis and ALK gene rearrangement are important for treatment management. Activating mutations in EGFR gene are clustered in exons 18–21. The two most common EGFR gene mutations are in-frame deletions in exon 19 (45%), followed by point mutation (CTG to CGC) in exon 21 at nucleotide 2573, which result in substitution of leucine by arginine at codon 858 (L858R)(41%). EML4-ALK fusion accounts for >90% of ALK gene rearrangements in lung adenocarcinoma. EGFR gene mutation and ALK gene rearrangement are more commonly found in never-smokers with adenocarcinoma. EGFR gene mutations are more common in Asian patients and women. KRAS gene mutations in codons 12, 13, or 61 are present in 30% of adenocarcinomas and are particularly common in smokers.
Prognosis	ACYSCs are in general characterized by long survival, with multiple local recurrences and late metastases over a 10–15-y period following resection. Surgical resection with or without radiation is the typical treatment. Poor prognosis is related to advanced stage of tumor at diagnosis, positive margins at surgery, and solid growth pattern predominance.	Never-smoking status and female sex are favorable prognostic factors independent from the tumor stage. Tumor size ≥2.5 cm, solid and micropapillary subtypes, and a maximum standardized uptake value (SUV) of ≥7 are predictors of poor disease-free survival. The prognosis for stage I lepidic predominant adenocarcinoma is usually good, unless associated with close margin in limited resection, visceral pleural, and/or angiolymphatic invasion or the presence of micropapillary growth pattern component. Tumors with EFGR gene mutation may respond favorably to epidermal growth factor tyrosine kinase inhibitors (EGFR TKIs) such as gefitinib and erlotinib. Tumors with ALK gene rearrangement may respond favorably to ALK blockade with crizotinib. Of note, mutations of in-frame insertions in EGFR gene exon 20 is associated with primary resistance to EGFR TKI. Acquisition of an additional T790M mutation is the most common cause of secondary resistance to EGFR TKI. However, using more sensitive mutation-detection techniques, it was shown that T790M EGFR mutation may coexist with L858R mutations, which might confer pretreatment (primary) resistance to EGFR TKIs. Amplification of MET gene is another mechanisms of EGFR TKIs resistance. The presence of KRAS gene mutation is usually associated with resistance to EGFR TKIs.

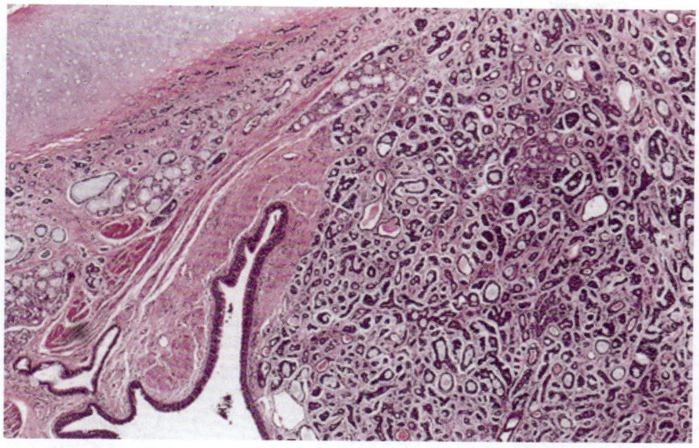

Figure 79.1 ACYSC growing in the characteristic cribriform and tubular growth patterns in the airway submucosa. Note the intact respiratory mucosa (*left*).

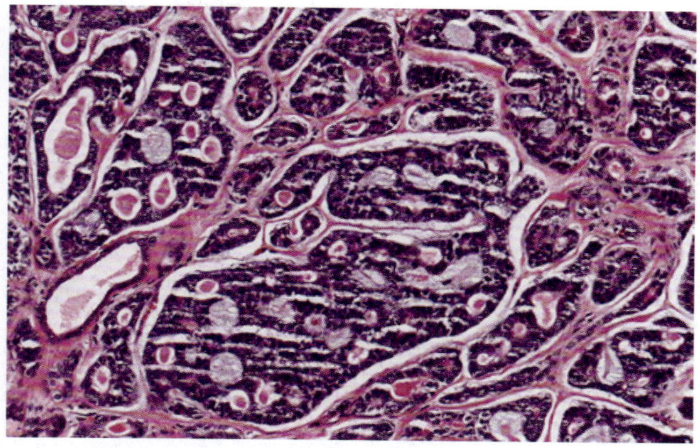

Figure 79.2 ACYSC: The cribriform growth pattern is the most typical architecture characterized by the presence of nests of cells arranged around spaces filled with eosinophilic (basement membrane-like) or basophilic-to-mucoid material.

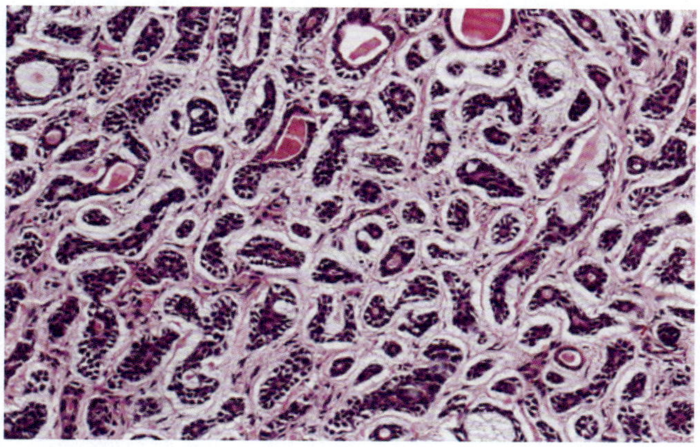

Figure 79.3 ACYSC showing tubular growth pattern.

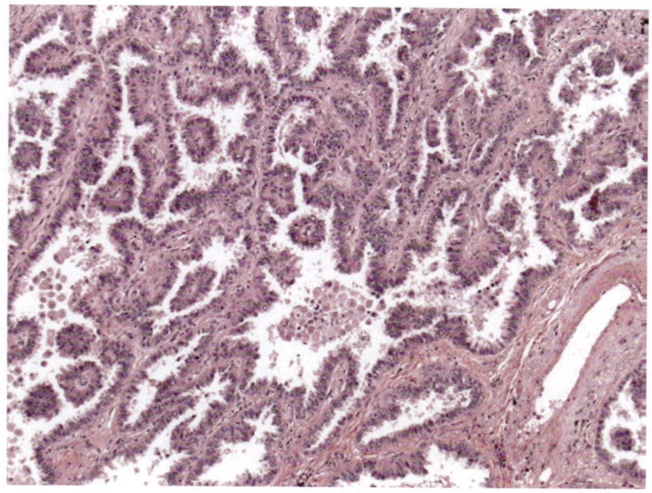

Figure 79.4 Lepidic adenocarcinoma: The tumor cells grow along the alveolar walls surface.

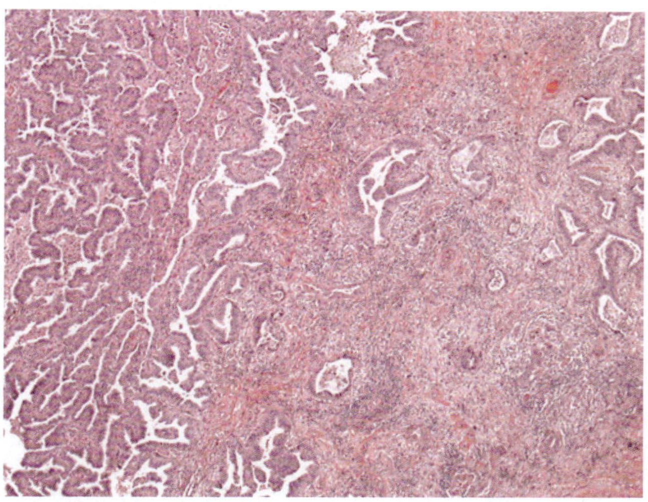

Figure 79.5 Adenocarcinoma: Lepidic growth pattern (*left*) and acinar growth pattern composed of malignant glands within a fibroinflammatory stroma (*right*).

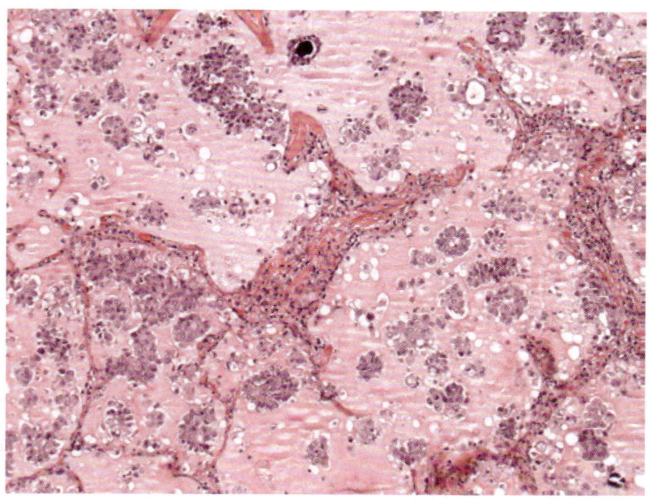

Figure 79.6 Micropapillary adenocarcinoma: Dyscohesive papillary clusters of cytologically malignant cells "float" within the air spaces. The tumor cells form papillae that lack a fibrovascular core.

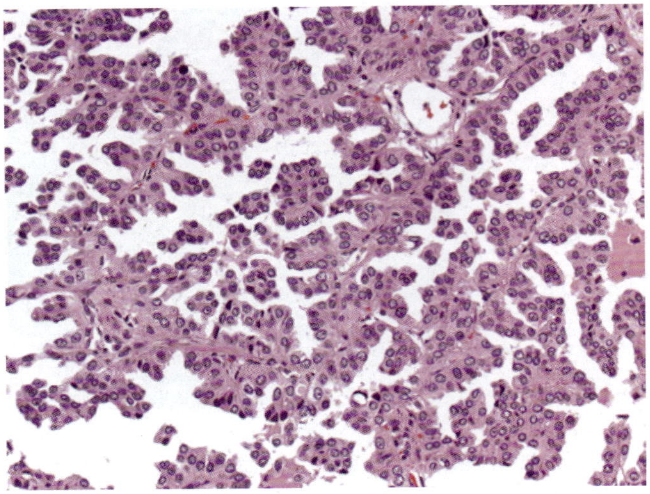

Figure 79.7 Papillary adenocarcinoma: The tumor cells form true papillary structures, with papillae lined by glandular epithelium surrounding a fibrovascular core.

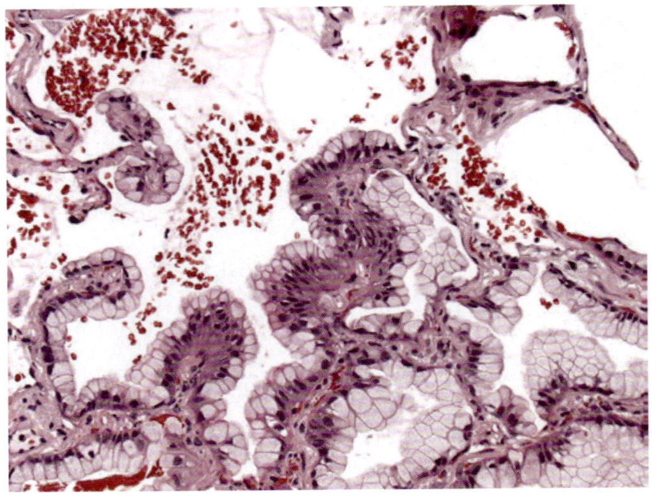

Figure 79.8 Mucinous adenocarcinoma: The columnar mucinous tumor cells grow in a lepidic growth pattern.

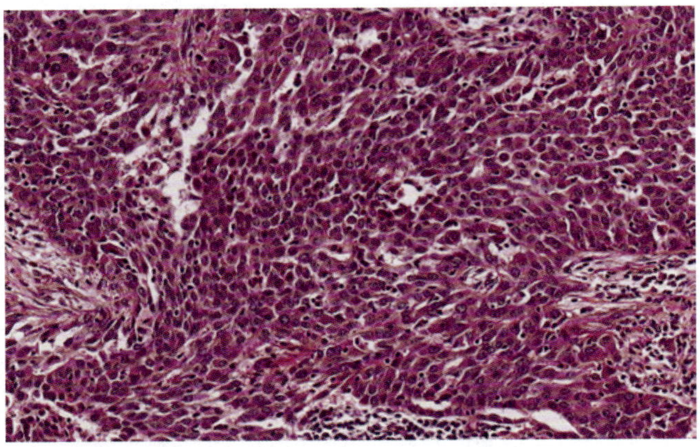

Figure 79.9 Solid adenocarcinoma: In this poorly differentiated carcinoma with solid growth pattern, immunoperoxidase stains are of paramount importance. In this case, the tumor cells expressed TTF-1, Napsin-A, and cytokeratin 7 and failed to express myoepithelial markers, supporting the diagnosis of poorly differentiated adenocarcinoma with solid growth pattern/solid adenocarcinoma.

80 EPITHELIOID MALIGNANT MESOTHELIOMA VS. BENIGN REACTIVE MESOTHELIAL HYPERPLASIA

	Epithelioid Malignant Mesothelioma (EMM)	Benign Reactive Mesothelial Hyperplasia (RMH)
Age	EMM occurs over a wide age range, but the vast majority of tumors are seen in patients between 50 and 70 y of age.	Benign RMH occurs over a wide age range, most commonly seen in adults.
Location	Right side involvement is more common than left side, with a ratio of 3:2.	No specific pleural location/side involvement.
Symptoms	Chest pain, dyspnea, and progressive shortness of breath.	Chest pain, dyspnea, shortness of breath, and constitutional symptoms, depending on the underlying cause.
Signs	Wide range of image abnormalities, with the most classic being the presence of diffuse circumferential and/or nodular pleural thickening that compresses the underlying lung and is usually associated with ipsilateral volume loss and pleural effusion. Caution is required in diagnosing malignant mesothelioma in the absence of pleural thickening on CT. Other abnormalities include localized pleural mass, calcified pleural plaques, and round atelectasis.	Variable amounts of pleural effusion and pleural thickening may be present.
Etiology	The most common cause of EMM is exposure to asbestos, particularly occupational exposure. EMM is also seen as a result of household contact exposure, such as washing asbestos-contaminated workclothes. Other causes include exposure to the mineral fiber erionite (in a localized area of Turkey), therapeutic radiation for other malignant neoplasms, or idiopathic.	RMH is associated with a number of underlying pathologic conditions, including asbestos exposure, benign pleural effusions, a variety of chronic pleural infections, underlying connective tissue diseases, prior radiation, reactions to subpleural bronchogenic carcinomas or pleural metastases, recurrent pneumothoraces, pulmonary infarcts, drug reactions, surgery, and trauma.
Histology	*Cellularity:* Dense (noninflammatory) cellularity in stroma. Most epithelioid mesotheliomas are composed of cuboidal or polygonal to flattened, cytologically bland cells and show a wide range of growth patterns, including solid, tubulopapillary, and trabecular. Less common patterns include micropapillary, pseudoglandular, adenomatoid (microcystic), clear cell, transitional, and deciduoid. The tumor cells usually have round nuclei, bland vesicular chromatin, prominent nucleoli, and moderate amounts of eosinophilic cytoplasm *(Figs. 80.1 and 80.2)*.	*Cellularity:* It may be densely cellular (including intense inflammatory cells infiltrate) in the pleural space, but not in the stroma. The mesothelial cells form piled-up accumulations to confluent sheets of cells along the pleural surface, which may be associated with papillary excrescences with tufts of cells with bland, tubule-like, nonbranching structures with no true fibrovascular cores. Complex branching papillary proliferations tubules or glands favor malignancy. The cells are cuboidal to elongated, may have enlarged nuclei, and often have prominent nucleoli, with significant cell-to-cell variation *(Figs. 80.6–80.8)*.

Epithelioid Malignant Mesothelioma (EMM)	Benign Reactive Mesothelial Hyperplasia (RMH)
Zonation: There is no zonation. The cellularity of the atypical cells is present throughout the full thickness of the pleura *(Fig. 80.3)*, and the process is often more cellular away from the effusion.	*Zonation:* There is zonation *(Fig. 80.9)*. The cellularity, including intense inflammatory cells infiltrate, is greatest toward the pleural surface immediately under the effusion, and becomes more fibrotic away from the effusion. Other features include vascular proliferation with few associated spindle cells. The capillaries are parallel to each other and perpendicular to pleural surface (in malignancy, the capillaries are usually inconspicuous and arranged in a haphazard fashion).
Cytologic atypia: In general, the EMM cells are usually deceptively bland and relatively monotonous but cytologic atypia (e.g., high N/C ratio, irregularity of the nuclear membranes, coarsely clumped chromatin) may be present in any area.	*Cytologic atypia:* Pleomorphism is more common in reactive mesothelial proliferations than typical EMM. However, cytologic atypia, when present, is usually confined to an area of organizing effusion. Cells immediately under effusion can be very atypical, particularly when mesothelial cells are mixed with fibrin.
Mitosis: Mitosis is infrequent. Many EMMs show very few mitoses , but the presence of atypical mitoses favors malignancy.	*Mitosis:* Mitoses may be numerous, with lack of atypical mitoses.
Necrosis: When present, is typically bland, unassociated with significant inflammation or cellular debris and a sign of malignancy.	*Necrosis:* Rare; when present, is typically associated with inflammatory cells and cellular debris.
Stromal invasion: There is stromal invasion *(Figs. 80.4 and 80.5)*. The presence of mesothelial cells invading into the adipose tissue of parietal pleura, underlying stroma *(Fig. 80.4)*, connective tissue, lung parenchyma, chest wall muscle, or soft tissue is the most reliable indicator of malignancy in mesothelial proliferations. These features can be identified only in an adequate tissue sample. Cytokeratin immunostain is useful to demonstrate invasion of the cells into underlying tissues *(Fig. 80.5)*.	*Stromal invasion:* No true invasion of the stroma *(Figs. 80.8, 80.10–80.12)*. Entrapment of benign reactive mesothelial cells is common and can occur with any type of inflammatory reaction, particularly within areas of organization, mimicking tissue invasion. This is characterized by the presence of superficial entrapment of nests of mesothelial cells *(Fig. 80.10)* in the pleural stroma or lines *(Figs. 80.11 and 80.12)* of mesothelial cells or small glands arranged parallel to the pleural surface, which may be located deep in a thickened pleura. A helpful hint in circumstances in which there are proliferating mesothelial cells but no inflammation is the distribution of the mesothelial cells. Benign process tend to be sharply circumscribed, with a few glands evident beneath the pleural surface *(Fig. 80.10)*, or with a sharp line *(Fig. 80.12)* beyond which no mesothelial cells are found. This is well demonstrated with keratin stains. In contrast, mesotheliomas are always invasive. En face cuts of poorly oriented pleural biopsies *(Figs. 80.6 and 80.8)* may also give the false impression of invasion *(Fig. 80.8)*. Sections cut parallel to the serosal surface may give the impression that benign surface-reactive mesothelial cells are surrounded by connective tissue *(Fig. 80.8)*. The presence of mesothelial cells on two surfaces is a clue that a specimen has been cut en face. When there is any doubt whether one is dealing with invasion, entrapment, or en face cuts of the surface on a

	Epithelioid Malignant Mesothelioma (EMM)	Benign Reactive Mesothelial Hyperplasia (RMH)
		pleural biopsy, the term *atypical mesothelial proliferation* or *atypical mesothelial hyperplasia* is recommended for the diagnosis, with a comment that additional tissue sampling should be obtained if clinically indicated.
Special studies	Both EMM and RMH cell populations express keratin and the mesothelial markers calretinin, CK5/6, WT-1, and D2-40. These immunostains may be useful for demonstrating invasion of the cells into underlying tissues and particularly for detecting subtle invasion of fat by few cells that may not be readily apparent on hematoxylin–eosin (H&E) staining. It has been demonstrated that EMM exhibit deletions or mutations in BAP 1 (BRCA1-associated protein) gene, located in chromosome 3p21, which leads to loss of detectable protein expression by immunohistochemical (IHC) staining. Although significant proportion of EMMs will not show BAP1 loss, the demonstration of loss of BAP1 staining by IHC is diagnostic of EMM. It has also been demonstrated that EMM exhibits loss of p16/CDKN2A (cyclin-dependent kinase inhibitor-2A) gene, located on chromosome 9p21, while reactive benign mesothelium shows retention of at least one copy of the gene. p16 homozygous deletion can be demonstrated by fluorescence in situ hybridization (FISH). Of note, in contrast to BAP1, p16 IHC stain cannot replace p16 FISH molecular testing. Although the markers p53, epithelial membrane antigen (EMA), and GLUT-1 have been proposed to provide support for the diagnosis of malignancy on pleural biopsy, none of these markers are absolutely specific or sensitive and therefore cannot be relied on to make a diagnosis.	Reactive mesothelial cells express pancytokeratin, and the mesothelial markers calretinin, CK5/6, WT-1, and D2-40, show retention of at least one copy of the p16/CDKN2A (cyclin-dependent kinase inhibitor-2A) gene (demonstrated by FISH) and express BPA1 (demonstrate by IHC). Although desmin has been proposed to provide support for the diagnosis of reactive mesothelial hyperplasia, some studies found that mesotheliomas stained for desmin. Therefore, we do not recommend its use.
Prognosis	The long-term survival rate of patients with malignant mesothelioma is poor, with average survival of less than 1 y. Younger age, epithelioid type (vs. sarcomatoid or biphasic types), and early TNM staging are indicators of longer median survival.	It depends on the underlying cause.

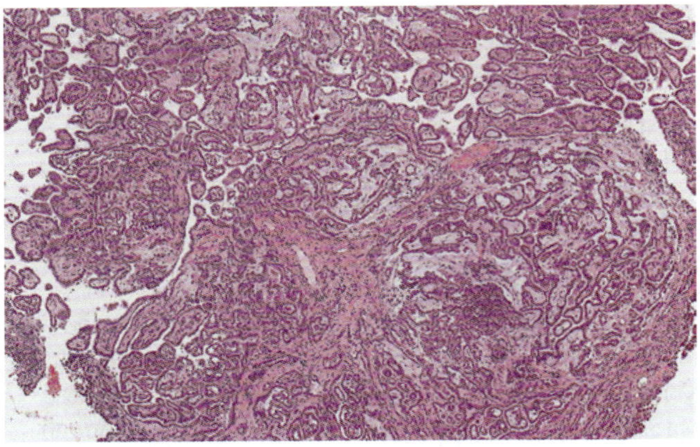

Figure 80.1 EMM: Epithelioid mesothelioma showing complex surface mesothelial proliferation composed of cuboidal cytologically bland cells showing tubulopapillary and trabecular growth patterns.

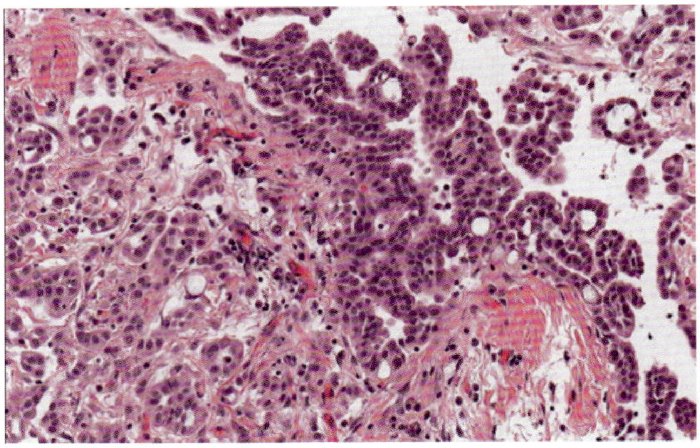

Figure 80.2 EMM: The tumor cells have round nuclei, bland vesicular chromatin, prominent nucleoli, and moderate amounts of eosinophilic cytoplasm.

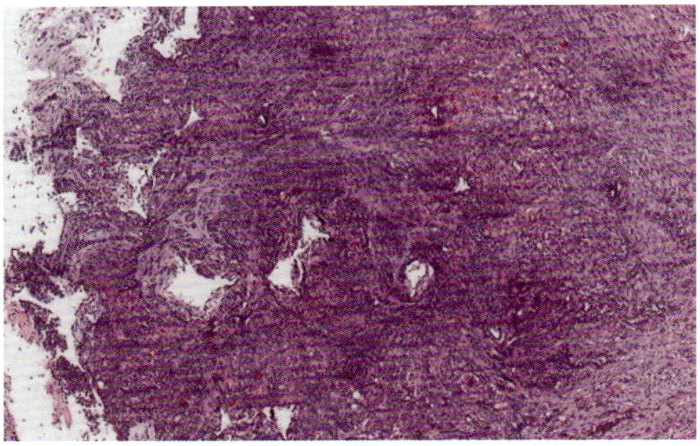

Figure 80.3 EMM: There is no zonation. The tumor cells are present throughout the full thickness of the pleura.

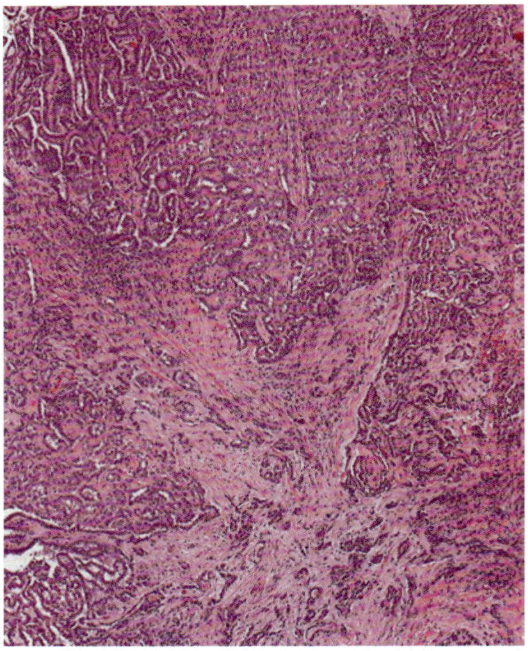

Figure 80.4 EMM: Disease with underlying stroma invasion. Invasion is the most reliable indicator of malignancy in mesothelial proliferations.

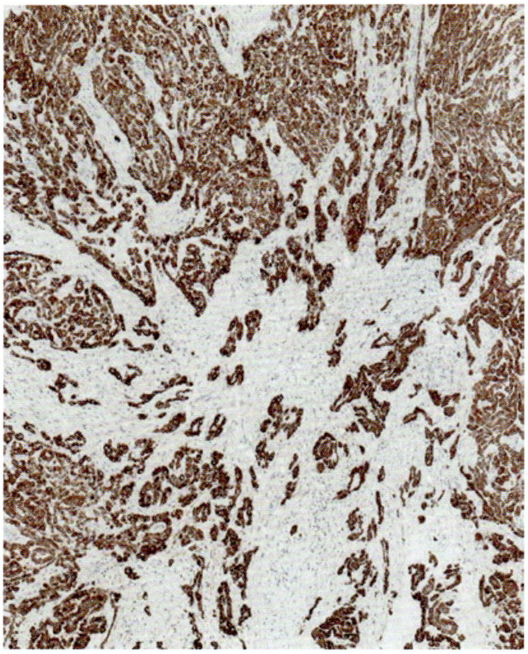

Figure 80.5 EMM: Invasion highlighted by cytokeratin immunoperoxidase stain. Both EMM and RMH cell populations express cytokeratin. This marker does not differentiate EMM from RMH but is useful to demonstrate invasion.

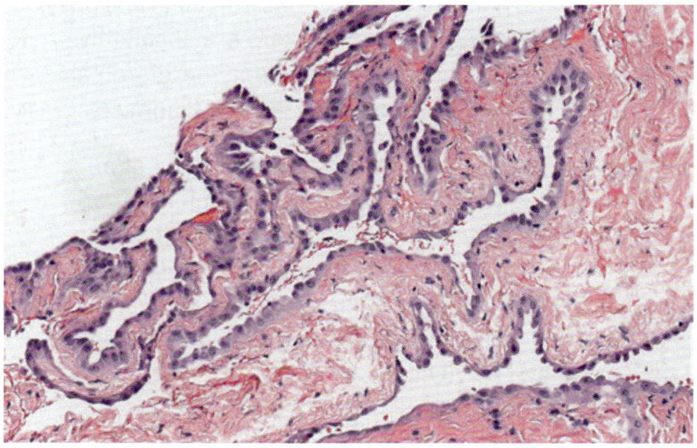

Figure 80.6 RMH: Simple mesothelial hyperplasia showing a more pronounced layer of relatively bland cuboidal cells along the pleural surface. Note that the presence of mesothelial cells on two surfaces is a clue that a specimen has been cut en face.

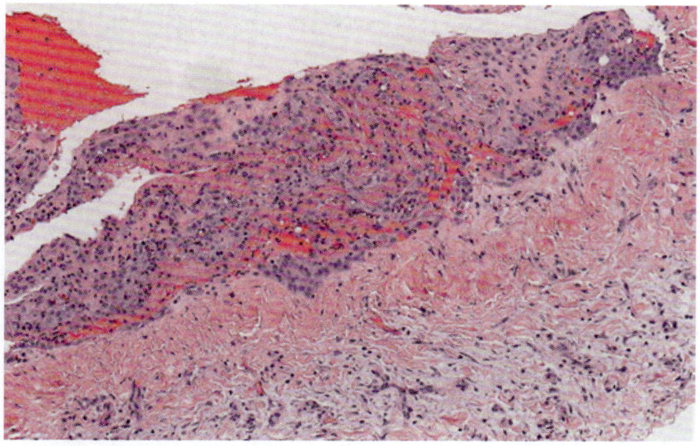

Figure 80.7 RMH: The reactive mesothelial cells form piled-up accumulations to confluent sheets of cells along the pleural surface, but not in the underlying stroma.

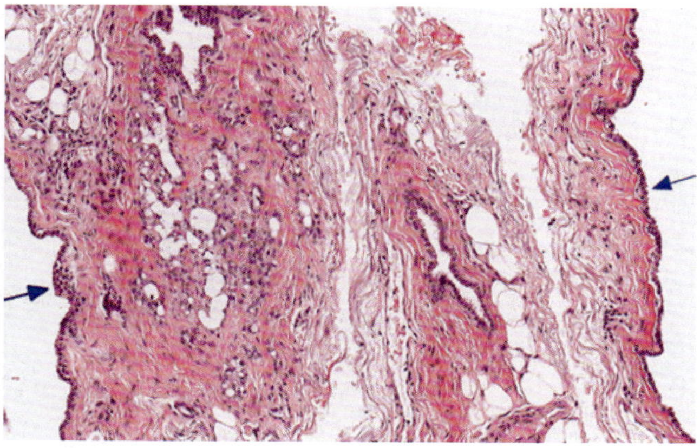

Figure 80.8 RMH: En face cuts of pleural biopsies, cut parallel to the serosal surface, may show entrapped reactive mesothelial cells surrounded by connective tissue (*middle and right*), and may give the false impression of invasion. The presence of mesothelial cells on 2 surfaces (*arrows*) is a clue that a specimen has been cut en face.

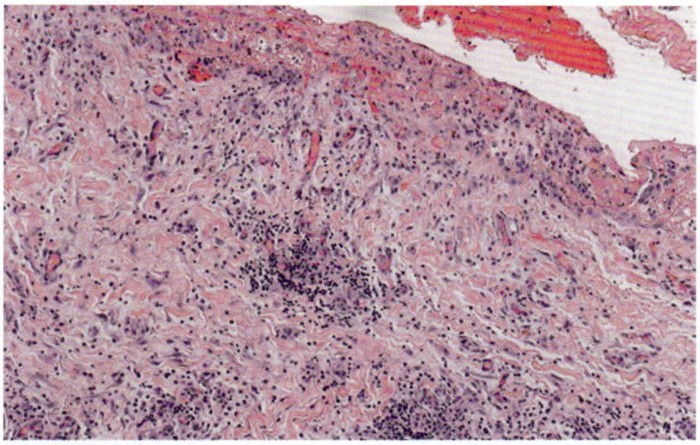

Figure 80.9 RMH: There is zonation characterized by reactive mesothelial cells and inflammatory cells, which is greatest toward the pleural surface immediately under the effusion (upper field), which becomes more fibrotic away from the effusion (lower field). Note capillaries parallel to each other and perpendicular to pleural surface (in malignancy, the capillaries are usually inconspicuous and arranged in a haphazard fashion).

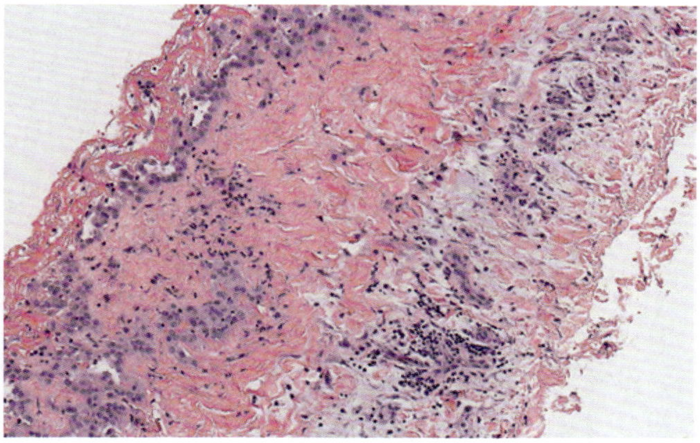

Figure 80.10 RMH: Entrapment of benign reactive mesothelial cells characterized by the presence of superficial entrapment of nests of mesothelial cells in the pleural stroma.

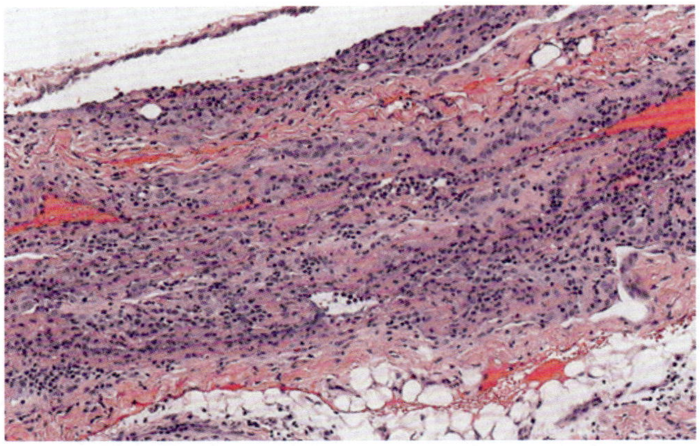

Figure 80.11 RMH: Entrapment of benign reactive mesothelial cells characterized by the presence of lines of mesothelial cells arranged parallel to the pleural surface. Note lack of invasion into the fat.

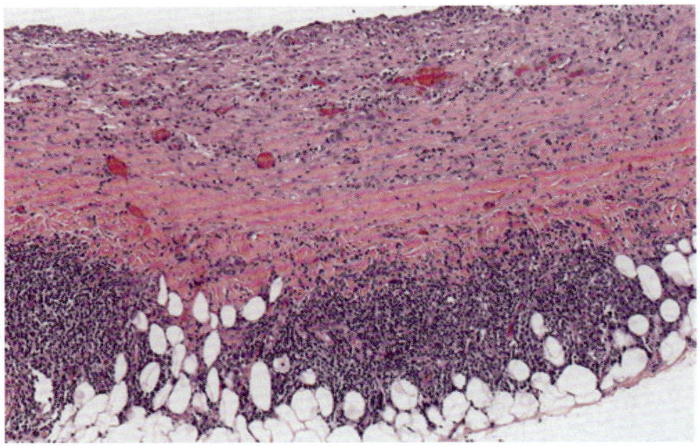

Figure 80.12 RMH: Entrapment of lines of benign reactive mesothelial arranged parallel to the pleural surface, which may be located deep in a thickened pleura, but lack invasion into the fat. Cytokeratin stain is helpful in cases like this, demonstrating the distribution of the mesothelial cells. Benign process tends to be sharply circumscribed, forming a sharp line (well demonstrated by cytokeratin stain), beyond which no mesothelial cells are found, whereas mesotheliomas are always invasive.

81 SARCOMATOID MALIGNANT MESOTHELIOMA VS. SOLITARY FIBROUS TUMOR

	Sarcomatoid Malignant Mesothelioma (SMM)	Solitary Fibrous Tumor (SFT)
Age	SMM occurs over a wide age range, but the vast majority of tumors are seen in patients between 50 and 70 y of age. SMM accounts for less than 10% of all mesotheliomas.	SFT can occur at any age, but it is more common in the sixth and seventh decades of life, with no sex predilection.
Location	Right-side involvement is more common than left side, with a ratio of 3:2.	SFTs of the pleura most often arise in the visceral pleura, but are widely distributed throughout the pleural cavity.
Symptoms	Chest pain, dyspnea, and progressive shortness of breath.	Many lesions are asymptomatic and discovered incidentally, but they may present with cough, dyspnea, chest pain, general malaise, or hypoglycemia (secondary to insulin-like growth factor production).
Signs	Wide range of image abnormalities, with the most classic being diffuse circumferential and/or nodular pleural thickening that compresses the underlying lung and is usually associated with ipsilateral volume loss and pleural effusion. Caution is required in diagnosing malignant mesothelioma in the absence of pleural thickening on CT. Other abnormalities include localized pleural mass, calcified pleural plaques, and round atelectasis.	Image studies usually demonstrate sharply demarcated, pleural-based soft tissue masses with no chest wall abnormality.
Etiology	The most common cause of SMM is exposure to asbestos, particularly occupational exposure. SMM is also seen as a result of household contact exposure, such as washing asbestos-contaminated work clothes. Other causes include exposure to the mineral fiber erionite (in a localized area of Turkey), therapeutic radiation for other malignant neoplasms, or idiopathic.	Unknown. There is no link with asbestos exposure.
Histology	SMM is characterized by a proliferation of spindle cells arranged in fascicles or in a haphazard pattern, with invasion into the adipose tissue of parietal pleura *(Figs. 81.1 and 81.2)*, underlying stroma, connective tissue, lung parenchyma, chest wall muscle, or soft tissue. Nuclear atypia and mitotic activity vary from minimal to moderate or marked. Heterologous (rhabdomyosarcomatous, osteosarcomatous, or chondrosarcomatous) elements may be present *(Fig. 81.3)*. The presence of necrosis and the degree of atypia and mitosis parallels the aggressiveness of the tumor.	SFT is typically characterized by the presence of hypo- and hypercellular areas, and branching hemangiopericytoma-like vessels of varying sizes and numbers. The hypercellular areas are composed of uniform elongate-to-spindle shaped cells with bland nuclear features arranged in fascicular, storiform, herringbone, or patternless architecture, with variable prominent stromal hyalinization *(Figs. 81.4–81.7)*. Rarely the stroma is myxoid. Necrosis is infrequent. Usually, there are less than 3 mitoses/2 mm^2 area of tumor *(Fig. 81.8)*. Malignant SFTs are usually hypercellular and show more than 4 mitoses per/2 mm^2 area of tumor.

	Sarcomatoid Malignant Mesothelioma (SMM)	Solitary Fibrous Tumor (SFT)
Special studies	SMM almost invariably stains, at least focally, with keratin markers such as AE1/AE3. However, keratin negativity may be encountered in 5% of cases and in 10% of tumors with heterologous (rhabdomyosarcomatous, osteosarcomatous, or chondrosarcomatous) elements. Keratin immunostaining can be very helpful for identifying tumor cells and for demonstrating invasion into underlying tissues. About 30% of SMMs express calretinin and D2-40. Other mesothelial markers, including CK5/6 and WT1, appear to be relatively insensitive. SMMs are often vimentin positive and occasionally express actin, desmin, or S100. It has been demonstrated that SMMs exhibit deletions or mutations in BAP 1 (BRCA1-associated protein) gene, located in chromosome 3p21, which lead to loss of detectable protein expression by immunohistochemical (IHC) stain. The presence of loss of BAP1 staining by IHC is diagnostic of SMM. It has also been demonstrated that SMM exhibits loss of p16/CDKN2A (cyclin-dependent kinase inhibitor-2A) gene, located on chromosome 9p21. p16 homozygous deletion can be demonstrated by fluorescence in situ hybridization (FISH). Of note, in contrast to BAP1, p16 IHC stain cannot replace p16 FISH molecular testing.	SFTs express CD34, Bcl2, CD99, and STAT 6. STAT 6 is the most specific, and positive in more than 95% of cases. Keratin markers are usually negative and rarely focally positive. Some cases are smooth muscle actin (SMA) positive, and occasional cases may stain for S100 or desmin. SFT harbors the specific (to date) gene fusion NAB2-STAT6, which results from the intrachromosomal inversion inv(12)(q13q13), and leads to overexpression of STAT6.
Prognosis	The long-term survival rate of patients with SMM is poor, with worse prognosis than the epithelioid subtype.	Complete surgical excision is the main therapy. Local recurrence occurs in about 10% of cases and metastasis in 5%–10%. More than 4 mitoses/ 2 mm^2 area of tumor is the most reliable indicator of aggressive behavior. However, cases having benign morphology may also give rise to metastasis.

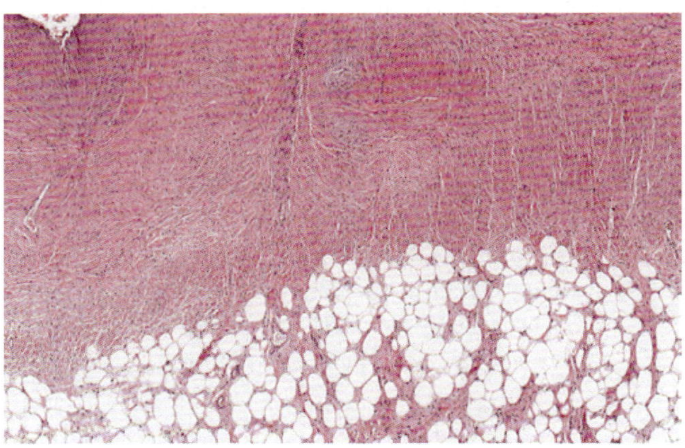

Figure 81.1 SMM: Full-thickness cellularity with invasion into the chest wall adipose.

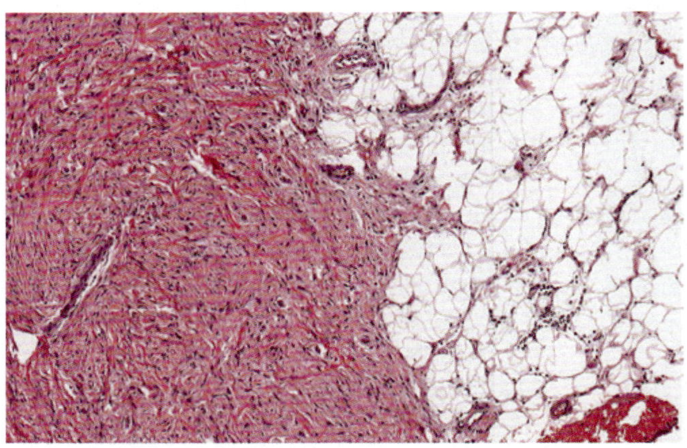

Figure 81.2 SMM: Proliferation of spindle cells arranged in a haphazard pattern, with invasion into the adipose tissue of parietal pleura. SMM usually express keratin but show low expression of mesothelial markers. Loss of BAP1 staining by IHC and p16 homozygous deletion by FISH supports the diagnosis of SMM.

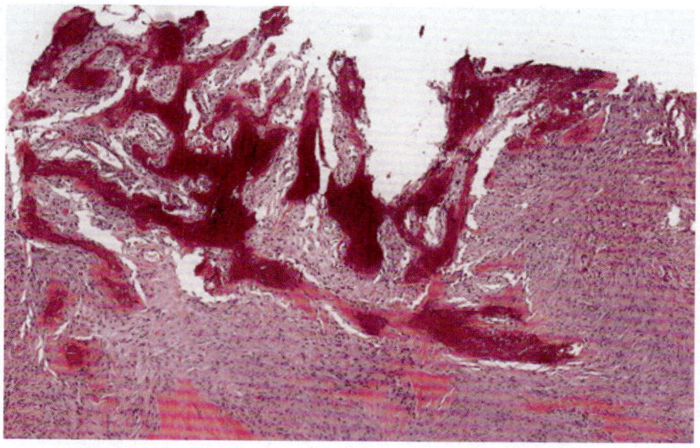

Figure 81.3 SMM: Note the presence of heterologous (osteosarcomatous) elements.

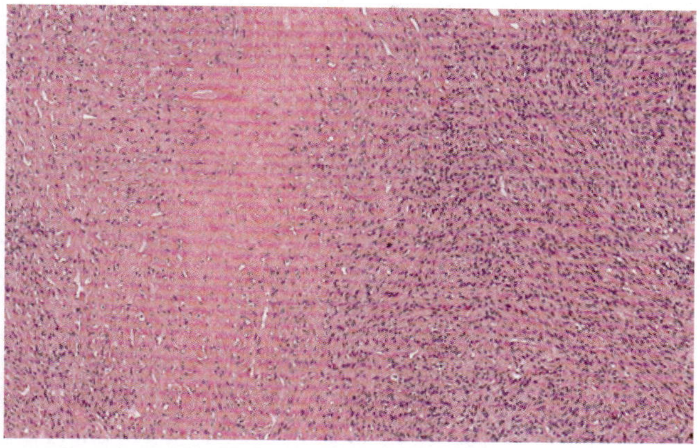

Figure 81.4 SFT: Hypocellular and hypercellular areas associated with vessels of variable sizes and numbers and collagenous stroma composed of thick collagen bundles are seen.

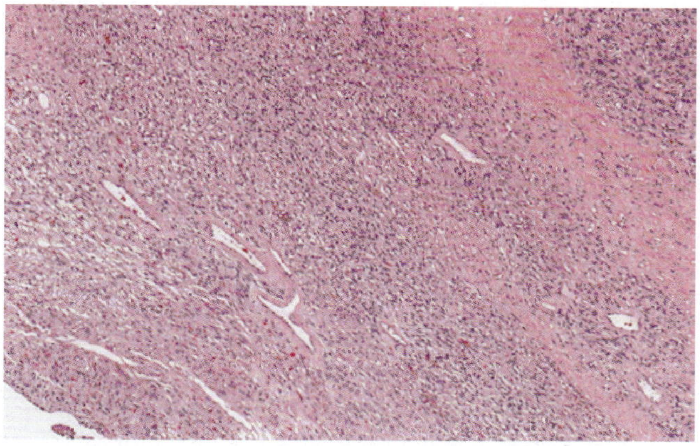

Figure 81.5 SFT: Hypercellular area with patternless architecture and branching hemangiopericytoma-like vessels.

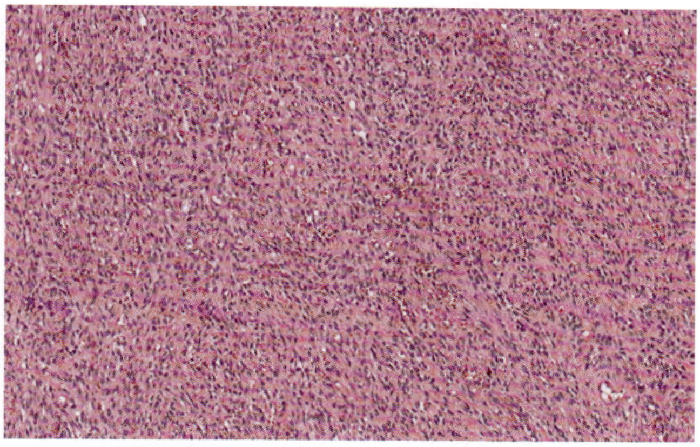

Figure 81.6 SFT: The hypercellular areas are composed of uniform, elongate-to-spindle shaped cells with bland nuclear features.

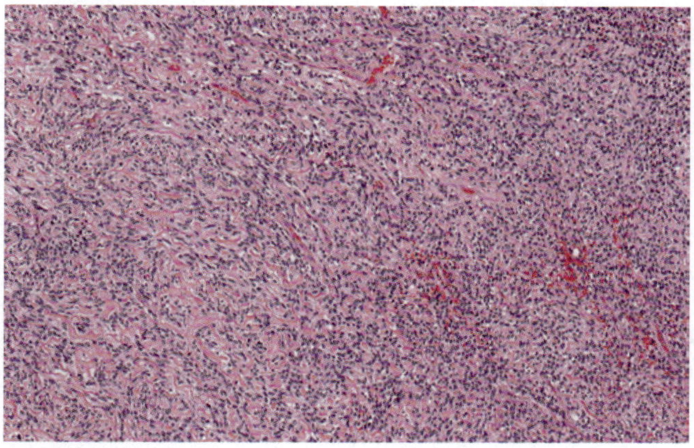

Figure 81.7 SFT: Hypercellular area showing cells with bland nuclear features arranged in a patternless architecture within a collagenous stroma. SFT is usually keratin negative, expresses CD34 and BCL2, and harbors the specific (to date), gene fusion NAB2-STAT6, which leads to overexpression of STAT6 by IHC.

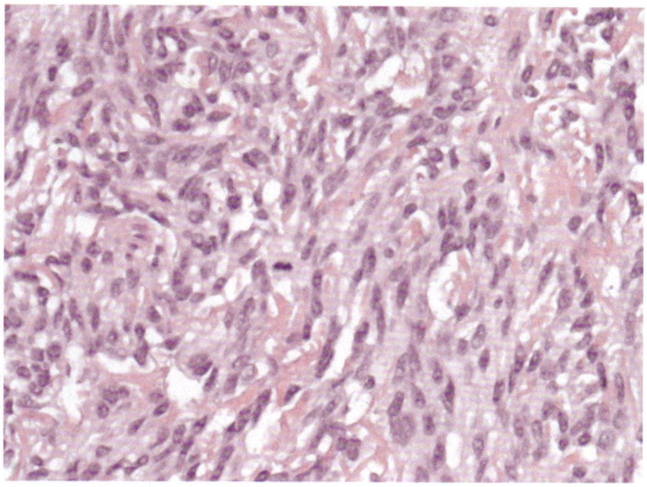

Figure 81.8 SFT: Note a mitotic figure (*center*). More than 4 mitoses/2 mm^2 area of tumor is the most reliable indicator of aggressive behavior.

82 INFLAMMATORY MYOFIBROBLASTIC TUMOR VS. SPINDLE CELL CARCINOMA

	Inflammatory Myofibroblastic Tumor (IMT)	Spindle Cell Carcinoma (SpCC)
Age	IMT has a wide age distribution, with the average age of presentation ranging from 8 to 44 y, and no gender predilection.	SpCC is a subtype of sarcomatoid carcinoma. The average age at diagnosis is 60 y.
Location	It can be peripherally or centrally located in the lung. Peripheral lesions can invade the pleura and mediastinum.	It can arise in the central or peripheral lung.
Symptoms	IMTs are frequently detected as an incidental finding on image studies, and approximately 50%–60% of the patients are asymptomatic. When present, symptoms include cough, chest pain, dyspnea, and hemoptysis. Some patients may present with fever, anemia, weight loss, elevated erythrocyte sedimentation rate, and hyperglobulinemia, and these abnormalities may stop when the mass is removed.	Symptoms depend on location. Central endobronchial tumors may present with cough, dyspnea, hemoptysis, or postobstructive pneumonia symptoms. Peripheral tumors may present with chest pain due to pleural or chest wall invasion.
Signs	Image studies typically demonstrate a solitary, well-demarcated, central or peripheral lung mass, but multifocal and bilateral masses can also occur. IMT can invade the pleura and mediastinum.	The most common presentation on image studies is a large peripheral mass, usually located in upper lobes, showing low central attenuation at CT, and frequently invading adjacent pleura.
Etiology	Unknown.	Most cases arise in tobacco smokers, although cases in never-smokers have also been described. Asbestos exposure, although uncommon, is another possible etiologic factor.
Histology	IMT is composed of spindle cells with fibroblastic and myofibroblastic differentiation and bland nuclear features arranged in fascicles or with storiform architecture. The spindle cells have ovoid nuclei, fine chromatin, inconspicuous nucleoli, and abundant eosinophilic cytoplasm. Nuclear atypia is usually absent or minimal. Admixed with the spindle cell proliferation, and often obscuring it, is a prominent inflammatory cell infiltrate composed of lymphocytes, plasma cells, foamy histiocytes, and Touton-type multinucleated giant cells *(Figs. 82.1–82.3)*. Plasma cells may be prominent. Areas of dense fibrosis can also be seen. The mitotic rate is variable but does not correlate with clinical behavior.	SpCC is composed of overtly malignant spindle cells arranged in fascicular or storiform pattern *(Fig. 82.4)*. The spindle cells have hyperchromatic nuclei, with nucleoli and granular chromatin. Background inflammation is common but prominent inflammatory infiltrates are unusual.
Special studies	IMT tumor spindle cells show variable positive expression of smooth muscle actin and desmin. Cytokeratin expression is unusual, but may be seen in approximately 30% of cases. About 50% of the cases show immunopositivity for ALK1 protein, and this usually correlates with clonal anaplastic lymphoma kinase (ALK) gene rearrangement at 2p23 locus. ALK gene rearrangement involves a variety of genes, especially tropomyosins TPM3 and TPM4. It can be identified by break-apart fluorescence in situ hybridization (FISH). It has been recently found that some cases lacking ALK gene rearrangement harbor ROS1 gene rearrangement.	The spindle cells usually express cytokeratin and epithelial membrane antigen (EMA) and show variable expression of Napsin A and thyroid transcription factor-1 (TTF-1), lacking smooth muscle actin, desmin, ALK1 expression, or ALK gene rearrangement.

	Inflammatory Myofibroblastic Tumor (IMT)	Spindle Cell Carcinoma (SpCC)
Prognosis	Treatment is based on surgical resection. Complete resection is necessary to avoid recurrence and metastasis, which occurs in approximately 55% and 10% of cases, respectively. Poor outcomes are seen with larger tumor size, invasion of adjacent structures (mediastinum, pleura, diaphragm), incomplete resection, metastasis, and nonsurgical treatments. ALK gene rearrangement-positive tumors may respond to crizotinib therapy, which may be useful in reducing tumor size before surgery.	SpCCs are aggressive tumors with poor prognosis even when the diagnosis is made in early-stage disease. Adjuvant chemotherapy and radiotherapy do not appear to be helpful. The 5-y survival rate is approximately 20%.

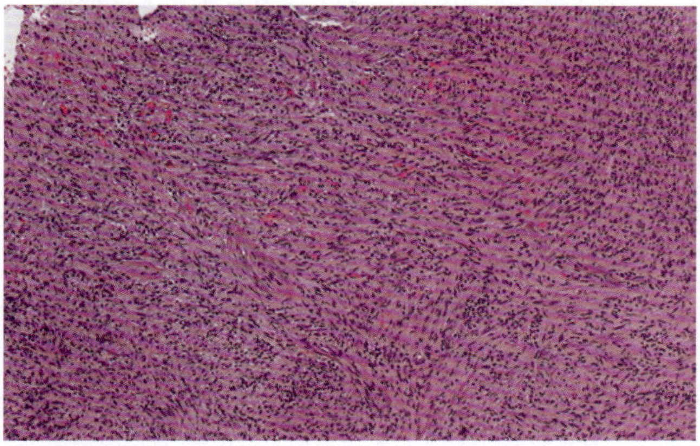

Figure 82.1 IMT: Cellular lesion composed of spindle myofibroblastic cells with bland nuclear features arranged in fascicles admixed with chronic inflammatory cells.

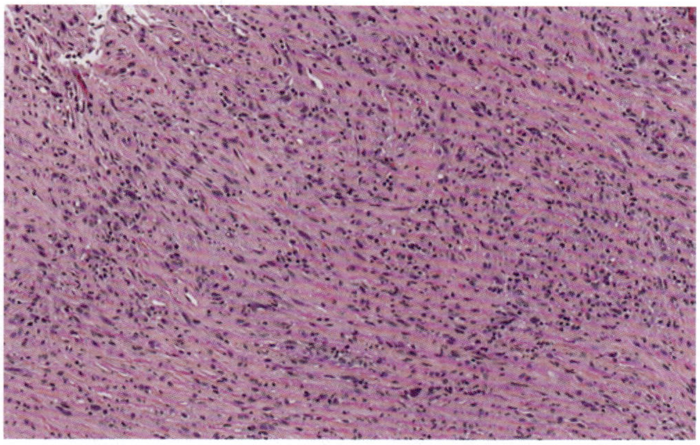

Figure 82.2 IMT: Spindle cells with minimal cytologic atypia admixed with chronic inflammatory cell infiltrate composed of lymphocytes and plasma cells.

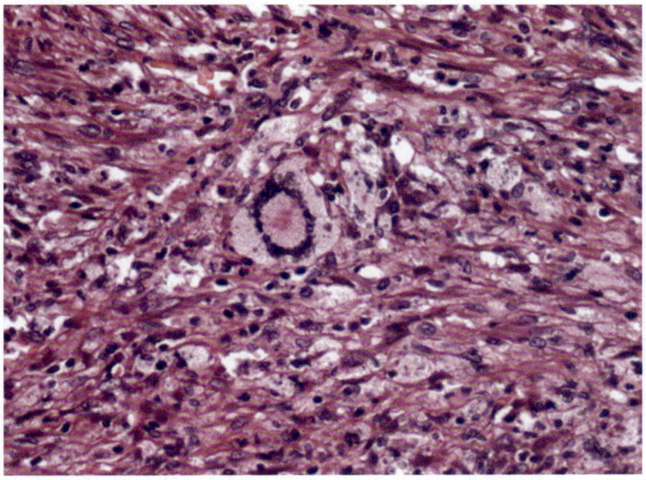

Figure 82.3 IMT: Foamy histiocytes and Touton-type multinucleated giant cells may be present in the inflammatory cell infiltrate.

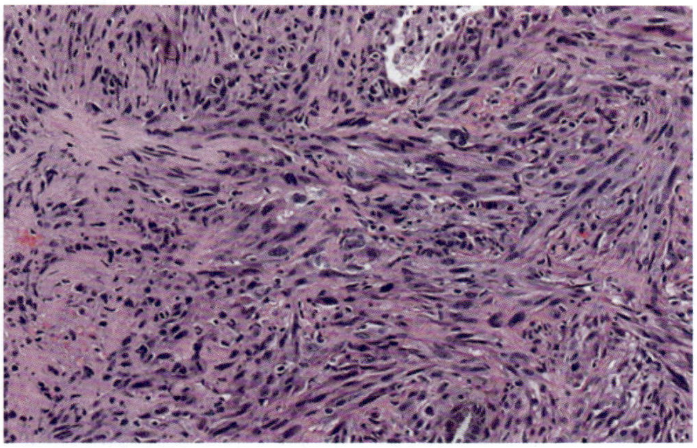

Figure 82.4 SpCC: Disease showing clearly malignant spindle cells arranged in fascicular pattern.

83 SOLITARY FIBROUS TUMOR VS. MONOPHASIC SYNOVIAL SARCOMA

	Solitary Fibrous Tumor (SFT)	Monophasic Synovial Sarcoma (MSS)
Age	SFT can occur at any age, but it is more common in the sixth and seventh decades of life, with no sex predilection.	Most patients are young or middle-aged adults, with a median age of 40 y and equal sex distribution.
Location	SFTs of the pleura most often arise in the visceral pleura, but are widely distributed throughout the pleural cavity.	MSS may be localized or present with diffuse pleural involvement. Pleural synovial sarcoma often involves the underlying lung. Intrapulmonary MSS can occur in any location.
Symptoms	Many lesions are asymptomatic and discovered incidentally, but patients may present with cough, dyspnea, chest pain, general malaise, or hypoglycemia (secondary to insulin-like growth factor production).	Chest pain, dyspnea, pleural effusion or hemothorax, hemoptysis, and constitutional symptoms.
Signs	Image studies usually demonstrate sharply demarcated pleural-based soft tissue masses.	Image studies of pleural MSS usually demonstrate large infiltrative pleural-based mass, which may have diffuse pleural thickening and growth along fissures, encasing the lung in a pattern that mimics malignant mesothelioma.
Etiology	Unknown.	Unknown.
Histology	SFT is typically characterized by the presence of hypo- and hypercellular areas, and branching hemangiopericytoma-like vessels of varying sizes and numbers. The hypercellular areas are composed of uniform elongate-to-spindle shaped cells with bland nuclear features arranged in fascicular, storiform, herringbone, or patternless architecture with variable prominent stromal hyalinization *(Figs. 83.1–83.4)*. Rarely the stroma is myxoid. Necrosis is infrequent. Usually, there are less than 3 mitoses/2 mm^2 area of tumor *(Fig. 83.5)*. Malignant SFTs are usually hypercellular and show more than 4 mitoses/2 mm^2 area of tumor.	MSS is composed of round-to-spindle shaped cells arranged in dense cellular sheets or vague fascicles with occasional herringbone pattern. The cells have ovoid-to-elongated nuclei, inconspicuous nucleoli, sparse cytoplasm, and indistinct cell borders *(Fig. 83.6)*. The amount of stromal collagen is variable and usually scant, but the tumor may contain strands of ropy and wiry collagen, bands of hyalinized collagen, or foci of dense fibrosis. Myxoid change is usually only focally present. Focal staghorn-shaped vessels may be seen, mimicking SFT *(Fig. 83.7)*. Mast cells can be abundant. Mitotic activity and necrosis is highly variable. Areas of calcification and ossification may be present.

	Solitary Fibrous Tumor (SFT)	Monophasic Synovial Sarcoma (MSS)
Special studies	SFTs express CD34, Bcl2, CD99, and STAT 6. STAT 6 is the most specific, and positive in more than 95% of cases. Keratin markers are usually negative and rarely focally positive. Some cases are smooth muscle actin (SMA) positive, and occasional cases may stain for S100 or desmin. SFT harbors the specific (to date) gene fusion NAB2-STAT6, which results from the intrachromosomal inversion inv(12)(q13q13), and leads to overexpression of STAT6.	MSS generally express at least one epithelial marker, such as epithelial membrane antigen (EMA) or cytokeratin, and often show nonspecific coexpression of vimentin, CD99, and Bcl2. Transducin-like enhancer of split-1 (TLE) is more specific, although may be seen in approximately 12% of SFT cases. Calretinin and S100 may be focally positive. Smooth muscle actin, desmin, and CD34 are immunonegative. The diagnostic translocation t(X;18)(p11;q11), which fuses the SS18 (also known as SYT) gene on chromosome 18 with either SSX1 or SSX2, both located at Xp11.2, are helpful in the diagnosis. Cytogenetics studies can demonstrate the t(X;18) translocation. Reverse transcriptase polymerase chain reaction (RT-PCR), and fluorescence in situ hybridization (FISH), can be used to show the SYT-SSX1 or SYT-SSX2 fusion gene, which is present in 90% of synovial sarcoma cases.
Prognosis	Complete surgical excision is the main therapy. Local recurrence occurs in about 10% of cases, and metastasis in 5%–10%. More than 4 mitoses/2 mm^2 area of tumor is the most reliable indicator of aggressive behavior. However, cases having benign morphology may also give rise to metastasis.	Complete surgical excision is the recommended therapy with adjuvant radiation treatment or chemotherapy. MSSs are aggressive tumors that commonly recur and metastasize after resection. The median survival is approximately 2 y.

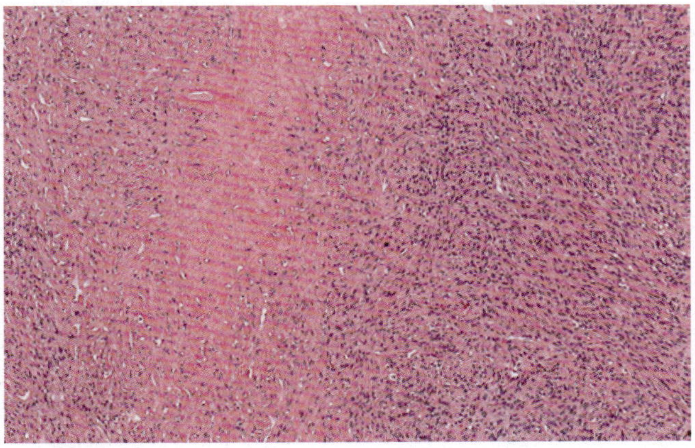

Figure 83.1 SFT: Hypocellular and hypercellular areas associated with vessels of variable sizes and numbers and collagenous stroma are seen.

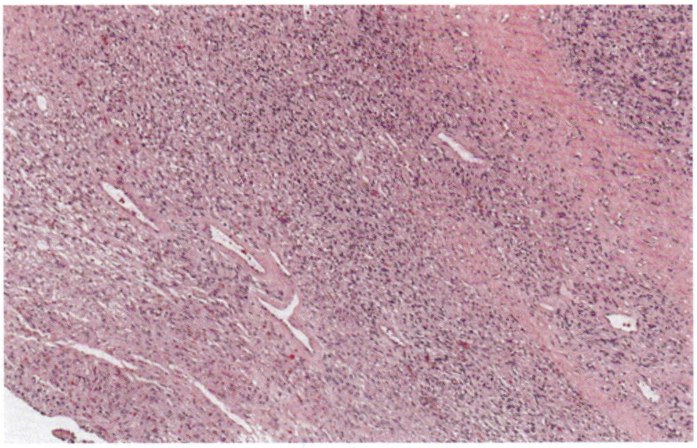

Figure 83.2 SFT: Hypercellular area with patternless architecture and branching hemangiopericytoma-like vessels.

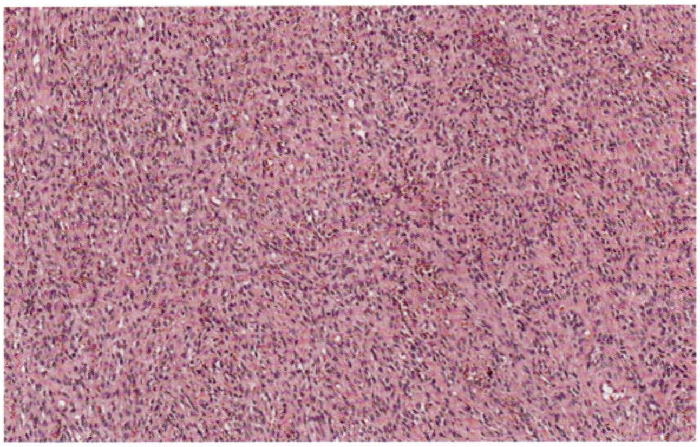

Figure 83.3 SFT: The hypercellular areas are composed of uniform elongate-to-spindle shaped cells with bland nuclear features.

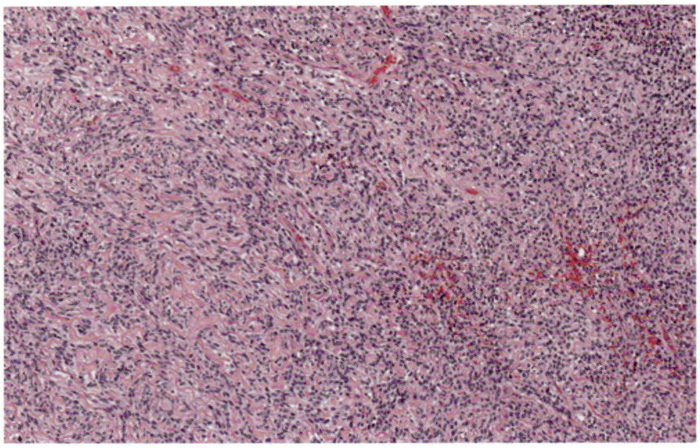

Figure 83.4 SFT: Hypercellular area showing cells with bland nuclear features arranged in a patternless architecture within a collagenous stroma.

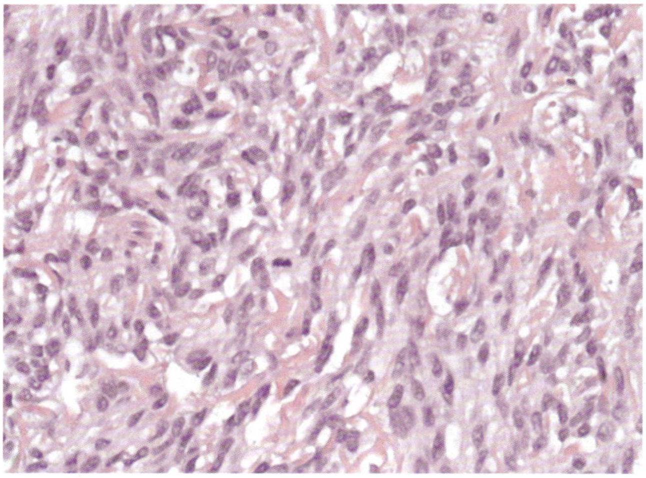

Figure 83.5 SFT: Note a mitotic figure (*center*). More than 4 mitoses/2 mm^2 area of tumor is the most reliable indicator of aggressive behavior.

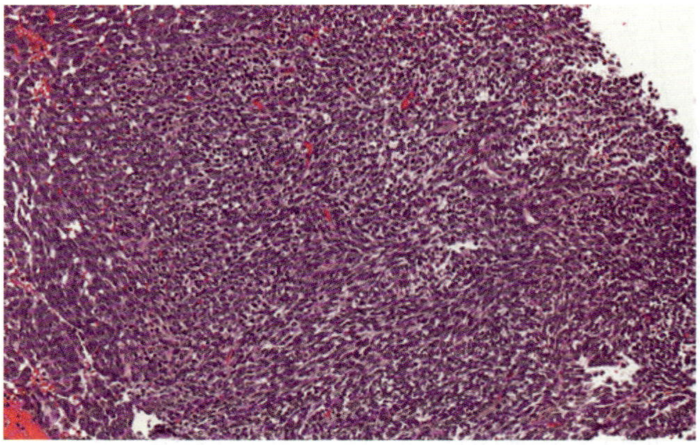

Figure 83.6 MSS: MSS showing round-to-spindle shaped cells arranged in dense cellular sheets and vague fascicles.

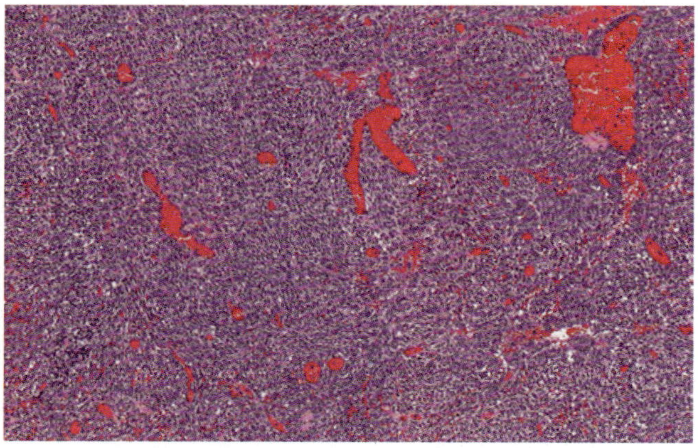

Figure 83.7 MSS: Staghorn-shaped vessels may be seen, mimicking SFT.

Suggested Readings

Abbondanzo SL, Rush W, Bijwaard KE, et al. Nodular lymphoid hyperplasia of the lung: a clinicopathologic study of 14 cases. *Am J Surg Pathol.* 2000;24(4):587–597.

Achcar R, Nikiforova M, Dacic S, et al. MAML2 11q21 gene rearrangement in bronchopulmonary mucoepidermoid carcinoma. *Hum Pathol.* 2009;40:854–860.

Achcar R, Nikiforova M, Yousem S. Micropapillary lung adenocarcinoma: EGFR, K-ras, and BRAF mutational profile. *Am J Clin Pathol.* 2009;131(5):694–700.

Aerni M, Vassallo R, Myers J, et al. Follicular bronchiolitis in surgical lung biopsies: clinical implications in 12 patients. *Respir Med.* 2008;102:307–312.

Allen T. Pathology of small airway disease. *Arch Pathol Lab Med.* 2010;134:702–718.

Anderson T, Zhang L, Hameed M, et al. Thoracic epithelioid malignant vascular tumors: a clinicopathologic study of 52 cases with emphasis on pathologic grading and molecular studies of WWTR1-CAMTA1 fusions. *Am J Surg Pathol.* 2015;39(1):132–139.

Arnaud L, Pierre I, Beigelman-Aubry C, et al. Pulmonary involvement in Erdheim–Chester disease: a single-center study of thirty-four patients and a review of the literature. *Arthritis Rheum.* 2010;62:3504–3512.

Beasley MB. The pathologist's approach to acute lung injury. *Arch Pathol Lab Med.* 2010;134:719–727.

Beasley MB, Franks TJ, Galvin JR, et al. Acute fibrinous and organizing pneumonia: a histopathologic pattern of lung injury and possible variant of diffuse alveolar damage. *Arch Pathol Lab Med.* 2002;126:1064–1070.

Bennett AK, Mills SE, Wick MR. Salivary-type neoplasms of the breast and lung. *Semin Diagn Pathol.* 2003;20(4):279–304.

Bergeron C, Tulic M, Hamid Q. Airway remodeling in asthma: from benchside to clinical practice. *Can Respir J.* 2010;17(4):85–93.

Bhardwaj H, Bhardwaj B, Levin D. Pulmonary adenocarcinoma in a young patient of pulmonary Langerhans cell histiocytosis (PLCH). *J Thorac Oncol.* 2013;8(8):e69–e70.

Boaq AH, Colby TV, Travis WD, et al. The pathology of interstitial lung disease in nylon flock workers. *Am J Surg Pathol.* 1999;23(12):1539–1545.

Bonfield TL, Russell D, Burgess S, et al. Autoantibodies against granulocyte macrophage colony-stimulating factor are diagnostic for pulmonary alveolar proteinosis. *Am J Respir Cell Mol Biol.* 2002;27:481–486.

Borzuck AC. Neoplastic and nonneoplastic benign mass lesions of the lung. *Arch Pathol Lab Med.* 2012;136:1227–1233.

Burgel P-R, Bergeron A, de Blic J, et al. Small airway diseases, excluding asthma and COPD: an overview. *Eur Respir Rev.* 2013;22(128):131–147.

Cagle PT, Allen TC, Dacic S, et al. *Advances in Surgical Pathology, Lung Cancer.* Philadelphia, PA: LWW; 2010.

Cagle PT, Churg A. Differential diagnosis of benign and malignant mesothelial proliferations on pleural biopsies. *Arch Pathol Lab Med.* 2005;129:1421–1427.

Chmielecki J, Crago AM, Rosenberg M, et al. Whole-exome sequencing identifies a recurrent NAB2-STAT6 fusion in solitary fibrous tumors. *Nat Genet.* 2013;45(2):131–132.

Chong S, Lee KS, Chung MJ, et al. Pneumoconiosis: comparison of imaging and pathologist findings. *Radiographics.* 2006;26:59–77.

Churg A, Cagle PT, Roggli VL. *Tumors of the Serosal Membranes.* AFIP Atlas of Tumor Pathology Series 4. Washington, DC: Armed Forces Institute of Pathology; 2006.

Churg A, Carrington CB, Gupta R. Necrotizing sarcoid granulomatosis. *Chest.* 1979;76:406–413.

Churg A, Galateau-Salle F. The separation of benign and malignant mesothelial proliferations. *Arch Pathol Lab Med.* 2012;136:1217–1226.

Churg A, Muller NL, Silva CI, et al. Acute exacerbation (acute lung injury of unknown cause) in UIP and other forms of fibrotic interstitial lung pneumonias. *Am J Surg Pathol.* 2007;31(2):277–284.

Churg A, Myers J, Suarez T, et al. Airway-centered interstitial fibrosis: a distinct form of aggressive diffuse lung disease. *Am J Surg Pathol.* 2004;28(1):62–68.

Churg A, Sheffield BS, Galateau-Salle F. New markers for separation benign from malignant mesothelial proliferations. *Arch Pathol Lab Med.* 2016;140:318–321.

Churg AM, Warnock ML. So-called "minute pulmonary chemodectoma": a tumor not related to paragangliomas. *Cancer.* 1976;37:1759–1769.

Colby TV. Current histological diagnosis of lymphomatoid granulomatosis. *Mod Pathol.* 2012;25:S39–S42.

Colby TV, Lombard C, Yousem SA, et al. *Atlas of Pulmonary Surgical Pathology.* Philadelphia, PA: W.B. Saunders; 1991.

Collins CE, Quismorio FP Jr. Pulmonary involvement in microscopic polyangiitis. *Curr Opin Pulm Med.* 2005;11:447–451.

Cordier JF. Cryptogenic organizing pneumonia. *Eur Respir J.* 2006;28:422–446.

Cordier JF, Loire R, Brune J. Amyloidosis of the lower respiratory tract. Clinical and pathologic features in a series of 21 patients. *Chest.* 1986;90:827–831.

Craig PJ, Wells AU, Doffman S, et al. Desquamative interstitial pneumonia, respiratory bronchiolitis and their relationship to smoking. *Histopathology.* 2004;45:275–282.

Craighead JE, Abraham JL, Churg A, et al. The pathology of asbestos-associated diseases of the lungs and pleural cavities: diagnostic criteria and proposed grading schema. Report of the Pneumoconiosis Committee of the College of American Pathologists and the National Institute for Occupational Safety and Health. *Arch Pathol Lab Med.* 1982;106(11):544–596.

Dacic S. *Current Concepts in Pulmonary Pathology, An Issue of Surgical Pathology Clinics, 1e (The Clinics: Internal Medicine).* Vol 3. Surgical Pathology Clinics. Philadelphia, PA: Saunders; 2010. ISBN-10:1437722660/ISBN-13:9781437722666.

Dacic S. Molecular diagnosis of lung carcinomas. *Arch Pathol Lab Med.* 2011;135:622–629.

Dacic S. Pulmonary preneoplasia. *Arch Pathol Lab Med.* 2008;132:1073–1078.

Dauriat G, Mal H, Thabut G, et al. Lung transplantation for pulmonary Langerhans' cell histiocytosis: a multicenter analysis. *Transplantation.* 2006;81(5):746–750.

Debelenko LV, Brambilla E, Agarwal SK, et al. Identification of MEN1 gene mutations in sporadic carcinoid tumors of the lung. *Hum Mol Genet.* 1997;6(13):2285–2290.

Debelenko LV, Swalwell JI, Kelley MJ, et al. MEN1 gene mutation analysis of high-grade neuroendocrine lung carcinoma. *Genes Chromosomes Cancer.* 2000;28(1):58–65.

Devouassoux-Shisheboran M, Hayashi T, Linnoila RI, et al. A clinicopathologic study of 100 cases of pulmonary sclerosing hemangioma with immunohistochemical studies: TTF-1 is expressed in both round and surface cells, suggesting an origin from primitive respiratory epithelium. *Am J Surg Pathol.* 2000;24(7):906–916.

Doyle LA, Vivero M, Fletcher CD, et al. Nuclear expression of STAT6 distinguishes solitary fibrous tumor from histologic mimics. *Mod Pathol.* 2014;27(3):390–395.

Elia D, Torre O, Cassandro R, et al. Pulmonary Langerhans cell histiocytosis: a comprehensive analysis of 40 patients and literature review. *Eur J Int Med.* 2015;26(5):351–356.

English JC, Mayo JR, Levy R, et al. Pleuroparenchymal fibroelastosis: a rare interstitial lung disease. *Respirol Case Rep.* 2015;3(2):82–84.

Epler G. Constrictive bronchiolitis obliterans: the fibrotic airway disorder. *Expert Rev Respir Med.* 2007;1(1):139–147.

Faber CN, Yousem SA, Dauber JH, et al. Pulmonary capillary hemangiomatosis: a report of three cases and a review of the literature. *Am Rev Respir Dis.* 1989;140:808–813.

Falk RJ, Gross WL, Guillevin L, et al. Granulomatosis with polyangiitis (Wegener's): an alternative name for Wegener's granulomatosis. *J Am Soc Nephrol.* 2011;22:587–588.

Feinstein MB, DeSouza SA, Travis WD, et al. A comparison of the pathological, clinical and radiographical, features of cryptogenic organizing pneumonia, acute fibrinous and organizing pneumonia and granulomatous organizing pneumonia. *J Clin Pathol.* 2015;68(6):441–447.

Feuillet S, Louis L, Bergeron A, et al. Pulmonary Langerhans cell histiocytosis associated with Hodgkin's lymphoma. *Eur Respir Rev.* 2010;19(115):86–88.

Finkelstein SD, Hasegawa T, Colby T, et al. 11q13 allelic imbalance discriminates pulmonary carcinoids from tumorlets. A microdissection-based genotyping approach useful in clinical practice. *Am J Pathol.* 1999;155(2):633–640.

Fraig M, Shreesha U, Savici D, et al. Respiratory bronchiolitis: a clinicopathologic study in current smokers, ex-smokers, and never-smokers. *Am J Surg Pathol.* 2002;26:647–653.

Frankel SK, Cool CD, Lynch DA, et al. Idiopathic pleuroparenchymal fibroelastosis: description of a novel clinicopathologic entity. *Chest.* 2004;126(6):2007–2013.

Fukuoka J, Franks TJ, Colby TV, et al. Peribronchiolar metaplasia: a common histologic lesion in diffuse lung disease and a rare cause of interstitial lung disease: clinicopathologic features of 15 cases. *Am J Surg Pathol.* 2005;29:948–954.

Gaffey MJ, Mills SE, Askin FB. Minute pulmonary meningothelial-like nodules. A clinicopathologic study of so-called minute pulmonary chemodectoma. *Am J Surg Pathol.* 1988;12:167–175.

Garcia BA, Goede T, Mohammed T-L. Acute fibrinous organizing pneumonia: a case report and literature review. *Curr Probl Diagn Radiol.* 2015;44(5):469–471.

Guarner J, Brandt ME. Histopathologic diagnosis of fungal infections in the 21st century. *Clin Microbiol Rev.* 2011;24:247–280.

Guinee DG Jr. Update on nonneoplastic pulmonary lymphoproliferative disorders and related entities. *Arch Pathol Lab Med.* 2010;134:691–701.

Haque A. Pathology of common pulmonary fungal infections. *J Thorac Imaging.* 1992;7:1–11.

Harari S, Torre O, Cassandro R, et al. Bronchoscopic diagnosis of Langerhans cell histiocytosis and lymphangioleiomyomatosis. *Respir Med.* 2012;106:1286–1292.

Herbst JB, Myers JL. Hypersensitivity pneumonia: role of surgical lung biopsy. *Arch Pathol Lab Med.* 2012;136:889–895.

Hogg JC. The pathology of asthma. *APMIS.* 1997;105:735–745.

Hoon V, Thung SN, Kaneko M, et al. HMB-45 reactivity in renal angiomyolipoma and lymphangioleiomyomatosis. *Arch Pathol Lab Med.* 1994;118:732–734.

Hull MJ, Abraham JL. Aluminum welding fume-induced pneumoconiosis. *Hum Pathol.* 2002;33(8):819–825.

Hwang HC, Sheffield BS, Rodriguez S, et al. Utility of BAP1 immunohistochemistry and p16 (CDKN2A) FISH in the diagnosis of malignant mesothelioma in effusion cytology specimens. *Am J Surg Pathol.* 2016;40(1):120–126.

Ichinose H, Hewitt RL, Drapanas T. Minute pulmonary chemodectoma. *Cancer.* 1971;28:692–700.

Ionescu DN, Pierson DM, Qing G, et al. Pulmonary crystal-storing histiocytoma. *Arch Pathol Lab Med.* 2005;129(9):1159–1163.

Ionescu DN, Sasatomi E, Aldeeb D, et al. Pulmonary meningothelial-like nodules: a genotypic comparison with meningiomas. *Am J Surg Pathol.* 2004;28:207–214.

Jennette JC, Falk RJ, Bacon PA, et al. 2012 Revised International Chapel Hill Consensus Conference Nomenclature of Vasculitides. *Arthritis Rheum.* 2013;65:1–11.

Jennette JC, Thomas DB, Falk RJ. Microscopic polyangiitis (microscopic polyarteritis). *Semin Diagn Pathol.* 2001;18:3–13.

Katzenstein AL. Diagnostic features and differential diagnosis of Churg–Strauss syndrome in the lung. A review. *Am J Clin Pathol.* 2000;5:767–772.

Katzenstein AL. *Katzenstein and Askin's Surgical Pathology of Non-Neoplastic Lung Disease.* 4th ed. Philadelphia, PA: W.B. Saunders; 2006.

Katzenstein AL. Smoking-related interstitial fibrosis (SRIF), pathogenesis and treatment of usual interstitial pneumonia (UIP), and transbronchial biopsy in UIP. *Mod Pathol.* 2012;25(Suppl 1):S68–S78.

Katzenstein AL. Smoking-related interstitial fibrosis (SRIF): pathologic findings and distinction from other chronic fibrosing lung diseases. *J Clin Pathol.* 2013;66(10):882–887.

Katzenstein AL, Doxtader E, Narendra S. Lymphomatoid granulomatosis: insights gained over 4 decades. *Am J Surg Pathol.* 2010;34:e35–e48.

Katzenstein AL, Gmelich JT, Carrington CB. Sclerosing hemangioma of the lung: a clinicopathologic study of 51 cases. *Am J Surg Pathol.* 1980;4(4):343–356.

Katzenstein AL, Liebow AA, Friedman PJ. Bronchocentric granulomatosis, mucoid impaction, and hypersensitivity reactions. *Am Rev Respir Dis.* 1975;111(4):497–537.

Katzenstein AL, Mukhopadhyay S, Zanardi C, et al. Clinically occult interstitial fibrosis in smokers: classification and significance of a surprisingly common finding in lobectomy specimens. *Hum Pathol.* 2010;41(3):316–325.

Keylock JB, Galvin JR, Franks TJ. Sclerosing hemangioma of the lung. *Arch Pathol Lab Med.* 2009;133:820–825.

Kim DS, Park JH, Park BK, et al. Acute exacerbation of idiopathic pulmonary fibrosis: frequency and clinical features. *Eur Respir J.* 2006;27:143–150.

King MS, Eisenberg R, Miler RF, et al. Constrictive bronchiolitis in soldiers returning from Iraq and Afghanistan. *N Engl J Med.* 2011;365:222–230.

Kobashi Y, Sugiu T, Mouri K, et al. Multifocal micronodular pneumocyte hyperplasia associated with tuberous sclerosis: differentiation from multiple atypical adenomatous hyperplasia. *Jpn J Clin Oncol.* 2008;38(6):451–454.

Korn D, Bensch K, Liebow AA, et al. Multiple minute pulmonary tumors resembling chemodectomas. *Am J Pathol.* 1960;37:641–672.

Koss MN, Hochholzer L, Langloss JM, et al. Lymphoid interstitial pneumonia: clinicopathological and immunopathological findings in 18 cases. *Pathology.* 1987;19:178–185.

Kuhn C III, Askin FB. The fine structure of so-called minute pulmonary chemodectomas. *Hum Pathol.* 1975;6:681–691.

Kuranishi LT, Leslie KO, Ferreira RG, et al. Airway-centered interstitial fibrosis: etiology, clinical findings and prognosis. *Respir Res.* 2015;16:55.

Kwon KY, Colby TV. *Rhodococcus equi* pneumonia and pulmonary malakoplakia in acquired immunodeficiency syndrome. Pathologic features. *Arch Pathol Lab Med.* 1994;118(7):744–748.

Ladanyi M, Antonescu CR, Leung DH, et al. Impact of SYT-SSX fusion type on the clinical behavior of synovial sarcoma: a multi-institutional retrospective study of 243 patients. *Cancer Res.* 2002;62(1):135–140.

Lawrence B, Perez-Atayde A, Hibbard MK, et al. TPM3-ALK and TPM4-ALK oncogenes in inflammatory myofibroblastic tumors. *Am J Pathol.* 2000;157(2):377–384.

Le Pavec J, Lorillon G, Jais X, et al. Pulmonary Langerhans cell histiocytosis associated pulmonary hypertension: clinical characteristics and impact of pulmonary arterial hypertension therapies. *Chest.* 2012;142(5):1150–1157.

Leslie KO. My approach to interstitial lung disease using clinical, radiologic and histopathological patterns. *J Clin Pathol.* 2009;62:387–401.

Leslie KO, Gruden JF, Parish JM, et al. Transbronchial biopsy interpretation in the patients with diffuse parenchymal lung disease. *Arch Pathol Lab Med.* 2007;131:407–423.

Leslie KO, Wick MR. *Practical Pulmonary Pathology, A Diagnostic Approach.* 2nd ed. Philadelphia, PA: Elsevier Saunders; 2011.

Liebow AA, Carrington CR, Friedman PJ. Lymphomatoid granulomatosis. *Hum Pathol.* 1972;3:457–558.

Lindeman NI, Cagle PT, Beasley MB, et al. Molecular testing guideline for selection of lung cancer patients for EGFR and ALK tyrosine kinase inhibitors: Guideline from the College of American Pathologists, International Association for the Study of Lung Cancer, and Association for Molecular Pathology. *Arch Pathol Lab Med.* 2013;137:828–860.

Lino-Silva LS, Flores-Gutiérrez JP, Vilches-Cisneros N, et al. TLE1 is expressed in the majority of primary pleuropulmonary synovial sarcomas. *Virchows Arch.* 2011;459(6):615–621.

Liu X, Adams A. Mucoepidermoid carcinoma of the bronchus: a review. *Arch Pathol Lab Med.* 2007;131:1400–1404.

Lohr RH, Boland BJ, Douglas WW, et al. Organizing pneumonia: features and prognosis of cryptogenic, secondary, and focal variants. *Arch Intern Med.* 1997;157(12):1323–1329.

Lovly CM, Gupta A, Lipson D, et al. Inflammatory myofibroblastic tumors harbor multiple potentially actionable kinase fusions. *Cancer Discov.* 2014;4(8):889–895.

Ma Y, Gal A, Koss MN. The pathology of pulmonary sarcoidosis: update. *Semin Diagn Pathol.* 2007;24:150–161.

Mendez JL, Nadrous HF, Vassallo R, et al. Pneumothorax in pulmonary Langerhans cell histiocytosis. *Chest.* 2004;125(3):1028–1032.

Minami Y, Matsuno Y, Iijima T, et al. Prognostication of small-sized primary pulmonary adenocarcinomas by histopathological and karyometric analysis. *Lung Cancer.* 2005;48:339–348.

Miyagawa-Hayashino A, Tazalar HD, Langel DJ, et al. Pulmonary sclerosing hemangioma with lymph node metastases: report of 4 cases. *Arch Pathol Lab Med.* 2003;127:321–325.

Montani D, Price LC, Dorfmuller P, et al. Pulmonary veno-occlusive disease. *Eur Respir J.* 2009;33:189–200.

Moro-Sibilot D, Lantuejoul S, Diab S, et al. Lung carcinomas with a basaloid pattern: a study of 90 cases focusing on their poor prognosis. *Eur Respir J.* 2008;31:854–859.

Muir TE, Leslie KO, Popper H, et al. Micronodular pneumocyte hyperplasia. *Am J Surg Pathol.* 1998;22:465–472.

Mukhopadhyay S, Farver CF, Vaszar LT, et al. Causes of pulmonary granulomas: a retrospective study of 500 cases from seven countries. *J Clin Pathol.* 2012;65(1):51–57.

Mukhopadhyay S, Gal A. Granulomatous lung disease: an approach to the differential diagnosis. *Arch Pathol Lab Med.* 2010;134:667–690.

Myers JL. Bronchocentric granulomatosis. Disease or diagnosis? *Chest.* 1989;96(1):3–4.

Myers JL. Hypersensitivity pneumonia: the role of lung biopsy in diagnosis and management. *Mod Pathol.* 2012;25:S58–S67.

Myers JL, Veal CF Jr, Shin MS, et al. Respiratory bronchiolitis causing interstitial lung disease. A clinicopathologic study of six cases. *Am Rev Respir Dis.* 1987;135:880–884.

Naqvi AH, Hunt A, Burnett BR, et al. Pathologic spectrum and lung dust burden in giant cell interstitial pneumonia (hard metal disease/cobalt pneumonitis): review of 100 cases. *Arch Environ Occup Health.* 2008;63:51–70.

Nasu M, Emi M, Pastorino S, et al. High incidence of Somatic BAP1 alterations in sporadic malignant mesothelioma. *J Thorac Oncol.* 2015;10(4):565–576.

National Asthma Education and Prevention Program. *Expert Panel Report 3: Guidelines for the Diagnosis and Management of Asthma.* Publication No. 07-4051. Bethesda, MD: National Institute of Health; 2007.

Niho S, Yokose T, Nishiwaki Y, et al. Immunohistochemical and clonal analysis of minute pulmonary meningothelial-like nodules. *Hum Pathol.* 1999;30:425–429.

Ohori NP, Yousem SA, Sonmez-Alpan E, et al. Estrogen and progesterone receptors in lymphangioleiomyomatosis, epithelioid hemangioendothelioma, and sclerosing hemangioma of the lung. *Am J Clin Pathol.* 1991;96:529–535.

Okamoto S, Hisaoka M, Daa T, et al. Primary pulmonary synovial sarcoma: a clinicopathologic, immunohistochemical, and molecular study of 11 cases. *Hum Pathol.* 2004;35(7):850–856.

Parambil JG, Myers JL, Ryu JH. Histopathologic features and outcome of patients with acute exacerbation of idiopathic pulmonary fibrosis undergoing surgical lung biopsy. *Chest.* 2005;128(5):3310–3315.

Parambil JG, Savci CD, Tazelaar HD, et al. Causes and presenting features of pulmonary infarctions in 43 cases identified by surgical lung biopsy. *Chest.* 2005;127:1178–1183.

Pelosi G, Maffini F, Decarli N, et al. Progesterone receptor immunoreactivity in minute meningothelioid nodules of lung. *Virchows Arch.* 2002;440:543–546.

Poletti V, Casoni G, Chilosi M, et al. Diffuse panbronchiolitis. *Eur Respir J.* 2006;28:862–871.

Popper HH, Klemen H, Colby TV, et al. Necrotizing sarcoid granulomatosis: is it different from nodular sarcoidosis? *Pneumologie.* 2003;57:268–271.

Raparia K, Villa C, DeCamp MM, et al. Molecular profiling in non–small cell lung cancer. *Arch Pathol Lab Med.* 2013;137:481–491.

Rekhtman N. Neuroendocrine tumors of the lung: an update. *Arch Pathol Lab Med.* 2010;134:1628–1638.

Rizvi SM, Goodwill J, Lim E, et al. The frequency of neuroendocrine cell hyperplasia in patients with pulmonary neuroendocrine tumours and non-neuroendocrine cell carcinomas. *Histopathology.* 2009;55(3):332–337.

Roberts KE, Hamele-Bena D, Saqi A, et al. Pulmonary tumor embolism: a review of the literature. *Am J Med.* 2003;115:228–232.

Robinson DR, Wu YM, Kalyana-Sundaram S, et al. Identification of recurrent NAB2-STAT6 gene fusions in solitary fibrous tumor by integrative sequencing. *Nat Genet.* 2013;45(2):180–185.

Roden AC, Yi ES. Pulmonary Langerhans cell histiocytosis: an update from the pathologists' perspective. *Arch Pathol Lab Med.* 2016;140:230–240.

Rosen Y. Four decades of necrotizing sarcoid granulomatosis: what do we know now. *Arch Pathol Lab Med.* 2014;139:252–263.

Rubinstein I, Mullen JB, Hoffstein V. Morphologic diagnosis of idiopathic pulmonary alveolar lipoproteinosis-revisited. *Arch Intern Med.* 1988;148:813–816.

Rush WL, Andriko JA, Galateau-Salle F, et al. Pulmonary pathology of Erdheim–Chester disease. *Mod Pathol.* 2000;13:747–754.

Ryu JH, Moss J, Beck GJ, et al. The NHLBI lymphangioleiomyomatosis registry: characteristics of 230 patients at enrollment. *Am J Respir Crit Care Med.* 2006;173:105–111.

Sakamoto K, Tanigushi H, Kondoh Y, et al. Acute exacerbation if idiopathic pulmonary fibrosis as the initial presentation of the disease. *Eur Respir Rev.* 2009;18(112):129–132.

Sauler M, Gulati M. Newly recognized occupational and environmental causes of chronic terminal airways and parenchymal lung disease. *Clin Chest Med.* 2012;33(4):667–680.

Scannell KA, Portoni EJ, Finkle HI, et al. Pulmonary malacoplakia and *Rhodococcus equi* infection in a patient with AIDS. *Chest.* 1990;97:1000–1001.

Schwaiblmair M, Behr W, Haeckel T, et al. Drug induced interstitial lung disease. *Open Respir Med J.* 2012;6:63–74.

Sholl LM. Biomarkers in lung adenocarcinoma. *Arch Pathol Lab Med.* 2015;139:469–480.

Smith M, Dalurzo M, Panse P, et al. Usual interstitial pneumonia-pattern fibrosis in surgical lung biopsies. Clinical, radiological and histopathological clues to aetiology. *J Clin Pathol.* 2013;66:896–903.

Soares FA, Pinto AP, Landell GA, et al. Pulmonary tumor embolism to arterial vessels and carcinomatous lymphangitis. A comparative clinicopathological study. *Arch Pathol Lab Med.* 1993;117:827–831.

Soler P, Chollet S, Jacque C, et al. Immunocytochemical characterization of pulmonary histiocytosis X cells in lung biopsies. *Am J Pathol.* 1985;118:439–451.

Spain DM. Intrapulmonary chemodectomas in subjects with organizing pulmonary thromboemboli. *Am Rev Respir Dis.* 1967;96:1158–1164.

Stacher E, Graham BB, Hunt JM, et al. Modern age pathology of pulmonary arterial hypertension. *Am J Respir Crit Care Med.* 2012;186:261–272.

Suda T, Kaida Y, Nakamura Y, et al. Acute exacerbation of interstitial pneumonia associated with collagen vascular diseases. *Respir Med.* 2009;103(6):846–853.

Takemura T, Akashi T, Ohtani Y, et al. Pathology of hypersensitivity pneumonitis. *Curr Opin Pulm Med.* 2008;14:440–454.

Tashtoush B, Okafor NC, Ramirez JF, et al. Follicular bronchiolitis: a literature review. *J Clin Diagn Res.* 2015;9(9):OE01–OE05.

Templeton PA, McLoud TC, Müller NL, et al. Pulmonary lymphangioleiomyomatosis: CT and pathologic findings. *J Comput Assist Tomogr.* 1989;13:54–57.

Terry J, Saito T, Subramanian S, et al. TLE1 as a diagnostic immunohistochemical marker for synovial sarcoma emerging from gene expression profiling studies. *Am J Surg Pathol.* 2007;31(2):240–246.

Tochigi N, Attanoos R, Chirieac LR, et al. p16 Deletion in sarcomatoid tumors of the lung and pleura. *Arch Pathol Lab Med.* 2013;137:632–636.

Tochigi N, Dacic S, Nikiforova M, et al. Adenosquamous carcinoma of the lung: a microdissection study of KRAS and EGFR mutational and amplification status in a Western patient population. *Am J Clin Pathol.* 2011;135(5):783–789.

Tomashefski JF, Khiyami A, Kleinerman J. Neoplasms associated with pulmonary eosinophilic granuloma. *Arch Pathol Lab Med.* 1991;115(5):499–506.

Trahan S, Hanak V, Ryu JH, et al. Role of surgical lung biopsy in separating chronic hypersensitivity pneumonia from usual interstitial pneumonia/idiopathic pulmonary fibrosis: analysis of 31 biopsies from 15 patients. *Chest.* 2008;134:126–132.

Travis WD. Advances in neuroendocrine tumors. *Ann Oncol.* 2010;21(7):vii65–vii71.

Travis WD. Non-neoplastic pulmonary lymphoid lesions. *Thorax.* 2001;56:964–971.

Travis WD. Sarcomatoid neoplasms of the lung and pleura. *Arch Pathol Lab Med.* 2010;134:1645–1658.

Travis WD. Update on small cell carcinoma and its differentiation from squamous cell carcinoma and other non-small cell carcinomas. *Mod Pathol.* 2012;25:S18–S30.

Travis WD, Brambilia E, Burke AP, et al. *WHO Classification of Tumors of the Lung, Pleura, Thymus and Heart.* Lyon, France: IARC Press; 2015.

Travis WD, Carpenter HA, Lie JT. Diffuse pulmonary hemorrhage. An uncommon manifestation of Wegener's granulomatosis. *Am J Surg Pathol.* 1987;9:702–708.

Travis WD, Colby TV, Koss MN, et al. *Non-Neoplastic Disorders of the Lower Respiratory Tract.* AFIP Atlas of Nontumor Pathology Series. Washington, DC: Armed Forces Institute of Pathology; 2002.

Travis WD, Colby TV, Lombard C, et al. A clinicopathologic study of 34 cases of diffuse pulmonary hemorrhage with lung biopsy confirmation. *Am J Surg Pathol.* 1990;14:1112–1125.

Travis WD, Costabel U, Hansell DM, et al. An Official American Thoracic Society (ATS)/European Respiratory Society (ERS) Statement: Update of the International Multidisciplinary Classification of the Idiopathic Interstitial Pneumonias. This official statement of the ATS and ERS was approved by the ATS Board of Directors, June 2013, and by the ERS Steering Committee, March 2013. *Am J Respir Crit Care Med.* 2013;188:733–748.

Travis WD, Fox CH, Devaney KO, et al. Lymphoid pneumonitis in 50 adult patients infected with the human immunodeficiency virus: lymphocytic interstitial pneumonitis versus nonspecific interstitial pneumonitis. *Hum Pathol.* 1992;23:529–541.

Travis WD, Hoffman GS, Leavitt RY, et al. Surgical pathology of the lung in Wegener's granulomatosis. Review of 87 open lung biopsies from 67 patients. *Am J Surg Pathol.* 1991;15(4):315–333.

Tuder RM, Abman SH, Braun T, et al. Development and pathology of pulmonary hypertension. *J Am Coll Cardiol.* 2009;54:S3–S9.

Turner RR, Colby TV, Doggett RS. Well-differentiated lymphocytic lymphoma. A study of 47 patients with primary manifestation in the lung. *Cancer.* 1984;54:2088–2096.

von Ahsen I, Rogalia P, Bullerdiek J. Expression patterns of the LPP-HMGA2 fusion transcript in pulmonary chondroid hamartomas with t(3;12)(q27~28;q14~15). *Cancer Genet Cytogenet.* 2005;163(1):68–70.

Wiedemann HP, Matthay RA. Pulmonary manifestations of the collagen vascular diseases. *Clin Chest Med.* 1989;10:677–722.

Yi E, Aubry M-C. Pulmonary pseudoneoplasms. *Arch Pathol Lab Med.* 2010;134:417–426.

Yi ES, Kim H, Ahn H, et al. Distribution of obstructive intimal lesions and their cellular phenotypes in chronic pulmonary hypertension. *Am J Respir Crit Care Med.* 2000;162:1577–1586.

Yoshida A, Tsuta K, Ohno M, et al. STAT6 immunohistochemistry is helpful in the diagnosis of solitary fibrous tumors. *Am J Surg Pathol.* 2014;38(4):552–559.

Yoshikawa Y, Sato A, Tsujimura T, et al. Frequent inactivation of the BAP1 gene in epithelioid-type malignant mesothelioma. *Cancer Sci.* 2012;103(5):868–874.

Yousem SA. Bronchocentric injury in Wegener's granulomatosis: a report of five cases. *Hum Pathol.* 1991;22:535–540.

Yousem SA. Pulmonary apical cap: a distinctive but poorly recognized lesion in pulmonary surgical pathology. *Am J Surg Pathol.* 2001;25(5):679–683.

Yousem SA. Respiratory bronchiolitis-associated interstitial lung disease with fibrosis is a lesion distinct from fibrotic nonspecific interstitial pneumonia: a proposal. *Mod Pathol.* 2006;19(11):1474–1479.

Yousem SA. Role of molecular studies in the diagnosis of lung adenocarcinoma. *Mod Pathol.* 2012;25(1):S11–S17.

Yousem SA. The surgical pathology of pulmonary infarcts: diagnostic confusion with granulomatous disease, vasculitis, and neoplasia. *Mod Pathol.* 2009;22:679–685.

Yousem SA, Colby TV, Carrington CB. Follicular bronchitis/bronchiolitis. *Hum Pathol.* 1985;16(7):700–706.

Yousem SA, Colby TV, Carrington CB. Lung biopsy in rheumatoid arthritis. *Am Rev Respir Dis.* 1985;131(5):770–777.

Yousem SA, Dacic S. Idiopathic bronchiolocentric interstitial pneumonia. *Mod Pathol.* 2002;15(11):1148–1153.

Yousem SA, Faber C. Histopathology of aspiration pneumonia not associated with food or other particulate matter: a clinicopathologic study of 10 cases diagnosed on biopsy. *Am J Surg Pathol.* 2011;35(3):426–431.

Yousem SA, Hochholzer L. Pulmonary hyalinizing granuloma. *Am J Clin Pathol.* 1987;87:1–6.

Zander DS, Farver CF. *Pulmonary Pathology.* A Volume in the Series Foundations in Diagnostic Pathology. Philadelphia, PA: Churchill Livingstone; 2008.

Index

Page numbers followed by *f* indicate figures.